End-Stage Renal Disease: An Issue of Nephrology Clinics

End-Stage Renal Disease: An Issue of Nephrology Clinics

Editor: Sienna Morrison

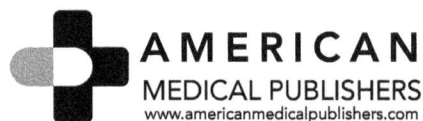

AMERICAN
MEDICAL PUBLISHERS
www.americanmedicalpublishers.com

AMERICAN
MEDICAL PUBLISHERS
www.americanmedicalpublishers.com

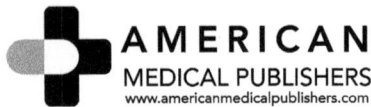

Cataloging-in-Publication Data

End-stage renal disease : an issue of nephrology clinics / edited by Sienna Morrison.
   p. cm.
Includes bibliographical references and index.
ISBN 978-1-63927-268-6
1. Chronic renal failure. 2. Kidneys--Diseases. 3. Nephrology. I. Morrison, Sienna.

RC918.R4 E53 2022

616.614--dc23

American Medical Publishers,
41 Flatbush Avenue,
1st Floor, New York,
NY 11217, USA

ISBN 978-1-63927-268-6 (Hardback)

Contents

Preface

End-stage renal disease refers to a condition in which the kidneys lose their function. It can be of two types-acute kidney failure and chronic kidney failure. Exhaustion, vomiting, confusion, leg swelling and loss of appetite are some of the symptoms of the disease. Complications such as high blood potassium, uremia or volume overload may occur in case of acute kidney failure. Chronic kidney failure may result in anemia, heart disease or high blood pressure. Blockage of the urinary tract, muscle breakdown, low blood pressure and hemolytic uremic syndrome are some causes of the acute condition. High blood pressure, diabetes, polycystic kidney disease and nephrotic syndrome are some of the causes of chronic kidney failure. The diagnosis of end-stage renal disease is established on the basis of an evaluation of glomerular filtration rate, urine production and serum creatinine level in blood. Treatment may include peritoneal dialysis, hemodialysis or a kidney transplant. If acute disease is indicated, the treatment tries to address the underlying cause of the disease. This book elucidates the concepts and innovative models around the diagnosis and treatment of end-stage renal disease. The topics included herein on this disease are of utmost significance and bound to provide incredible insights to readers. This book includes contributions of experts and scientists which will provide innovative insights into nephrology.

This book is the end result of constructive efforts and intensive research done by experts in this field. The aim of this book is to enlighten the readers with recent information in this area of research. The information provided in this profound book would serve as a valuable reference to students and researchers in this field.

At the end, I would like to thank all the authors for devoting their precious time and providing their valuable contribution to this book. I would also like to express my gratitude to my fellow colleagues who encouraged me throughout the process.

Editor

Soluble Erythropoietin Receptor Contributes to Erythropoietin Resistance in End-Stage Renal Disease

Eliyahu V. Khankin[1,⊙], Walter P. Mutter[1,⊙], Hector Tamez[1], Hai-Tao Yuan[1], S. Ananth Karumanchi[1,3]*, Ravi Thadhani[2]

1 Department of Medicine, Beth Israel Deaconess Medical Center and Harvard Medical School, Boston, Massachusetts, United States of America, 2 Department of Medicine, Massachusetts General Hospital and Harvard Medical School, Boston, Massachusetts, United States of America, 3 Howard Hughes Medical Institute, Beth Israel Deaconess Medical Center and Harvard Medical School, Boston, Massachusetts, United States of America

Abstract

Background: Erythropoietin is a growth factor commonly used to manage anemia in patients with chronic kidney disease. A significant clinical challenge is relative resistance to erythropoietin, which leads to use of successively higher erythropoietin doses, failure to achieve target hemoglobin levels, and increased risk of adverse outcomes. Erythropoietin acts through the erythropoietin receptor (EpoR) present in erythroblasts. Alternative mRNA splicing produces a soluble form of EpoR (sEpoR) found in human blood, however its role in anemia is not known.

Methods and Findings: Using archived serum samples obtained from subjects with end stage kidney disease we show that sEpoR is detectable as a 27kDa protein in the serum of dialysis patients, and that higher serum sEpoR levels correlate with increased erythropoietin requirements. Soluble EpoR inhibits erythropoietin mediated signal transducer and activator of transcription 5 (Stat5) phosphorylation in cell lines expressing EpoR. Importantly, we demonstrate that serum from patients with elevated sEpoR levels blocks this phosphorylation in *ex vivo* studies. Finally, we show that sEpoR is increased in the supernatant of a human erythroleukaemia cell line when stimulated by inflammatory mediators such as interleukin-6 and tumor necrosis factor alpha implying a link between inflammation and erythropoietin resistance.

Conclusions: These observations suggest that sEpoR levels may contribute to erythropoietin resistance in end stage renal disease, and that sEpoR production may be mediated by pro-inflammatory cytokines.

Editor: Vineet Gupta, All India Institute of Medical Sciences, India

Funding: This work was supported by Department of Medicine seed funds from the Beth Israel Deaconess Medical Center and the Massachusetts General Hospital. S.A.K. is an investigator of the Howard Hughes Medical Institute. Work was also funded by Satellite Research, Normon S. Coplon Grant to W.P.M. The funders had no role in study design, data collection and analysis, decision to publish, or preparation of the manuscript.

Competing Interests: Authors Eli Khankin, Walter Mutter, S. Ananth Karumanchi and Ravi Thadhani are listed as co-inventors on provisional patents filed by the Harvard Hospitals that is related to use of soluble epo receptor for the diagnosis and therapy of anemia.

* E-mail: sananth@bidmc.harvard.edu

⊙ These authors contributed equally to this work.

Introduction

Management of anemia with erythropoietin in patients with renal failure on dialysis has significantly changed clinical practice in nephrology. The widespread clinical use of recombinant erythropoietin has reduced the requirement for blood transfusions and is associated with improved left ventricular hypertrophy [1] as well as quality of life outcomes in dialysis patients [2–4]. Recent clinical studies, however, have suggested an excess of cardiovascular events in patients requiring elevated doses of erythropoietin [5–7] and a trend toward excess mortality in dialysis patients with higher hemoglobin targets [8]. It is not clear if this excess risk is related to erythropoietin dose or an absolute rise in hemoglobin concentration. As a result there is significant debate about optimal erythropoietin dose and hemoglobin targets. Nevertheless, erythropoietin therapy still remains a cornerstone in the management of anemia in chronic dialysis patients.

Erythropoietin is protein hormone produced by the kidney in response to hypoxia. Erythropoietin binds the membrane bound erythropoietin receptor (EpoR) located on erythroblasts in the bone marrow. Following receptor binding, an intracellular signaling cascade leads to the transcription of anti-apoptotic genes. This results in production of new red blood cells and improvement in anemia. While most patients respond well to erythropoietin, a subset of patients are considered resistant to erythropoietin, requiring 25–100% higher doses than the average patient to maintain acceptable hemoglobin levels [9–11]. This lack of response termed "Erythropoietin Resistance" or "Erythropoietin Hyporesponsiveness" is multifactorial but may be related to iron stores (both absolute and effective), renal osteodystrophy, and inflammation [9–11]. Generally patients who receive in excess of 400 IU/kg per week of erythropoietin and fail to achieve target hemoglobin are considered resistant although there is clearly a spectrum of erythropoietin sensitivity [9]. It remains clinically challenging to accurately predict which patients will be resistant to erythropoietin prior to initiating erythropoietin therapy. Chronic inflammation seems to play a role in some patients and there is evidence that inflammatory cytokines may down regulate the bone marrow response to erythropoietin [10,11]. In such cases there may be functional iron deficiency related to inadequate delivery of iron to the erythroid marrow in the face of adequate iron sores in the reticuloendothelial system [12]. Iron delivery may be inhibited by inflammatory cytokines and hormones such as hepcidin which may play a role in renal anemia [13–15]. In addition, markers of erythropoiesis such as the soluble transferrin receptor (sTfR) may be useful in determining appropriate iron management strategies [16–19].

EpoR is a membrane-bound receptor present in erythroblasts and is a member of the cytokine superfamily of type 1 transmembrane proteins [20,21]. Erythropoietin binding results in phosphorylation of intracellular messengers such as Stat-5 that bind tyrosine residues, become phosphorylated and translocate to the nucleus to initiate gene transcription [22]. Other intracellular signaling cascades may be activated as well including phospho-inositide 3-kinase, IkappaB kinase, and heat shock protein 70 [22], leading to transcription of anti-apoptotic factors [22]. Importantly, alternative mRNA splicing produces a soluble form of EpoR (sEpoR) that is present in human blood [23–25]. Soluble EpoR consists of the extracellular domain only and has a reported molecular weight of between 27 and 34 kDa with differences presumed related to glycosylation, although sEpoR protein has not yet been purified from serum or sequenced [23,25–27]. It is also possible that there is more than one form of circulating sEpoR [28] as more than one splice variant have been identified [29]. The function of sEpoR is unknown, but levels are thought to correlate with the amount of erythropoiesis, raising the possibility of a physiologic role for this soluble receptor [25,30]. Soluble EpoR has been identified in human serum and plasma as well as a number of tissues including brain, liver, spleen, kidney, heart and bone marrow [30,31]. It has also been identified as a secreted product from several cancer cell lines [29]. It is well known that soluble receptors often play an important role in cytokine signaling by stabilizing their ligand, changing concentrations of active ligand or by altering the interaction between endogenous cytokine and membrane bound ligand [32,33]. Although it has been shown that secreted sEpoR is able to bind erythropoietin, the role of circulating sEpoR in humans remains largely unknown [25,30,34].

We hypothesized that circulating sEpoR competes with erythropoietin for receptor binding and that elevated levels of sEpoR at initiation of hemodialysis portend increased erythropoietin dose requirements needed to sustain target hemoglobin levels. Furthermore we hypothesized that sEpoR production may be mediated by inflammatory cytokines present in the uremic milieu.

Materials and Methods

Immunoprecipitation

Human serum samples from ESRD subjects (approximately 1 ml) were mixed in a 1:1 ratio with IP lysis buffer (150 mM NaCl, 10 mM Tris pH 7.5, 1 mM EDTA, 50 nM NaF, 1%Triton X, 0.5% NP40, Na Orthovanadate 200 µM, PMSF 10 µg/ml, protease Inhibitor and phosphatase inhibitor at 4°C. Primary antibody directed against EpoR (R&D Systems, AF-322-PB goat anti-human polyclonal or R&D Systems, MAB307 mouse anti-human monoclonal (approximately 0.5 µg/reaction) was added to each tube and incubated over night at 4°C.followed by precipitation with Protein G coated magnetic beads, then pelleted and supernatant discarded. Beads were washed three times with lysis buffer. Bound proteins were eluted with 2X loading buffer (Laemmli's SDS–sample buffer 4x reducing, Boston BioProducts No. BP-110R) according to manufacturer's recommendations. The supernatant was retained and the beads discarded. Equal

amounts of eluted proteins were separated on an acrylamide 4–12% gradient gel. Protein was transferred to PDVF using a semi-dry transfer and western blotting performed using either of the two EpoR antibodies at concentrations of 1/1,000 (R&D Systems, MAB307 mouse anti-human monoclonal or R&D Systems, AF-322-PB goat anti-human polyclonal).

Protein Sequencing/Mass Spectrometry

Immunoprecipitation was performed as described above with the exception that 30 ml of pooled serum from uremic subjects were used. Denaturing acrylamide gels were stained with 0.1% Coomassie Brilliant Blue. A band of appropriate size and a section of gel for negative control were cut out and rinsed in 1% acetonitrile. Gel fragments were subject to trypsin digest and mass spectrometry at the Beth Israel Deaconess proteomics core laboratory. Briefly, the samples were treated with trypsin (1:100) and resuspended in 1% trifluoroacetic acid and injected it into a CapLC (Waters) high performance liquid chromatography instrument. The peptides were separated using a 75 µm Nano Series column (LC Packings) and analyzed them using a Qstar XL MS/MS system. The peptides were searched using the Mascot search engine (Matrix Science) against the human protein database NCBInr.

sEpoR ELISA

ELISA testing of serum samples and cell culture supernatants was performed using an Erythropoietin Receptor DuoSet ELISA (DY307, R&D Systems, Minneapolis, MN). On the day of the ELISA assay, frozen serum or cell culture supernatant samples were thawed at room temperature and 100 µl (100%) serum was added to each well. A standard curve was generated using serial dilutions of recombinant sEpoR (R&D Systems 307-ER/CF) at concentrations ranging from 4 ng/ml to 62.5 pg/ml in Reagent Diluent (1% BSA/Phosphate Buffered Saline, R&D Systems DY995). All reactions were carried out at room temperature. Plates were coated overnight with primary mouse anti-human EpoR antibody in PBS 1 µg/mL (100 µl/well). On the day of the assay each well was washed three times with wash buffer (0.05% Tween 20/Phosphate Buffered Saline, R&D Systems WA126) 400 µl/well using a Columbus Pro washer (Tecan, Inc). Reagent Diluent 300 µl/well was added and plates incubated for 1 hour. Plates were then washed three times with wash buffer and 100 µl standard or sample was added to each well. Plates were incubated for 4 hours on a table top shaker and washed three times with 400 µl/well Wash Buffer. Secondary biotinylated mouse anti-human EpoR antibody 500 ng/ml (100 µl/well) was added and plates were incubated for 2 hours on a table top shaker. Plates were washed again with Wash Buffer three times and Streptavidin conjugated to Horseradish-Peroxidase (100 µl/well) was added for 20 minutes. Plates were washed three times in wash buffer and color reagent containing H_2O_2 and tetramethylbenzidine (100 µl/well) was added (R&D Systems DY993). Plates were incubated for 20 minutes and Stop Solution 2N H_2SO_4 50 µl (R&D Systems DY994) was added to each well. Optical density was measured using a Microplate Reader (BioRad, Model 660). Optical density at 550 nm was subtracted from optical density at 450 nm and serum concentrations were determined using a standard curve generated by a quadratic plot of the standard sample concentrations versus the measured optical density. We ran the assay in duplicate for all samples with the exception of 18 serum samples which were measured only once as we were limited by sample volume. The operator was blinded to the clinical data.

The antibodies used in the R&D Systems DuoSet ELISA have proprietary epitopes that target the extracellular region of the receptor (AA 25 to 225). The ELISA was able to detect two alternative recombinant sEpoRs (Sigma-Aldrich E0643 and R&D Systems 963-ER) in addition to the sEpoR (R&D Systems 307-ER/CF) used to generate the standard curve. We calculated intra and inter-assay coefficients of variance using 3 serum samples run in triplicate on three separate plates. The mean intra assay coefficient of variance for the three samples was 4.71% range (1.10% to 9.49%) and the mean inter assay coefficient of variance was 4.74% range (1.20% to 9.27%). We also tested for erythropoietin interference by spiking both serum and control wells with recombinant erythropoietin up to 10,000 mU/ml and observed no significant alteration in EpoR measurements suggesting the assay measures total sEpoR rather than free sEpoR.

BaF3/EpoR Stat-5 Signaling Assay

BaF3/EpoR cells stably expressing the EpoR receptor were obtained from Dr. Laurie Feldman, Beth Israel Deaconess Medical Center [35,36]. Cells were plated at 500,000 cells per well in a 24 well dish and grown overnight in RPMI with 1% FCS. Media was replaced with serum free media and incubated for 12 hours. Vehicle, recombinant erythropoietin (Amgen), human serum, and recombinant receptor (R&D Systems) was added to wells to a total volume of 500 µl (50 µl serum per well) with erythropoietin 50 mU/ml and recombinant receptor. Cells were incubated for 10 minutes at 37°, and immediately lysed in RIPA buffer with protease inhibitors and samples frozen at −80°C for further analysis by western blots using phospho-Stat-5 and Stat-5 antibodies (Stat-5 antibody (No. 9363), phospho-Stat-5, Thyr694, antibody (No. 9351) both from Cell Signaling Technology, Danvers MA.

Statistical Considerations for In Vitro Data

Standard statistical analysis was performed on all data. Individual values were collated as means +/− S.E.M. Comparisons between multiple groups were by a two way ANOVA test followed by a Mann-Whitney nonparametric test or a paired t test when appropriate. Statistical significance was considered if $p < 0.05$.

Human Subjects

In order to test if sEpoR levels at the initiation of chronic hemodialysis are correlated with subsequent erythropoietin requirements, we selected consecutive chronic hemodialysis (CHD) patients from the Accelerated Mortality on Renal Replacement (ArMORR) cohort study which has been described in detail [37–41]. This study was approved by the Institutional Review Board of the Massachusetts General Hospital and informed consent was waived by the Institutional Review board as only archived samples were used in this study. ArMORR includes 10,044 subjects who initiated CHD at any one of the 1056 U.S. dialysis centers operated by Fresenius Medical Care North America (Waltham, MA) between 2004 and 2005. All the subjects underwent 1 year follow-up except for those who died (15%), underwent kidney transplant (3%), recovered renal function (4%), or transitioned to a dialysis unit outside the Fresenius Medical Care North America system before completing 1 year of hemodialysis treatment (12%).

Within this cohort we targeted 500–1000 consecutive patients with adequate baseline blood samples and who survived at least 6 months so as to examine erythropoietin requirements during this time period. This sample size was chosen based on our previous studies examining baseline levels of other parameters and subsequent outcomes [37,39], and because no prior human data were available to provide us with an estimate of effect size and appropriate sample size to achieve adequate power. Of these, 697 subjects representing over 400 CHD units in the U.S. had

adequate remnant volumes of baseline samples with complete erythropoietin dosing information (amount of erythropoietin administered at each dialysis session). Specifically, each subject had a blood sample collected within 14 days of initiating CHD and each subject was new to CHD. No subject had ever undergone CHD or peritoneal dialysis in the past, and no subject had ever undergone a renal transplantation prior to enrollment or recovered renal function during the study period. We measured sEpoR levels by ELISA assay and the distribution plot suggested that approximately 5% of ESRD subjects had high circulating levels of EpoR (>2 standard deviations from the mean). We therefore divided the 697 patients into two groups based on sEpoR levels at CHD start. The High sEpoR group had sEpoR levels ≥800 pg/ml (n = 36), and the Low sEpoR group (n = 661) included the remainder.

Statistical Considerations for Clinical Study

Categorical and continuous variables were examined using standard univariate tests for comparison. Longitudinal analysis was used to test the group (sEpoR Low vs. High) differences over time. Cumulative erythropoietin dose was categorized as follows: mean weekly dose administered between days 0 and 14 (14d) after initiating CHD; mean weekly dose administered between days 14 and 90 (90d); and mean weekly dose administered between days 90 and 180 (180d). Mean hemoglobin levels were categorized in a similar fashion. We performed repeated measures ANOVA to examine within and between sEpoR group comparisons. The interaction between time and sEpoR group status was tested to determine whether the relationship with erythropoietin requirements and hemoglobin levels differed between groups over time. Logistic and linear regression analyses were used to adjust for potential confounders. All analyses were performed using SAS version 9.1 for Windows (SAS Institute Inc., Cary, NC, USA). Two-sided P values <0.05 were considered statistically significant.

Cell Culture, Stimulation of K562 Cells and Assay of sEpoR in Supernatants

K562 cells (ATCC, Virginia, CCL-243) were maintained in IMDM media +10% FCS were plated at 500,000 cells per well in a 12 well plate without serum. At time zero cells were exposed to vehicle, phorbol ester 500 nM and 1000 nM, TNF-α 50 ng/ml, IL-6 10 ng/ml, and IL-8 10 ng/ml, in triplicate for 48 hours. At the end of 48 hours cells were pelleted at 4°C. The supernatant was collected and stored at −80°C. EpoR ELISA was performed on the supernatants as described above. Protein assay was performed as follows using BCA protein assay (Pierce, Thermo Fisher Scientific, Rockford IL) according to manufacturer's standard protocol.

IL-6 Levels

Serum IL-6 was measured using a commercially available ELISA kit (Catalog # DY6050, R&D Systems, MN) and manufacturer's instructions were followed. All 32 subjects with high sEpoR (>800 pg/ml) who had remaining serum available and an equal number of randomly chosen subjects with low sEpoR (≤62.5 pg/ml) were included for this substudy. Data are depicted as mean IL-6 levels in pg/ml +/− S.E.M for both groups.

Results

sEpoR Is Present in the Serum of Dialysis Patients

We initially attempted to characterize sEpoR in uremic serum using two different antibodies by western blot and were unable to detect any specific band that was consistent with the expected size of sEpoR. However, immunoprecipitation with goat anti-human erythropoietin receptor followed by western blotting with mouse anti-human erythropoietin receptor revealed a clear band of approximately 27 kDa consistent with the expected size of sEpoR in 6 representative dialysis patient samples (**Figure 1a**). A band of similar size was also detected when immunoprecipitation and western blotting was performed with the same antibodies in reverse order (**Figure 1b**). Purification of the 27 kDA protein from sera of uremic subjects and analysis by mass spectrometry revealed at least 2 different peptides (GPEELLCFTERL and YEVDVSAGNGAGSVQR) corresponding to the N-terminal extracellular region of the EpoR. Taken together with the immunoprecipation studies (**Figure 1a, 1b**), these data suggest that dialysis subjects have sEpoR in their serum.

Elevated sEpoR Levels at Initiation of Dialysis Predict Subsequent Erythropoietin Dose

We measured sEpoR levels by ELISA in representative group of 697 incident dialysis patients. The distribution of sEpoR levels is shown in **Figure 2a**. Most of the patients had low levels of sEpoR (less than or equal to 100 pg/ml). However, a subset of patients demonstrated significantly elevated values. The distribution plot suggested that approximately 5–6% of end-stage renal disease (ESRD) subjects had high circulating levels of EpoR (>2 standard deviations from the mean), and the subjects were divided accordingly The mean levels of sEpoR at the initiation of chronic hemodialysis were 2437±1299 pg/ml in the *High* group (n = 36) and 112±111 pg/ml in the *Low* group (n = 661) (p<0.001). Median values were 2147 pg/ml (inter-guartile range 1400–3445) and 69 pg/ml (inter-quartile range 62.5–101), respectively.

Table 1 shows the baseline characteristics of the Low and High sEpoR groups. We found no difference between the two groups with respect to age, race, gender, body mass index (BMI), or blood pressure. Importantly ferritin, iron saturation and hemoglobin were not different. In addition correlations between baseline sEpoR and ferritin, iron saturation, and hemoglobin levels were also not significant (p>0.05). Erythropoietin resistance has been associated with osteodystrophy and elevated parathyroid hormone (PTH) [9,10], but PTH was also not different between the groups,

and the correlation with PTH in the entire group was not significant as well (r = −0.03, p = 0.33). Bone biopsies were not available for these subjects to confirm osteodystrophy. Hypertension as an etiology of ESRD was slightly over represented in the Low sEpoR group. Nevertheless, standard clinical parameters did not appear to be associated with sEpoR levels.

To determine if sEpoR levels at the initiation of chronic dialysis are associated with subsequent erythropoietin dose, we compared longitudinal weekly erythropoietin administration in our Low and High sEpoR groups (**Figure 2b**). Erythropoietin administration not only differed with time (P<0.001), but also according to sEpoR status by 90 and most notably by 180 days following hemodialysis initiation (P = 0.038). We next examined respective mean hemoglobin levels over the same time period because erythropoietin resistance has been associated with increasing erythropoietin administration in the face of lower hemoglobin levels [42]. By day 180, the Low sEpoR group had slightly higher hemoglobin levels despite receiving lower weekly erythropoietin doses (**Figure 2c**). Next, rather than categorize the cohort according to baseline sEpoR levels, we examined the cumulative erythropoietin administration as measure of erythropoietin resistance suggested by previous investigators [43]. The mean cumulative erythropoietin administration over 180 days following hemodialysis initiation was 542,102±330,308 IU. We categorized the entire cohort into quintiles of cumulative erythropoietin administration and within each quintile examined the mean baseline sEpoR levels (**Figure 2d**). Those that received higher cumulative erythropoietin doses over the study period had progressively higher baseline sEpoR levels. We then performed logistic regression analyses to determine the independent baseline variables associated with the highest cumulative erythropoietin administration (Quintile 5). In addition to High vs. Low sEpoR levels, we adjusted for characteristics previously linked with erythropoietin administration including age, race, sex, cause of end-stage renal failure (diabetes, hypertension, glomerulonephritis, other), and baseline exposures such as arterio-venous access (fistula, graft, catheter), weight, serum ferritin, transferrin saturation, and PTH levels [42–44]. The risk for requiring the highest

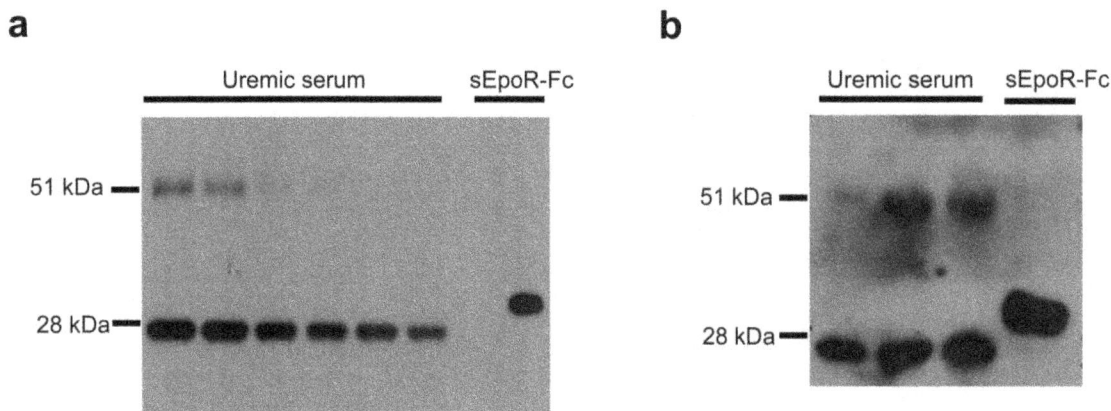

a

b

Figure 1. sEpoR characterization in uremic serum. 1a. Soluble EpoR is detectable in serum from dialysis patients by western blot. Human serum was subjected to immunoprecipitation with goat anti-human erythropoietin receptor antibody (R&D Systems, AF-322-PB) followed by western blotting with mouse monoclonal anti-human erythropoietin receptor (R&D Systems, MAB307). Both antibodies recognize the extracellular domain of the receptor. Lanes 1–6 are serum from 6 representative dialysis patients, lane 7 is blank and lane 8 is recombinant sEpoR (Sigma Aldrich E0643, Saint Louis MI). Shown in the serum samples is a band of expected molecular weight of approximately 27 kDa. The control sEpoR with Fc tag is consistent with the manufacturers reported molecular weight of 32 kDa. **1b.** Soluble EpoR is also detected using the same dialysis patient serum samples by performing immunoprecipitation in reverse order. In this experiment immunoprecipitation was done with mouse monoclonal anti-human erythropoietin receptor (R&D Systems, MAB307) followed by western blotting with goat anti-human erythropoietin receptor (R&D Systems, AF-322-PB). Lanes 1 to 3 are serum from 3 dialysis patients, and lane 4 is recombinant sEpoR-Fc (Sigma, 307) as positive control.

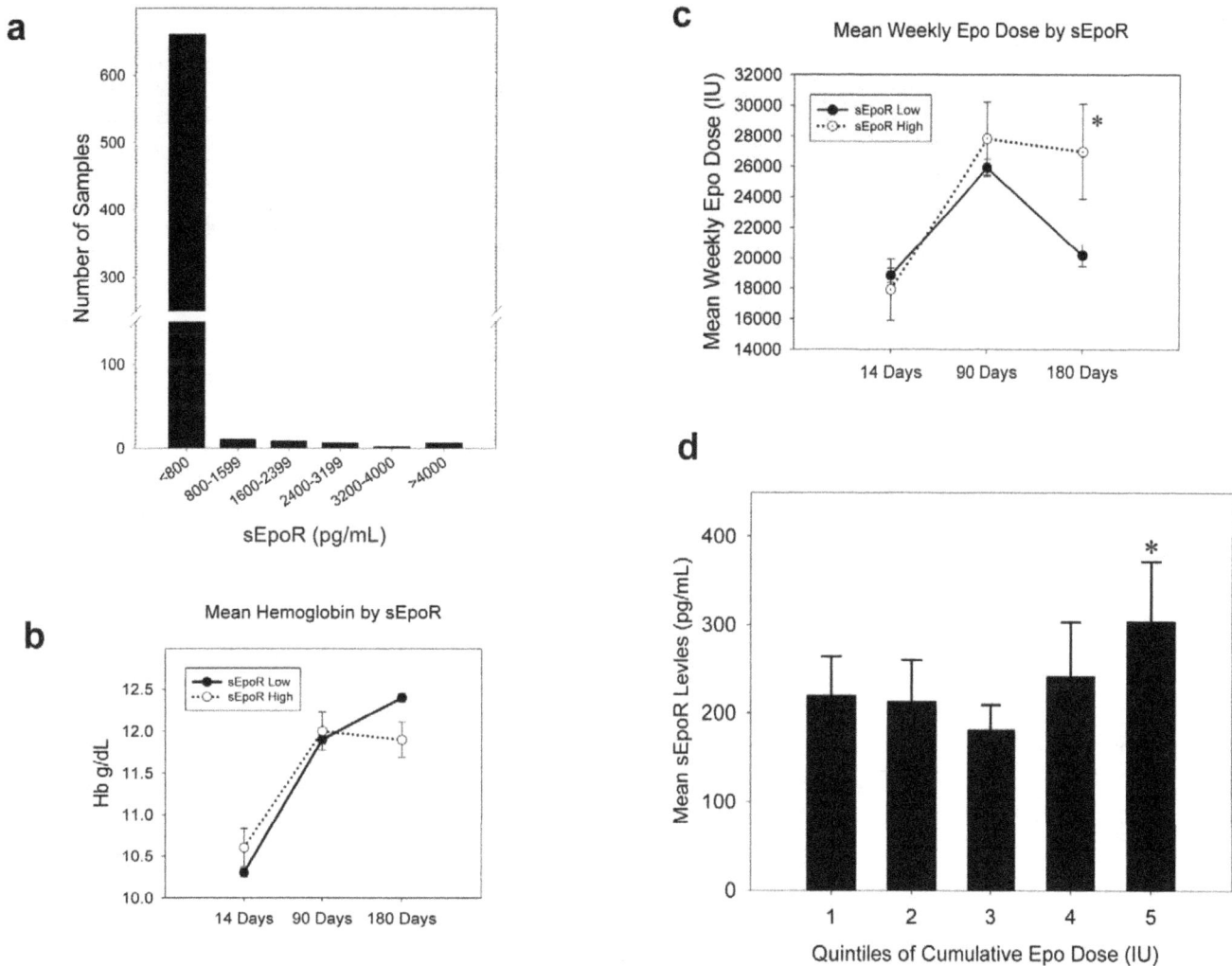

Figure 2. Relationship of sEpoR and erythropoietin dosage in human ESRD subjects. 2a. This figure shows the distribution of sEpoR levels as measured by ELISA in our sample of 697 dialysis patients. **2b.** Erythropoietin dose over time for the Low and High sEpoR groups. Erythropoietin dose at the start of dialysis (Days 0 to14) was the same in both groups, 17,908 IU/week in the High sEpoR group vs. 18,851 IU/week in the Low sEpoR group. Between days 14 and 90 the High group received 27,819 IU/week vs. 25,906 IU/week in the Low group. By days 90 and 180 the High sEpoR group required a significantly greater dose of erythropoietin then the Low sEpoR group (26,977 IU/week vs. 20,173 IU/week, p = 0.038). It is notable that the average dose rose in both groups over the period 14 to 90 days but then fell again over the 90 to 180 day period as might be expected in patients starting erythropoietin therapy. **2c.** Mean hemoglobin was compared for the Low and High sEpoR groups at three time points (Days 0 to14, 14 to 90 and 90 to 180). Hemoglobin at the start of dialysis (Days 0-14) was not statistically different between the High and Low sEpoR groups (10.5 vs. 10.3 mg %). Between 90 and 180 day there was a trend toward lower hemoglobin in the High sEpoR group 12.4 vs. 11.9 that approached statistical significance (p = 0.054). This suggests that even though both groups likely had identical hemoglobin targets, the high sEpoR group may have impaired erythropoietin response even with significantly higher erythropoietin dose. **2d.** The cohort was divided according to quintiles of cumulative EPO dose during the study period, and within each quintile examined the mean sEpoR level. The mean sEpoR values according to quintile were: Quintile 1: 220±44 pg/ml; Quintile 2: 213±47 pg/ml; Quintile 3: 181±28 pg/ml; Quintile 4: 242±61 pg/ml; Quintile 5: 304±67 pg/ml, p value for trend = 0.038. The mean cumulative Epo doses in units according to quintile were: Quintile 1: 209,004±4863, Quintile 2: 347,019±2655, Quintile 3: 459,719±3362, Quintile 4: 622,460±5334, Quintile 5: 1,077,666±25,576.

erythropoietin administration in the High vs. Low sEpoR groups was approximately 3-fold higher (OR 2.8, 95% CI 1.3–6.4).

sEpoR Blocks EPO Mediated Signaling *In Vitro*

We next sought to test the hypothesis that circulating sEpoR may block erythropoietin mediated signaling via the membrane bound receptor *in vitro*. We selected the BaF3/EPOR cell line which is a murine pro B cell line stably transfected with EPOR. This cell line is well characterized and responds to erythropoietin by increasing intracellular signaling via the Stat-5 and Janus kinase 2 (Jak2) pathways resulting in cell proliferation [35,36,45,46].

Using the BaF3/EpoR cells we established an *in vitro* system in which to test Stat-5 phosphorylation in response to erythropoietin. **Figure 3a** is a dose-response curve demonstrating increased Stat-5 phosphorylation in response to increasing erythropoietin. **Figure 3b** shows that addition of recombinant sEpoR blocks erythropoietin mediated Stat-5 phosphorylation in this system at concentrations ranging from 50 ng/mL to 5,000 ng/mL. Quantification of this inhibition is shown in **Figure 3c** as the ratio of phospho-Stat-5 to total Stat-5.

We next tested whether serum from patients with high levels of sEpoR blocks erythropoietin mediated signaling when compared

Table 1.

	sEpoR Low	sEpoR High	p-value
N	661	36	
Age (Years)	67±13	68±15	0.76
Female (%)	51	36	0.09
Race (%)			0.30
White	63	72	
Black	33	28	
Other	4	0	
[a]BMI (kg/m2)	26±6	27±7	0.66
Etiology of renal failure (%)			0.03
Diabetes Mellitus	47	47	
Hypertension	37	22	
Glomerulonephritis	8	8	
Polycystic Kidney Disease	2	8	
Other	6	15	
Vascular Access			0.76
Fistula	22	20	
Graft	13	17	
Catheter	65	63	
Systolic blood pressure (mmHg)	144±22	140±18	0.81
Diastolic blood pressure (mmHg)	72±13	71±10	0.31
[b]PTH (bio-intact; pg/ml)	297±302	278±268	0.81
Calcium (mg/dl)	8.5±0.7	8.7±0.6	0.31
Phosphorus (mg/dl)	4.5±1.5	4.3±1.8	0.46
Ferritin (ng/ml)	297±512	318±273	0.25
Iron saturation (%)	20±10	18±8	0.25
White blood cell count (cells/µl)	8±3	8±3	0.69
Platelets (cells/dl)	239±94	211±81	0.81

Results are expressed as mean ± standard deviation.
[a]BMI–body mass index.
[b]PTH–parathyroid hormone.

to serum from patients with low sEpoR levels. For this assay BaF3/EpoR were stimulated with 50 mU/ml erythropoietin in the presence and absence of 10% human serum from patients with high and low levels of sEpoR. **Figure 3d** shows a representative western blot from this experiment. Quantification by densitometry (**Figure 3e**) shows a significant (p<0.05) decrease in Stat-5 phosphorylation when BaF3/EpoR cells were exposed to serum from patients with high (>4000 pg/ml) sEpoR as compared to serum from patients with sEpoR levels ≤62.5 pg/ml).

sEpoR Is Increased by Pro-Inflammatory Cytokines IL-6 and TNF-α

The source of circulating sEpoR is also unknown. It is plausible that sEpoR levels are regulated, and that sEpoR has physiologic function in some tissues. Some have noted a positive correlation between sEpoR levels and the degree of erythropoiesis [25] while others have not observed an association [28]. In addition, recent data shows a correlation between elevated TNF-α, IL-6 and IL-8 levels and anemia in patients with chronic kidney disease [47]. We hypothesized that sEpoR may be stimulated by inflammatory cytokines present in the uremic patients. In order to test this hypothesis we selected K562 cells a cell line known to express

EpoR [48,49]. We used phorbol ester (PMA) as a positive control as it has been shown to induce secretion of soluble growth factor receptors in other cell lines [50]. We found that sEpoR in the cell supernatant was increased significantly over baseline by exposure to PMA, IL-6 and TNF-α but not IL-8 (**Figure 4a**). We then measured circulating levels of IL-6 in a subset of patients with high sEpoR and low sEpoR and found that IL-6 levels were on average 2.5 times higher in subjects with high circulating levels of sEpoR than in subjects with low sEpoR levels (**Figure 4b**).

Discussion

In this study we demonstrate that sEpoR is present in the serum of patients at the initiation of CHD, and that higher levels at the start of dialysis are independently associated with subsequent erythropoietin dose administered in the ensuing 6 months from start of treatment. We also demonstrate that sEpoR is a functional protein and inhibits erythropoietin mediated Stat-5 phosphorylation. We further show that serum with high levels of sEpoR decreases erythropoietin mediated Stat-5 phosphorylation compared with serum from patients with low sEpoR levels suggesting that sEpoR may compete with membrane bound EPOR and inhibit erythropoietin stimulated erythropoiesis. Additionally, we suggest a mechanism for elevated sEpoR by showing that IL-6 and TNF-α can increase sEpoR production in the supernatant of cell lines expressing endogenous EpoR. Importantly, we also demonstrate that subjects with high sEpoR on average had higher circulating levels of IL-6 than subjects with low sEpoR.

The hypothesis that sEpoR may modulate erythropoietin signaling has biologic plausibility for several reasons. First, other investigators have shown that sEpoR may block EpoR signaling in vitro [25,51]. Second there is recent data to suggest that sEpoR may inhibit erythropoietin signaling *in vivo*. Soluble EpoR is expressed in the brain and is down-regulated in response to chronic hypoxia in a recently described murine model [30]. This down-regulation contributes to increased minute ventilation. Infusion of exogenous sEpoR decreases endogenous erythropoietin signaling and blocks the increase in minute ventilation [30]. Also, transgenic expression of sEpoR can block erythropoietin in a rat model [52]. Furthermore, many cytokines of the superfamily type 1 transmembrane proteins (of which EpoR is a member) are synthesized in soluble forms, and alter native ligand receptor binding [26,27,53]. Two other groups have reported sEpoR levels in patients with chronic kidney disease or on dialysis but they were not able to show a physiologic role for this protein [25,26]. Here we confirm the presence of sEpoR by immunoprecipitation and ELISA of serum and show that serum enriched in sEpoR inhibits erythropoietin mediated Stat-5 phosphorylation suggesting that sEpoR may have a physiologic role rather than being an epiphenomenon related to the degree of erythropoiesis.

We speculated that sEpoR levels may be modulated by cytokines present in the chronic inflammatory state present in many dialysis patients. Data regarding the regulation of sEpoR is limited, although membrane bound EpoR is known to be regulated by several cytokines such as TNF-α, IL-1β, and IL-6 [54,55]. Hypoxia and erythropoietin may also stimulate EpoR expression. EpoR is regulated by hypoxia-inducible factor 1 [56] and recent data shows increased EpoR expression in primary human venous endothelial cells and bone marrow vascular endothelial cells under hypoxic conditions and in response to erythropoietin [57]. It is unknown if sEpoR is produced in proportion to EpoR of if it is independently regulated. Lysosomal degradation plays an important role in altering the cell surface expression of many cytokine receptors [58]. Interestingly, blocking

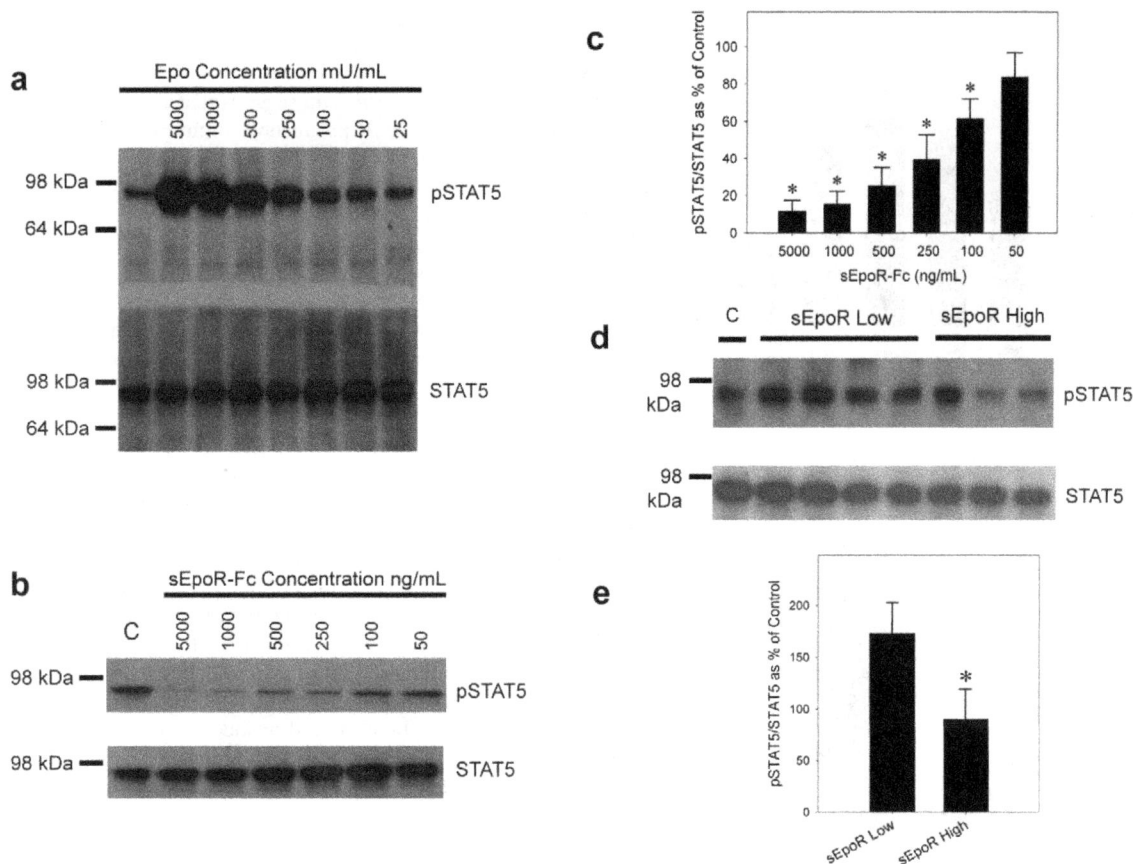

Figure 3. Functional characterization of sEpoR. 3a. Western blot showing increasedphospho-Stat-5 in the presence of increasing erythropoietin (25 to 5000 mU/ml) in BaF3/EpoR cell lysates. **3b.** Representative western blot showing total phospho-Stat-5 and Stat-5 in the presence of erythropoietin 5000 mU/ml and varying concentrations of recombinant sEpoR-Fc (50 -5000 ng/ml). Phospho-Stat-5 decreases with increasing recombinant sEpoR. **3c.** Quantification of sEpoR-Fc inhibition of phospho-Stat 5 (Figure 3b). Ratios of phospho/total Stat-5 (mean $\pm$ SD, n = 3) represented as a percentage of control (Epo alone). *represents p<0.05. **3d.** Serum from patients with high sEpoR blocks erythropoietin mediated Stat-5 phosphorylation. Shown is the ratio of phospho-Stat-5 to Stat-5 as measured by densitometry. Serum starved BaF3/EpoR cells were exposed to vehicle (negative control), erythropoietin at 50 mU/ml (positive control) and erythropoietin plus 10% serum with Low sEpoR ($\leq$62.5 pg/ml) or serum with high sEpoR ($\geq$4000 pg/ml) for 10 minutes. Cells were lysed in RIPA buffer and 10 ug protein/lane was run on a 4-12% denaturing gel. Gels were transferred and blotted with anti-Stat-5 and anti-phospho-Stat 5. **3e.** Quantification of western data (Figure 3d). Ratios of phospho/total Stat-5 (mean $\pm$ SD, n = 5 individual patient samples each for low sEpoR and high sEpoR) represented as a percentage of control (Epo alone). *represents p<0.05.

lysosomal degradation of EpoR with calpain inhibitors increased sEpoR by 2 to 5 fold but only increased membrane bound EpoR 1.5 fold arguing for differential regulation of the two proteins [59]. Here we provide evidence that IL-6 and TNF-α can increase sEpoR in the supernatant of cells known to express the native receptor and that subjects with high sEpoR on average had higher circulating levels of IL-6. This suggests one possible mechanistic link between inflammation and erythropoietin resistance.

Our preliminary data suggest that elevated sEpoR levels at initiation of CHD identify those that require higher erythropoietin doses over the ensuing 6 months. Importantly, sEpoR levels were not correlated with other parameters considered linked to erythropoietin resistance such as ferritin, iron saturation, and parathyroid hormone levels. Higher erythropoietin doses were received in the context of achieving lower hemoglobin values compared to those with lower sEpoR levels. It is interesting to find that mean weekly erythropoietin doses differed most markedly between days 90 and 180. This may be because starting doses of erythropoietin are usually similar when patients initiate CHD (as seen in **Figure 2b**) given the low hemoglobin levels at the

initiation of hemodialysis and the ease of administration of standard doses in busy dialysis units. In this context, it is likely that only later is erythropoietin resistance (even in a subtle form) uncovered. Furthermore, since the half-life of red blood cells is 120 days, it is likely that the effects of sEpoR are more prominent at 180 days rather than at 90 days. There are recent data showing that higher erythropoietin dose is associated with increased mortality, and a subset of patients require significantly higher amounts of erythropoietin to sustain adequate hemoglobin levels [60]. It is not clear if this is related to erythropoietin itself, or is associated with risk factors such as chronic inflammation. For this study we chose to closely examine the link between sEpoR levels and subsequent erythropoietin dose, hence we required all subjects to remain alive during the study period. Future studies should examine whether there may be a link between sEpoR levels and outcomes including death.

In this initial description sEpoR levels independently identified those that required higher doses of erythropoietin in the ensuing 6 months even after accounting for standard baseline clinical characteristics and laboratory measures. In these analyses we

a

b

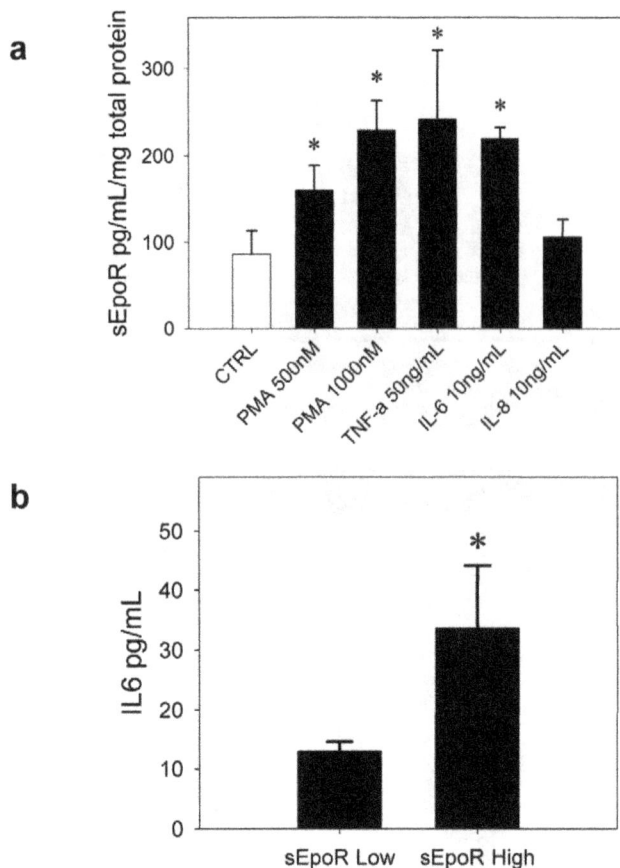

Figure 4. sEpoR is regulated by proinflammatory cytokines. 4a.
IL-6, TNF-α and PMA increase sEpoR in the supernatant of K562 cells. K562 were plated in serum free media and exposed for 48 h to vehicle, PMA, IL-6 and TNF-α. At the end of the incubation cells were pelleted and the supernatant subjected to ELISA for sEpoR. sEpoR measurements were corrected for total protein concentration. * represents p value of <0.05 when compared to the control group. **4b.** Mean IL-6 levels in subjects with low (n = 32) and high sEpoR (n = 32) are shown. * represents p value of <0.05 when compared to low sEpoR group.

controlled for routinely measured factors previously linked with erythropoietin resistance, including PTH, iron status, and measures of inflammation such as ferritin. However, we did not measure novel circulating markers associated with erythropoietin resistance such as pro-hepcidin which may be a marker for inflammation and alter iron availability [13–15], soluble transferrin receptor which has been shown to be decreased in chronic kidney disease [16–19], and C-reactive protein (CRP). Patients with elevated CRP require higher erythropoietin dose and there may be decreased clearance of inflammatory cytokines such as TNF-α, IL-1 and IL-6 [9,61]. At high levels these cytokines can

blunt erythropoietin action on bone marrow precursor cells [10]. It is also possible that some inflammatory cytokines may regulate sEpoR production themselves or they may both be associated with a common factor. Our *in vitro* data suggests that IL-6 and TNF-α may directly stimulate sEpoR production. In future work it would be reasonable to measure pro-hepcidin, soluble transferrin receptor, CRP, IL-6 and TNF-α to see if any of these factors are associated with sEpoR levels.

We studied subjects representative of incident US dialysis patients. However, erythropoietin dosing varies significantly by country with most studies showing the highest doses in the United States [62]. A recent review of erythropoietin dosing patterns in 12 countries showed that average weekly erythropoietin dose among chronic stable dialysis patients in the US was highest at 17,360 IU per week compared with a low of 5,297 per week in Japan [63]. In this study greater erythropoietin dose was associated with greater mean hemoglobin concentration. Our findings would need to be validated in other patient populations, including European and Asian groups to assess generalizability. Our data may have particular relevance to cancer subjects as several tumor cell lines have been shown to secret sEpoR [26] and in whom higher doses of erythropoietin have been associated with mortality [64].

The data presented showing increased sEpoR in response to IL-6 and TNF-α is preliminary. Future work includes a full analysis of sEpoR in response to these and other potential inflammatory cytokines. Questions to be answered include what is the effect on membrane bound EpoR, what is the time course for sEpoR release, and is sEpoR regulated at a translational, transcriptional, or post-transcriptional level? Importantly, we also do not know whether sEpoR may also be involved in the pathogenesis of anemia of chronic disease, which is also thought to be secondary to chronic inflammation [65].

In summary, our findings suggest that sEpoR may play a role in the response of dialysis patients to exogenous erythropoietin and sEpoR may be produced in response to inflammatory cytokines. A better understanding of sEpoR regulation and it association with other factors known to contribute to erythropoietin resistance may lead to more strategic and effective erythropoietin dosing protocols. If sEpoR can be shown in further studies to inhibit erythropoietin effectiveness in dialysis patients then therapeutic strategies aimed at decreasing sEpoR may be useful.

Acknowledgments

We thank Dr. Samir Parikh and Dr. Laurie Feldman for helpful discussions.

Author Contributions

Conceived and designed the experiments: EK WM SAK RT. Performed the experiments: EK WM. Analyzed the data: EK WM HT HTY SAK RT. Contributed reagents/materials/analysis tools: RT. Wrote the paper: EK WM SAK RT.

References

1. Chen HH, Tarng DC, Lee KF, Wu CY, Chen YC (2008) Epoetin alfa and darbepoetin alfa: effects on ventricular hypertrophy in patients with chronic kidney disease. J Nephrol 21: 543–549.
2. Navaneethan SD, Bonifati C, Schena FP, Strippoli GF (2006) Evidence for optimal hemoglobin targets in chronic kidney disease. J Nephrol 19: 640–647.
3. Paoletti E, Cannella G (2006) Update on erythropoietin treatment: should hemoglobin be normalized in patients with chronic kidney disease? J Am Soc Nephrol 17: S74–77.
4. Strippoli GF, Navaneethan SD, Craig JC (2006) Haemoglobin and haematocrit targets for the anaemia of chronic kidney disease. Cochrane Database Syst Rev. CD003967.
5. Coyne DW (2008) From anemia trials to clinical practice: understanding the risks and benefits when setting goals for therapy. Semin Dial 21: 212–216.
6. Drueke TB, Locatelli F, Clyne N, Eckardt KU, Macdougall IC, et al. (2006) Normalization of hemoglobin level in patients with chronic kidney disease and anemia. N Engl J Med 355: 2071–2084.
7. Singh AK, Szczech L, Tang KL, Barnhart H, Sapp S, et al. (2006) Correction of anemia with epoetin alfa in chronic kidney disease. N Engl J Med 355: 2085–2098.
8. Besarab A, Bolton WK, Browne JK, Egrie JC, Nissenson AR, et al. (1998) The effects of normal as compared with low hematocrit values in patients with cardiac disease who are receiving hemodialysis and epoetin. N Engl J Med 339: 584–590.

9. Johnson DW, Pollock CA, Macdougall IC (2007) Erythropoiesis-stimulating agent hyporesponsiveness. Nephrology (Carlton) 12: 321–330.
10. Stenvinkel P, Barany P (2002) Anaemia, rHuEPO resistance, and cardiovascular disease in end-stage renal failure; links to inflammation and oxidative stress. Nephrol Dial Transplant 17 Suppl 5: 32–37.
11. Priyadarshi A, Shapiro JI (2006) Erythropoietin resistance in the treatment of the anemia of chronic renal failure. Semin Dial 19: 273–278.
12. Goodnough LT (2007) Erythropoietin and iron-restricted erythropoiesis. Exp Hematol 35: 167–172.
13. Tsuchihashi D, Abe T, Komaba H, Fujii H, Hamada Y, et al. (2008) Serum pro-hepcidin as an indicator of iron status in dialysis patients. Ther Apher Dial 12: 226–231.
14. Kato A, Tsuji T, Luo J, Sakao Y, Yasuda H, et al. (2008) Association of prohepcidin and hepcidin-25 with erythropoietin response and ferritin in hemodialysis patients. Am J Nephrol 28: 115–121.
15. Eleftheriadis T, Kartsios C, Liakopoulos V, Antoniadi G, Ditsa M, et al. (2006) Does hepcidin affect erythropoiesis in hemodialysis patients? Acta Haematol 116: 238–244.
16. Tarng DC, Huang TP (2002) Determinants of circulating soluble transferrin receptor level in chronic haemodialysis patients. Nephrol Dial Transplant 17: 1063–1069.
17. Ahluwalia N, Skikne BS, Savin V, Chonko A (1997) Markers of masked iron deficiency and effectiveness of EPO therapy in chronic renal failure. Am J Kidney Dis 30: 532–541.
18. Daschner M, Mehls O, Schaefer F (1999) Soluble transferrin receptor is correlated with erythropoietin sensitivity in dialysis patients. Clin Nephrol 52: 246–252.
19. Chiang WC, Tsai TJ, Chen YM, Lin SL, Hsieh BS (2002) Serum soluble transferrin receptor reflects erythropoiesis but not iron availability in erythropoietin-treated chronic hemodialysis patients. Clin Nephrol 58: 363–369.
20. Winkelmann JC, Penny LA, Deaven LL, Forget BG, Jenkins RB (1990) The gene for the human erythropoietin receptor: analysis of the coding sequence and assignment to chromosome 19p. Blood 76: 24–30.
21. Jones SS, D'Andrea AD, Haines LL, Wong GG (1990) Human erythropoietin receptor: cloning, expression, and biologic characterization. Blood 76: 31–35.
22. Rossert J, Eckardt KU (2005) Erythropoietin receptors: their role beyond erythropoiesis. Nephrol Dial Transplant 20: 1025–1028.
23. Barron C, Migliaccio AR, Migliaccio G, Jiang Y, Adamson JW, et al. (1994) Alternatively spliced mRNAs encoding soluble isoforms of the erythropoietin receptor in murine cell lines and bone marrow. Gene 147: 263–268.
24. Todokoro K, Kuramochi S, Nagasawa T, Abe T, Ikawa Y (1991) Isolation of a cDNA encoding a potential soluble receptor for human erythropoietin. Gene 106: 283–284.
25. Baynes RD, Reddy GK, Shih YJ, Skikne BS, Cook JD (1993) Serum form of the erythropoietin receptor identified by a sequence-specific peptide antibody. Blood 82: 2088–2095.
26. Westphal G, Braun K, Debus J (2002) Detection and quantification of the soluble form of the human erythropoietin receptor (sEpoR) in the growth medium of tumor cell lines and in the plasma of blood samples. Clin Exp Med 2: 45–52.
27. Harris KW, Winkelmann JC (1996) Enzyme-linked immunosorbent assay detects a potential soluble form of the erythropoietin receptor in human plasma. Am J Hematol 52: 8–13.
28. Yoshida S, Bessho M, Sakate K, Hirasawa I, Murayoshi M, et al. (1996) Lack of relationship between soluble erythropoietin receptor levels and erythroid parameters in anemic patients. Blood 88: 3246–3247.
29. Arcasoy MO, Jiang X, Haroon ZA (2003) Expression of erythropoietin receptor splice variants in human cancer. Biochem Biophys Res Commun 307: 999–1007.
30. Soliz J, Gassmann M, Joseph V (2007) Soluble erythropoietin receptor is present in the mouse brain and is required for the ventilatory acclimatization to hypoxia. J Physiol 583: 329–336.
31. Ferro FE Jr, Kozak SL, Hoatlin ME, Kabat D (1993) Cell surface site for mitogenic interaction of erythropoietin receptors with the membrane glycoprotein encoded by Friend erythroleukemia virus. J Biol Chem 268: 5741–5747.
32. Maynard SE, Min JY, Merchan J, Lim KH, Li J, et al. (2003) Excess placental soluble fms-like tyrosine kinase 1 (sFlt1) may contribute to endothelial dysfunction, hypertension, and proteinuria in preeclampsia. J Clin Invest 111: 649–658.
33. Venkatesha S, Toporsian M, Lam C, Hanai J, Mammoto T, et al. (2006) Soluble endoglin contributes to the pathogenesis of preeclampsia. Nat Med 12: 642–649.
34. Yet MG, Jones SS (1993) The extracytoplasmic domain of the erythropoietin receptor forms a monomeric complex with erythropoietin. Blood 82: 1713–1719.
35. Chen C, Sytkowski AJ (2004) Erythropoietin regulation of Raf-1 and MEK: evidence for a Ras-independent mechanism. Blood 104: 73–80.
36. Chen C, Sytkowski AJ (2001) Erythropoietin activates two distinct signaling pathways required for the initiation and the elongation of c-myc. J Biol Chem 276: 38518–38526.
37. Gutierrez OM, Mannstadt M, Isakova T, Rauh-Hain JA, Tamez H, et al. (2008) Fibroblast growth factor 23 and mortality among patients undergoing hemodialysis. N Engl J Med 359: 584–592.
38. Lee PS, Sampath K, Karumanchi SA, Tamez H, Bhan I, et al. (2009) Plasma gelsolin and circulating actin correlate with hemodialysis mortality. J Am Soc Nephrol 20: 1140–1148.
39. Wolf M, Shah A, Gutierrez O, Ankers E, Monroy M, et al. (2007) Vitamin D levels and early mortality among incident hemodialysis patients. Kidney Int 72: 1004–1013.
40. Wolf M, Betancourt J, Chang Y, Shah A, Teng M, et al. (2008) Impact of activated vitamin D and race on survival among hemodialysis patients. J Am Soc Nephrol 19: 1379–1388.
41. Brunelli SM, Lynch KE, Ankers ED, Joffe MM, Yang W, et al. (2008) Association of hemoglobin variability and mortality among contemporary incident hemodialysis patients. Clin J Am Soc Nephrol 3: 1733–1740.
42. Kalantar-Zadeh K, Lee GH, Miller JE, Streja E, Jing J, et al. (2009) Predictors of hyporesponsiveness to erythropoiesis-stimulating agents in hemodialysis patients. Am J Kidney Dis 53: 823–834.
43. Kaysen GA, Muller HG, Ding J, Chertow GM (2006) Challenging the validity of the EPO index. Am J Kidney Dis 47: 166.
44. Lacson E Jr, Rogus J, Teng M, Lazarus JM, Hakim RM (2008) The association of race with erythropoietin dose in patients on long-term hemodialysis. Am J Kidney Dis 52: 1104–1114.
45. Leist M, Ghezzi P, Grasso G, Bianchi R, Villa P, et al. (2004) Derivatives of erythropoietin that are tissue protective but not erythropoietic. Science 305: 239–242.
46. Krosl J, Damen JE, Krystal G, Humphries RK (1996) Interleukin-3 (IL-3) inhibits erythropoietin-induced differentiation in Ba/F3 cells via the IL-3 receptor alpha subunit. J Biol Chem 271: 27432–27437.
47. Keithi-Reddy SR, Addabbo F, Patel TV, Mittal BV, Goligorsky MS, et al. (2008) Association of anemia and erythropoiesis stimulating agents with inflammatory biomarkers in chronic kidney disease. Kidney Int 74: 782–790.
48. Lozzio CB, Lozzio BB (1975) Human chronic myelogenous leukemia cell-line with positive Philadelphia chromosome. Blood 45: 321–334.
49. Kubota Y, Tanaka T, Kitanaka A, Ohnishi H, Okutani Y, et al. (2001) Src transduces erythropoietin-induced differentiation signals through phosphatidylinositol 3-kinase. EMBO J 20: 5666–5677.
50. Hornig C, Barleon B, Ahmad S, Vuorela P, Ahmed A, et al. (2000) Release and complex formation of soluble VEGFR-1 from endothelial cells and biological fluids. Lab Invest 80: 443–454.
51. Kuramochi H, Motegi A, Maruyama S, Okamoto K, Takahashi K, et al. (1990) Factor analysis of in vitro antitumor activities of platinum complexes. Chem Pharm Bull (Tokyo) 38: 123–127.
52. Maruyama H, Higuchi M, Higuchi N, Kameda S, Saito M, et al. (2004) Post-secretion neutralization of transgene-derived effect: soluble erythropoietin receptor/IgG1Fc expressed in liver neutralizes erythropoietin produced in muscle. J Gene Med 6: 228–237.
53. Nagao M, Masuda S, Abe S, Ueda M, Sasaki R (1992) Production and ligand-binding characteristics of the soluble form of murine erythropoietin receptor. Biochem Biophys Res Commun 188: 888–897.
54. Maiese K, Li F, Chong ZZ (2005) New avenues of exploration for erythropoietin. JAMA 293: 90–95.
55. Buck I, Morceau F, Cristofanon S, Heintz C, Chateauvieux S, et al. (2008) Tumor necrosis factor alpha inhibits erythroid differentiation in human erythropoietin-dependent cells involving p38 MAPK pathway, GATA-1 and FOG-1 downregulation and GATA-2 upregulation. Biochem Pharmacol 76: 1229–1239.
56. Joyeux-Faure M (2007) Cellular protection by erythropoietin: new therapeutic implications? J Pharmacol Exp Ther 323: 759–762.
57. Beleslin-Cokic BB, Cokic VP, Yu X, Weksler BB, Schechter AN, et al. (2004) Erythropoietin and hypoxia stimulate erythropoietin receptor and nitric oxide production by endothelial cells. Blood 104: 2073–2080.
58. Sorkin A, Waters CM (1993) Endocytosis of growth factor receptors. Bioessays 15: 375–382.
59. Neumann D, Yuk MH, Lodish HF, Lederkremer GZ (1996) Blocking intracellular degradation of the erythropoietin and asialoglycoprotein receptors by calpain inhibitors does not result in the same increase in the levels of their membrane and secreted forms. Biochem J 313 (Pt 2): 391–399.
60. Zhang Y, Thamer M, Stefanik K, Kaufman J, Cotter DJ (2004) Epoetin requirements predict mortality in hemodialysis patients. Am J Kidney Dis 44: 866–876.
61. Horl WH (2002) Non-erythropoietin-based anaemia management in chronic kidney disease. Nephrol Dial Transplant 17 Suppl 11: 35–38.
62. Greenwood RN, Ronco C, Gastaldon F, Brendolan A, Homel P, et al. (2003) Erythropoeitin dose variation in different facilities in different countries and its relationship to drug resistance. Kidney Int Suppl. S78–86.
63. Pisoni RL, Bragg-Gresham JL, Young EW, Akizawa T, Asano Y, et al. (2004) Anemia management and outcomes from 12 countries in the Dialysis Outcomes and Practice Patterns Study (DOPPS). Am J Kidney Dis 44: 94–111.
64. Bennett CL, Silver SM, Djulbegovic B, Samaras AT, Blau CA, et al. (2008) Venous thromboembolism and mortality associated with recombinant erythropoietin and darbepoetin administration for the treatment of cancer-associated anemia. JAMA 299: 914–924.
65. Weiss G, Goodnough LT (2005) Anemia of chronic disease. N Engl J Med 352: 1011–1023.

2

The Role of Serum Magnesium and Calcium on the Association between Adiponectin Levels and All-Cause Mortality in End-Stage Renal Disease Patients

Anastasia Markaki[1], John Kyriazis[2]*, Kostas Stylianou[3], George A. Fragkiadakis[1], Kostas Perakis[3], Andrew N. Margioris[4], Emmanuel S. Ganotakis[5], Eugene Daphnis[3]

1 Department of Nutrition and Dietetics, Technological Educational Institute of Crete, Crete, Greece, **2** Department of Nephrology, General Hospital of Chios, Chios, Greece, **3** Department of Nephrology, University Hospital of Heraklion, Heraklion, Crete, Greece, **4** Department of Clinical Chemistry, School of Medicine, University of Crete, Heraklion, Crete, Greece, **5** Department of Internal Medicine, University Hospital of Heraklion, Heraklion, Crete, Greece

Abstract

Background: Adiponectin (ADPN) is the most abundant adipocyte-specific cytokine that plays an important role in energy homeostasis by regulating lipid and glucose metabolism. Studies of the impact of ADPN on clinical outcomes have yielded contradictory results so far. Here, we examined the association of ADPN with serum magnesium (s-Mg) and calcium (s-Ca) levels and explored the possibility whether these two factors could modify the relationship between ADPN and all-cause mortality in patients with end-stage renal disease.

Methodology/Principal Findings: After baseline assessment, 47 hemodialysis and 27 peritoneal dialysis patients were followed- up for a median period of 50 months. S-Mg and s-Ca levels emerged as positive and negative predictors of ADPN levels, respectively. During the follow-up period 18 deaths occurred. There was a significant 4% increased risk for all-cause mortality for each 1-μg/ml increment of ADPN (crude HR, 1.04; 95% CI, 1.01–1.07), even after adjustment for s-Mg and s-Ca levels, dialysis mode, age, albumin and C-reactive protein. Cox analysis stratified by s-Mg levels (below and above the median value of 2.45 mg/dl) and s-Ca levels (below and above the median value of 9.3 mg/dl), revealed ADPN as an independent predictor of total mortality only in the low s-Mg and high s-Ca groups. Furthermore, low s-Mg and high s-Ca levels were independently associated with malnutrition, inflammation, arterial stiffening and risk of death.

Conclusions/Significance: The predictive value of ADPN in all-cause mortality in end-stage renal disease patients appears to be critically dependent on s-Mg and s-Ca levels. Conversely, s-Mg and s-Ca may impact on clinical outcomes by directly modifying the ADPN's bioactivity.

Editor: Leighton R. James, University of Florida, United States of America

Funding: No current external funding sources for this study.

Competing Interests: The authors have declared that no competing interests exist.

* E-mail: jks@otenet.gr

Introduction

Adipose tissue is not merely a fuel storage organ but an active endocrine organ, producing a variety of bioactive substances termed adipocytokines. Adiponectin (ADPN), the most abundant adipocyte-derived adipocytokine, appears to serve as a central regulatory protein in many of the physiologic pathways controlling lipid and carbohydrate metabolism and to mediate various vascular processes [1]. ADPN displays insulin sensitizing, anti-inflammatory and antiatherogenic properties [2] and it has been associated with better glycemic control, improved lipid profiles and reduced inflammation in diabetic patients [3]. Accordingly, high ADPN concentrations are associated with a favorable cardiovascular risk (CV) profile [4], [5]; however, high ADPN concentrations have also been associated with increased all-cause and CV mortality [6], [7]. Things become more complex when analyzing ADPN concentrations in relation to CV outcomes in chronic kidney disease (CKD) patients. ADPN levels are

consistently elevated among patients with CKD and end-stage renal disease (ESRD) [8], [9], being negatively correlated to glomerular filtration rate. However, since ADPN remains elevated after kidney transplantation, other factors in addition to impaired clearance may contribute [10]. Studies in predialysis [11], [12] and hemodialysis (HD) [13], [14], [15] patients showed that low ADPN levels predict worse clinical outcomes. However, more recent and better-powered studies in predialysis [16] and HD [17] patients showed that high, not low, ADPN levels were associated with worse overall and CV mortality. Similarly, high ADPN levels were associated with poor outcomes in patients with coronary artery disease and congestive heart failure [18], [19], [20]. Taken together, while ADPN may be a potential modulator of CV risk, both directly and through the metabolic processes that elevate this risk, epidemiological evidence has not consistently supported elevated levels being protective for adverse outcomes.

The conflicting data concerning the effects of ADPN on outcomes may be caused by differences in study design, inclusion criteria, sex and ethnic background. Also, ADPN's contradictory role may relate to its concomitant associations with wasting, inflammation, insulin resistance and vascular injuries [21], signifying that differences in mortality may be attributable to differences in the variables that were adjusted for in multivariate analyses. More interestingly, there are factors, such as waist circumference [22] and gender [23], capable of modifying the relationship between ADPN and outcome. In this regard, based on published evidence linking serum magnesium (s-Mg) and calcium (s-Ca) to ADPN in healthy individuals and outcomes in ESRD, we hypothesized that both these two factors could modulate the association between ADPN and outcomes in uremic subjects. Dietary intake of Mg has been associated with increased ADPN levels in the general population [24], [25]. In a recent study [26], both ADPN and intracellular Mg, strongly correlated with each other, were lower in infants with small compared to those with appropriate gestational age, and thus, were both proposed as markers of early fetal growth and insulin resistance in adulthood. Regarding s-Ca, in a population based study, where the associations of s-Ca with cardio-metabolic risk factors were examined, adiponectin had the strongest negative association with corrected s-Ca [27]. Moreover, reduced ADPN levels were detected in patients with primary hyperparathyroidism [28], [29], a state characterized by high s-Ca and insulin resistance. Finally, the adverse impact of low s-Mg [30] and elevated s-Ca [31] or high dialysate calcium (dCa) [32] on clinical outcomes has been well documented in ESRD. Considering all the above, a more thorough examination of the interrelationships of ADPN with s-Mg and s-Ca on all-cause mortality in the ESRD setting is warranted.

The current study was undertaken in ESRD patients to examine a) the existing relationships of ADPN with s-Mg and s-Ca, b) the relationship of ADPN levels with all cause mortality and c) the possible modification effects of s-Mg and s-Ca on the association between ADPN levels and all-cause mortality. Since manipulations of dCa concentrations impact on s-Ca, as they enable alterations on Ca load, the role of dCa itself in relation to ADPN and mortality was also examined.

Materials and Methods

Ethics Statement

The study was performed in strict accordance with the ethical guidelines of the Helsinki Declaration and was approved by the Ethical Scientific Committee of the University Hospital of Heraklion, Greece. All study participants provided written informed consent.

Study Population

The study was performed at the dialysis unit of the University Hospital of Heraklion, Greece. Patients were included when they had been on renal replacement therapy (RRT) for at least 6 months and were 18 years or older. Exclusion criteria included malignant disease, concurrent inflammatory illness and unwillingness to participate. Forty-seven HD and 27 peritoneal dialysis (PD) eligible patients were recruited between October 2007 and November 2008. The etiology of renal failure was hypertensive nephrosclerosis in 20 patients (27%), diabetic nephropathy in 14 (18.9%), glomerulonephritis in 11 (14.9%), interstitial nephritis in 9 (12.2%), polycystic kidney disease in 9 (12.2%) and undetermined in 11 (14.9%). Enrolled HD patients were on standard 4 hours, 3 times weekly dialysis program, using bicarbonate dialysate and high-flux (32%) or low flux (68%) dialysis membranes and aiming for a minimum target KT/V of 1.3. All HD patients were dialyzed against a 0.5 mmol/l Mg dialysate bath, whereas 13 and 34 patients were treated with a low dCa (LdCa) of 1.25 mmol/l and high dCa (HdCa) of

1.75 mmol/l, respectively. PD patients were on a standard continuous ambulatory PD program (4–5 exchanges per day) aiming to a weekly KT/V of 1.7 and creatinine clearance of 70 L/ week. All PD patients were treated with a dialysis solution containing Mg at 0.5 mmol/l, whereas 18 and 9 patients were treated with a LdCa of 1.25 mmol/l and HdCa of 1.75 mmol/l, respectively. dCa was selected, aiming at maintaining normal serum calcium and serum parathyroid hormone, after taking into account factors related to Ca load, such as type of phosphorus binder, vitamin D and calcimimetic prescription. In patients prone to intradialytic hypotension, a HdCa of 1.75 mmol/l was frequently used, as a means to improve intradialytic blood pressure instability. dCa prescription remained constant during the follow-up period. Data pertaining to history of CVD, diabetes, arterial hypertension and antihypertensive drugs were retrieved from patients' medical charts.

Body Composition

On the day of blood collection, body composition was assessed with bioimpedance analysis (BIA-101; RJL/Akern Systems, Clinton Township, MI, USA). Fat mass and fat free mass were standardized by squared height (m^2), and expressed in kg/m^2 as fat mass index (FMI) and fat free mass index, respectively.

Anthropometric Evaluation

Anthropometric measurements involved body mass index (BMI), waist circumference, triceps skinfold thickness, mid-arm circumference (MAC), mid arm muscle circumference (MAMC) and arm muscle area (AMA). MAMC and AMA were calculated using the formulas:

MAMC (cm) = MAC (cm) −3.14×Triceps Skinfold Thickness (cm).

AMA (cm^2) = MAMC (cm) ^{2}/12.56.

Laboratory Measurements

For laboratory testing, blood sample was drawn from a peripheral vein under fasting conditions. Blood samples for determination of interleukin-6 (IL-6), interleukin-8 (IL-8), and ADPN levels were centrifuged, separated and stored at $-80°C$ until analysis. IL-6 and IL-8 were measured with a chemiluminescent immunometric assay, using an Immulite 1000 analyzer (Siemens Medical Solutions Diagnostics Limited, UK). Total human ADPN was measured in serum samples using commercially available enzyme-linked immunosorbent assay kits (R&D System, Minneapolis, MN, USA) according to the manufacturer's protocol. The lower limit of detection for ADPN was 0.246 μg/ml and the inter- and intra-assay coefficients of variation were 5.8–6.9% and 2.5–4.7%, respectively.

Hemoglobin, serum albumin, prealbumin, transferrin, creatinine, parathormone, total cholesterol, high-density lipoprotein (HDL) and low-density lipoprotein (LDL) cholesterol, triglycerides, Ca and Mg were determined using standard laboratory techniques. C-reactive-protein (CRP) was measured by nephelometry.

Follow-up

Follow-up data were retrieved from clinical records and/or death certificates by personnel blind to anthropometric, body composition and laboratory assessments. Follow-up began on the date of enrolment and finished upon the death from all causes or 31 December 2011, whichever came first. No patient was lost to follow-up.

Statistical Analysis

For all statistical analyses, the SPSS/PC 18 statistical package (Chicago, IL) was used. Normally distributed variables were

Table 1. Characteristics of the patients classified into low- and high- adiponectin levels.

Characteristic	Low adiponectin (n = 25)	High adiponectin (n = 49)	P	Adjusted* R	P
Epidemiologic and clinical					
Age (yr)	58±13	62±15	0.240	–	–
Sex (males/females %)	56/44	55.1/44.9	0.941	–	–
Diabetes (%)	16	20.4	0.647	–	–
CVD (%)	24	18.4	0.569	–	–
Dialysis mode (HD/PD %)	60/40	65.3/34.7	0.654	–	–
RRT vintage (months)	61±56	68±44	0.556	–	–
Dialysate Ca (Low/High %)	36/49.9	64/53.1	0.369	–	–
Mean arterial pressure (mmHg)	94±14	94±17	0.978	–	–
Hypertension (%)	56	63.3	0.545	–	–
β-Blockers (%)	16	6.1	0.170	–	–
ACEIs +ARBs (%)	44.4	28.6	0.184	–	–
CCB (%)	24	26.5	0.814	–	–
Death from all causes (%)	8	32.7	0.023		
Anthropometric					
Body mass index (Kg/m^2)	28.1±2.7	24.7±3.1	<0.001	−0.120	0.311
Fat mass index (Kg/m^2)	10.7±2.5	8.5±3.0	0.003	–	–
Fat-free mass index (Kg/m^2)	17.4±1.7	16.2±2.2	0.016	−0.120	0.312
Waist circumference (cm)	102.4±9.9	90.9±9.6	0.000	−0.317	0.006
Triceps skinfold thickness (cm	1.8±0.8	1.4±0.7	0.049	0.002	0.984
Mid-arm circumference (cm)	30.9±3.6	27.9±4.1	0.003	−0.232	0.048
Mid-arm muscle circumference (cm)	25.3±3.6	23.4±3.4	0.034	−0.246	0.036
Arm muscle area (cm^2)	51.9±15.8	44.7±13.2	0.042	−0.238	0.042
Inflammatory					
C-reactive protein (mg/dl)	0.37 (0.3–1.3)	0.46 (0.3–1.2)	0.909	−0.131	0.268
Interleukin-6 (pg/ml)	5.3(3.2–9.0)	5.8 (4.3–11.3)	0.346	0.011	0.926
Interleukin-8 (pg/ml)	10.5 (6.9–19)	13.8 (10–22.4)	0.141	0.266	0.023
Nutritional and biochemical					
Albumin (g/dl)	4.0±0.36	3.85±0.46	0.156	−0.331	0.004
Prealbumin (mg/dl)	30±12	27±9	0.197	−0.109	0.357
Transferrin (mg/dl)	173±41	164±34	0.329	−0.004	0.970
Hemoglobin (g/dl)	11.9±1.2	11.8±1.4	0.883	−0.056	0.643
Creatinine (mg/dl)	8.2±2.7	8.9±2.7	0.924	−0.166	0.159
Total Cholesterol (mg/dl)	174±3.3	171±41	0.407	0.199	0.091
HDL cholesterol (mg/dl)	42±14	50±1 5	0.044	0.207	0.079
LDL cholesterol (mg/dl)	84±25	85±37	0.920	0.251	0.032
Triglycerides (mg/dl)	207 (160–311)	166 (99–216)	0.001	−0.137	0.285
Parathormone (pg/ml)	121 (61–205)	121 (58–169)	0.773	−0.101	0.395
Calcium (mg/dl)	9.3±0.8	9.2±0.8	0.560	−0.293	0.012
Magnesium (mg/dl)	2.4±0.4	2.6±0.5	0.247	0.288	0.014
Phosphorus (mg/dl)	5.2±1.2	5.1±1.1	0.701	−0.076	0.581
Adiponectin (μg/ml)	11.7 (9.7–14.3)	23.5 (20–34.1)	<0.001	–	

Values expressed as mean ± SD or median (interquartile range).
CVD, cardiovascular disease; HD, hemodialysis; PD, peritoneal dialysis; RRT, renal replacement therapy; ACEI's, angiotensin-converting enzyme inhibitors; ARBs, angiotensin receptor blockers; CCB, calcium channel blockers.
*Partial coefficients of correlations between adiponectin and baseline characteristics (anthropometric, inflammatory and nutritional) after correction for fat mass index.

expressed as mean ±SD and non-normally distributed variables were expressed as median (interquartile range). ADPN was examined both as continuous and as dichotomous variable, in the latter case comparing the lowest sex-specific tertile of ADPN (low ADPN group) to the higher (middle and highest) tertiles (high ADPN group). ADPN tertile cut-off points for men were 14.0 and

22.9 μg/ml and 18.0 and 27.3 μg/ml for women, respectively. Differences in baseline characteristics between the groups were tested using the χ^2 test and the Kruskall-Wallis test as appropriate. Univariate and multivariate regression analyses were used to determine associations between variables. Kaplan-Meier analysis was used to compare survival according to ADPN levels. Cox proportional hazards models were used to evaluate the relationship between ADPN and all-cause mortality initially without adjustment and subsequently adjusting for variables related to ADPN at baseline (s-Mg, s-Ca and dialysis mode) and traditional risk factors (age, albumin, CRP) univariately associated with all-cause mortality at the P<0.05 level. In these models, both Mg and Ca were analyzed as categorical variables. Regarding Mg, patients were classified into two groups based on those who were below the median value (Low Mg group) of s-Mg (2.45 mg/dl) and those above the median value (High Mg group). Regarding Ca, patients were classified into two groups based on those who were below the median value (Low Ca group) of s-Ca (9.3 mg/dl) and those above the median value (High Ca group). Since dCa is the most important prescribed determinant of calcium balance in patients receiving dialysis and, as a consequence, s-Ca is strongly dependent on dCa, as it was in the present study (rho = 0.362; p<0.002), a separate Cox analysis was done by stratifying patients into two groups based on dCa, LdCa and HdCa, as defined previously. Because both these Cox analyses produced almost identical results, we present only the Cox model accounting for s-Ca. Statistical significance was set at the level of P<0.05 (two sides).

Results

General Characteristics

The study cohort consisted of 74 patients with a mean age of 65±15 (range 18–83) years. Forty-seven patients (28 men and 19 women, mean age 63±14 years) were undergoing HD treatment and 27 patients (13 men and 14 women, mean age 58±16 years) were treated with PD. Diabetes and CVD were detected in 14 (18.9%) and 15 (20.3%) patients, respectively. There were 45 (60.1%) hypertensive patients and most of them (n = 41) were on antihypertensive drugs [b-blockers, n = 7; calcium channel blockers, n = 19 and angiotensin-converting enzyme inhibitors/angiotensin receptor blockers, n = 25]. RRT was shorter in PD than HD patients (44±37 vs.78±50 months; p<0.05).

Patients with Low versus High Adiponectin Levels

Twenty five patients had low ADPN levels, as defined in the Methods section, while 49 patients had high ADPN levels. The baseline characteristics of the two groups are shown in Table 1.The two groups did not differ significantly from each other in terms of age, sex and dialysis mode, dCa, RRT vintage, mean arterial pressure, prevalence of diabetes, CVD and hypertension, antihypertensive agent class use and cause of ESRD (data not shown). There was no difference in mean ADPN concentrations between men (n = 41) and women (n = 33) in the study (22±15 vs.25±13 μg/ml), whereas ADPN was lower in HD compared to that in PD patients (21±12 vs.28±16 μg/ml; p<0.05).

All anthropometric mesurements were lower in the high ADPN group, while no significant differences were found in any of the inflammatory parameters in the two groups. With regard to nutritional parameters, higher HDL cholesterol and lower triglycerides levels were seen in patients with high compared to those with low ADPN.

Determinants of Serum Adiponectin Levels

Adiponectin adjusted for FMI was inversely associated with almost all anthropometric measurements, serum albumin and s-Ca and positively associated with IL-8, LDL cholesterol and s-Mg (Table 1). In multiple regression analysis, where variables significant in univariate analysis were included, lower BMI, albumin and s-Ca and higher s-Mg and IL-8 were associated with higher ADPN levels (Table 2). HDL cholesterol and sex did not emerge as independent determinants of ADPN levels. This model explained 43% of the variability in adiponectin levels. When dCa was entered instead of serum Ca and FMI instead of BMI, each was significant (data not shown).

s-Mg was inversely correlated with inflammation (IL-6, CRP) markers and arterial stiffness (pulse pressure) and positively with nutritional (transferrin, creatinine) markers, whereas the opposite correlations was observed between s-Ca and these markers (Table 3). Finally, the HdCa group had higher CRP [(0.46 (0.30–1.47) vs. 0.38 (0.30–0.94)] mg/dl; p = 0.040] than the LdCa group.

Adiponectin and Mortality

During a median follow-up period of 50 months, 18 deaths occurred. Causes of death were CVD (n = 7), infectious complications (n = 6), malignancies (n = 2), intestinal rupture (n = 2) and cirrhosis (n = 1). Patients who died had higher ADPN compared with surviving patients (29±16 vs. 22±12 μg/ml; p = 0.040). Kaplan-Meier analysis (Figure 1) showed that patients in the high ADPN group had a shorter survival rate compared to those in the low ADPN group (67% vs. 92%; p = 0.020). In unadjusted Cox regression analysis (Table 4), every 1 μg/ml of increase in serum ADPN concentration increased the all-cause mortality risk by 4% (crude HR, 1.04; 95% CI, 1.01–1.07). This elevated risk persisted even after adjustment for potential mediators and confounders (HR, 1.07; 95% CI, 1.02–1.12). Results remained similar when dCa (LdCa/HdCa) replaced s-Ca (Low/High Ca groups) in the model; the same was true when BMI replaced albumin, as an index of wasting (data not shown). It is worth mentioning that in the final model, high s-Ca levels and/or HdCa emerged as independent predictors of all-cause mortality, whereas the significant inverse association detected between s-Mg levels and all-cause mortality was lost only after adjustment for age.

Table 2. Multiple regression analysis for assessing the predictors of serum adiponectin levels.

Parameter	B	Std error	Std beta	P	Partial r
Constant	97.268	22.221		<0.000	
BMI (Kg/m²)	−1.050	0.359	−0.287	0.005	−0.334
Mg (mg/dl)	7.996	3.065	0.260	0.011	0.302
Ca (mg/dl)	−4.914	1.922	−0.270	0.013	−0.296
Interleukin-8 (pg/ml)	0.318	0.136	0.244	0.022	0.273
Albumin (g/dl)	−6.876	3.421	−0.214	0.048	−0.237

Std beta, standardized regression coefficients; r, correlation coefficient; BMI, body mass index;

Table 3. Correlations of serum magnesium and calcium with selected baseline parameters.

Parameter	Magnesium		Calcium	
	rho	P	rho	P
Age (ys)	−0.283	0.014	0.194	0.098
Dialysate Ca (LdCa/HdCa)	−0.139	0.236	0.361	0.002
Pulse pressure (mmHg)	−0.274	0.018	0.248	0.033
Transferrin (mg/dl)	0.259	0.026	−0.279	0.016
Creatinine (mg/dl)	0.261	0.021	0.043	0.713
Interleukin-6 (pg/ml)	−0.277	0.017	0.101	0.391
Interleukin-8 (pg/ml)	0.076	0.516	0.232	0.047
CRP (mg/dl)	−0.251	0.031	0.095	0.418

LdCa, low dialysate calcium; HdCa, high dialysate calcium; CRP, C-reactive protein.

Serum Mg Levels and Dialysate Ca levels Influence the Relationship between Adiponectin and All-cause Mortality

Next, we examined whether adiponectin interacted with s-Mg levels (Low/High Mg groups) and s-Ca (Low/High Ca groups) to modify its association with all-cause mortality. An interaction term between ADPN concentration and s-Mg levels was significant ($p = 0.002$), after controlling for the main effects, albumin, CRP, and dialysis mode. The same was true ($p = 0.001$) for the interaction between ADPN and s-Ca. Then, the association between ADPN (per 1 μg/ml) and all-cause mortality by

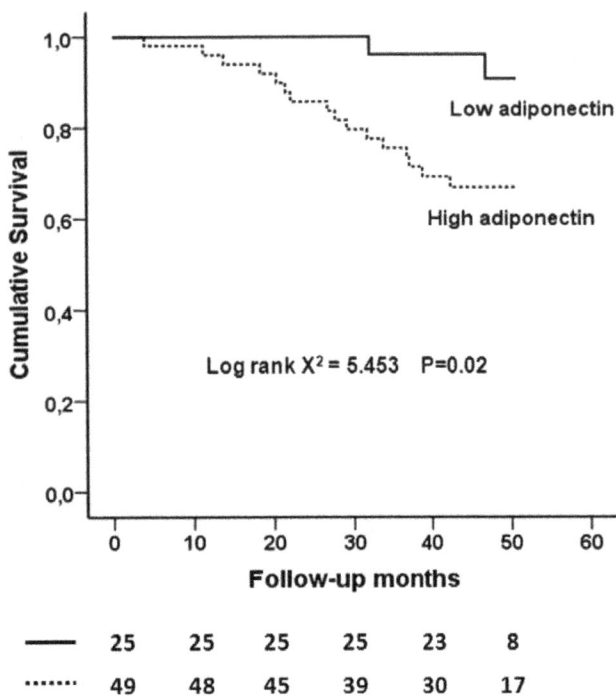

Figure 1. Kaplan-Meier analyses comparing the lowest sex-specific tertile of adiponecting (<14 for men and <18 μg/ml for women) to the higher (middle and highest) tertiles. The number of patients at risk are given below the plot.

subgroups of s-Mg and s-Ca was examined (Table 5). In the low Mg and high Ca groups, ADPN was a significant predictor of all-cause mortality, even after adjustment for age, CRP and albumin. On the contrary, in the high Mg and low Ca groups, ADPN levels were not predictive of outcome in either crude or the adjusted models. Of note, a significant ($p = 0.001$) interaction between ADPN and dCa (LdCa/HdCa) was also observed; the effect modification of dCa on the ADPN-mortality association in magnitude and direction was similar to that observed with s-Ca (data not shown).

Discussion

The present study showed that both s-Mg and s-Ca are major determinants of ADPN levels in ESRD patients. ADPN was positively associated with s-Mg and negatively with s-Ca. In addition, a strong association was demonstrated between high ADPN levels and all-cause mortality, which persisted after multivariate adjustment for possible confounders. Our main finding was that the predictive value of the effect of ADPN levels on mortality was critically dependent on s-Mg and s-Ca concentrations, since high ADPN levels were not predictive of all-cause mortality in patients having high s-Mg and low s-Ca levels.

In this study, we confirm many of the metabolic associations reported previously with ADPN in non-renal [2], [18], [19] and renal patients [13], [16], [17]. Specifically, in our study, lower BMI, albumin, triglycerides and higher HDL cholesterol were associated with higher ADPN levels. In this regard, our findings are in accord with the literature and support the validity of our dataset. Most importantly, this study documents for first time the existence of strong positive and negative associations of ADPN with s-Mg and s-Ca, respectively, in ESRD patients. These associations were independent of each other and independent of body composition, nutritional and inflammatory status. Thus, our data confirm the results of previously reported associations of ADPN with s-Mg [24], [25], [26] and s-Ca [27], [28], [29] in non-renal populations and further extent these findings in the ESRD population, where s-Mg [30] and s-Ca [31] strongly impact on outcomes. The exact mechanisms underlying these associations are not clear, but the fact that common defects in Mg and Ca metabolism are reportedly [33] related to glucose metabolism, provides a possible explanation for this. Indeed, there is enough evidence to indicate that both hypomagnesemia [34], [35] and hypercalcemia [36], [37] are closely associated with insulin resistance. These findings, in concert with the observation that ADPN levels are decreased in patients with type 2 diabetes and in insulin resistance states may at least partially explain the positive and negative associations of ADPN with s-Mg and s-Ca, respectively.

Our results indicated that high ADPN levels were an independent predictor of total mortality in ESRD patients. There was a significant 7% increased risk for death from any cause for each 1-μg/ml increment of ADPN. In addition, the survival rate was significantly lower in patients in the higher sex-specific tertiles compared to those in the lower tertile of ADPN. These data are consistent with recent studies, where there was a 3% to 10.3% increased risk for all-cause mortality for each 1-μg/ml increment of ADPN in CKD [16] and ESRD patients [17]. Since ADPN is presumed to possess antiatherogenic and cardioprotective properties, the association of high ADPN levels with adverse clinical outcomes may be explained by an increased counter-regulatory secretion of ADPN to mitigate inflammation, malnutrition and to protect against endothelial damage and atherogenesis. Although,

Table 4. Crude and adjusted hazard ratios of serum adiponectin (per 1 µg/ml) for prediction of all-cause mortality in 74 prevalent ESRD patients.

VariableUnints of increase)	Model 1 (unadjusted)		Model 2		Model 3	
	HR (CI, 95%)	P	HR (CI, 95%)	P	HR (CI, 95%)	P
Adiponectin (1 µg/ml)	1.04 (1.01–1.07)	0.013	1.08 (1.3–1.12)	0.000	1.07 (1.02–1.12)	0.005
Factors related to ADPN						
Low Mg (vs High Mg)			4.04 (1.27–12.8)	0.018	1.16 (0.34–3.96)	0.813
High Ca (vs Low Ca)			5.82 (1.66–20.3)	0.006	5.39 (1.33–21.87)	0.018
PD (vs. HD)			2.93 (1.05–8.19)	0.040	3.14 (0.96–10.31)	0.059
Traditional risk factors						
Albumin (1 g/dl)					0.27 (0.06–1.30)	0.102
CRP (1 mg/dl)					1.51 (0.99–2.30)	0.056
Age (1 yr)					1.09 (1.03–1.16)	0.005

Data adjustment for variables related to adiponectin (model 2), as well as for traditional risk factors (model 3), did not modify the relationship between adiponectin levels and all-cause mortality.
ADPN, adiponectin; PD, peritoneal dialysis; HD, hemodialysis.

nutritional and inflammatory statuses were independent determinants of ADPN at baseline, they did not affect the ADPN-mortality association in our study. Alternatively, the existence of a state of adiponectin resistance [38] perhaps due to reduced ligand/receptor activities or down regulation of adiponectin receptors or both may trigger a counter-regulatory increase of ADPN secretion in high risk ESRD patients. Another consideration is that a higher adiponectin level may induce protein energy wasting, a condition associated with malnutrition and inflammation [21]. Reportedly, ADPN may increase energy expenditure and induce weight loss through a direct effect on the brain [39], thus, linking increased ADPN levels to increased mortality in patients with ESRD. Conversely, due to the inverse relationship between adiponectin and fat mass or BMI, weight loss increases plasma adiponectin levels [40] and thus, high ADPN levels in ESRD patients may be a marker of wasting processes and poor prognosis. However, in the present study, adjusting for body composition (BMI) did not alter the effect of high ADPN on mortality.

However, there are also studies, carried out in the general [6], [7], CKD [11], [12], [13] and ESRD [14], [15] [41] populations, in which the lowest levels of ADPN had the worst outcome.

Table 5. Association of adiponectin with all-cause mortality stratified by serum Mg and dialysate calcium.

Per 1 µg/ml increase of adiponectin					
	E/P	Unadjusted		Adjusted*	
		HR (CI, 95%)	P	HR (CI, 95%)	P
Stratified by s-Mg					
Low Mg group	12/37	1.08 (1.03–1.13)	0.003	1.09 (1.02–1.17)	0.011
High Mg group	6/37	1.04 (0.99–1.09)	0.114	1.03 (0.98–1.07)	0.273
Stratified by s-Ca					
Low Ca group	6/30	1.02 (0.98–1.07)	0.346	1.05 (0.98–1.13)	0.174
High Ca group	11/38	1.09 (1.03–1.15)	0.001	1.08 (1.01–1.16)	0.022

*adjusted for age, C- reactive protein and albumin.
E/P, events/patients.

Discrepancies among studies in ESRD patients might be explained by differences in the populations studied, inclusion criteria, method of dialysis, confounding influences of covariates, different retention of the different ADPN isoforms in kidney disease [42] and post-translational modifications in the ADPN molecule [23]. In the study by Diez et al [41], comprised of 98 HD and 86 PD patients, an inverse relationship between ADPN levels and all-cause and CVD mortality was reported. Beside a shorter mean follow-up period of 31.2 months, the dialysis vintage was 2.5 (1.7–11.5) months in PD and 12.2 (4.8–43) months in HD patients, whereas the corresponding figures in our study were 36 (18–54) and 80 (36–108) months in PD and HD patients, respectively. In addition PD patients had a mean residual renal function of 3.3 (0.5–6.9) ml/min. It cannot be excluded that the beneficial effect s of ADPN during the early period of renal replacement treatment become harmful over time, particularly when the compensatory increase of ADPN is overwhelming. This assumption is further supported by a population-based cohort of 2484 participants [43], aged 50–75 year, where a higher ADPN was associated with an increased risk of CVD mortality in people with prevalent CVD [HR 1.27 (0.98–1.63)] and with reduced risk in people without CVD [HR 0.90 (0.73–1.11)]. In addition, data regarding s-Mg and s-Ca levels and dialysis prescription were not reported. In contrast, the inverse relationship between ADPN levels and CVD events in a cohort of 227 HD patients [13] can be potentially explained by the Mg and Ca dialysate concentrations used in concert with the findings of the present study, a topic which will be discussed later.

In this study, s-Mg levels were directly correlated with nutritional factors and inversely with pulse pressure, a gross estimate of arterial stiffness, inflammatory markers and age. Furthermore, s-Mg levels predicted total mortality, but this association was largely dependent on age. These findings confirm the results of previous studies supporting a link between low s-Mg levels and atherogenesis [44] or arterial calcification [45], malnourishment and increased risk of death in HD patients [46].

Elevated s-Ca levels and treatment with HdCa, both associated with an increased risk of Ca overload, have also been linked with morbidity and mortality [32], [47], [48]. Our data agree with these reports showing that both increased s-Ca levels and the use of HdCa are associated with adverse clinical outcomes. Indeed, elevated s-Ca levels were associated with a more disadvantageous metabolic risk profile, in terms of increased pulse pressure and IL-8 and lower transferrin, while treatment with a HdCa of 1.75 mmol/l was associated with increased CRP. Both increased s-Ca levels and HdCa predicted independently total mortality. Thus, we provide solid evidence suggesting that Mg deficiency and Ca overload may contribute significantly to malnutrition, inflammation, arterial stiffening and increased CVD death in ESRD patients [30], [31], [46], [47], [48].

The most important finding of this study is that the association between ADPN and mortality varied among subgroups of patients stratified by s-Mg and s-Ca (and/or dCa). In contrast to low s-Mg and high s-Ca (and/or HdCa) groups, ADPN levels were not predictive of death in the high s-Mg and low s-Ca (and/or LdCa) groups. We speculated that the presence of ADPN resistance could be more pronounced in the former groups, due to a worse CVD risk profile, as discussed above. Alternatively, ADPN may not directly affect death risk, but may be a marker of other risks. Another possibility is that s-Mg and s-Ca may impact directly on the bioactivity of ADPN isomers in uremia. ADPN circulates in plasma as a low-molecular-weight (LMW) adiponectin (trimer), middle-molecular-weight (MMW) adiponectin (hexamer) and a high-molecular- weight (HMW) adiponectin (multimer). Although HMW is the most abundant isoform in ESRD patients [49], the distribution and role of each isoform in CKD remains largely unknown. However, emerging evidence suggest that LMW isoforms are associated with better clinical outcomes in both non-uremic and uremic populations, compared to the other isoforms. LMW isoforms were associated with lower CVD risk in children with CKD stage 2–4 [42], and as opposed to HMW isoforms, appear to exert a protective role in older adults with previous coronary heart disease [50] and lead to a reduction of liver cancer risk [51]. Most importantly, a recent study clearly demonstrated that the formation of the fully developed complex HMW structure of ADPN is influenced by the presence of Ca [52]. In both human and mice adipocyte cells, the presence of Ca led to a substantial increased formation of HMW adiponectin, with a corresponding decrease in MMW and LMW isomers, whereas the absence of Ca had the opposite result. These data indicate that low s-Ca and/or potentially high s-Mg levels may be associated with increased LMW isoforms and better outcomes, whereas high s-Ca and/or potentially low s-Mg levels may be associated with HMW isoforms and poor prognosis. This intriguing hypothesis needs to be confirmed in future studies.

This study may also have important clinical implications. Indeed, if s-Mg and s-Ca levels prove to be true effect modifiers of the association between ADPN and mortality, then these findings may impact on clinical practice in the management of ESRD patients, through modifications of dialysate prescriptions, particularly with regard to Mg and Ca and lead to improved guidelines for better outcomes in our high-risk patients. The median s-Mg concentration of 2.45 (2.3–2.7) mg/dl, above which a survival benefit was observed in this study, remained within normal range (1.7 to 2.67 mg/dl). Also, in a previous study [46] using the same dialysate Mg concentration of 0.5 mmol/l, survival was significantly higher in patients with a mean s-Mg concentration above 2.77 mg/dl, a value considered indicative of mild hypermagnesemia. It is possible that if higher Mg dialysate levels had been used, the ensuing higher degree of hypermagnesemia could have resulted in an even better outcome. Since dialysate Mg concentration is an important determinant of Mg balance in both HD and PD patients, a higher s-Mg can be achieved by using a higher dialysate Mg concentration (0.75 mmol/l) than the currently used (0.5 mmol/l) in most countries. We have previously reported [53] that after a four-week treatment with a dialysate Mg concentration

of 0.75, 0.5 and 0.25 mmol/l, mean s-Mg concentrations were 2.94, 2.57 and 2.21 mg/dl, respectively. Major guidelines do not comment on dialysate Mg concentrations and trials on this topic with morbidity and/or mortality end points are lacking. A recent review [54] of Mg in dialysis patients indicated that a Mg dialysate of 0.75 mmol/l is likely to cause mild hypermagnesemia, whereas s-Mg levels were mostly normal to low when 0.2 and 0.25 mmol/l Mg concentrations were used. Results were inconsistent (normo-magnesemia in most studies) with regard to Mg dialysate of 0.5 mmol/l. A higher survival rate was also observed in patients with a s-Ca concentration below the median 9.3 (8.8–9.7) mg/dl and/or using a LdCa of 1.25 mmol/l. Current guidelines [55] recommend the use of a dCa concentration of 1.25 to 1.5 mmol/l in both HD and PD patients. However a recent study [56] showed that the intradialytic Ca mass balance was nearly neutral using a dCa of 1.25 mmol/l, whereas treatment with a dCa of 1.50 mmol/l resulted in gain of Ca during HD. dCa concentrations as high as 1.75 mmol/l should be avoided to prevent calcium overload and the induction of adynamic bone disease. However, most studies [57] showed a positive effect of HdCa on haemodynamic stability during dialysis compared with LdCa concentrations. Taken all these data together, one could speculate that by increasing dialysate Mg concentration up to 0.75 mmol/l and decreasing dCa concentration from 1.75 or 1.50 to 1.25 mmol/l, the increased ADPN levels in uremia would have rather a beneficial effect on outcomes. Unfortunately, dialysate Mg and Ca levels are not reported in the relevant studies. In the study of Zocalli et al [13], where these were reported, the use of a high Mg dialysate of 0.75 mmol/l and a LdCa of 1.25 mmol/l were associated with a 3% CV risk reduction for each 1-µg/ml increase in plasma ADPN levels. Thus, we recommend that s-Mg and s-Ca levels should be taken into consideration when assessing the role of ADPN on outcomes in ESRD and the optimal s-Mg and s-Ca levels required for a survival advantage in relation to ADPN be established.

This study has several limitations. First, due to the small number of patients who died, specific mortality risk (i.e. CVD) could not be determined and generalizability of study results might have been compromised. Generalizability might also have been jeopardized by the low percentage of diabetics, low number of comorbid conditions, lack of other ethnic groups and the fact that a single center participated in the study. Nevertheless, this study enabled us to detect a strong ADPN-mortality association in ESRD patients, the magnitude and direction of which were comparable to those previously reported in relevant studies of the same [17] or larger populations [16]. In the study of Ohashi et al [17], with a sample size (n = 75), number of deaths (n = 15) and a threshold for assessing mortality (15 µg/ml) quite similar to ours, the magnitude of association between ADPN and total mortality was comparable to ours (10.3% vs. 7% adjusted risk increment for each 1-µg/ml increase in ADPN). The robustness of this association did not decrease after adjusting for potential confounder and/or mediators in both pooled and subgroup analyses. Second, we measured total ADPN and not its various isoforms, the reason being that the relevant methodology at the time of our measurements was not available. Notwithstanding, since this was generating hypothesis study, further assessment of ADPN isomers will be necessary to elucidate the difference in the effect of each ADPN isomer on clinical outcomes. In this regard, the first step in testing this intriguing hypothesis is to confirm the presumed positive and negative associations of LMW isoforms with s-Mg and s-Ca, respectively and the corresponding opposite associations regarding HMW isoforms in large cross-sectional studies, and b) then prospectively verify the favorable and unfavorable effects of LMW and HMW isoforms, respectively, on outcomes in relation to targeted s-Mg and s-Ca concentration, through appropriate use and manipulation of Mg and Ca concentration in the dialysis bath. Third, the use of a single baseline measurement to predict events several years in the future. However, serum concentrations of adiponectin seem stable during a period of 1 yr, with minimal short-term variation and high degree of reproducibility [58].

In conclusion, we showed that s-Mg and s-Ca levels can modify the effect of ADPN on all-cause mortality, aiding in unraveling the controversy which surround this association in the existing literature. High ADPN was an independent predictor of death risk only in patients with low s-Mg and high s-Ca levels, respectively, conditions highly associated with a worse CVD risk

profile and possibly a marked increase in ADPN resistance. Conversely, the better survival rates seen with high s-Mg and low s-Ca may be caused by altered ADPN bioactivities associated with death risk reduction. Future studies are needed to elucidate the exact roles of s-Mg and s-Ca on ADPN bioactivity in relation to clinical outcomes in ESRD.

Author Contributions

Conceived and designed the experiments: AM GF KP KS ESG ED. Performed the experiments: A. Markaki GF KP. Analyzed the data: JK KS ESG ED. Contributed reagents/materials/analysis tools: A. Markaki GF KP A. Margioris. Wrote the paper: A. Markaki JK KS A. Margioris ESG ED.

References

1. Rabin KR, Kamari Y, Avni I, Grossman E, Sharabi Y (2005) Adiponectin: linking the metabolic syndrome to its cardiovascular consequences. Expert Rev Cardiovasc Ther 3: 465–471.
2. Chandran M, Phillips SA, Ciaraldi T, Henry RR (2003) Adiponectin: more than just another fat cell hormone? Diabetes Care 26: 2442–2450.
3. Mantzoros CS, Li T, Manson JE, Meigs JB, Hu FB (2005) Circulating adiponectin levels are associated with better glycemic control, more favorable lipid profile, and reduced inflammation in women with type 2 diabetes. J Clin Endocrinol Metab 90: 4542–4548.
4. Sattar N, Wannamethee G, Sarwar N, Tchernova J, Cherry L, et al. (2006) Adiponectin and coronary heart disease. A prospective study and meta-analysis. Circulation 114: 623–629.
5. Pischon T, Girman CJ, Hotamisligil GS, Rifai N, Hu FB, et al. (2004) Plasma adiponectin levels and risk of myocardial infarction in men. JAMA 291: 1730–1737.
6. Wannamethee SG, Whincup PH, Lennon L, Sattar N (2007) Circulating adiponectin levels and mortality in elderly men with and without cardiovascular disease and heart failure. Arch Intern Med 167: 1510–1517.
7. Laughlin GA, Barrett-Connor E, May S, Langenberg C (2007) Association of adiponectin with coronary heart disease and mortality: the Rancho Bernardo study. Am J Epidemiol 165: 164–174.
8. Mallamaci F, Zoccali C, Cuzzola F, Tripepi G, Cutrupi S, et al. (2002) Adiponectin in essential hiypertension. J Nephrol 15: 507–511.
9. Stenvinkel P, Marchlewska A, Pecoits-Filho R, Heimbürger O, Zhang Z, et al. (2004) Adiponectin in renal disease: relationship to phenotype and genetic variation in the gene encoding adiponectin. Kidney Int 65: 274–281.
10. Chudek J, Adamczak M, Karkoszka H, Budziński G, Ignacy W, et al. (2003) Plasma adiponectin concentration before and after successful kidney transplantation. Transplant Proc 35: 2186–2189.
11. Becker B, Kronenberg F, Kielstein JT, Budziński G, Ignacy W, et al. (2005) Renal insulin resistance syndrome, adiponectin and cardiovascular events in patients with kidney disease: the mild and moderate kidney disease study. Am Soc Nephrol 16: 1091–1098.
12. Iwashima Y, Horio T, Kumada M, Budziński G, Ignacy W, et al. (2006) Adiponectin and renal function, and implication as a risk of cardiovascular disease. Am J Cardiol 98: 1603–1608.
13. Zoccali C, Mallamaci F, Tripepi G, Benedetto FA, Cutrupi S, et al. (2002) Adiponectin, metabolic risk factors, and cardiovascular events among patients with end-stage renal disease. J Am Soc Nephrol 13: 134–141.
14. Ignacy W, Chudek J, Adamczak M, Benedetto FA, Cutrupi S, et al. (2005) Reciprocal association of plasma adiponectin and serum C-reactive protein concentration in haemodialysis patients with end-stage kidney disease - a follow-up study. Nephron 101: c18–c24.
15. Nishimura M, Hashimoto T, Kobayashi H, Yamazaki S, Okino K, et al. (2006) Association of the circulating adiponectin concentration with in-stent restenosis in hemodialysis patients. Nephrol Dial Transplant 21: 1640–1647.
16. Menon V, Li L, Wang X, Greene T, Balakrishnan V, et al. (2006) Adiponectin and mortality in patients with chronic kidney disease. J Am Soc Nephrol 17: 2599–2606.
17. Ohashi N, Koto A, Misaki T, Sakakima M, Sakakima M, et al. (2008) Association of serum adiponectin levels with all-cause mortality in hemodialysis patients. Intern Med (Tokyo, Japan) 47: 485–491
18. Cavusoglu E, Ruwende C, Chopra V, Yanamadala S, Eng C, et al. (2006) Adiponectin is an independent predictor of all-cause mortality, cardiac mortality, and myocardial infarction in patients presenting with chest pain. Eur Heart J 27: 2300–2309.
19. Kistorp C, Faher I, Galatius S, Gustafsson F, Frystyk J, et al. (2005) Plasma adiponectin, body mass index, and mortality in patients with chronic heart failure. Circulation 112: 1756–1762.
20. Pills S, Mangge H, Wellnitz B, Seelhorst U, Winkelmann BR, et al. (2006) Adiponectin and mortality in patients undergoing coronary angiography. J Clin Endocrinol Metab 91: 4277–4286.
21. Park SH, Carrero JJ, Lindholm B, Stenvinkel P (2009) Adiponectin in chronic kidney disease has an opposite impact on protein-energy wasting and cardiovascular risk: two sides of the same coin. Clin Nephrol 72: 87–96.
22. Zoccali C, Postorino M, Marino C, Pizzini P, Cutrupi S, et al. (2011) Waist circumference modifies the relationship between the adipose tissue cytokines leptin andadiponectin and all-cause and cardiovascular mortality in haemodialysis patients. J Intern Med 269: 172–181.
23. Kollerits B, Fliser D, Heid IM, Ritz E, Kronenberg F; MMKD Study Group (2007) Gender-specific association of adiponectin as a predictor of progression of chronic kidney disease: the Mild to Moderate Kidney Disease Study. Kidney Int 71: 1279–1286.
24. Qi L, Rimm E, Liu S, Rifai N, Hu FB (2005) Dietary glycemic index, glycemic load, cereal fiber, and plasma adiponectin concentration in diabetic men. Diabetes Care 28: 1022–1028.
25. Cassidy A, Skidmore P, Rimm EB, Welch A, Fairweather-Tait S, et al. (2009) Plasma adiponectin concentrations are associated with body composition and plant-based dietary factors in female twins. J Nutr 139: 353–358.
26. Takaya J, Yamato F, Higashino H, Kaneko K (2007) Intracellular magnesium and adipokines in umbilical cord plasma and infant birth size. Pediatr Res 62: 700–703.
27. Guessous I, Bonny O, Paccaud, F Mooser V, Waeber G, et al. (2011) Serum calcium levels are associated with novel cardiometabolic risk factors in the population-based CoLaus study. Plos one 6: e18865.
28. Delfini E, Petramala L, Caliumi C, Cotesta D, De Toma G, et al. (2007) Circulating leptin and adiponectin levels in patients with primary hyperparathyroidism. Metabolism 56: 30–36.
29. Bollerslev J, Rosen T, Mollerup CL, Nordenström J, Baranowski M, et al. (2009) Effect of surgery on cardiovascular risk factors in mild primary hyperparathyroidism. J Clin Endocrinol Metab 94: 2255–2261.
30. Massy ZA, Drüeke TB (2012) Magnesium and outcomes in patients with chronic kidney disease: focus on vascular calcification, atherosclerosis and survival. Clin Kidney J 5[Suppl 1]: i52–i61.
31. Young EW (2007) Mineral metabolism and mortality in patients with chronic kidney disease. Adv Chronic Kidney Dis 14: 13–21.
32. Hsu CW, Lin JL, Lin-Tan DT, Yen TH, Chen KH, et al. (2010) High-calcium dialysate: a factor associated with inflammation, malnutrition and mortality in non-diabetic maintenance haemodialysis patients. Nephrology (Carlton) 15: 313–320.
33. Resnick LM (1989) Hypertension and abnormal glucose homeostasis. Possible role of divalent ion metabolism. Am J Med 87: 17S–22S.
34. Pham PC, Pham PM, Pham SV, Miller JM, Pham PT (2007) Hypomagnesemia in patients with type 2 diabetes. Clin J Am Soc Nephrol 2: 366–373.
35. Saris NE, Mervaala E, Karppanen H, Khawaja JA, Lewenstam A (2000) Magnesium. An update on physiological, clinical and analytical aspects. Clin Chim Acta 294: 1–26.
36. Sun G, Vasdev S, Martin GR, Gadag V, Zhang H (2005) Altered Calcium Homeostasis Is Correlated With Abnormalities of Fasting Serum Glucose, Insulin Resistance, and β-Cell Function in the Newfoundland Population. Diabetes 54: 3336–3369.
37. Ybarra J, Doñate T, Jurado J, Pou JM (2007) Primary hyperparathyroidism, insulin resistance, and cardiovascular disease: a review. Nurs Clin North Am 42: 79–85.
38. Kadowaki T, Yamauchi T (2005) Adiponectin and adiponectin receptors. Endocr Rev 26: 439–451.
39. Qi Y, Takahashi N, Hileman SM, Patel HR, Berg AH, et al. (2004) Adiponectin acts in the brain to decrease body weight. Nat Med 10: 524–529.
40. Yang WS, Lee WJ, Funahashi T, Tanaka S, Matsuzawa Y, et al. (2001) Weight reduction increases plasma levels of an adipose-derived anti-inflammatory protein, adiponectin. J Clin Endocrinol Metab 86: 3815–3819.
41. Diez JJ, Estrada P, Bajo MA, Fernández-Reyes MJ, Grande C, et al. (2009) High stable serum adiponectin levels are associated with a better outcome in prevalent dialysis patients. Am J Nephrol 30: 244–252.

42. Lo MM, Salisbury S, Scherer PE, Furth SL, Warady BA, et al. (2011) Serum adiponectin complexes and cardiovascular risk in children with chronic kidney disease. Pediatr Nephrol 26: 2009–2017.

43. Dekker JM, Funahashi T, Nijpels G, Pilz S, Stehouwer CD, et al. (2008) Prognostic value of adiponectin for cardiovascular disease and mortality. J Clin Endocrinol Metab 93: 1489–1496.

44. Tzanakis I, Virvidakis K, Tsomi A, Tanaka S, Matsuzawa Y, et al. (2004) Intra- and extracellular magnesium levels and atheromatosis in haemodialysis patients. Magnes Res 17: 102–108.

45. Salem S, Bruck H, Bahlmann FH, Peter M, Passlick-Deetjen J, et al. (2012) Relationship between magnesium and clinical biomarkers on inhibition of vascular calcification. Am J Nephrol 35: 31–39.

46. Ishimura E, Okuno S, Yamakawa T, Inaba M, Nishizawa Y (2007) Serum magnesium concentration is a significant predictor of mortality in maintenance hemodialysis patients. Magnes Res 20: 237–244.

47. Young EW, Albert JM, Satayathum S, Goodkin DA, Pisoni RL, et al. (2005) Predictors and consequences of altered mineral metabolism: the Dialysis Outcomes and Practice Patterns Study. Kidney Int 67: 1179–1187.

48. Tetta C, Gallieni M, Panichi V, Brancaccio D (2002) Vascular calcifications as a footprint of increased calcium load and chronic inflammation in uremic patients: a need for a neutral calcium balance during hemodialysis? Int J Artif Organs 25: 18–26.

49. Shen YY, Charlesworlh JA, Kelly JJ, Loi KW, Peake PW (2007) Up-regulation of adiponectin, its isoforms and receptors in end-stage kidney disease. Nephrol Dial Transplant 22: 171–178.

50. Rizza S, Gigli F, Galli A, Micchelini B, Lauro D, et al. (2010) Adiponectin isoforms in elderly patients with or without coronary artery disease. J Am Geriatr Soc 58: 702–706.

51. Kotani K, Wakai K, Shibata A, Fujita Y, Ogimoto I, et al.(2009) Serum adiponectin multimer complexes and liver cancer risk in a large cohort study in Japan. Asia J Cancer Prev 10 Suppl: 87–90.

52. Banga A, Bodies AM, Rasouli N, Ranganathan G, Kern PA, et al. (2008) Calcium is involved in formation of high molecular weight adiponectin. Metab Syndr Relat Disord 6: 103–111.

53. Kyriazis J, Kalogeropoulou K, Bilirakis L, Smirnioudis N, Pikounis V, et al. (2004) Dialysate magnesium level and blood pressure. Kidney Int 66: 1221–1231.

54. Cunningham J, Rodrıguez M, Messa P (2012) Magnesium in chronic kidney disease Stages 3 and 4 and in dialysis patients. Clin Kidney J 5 (suppl1): i39–i52i.

55. (2011) KDIGO clinical practice guideline for the diagnosis, evaluation, prevention, and treatment of Chronic Kidney Disease-Mineral and Bone Disorder (CKD-MBD). Kidney Int :76 (Suppl 113) S50–S99.

56. Bosticardo G, Malberti F, Basile C, Leardini L, Libbuti P, et al. (2012) Optimizing the dialysate calcium concentration in bicarbonate haemodialysis. Nephrol Dial Transplant 27: 2489–2496.

57. Kyriazis J, Glotsos J, Bilirakis L, Smirnioudis N, Tripolitou M, et al. (2002) Dialysate calcium profiling during hemodialysis: use and clinical implications. Kidney Int 61: 276–287.

58. Pischon T, Hotamisligil GS, Rimm EB (2003) Adiponectin: Stability in plasma over 36 hours and within-person variation over 1 year. Clin Chem 49: 650–652.

3

CUBN as a Novel Locus for End-Stage Renal Disease: Insights from Renal Transplantation

Anna Reznichenko[1]*, **Harold Snieder**[2], **Jacob van den Born**[1], **Martin H. de Borst**[1], **Jeffrey Damman**[3], **Marcory C. R. F. van Dijk**[4], **Harry van Goor**[4], **Bouke G. Hepkema**[5], **Jan-Luuk Hillebrands**[4], **Henri G. D. Leuvenink**[3], **Jan Niesing**[3], **Stephan J. L. Bakker**[1], **Marc Seelen**[1], **Gerjan Navis**[1], on behalf of the REGaTTA (REnal GeneTics TrAnsplantation) Groningen group

1 Division of Nephrology, Department of Internal Medicine, University Medical Center Groningen, University of Groningen, Groningen, The Netherlands, 2 Unit of Genetic Epidemiology & Bioinformatics, Department of Epidemiology, University Medical Center Groningen, University of Groningen, Groningen, The Netherlands, 3 Department of Surgery, University Medical Center Groningen, University of Groningen, Groningen, The Netherlands, 4 Department of Pathology and Medical Biology, University Medical Center Groningen, University of Groningen, Groningen, The Netherlands, 5 Department of Transplant Immunology, University Medical Center Groningen, University of Groningen, Groningen, The Netherlands

Abstract

Chronic kidney disease (CKD) is a complex disorder. As genome-wide association studies identified cubilin gene *CUBN* as a locus for albuminuria, and urinary protein loss is a risk factor for progressive CKD, we tested the hypothesis that common genetic variants in *CUBN* are associated with end-stage renal disease (ESRD) and proteinuria. First, a total of 1142 patients with ESRD, admitted for renal transplantation, and 1186 donors were genotyped for SNPs rs7918972 and rs1801239 (case-control study). The rs7918972 minor allele frequency (MAF) was higher in ESRD patients comparing to kidney donors, implicating an increased risk for ESRD (OR 1.39, $p = 0.0004$) in native kidneys. Second, after transplantation recipients were followed for 5.8 [3.8–9.2] years (longitudinal study) documenting ESRD in transplanted kidneys – graft failure (GF). During post-transplant follow-up 92 (9.6%) cases of death-censored GF occurred. Donor rs7918972 MAF, representing genotype of the transplanted kidney, was 16.3% in GF vs 10.7% in cases with functioning graft. Consistently, a multivariate Cox regression analysis showed that donor rs7918972 is a predictor of GF, although statistical significance was not reached (HR 1.53, $p = 0.055$). There was no association of recipient rs7918972 with GF. Rs1801239 was not associated with ESRD or GF. In line with an association with the outcome, donor rs7918972 was associated with elevated proteinuria levels cross-sectionally at 1 year after transplantation. Thus, we identified *CUBN* rs7918972 as a novel risk variant for renal function loss in two independent settings: ESRD in native kidneys and GF in transplanted kidneys.

Editor: Florian Kronenberg, Innsbruck Medical University, Austria

Funding: Funding was provided by GENECURE grant EU_FP-6 037697. The funder had no role in study design, data collection and analysis, decision to publish, or preparation of the manuscript.

Competing Interests: The authors have declared that no competing interests exist.

* E-mail: a.reznichenko@umcg.nl

Introduction

Chronic kidney disease (CKD) is a complex multifactorial disorder with an important genetic component [1–3]. A recent genome-wide association study (GWAS) identified the cubilin gene *CUBN* as a locus for albuminuria: a missense single-nucleotide polymorphism (SNP) rs1801239 (Ile2984Val) in this gene was associated with elevated urinary albumine-to-creatinine ratio and microalbuminuria in both the general population and in diabetic patients [4].

As albuminuria is a risk factor for progression of CKD up to end stage renal disease (ESRD) [5], we hypothesized that genetic variation in *CUBN* is associated with development of ESRD. To test this hypothesis we genotyped patients with ESRD, admitted for renal transplantation, with their donors as a control population, for SNPs in the *CUBN* locus and followed the recipients after transplantation documenting clinical parameters and occurrence of graft failure (GF).

Two *CUBN* SNPs were genotyped in our study: the previously published rs1801239 and a tagSNP rs7918972. The latter was selected based on its linkage disequilibrium with 9 other SNPs thus covering more variability in the locus and taking into account that one of the linked polymorphisms is a coding missense variant which might potentially be functional. Another selection criterion was the minor allele frequency (MAF); we targeted a lower part of the common variability range, with MAFs between 10 and 15%.

Within this cohort we performed essentially two independent analyses: 1) ESRD patients admitted for renal transplantation versus kidney donors (extreme case-control study) – to test for association with ESRD in native kidneys; and 2) long-term post-transplant follow-up for GF in the recipients (longitudinal study) – for association with ESRD in the transplanted kidney.

We also tested association of the *CUBN* SNPs with 24-h total urinary protein excretion as an intermediate phenotype.

Materials and Methods

Study population

From all renal transplantations carried out in our center between 1993 and 2008 we retrospectively selected 1142 first graft recipients and 1186 donors for the present genetic study. The exclusion criteria were: cases of re-transplantation, combined kidney/pancreas or kidney/liver transplantation, technical problems, absence of DNA and loss of follow-up. A flowchart of the study participants selection is shown in the *Figure 1*. After transplantation the recipients were followed up and immunosuppression regimen, clinical and laboratory parameters, and time to GF were documented. GF was defined as return to dialysis or re-transplantation and was censored for death with a functioning graft. Cases with post-transplant graft survival <1 year were excluded from the analyses, to decrease heterogeneity in the sample, as graft loss <1 year is to an important extent due to acute complications, such as technical surgical problems, delayed graft function and/or acute rejection episodes, whereas we wanted to focus on the process of chronic transplant dysfunction. Donor and recipient characteristics, transplantation-related parameters and clinical data (24 h urinary protein excretion, blood pressure, renal function) were retrieved from medical records. The Institutional Review Board of the University Medical Center Groningen approved the study protocol. Written informed consent was given by all recipients and living donors. For deceased donors, with research carried out after the organ removal and implantation, no consent was required. According to Dutch law general consent for organ donation and transplantation includes consent for research projects. The study was conducted according to the principles of the Declaration of Helsinki. All the genetic and clinical data were anonymized prior to analyses.

DNA isolation, tagSNP selection and genotyping

DNA was extracted from peripheral whole blood (in recipients and living donors) or lymph nodes/spleen lymphocytes (in deceased donors) using a commercial kit following the manufacturer's instructions, transferred into 2 ml Eppendorf tubes and stored at −20°C. Absorbance at 260 nm was measured with NanoDrop spectrophotometer (ND-1000, NanoDrop Technologies) and DNA concentration was calculated by the NanoDrop nucleic acid application module. As a measure of DNA purity 260/280 and 260/230 absorbance ratios were assessed. Where samples failed to meet the minimum DNA concentration and purity recommended for Illumina genotyping, repeated isolation attempts were made.

Two SNPs in the *CUBN* locus were genotyped: missense (Ile2984Val) rs1801239 and rs7918972. The latter is a tagSNP in the *CUBN* intron, which was selected using Genome Variation Server v5.11 (Seattle SNPs Program for Genomic Applications). This program utilizes the LDSelect algorithm [6]. All the SNPs within the *CUBN* gene including 500 bases at the gene flanking regions were submitted to the selection procedure. The following parameter settings were used: HapMap-CEU population (unrelated only, no HapMap 3), monomorphic sites excluded, r^2 threshold 0.8, minimal genotype coverage for tagSNPs 85%. Further, for our study we considered SNPs with MAFs 10–15%, tagging as many other variants as possible including the missense ones. Rationale for the arbitrary MAF cut-off was based on the general expectation that rarer variants have a slightly higher likelihood to be causal and may confer stronger effects. At the same time, as power to detect such effects depends on sample size, we were constrained by the moderate sample size of our study. That is why we set the cut-off in the range of 10–15%. Using these

settings, the SNP rs7918972 was the best tagSNP meeting all our criteria (minimal MAF – 10%, maximal number of the tagged SNPs – 9, tagging a missense variant) and therefore was ultimately chosen for this study. This SNP is in strong linkage disequilibrium with intronic SNPs rs4088454, rs7897625, rs7897716, rs7898076, rs11254232, rs11254238, rs7897442, rs7897705 and missense (Asn3552Lys) rs1801232, all of which map to the *CUBN* locus. The LD structure of the studied *CUBN* SNPs is shown in the *Supplemental Figure S1*.

Genotyping of the selected SNPs was performed using the Illumina VeraCode GoldenGate assay kit (Illumina, San Diego, CA, USA), according to the manufacturer's instructions. Genotype clustering and calling were performed using BeadStudio Software (Illumina). In five individuals genotyping was unsuccessful.

Statistical analysis

Analyses were performed with PASW Statistics 18.0 (SPSS Inc., Chicago, IL) and PLINK v1.07 (S. Purcell, http://pngu.mgh.harvard.edu/purcell/plink/) [7]. QUANTO v1.2.4 (http://hydra.usc.edu/gxe/) and PASS v11 were used for power estimation. PolyPhen2 [8] was used to predict functional consequences of the missense SNP. The studied *CUBN* SNPs LD structure plot was generated with SNAP v2.2 [9].

As a routine data quality control, alleles frequencies, Hardy-Weinberg equilibrium and case/control differential missingness were tested for. Subsequent statistical analyses were performed on a final sample of 2323 subjects in a case-control design (1141 recipients vs 1182 donors) and 962 renal transplant recipients in a longitudinal design. With two-sided p = 0.05, assuming an additive genetic model and MAF of 10–15%, we had 57% and 99% power to detect an OR of 1.2 and 1.4, respectively, in the ESRD case-control analysis, and 43% and 87% power to detect a HR of 1.5 and 2.0, respectively, in the Cox regression analysis of graft survival.

Genotype-phenotype associations were tested under an additive genetic model and results (regression coefficients and *p*-values) are reported per copy of the minor allele.

In the case-control analysis, the PLINK DFAM algorithm was used to account for donor-recipient relatedness within living-donor transplantation cases. Interaction between the SNPs was tested with the PLINK –*epistasis* function which includes the interaction term and the marginal effects of the SNPs into the interaction model. Subsequently, stratified logistic regression analyses were performed for each of the three groups of minor allele carriers of both SNPs using the group of non-carriers as the reference.

For the longitudinal study we included cases with post-transplant graft survival ≥1 year. The effect of SNPs on graft survival was investigated with Kaplan-Meier and Cox regression analyses including known predictors of GF (donor and recipient age and sex, donor type, cold and warm ischemia times, immunosuppressive therapy).

Association between genotypes and 24 h urinary protein excretion was studied cross-sectionally at 1 year after transplantation assuming stable graft function at this time-point. As proteinuria was considered a left-censored phenotype with 0 values in 24.4% of patients (due to the diagnostic assay detection limit and rounding of routinely reported values), it was analyzed with Tobit regression [10,11], both univariately and including relevant covariates (age, sex, systolic and diastolic blood pressure).

Results

Main patients characteristics are presented in *Table 1*.

The overall minor allele frequency was 13.1% for rs7918972 and 12.5% for rs1801239. There was no deviation from Hardy-

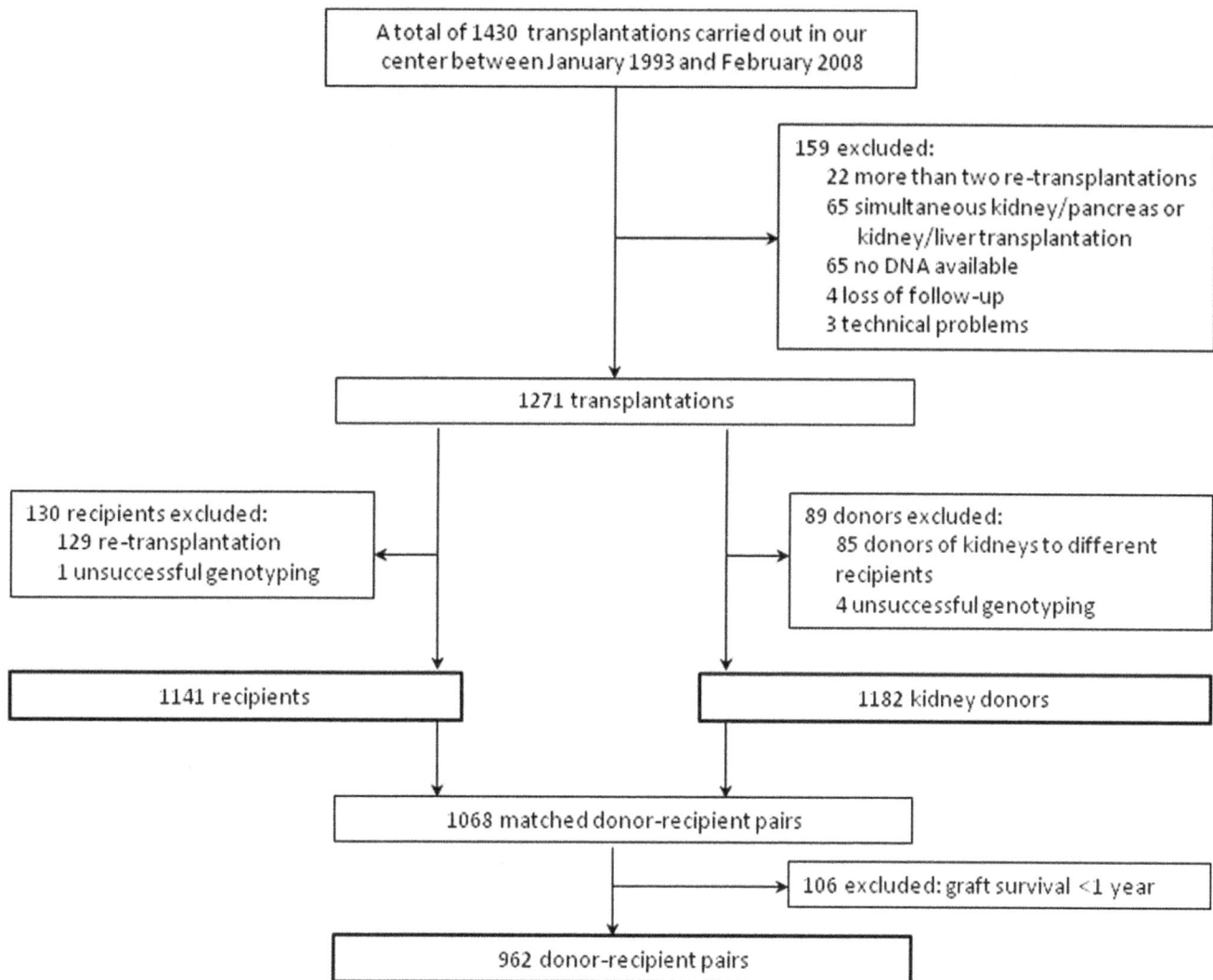

Figure 1. A flowchart of the study participants selection.

Weinberg equilibrium in controls ($p = 0.2908$ for rs7918972; $p = 0.4126$ for rs1801239). The missing genotypic data fraction was not different between cases and controls ($p = 1.000$ and $p = 0.625$ for rs7918972 and rs1801239, respectively). There was no linkage disequilibrium between rs7918972 and rs1801239 ($r^2 = 0.002$, $D' = 0.059$). The missense rs1801232 (Asn3552Lys), tagged by rs7918972, was predicted to be benign by PolyPhen2: score 0.011; sensitivity 0.96; specificity 0.72.

Case-control study: ESRD patients vs kidney donors

The minor allele frequency (MAF) for rs7918972 was significantly higher in ESRD patients as compared to kidney donors, implicating an increased risk of ESRD: OR [95% CI] 1.39 [1.16–1.65], $p = 0.0004$, in an additive model adjusted for age, sex and case-control relatedness *(Table 2)*; additional adjustment for diabetes status did not change the results. There was no association between rs7918972 genotype and any of the primary diseases (etiology of ESRD). The MAF for rs7918972 was not different between living and deceased donors and in the latter it was not significantly associated with the cause of death (mortality due to cerebro- or cardiovascular accident vs other reasons).

Genotype of rs1801239 was not associated with case/control status or any of the other traits studied.

The effects of the two SNPs were not independent as a case-control test for epistasis revealed an interaction between them ($p = 5 \times 10^{-10}$). A finer analysis showed that the rs7918972 minor allele requires a copy of the rs1801239 minor allele to express its risk phenotype (OR 3.15 [2.21–4.48], $p = 1.8 \times 10^{-10}$), whereas the minor allele of rs1801239 displays protective effect in the absence of rs7918972 minor allele (OR 0.65 [0.52–0.81], $p = 1.7 \times 10^{-4}$) *[Table 3]*.

Longitudinal study: post-transplant follow-up

A total of 92 (9.6%) cases of death-censored GF occurred and 151 (15.8%) patients died with a functioning graft during a median [IQR] of 5.8 [3.8–9.5] years of follow-up.

Donor MAF, representing genotype of the transplanted kidney, was higher in subjects that suffered death-censored GF as compared to cases with a functioning graft (16.3% vs 10.7%, respectively). Kaplan-Meier survival analysis revealed worse graft survival ($p = 0.067$) for the carriers of the minor allele *(Figure 2)*. Consistently, a multivariate Cox regression analysis showed that donor kidney rs7918972 is a predictor of GF yielding a HR of 1.53

Table 1. Main patients and transplantation-related characteristics.

ESRD patients, n = 1141	
Age, years	48.2±13.5
Sex: male, n (%)	662 (58.0)
Primary disease:	
- glomerulopathies, n (%)	292 (25.6)
- kidney cysts, n (%)	188 (16.5)
- tubulo-interstitial lesions, n (%)	135 (11.8)
- diabetes types I and II, n (%)	47 (4.1)
- renal hypoplasia, n (%)	23 (2.0)
- drug-induced nephritis, n (%)	15 (1.3)
- other/uncertain etiology, n (%)	488 (43)
Kidney donors, n = 1182	
Age, years	44.5±14.3
Sex: male, n (%)	603 (51.0)
Living donors, n (%)	282 (23.9)
- from which related donors, n (%)	164 (58.2)
Transplantation, n = 962 renal transplant recipients	
Cold ischemia time, minutes	1140 [869–1428]
Total warm ischemia time, minutes	40 [34–50]
Follow-up duration, years	5.8 [3.8–9.5]
Measured GFR at 1 year post-transplant, ml/min	54.8±19.2
Total proteinuria at 1 year post-transplant, g/24 h	0.20 [0.05–0.40]
Acute rejection episodes history, n (%)	324 (33.7)
Graft failure, n (%)	92 (9.6)
Death with a functioning graft, n (%)	152 (15.8)

Continuous normally distributed variables are presented as mean±SD, non-normally distributed – as median [IQR].

[0.99–2.37], $p = 0.055$, per copy of the minor allele, in a model adjusted for donor and recipient age and sex, donor type (living vs deceased), ischemia times, immunosuppressive drug use and acute rejection episodes *(Table 4)*. In contrast, recipient rs7918972 was not associated with development of GF (HR 1.00, $p = 0.992$). Neither donor nor recipient rs1801239 was significantly associated with GF. There was no statistically significant interaction between the two SNPs in the longitudinal analysis of GF.

Neither donor nor recipient genotypes were significantly associated with cardiovascular or all-cause mortality during post-transplant follow-up.

We found donor rs7918972 to be associated with proteinuria levels cross-sectionally at 1 year of post-transplant follow-up (beta 0.201, $p = 0.015$) [*Table 5*]. No association between the SNPs and renal function by measured GFR or creatinine clearance was observed at the same time-point; however, donor rs7918972 showed a directionally consistent, although not statistically significant, trend for association with an increased rate of GFR decline (data not shown).

Discussion

In the present study we followed up the results of a recent GWAS, which identified the cubilin gene *CUBN* as a locus for albuminuria [4]. As albuminuria is an established risk factor for progressive renal function loss, the GWAS findings raised the hypothesis that genetic variation in the *CUBN* locus could be associated with progressive renal function loss and finally end stage renal disease. To test this hypothesis we studied the cited top SNP as well as a tagSNP in *CUBN* in relation to final renal clinical outcomes, namely ESRD in native kidneys and GF in the transplanted kidney.

In a case-control design we studied rs7918972 and rs1801239 genotypes in ESRD patients versus kidney donors. The MAF for rs7918972 was significantly higher in ESRD patients as compared to kidney donors, imposing a 39% increased risk for ESRD per copy of the minor allele. Follow-up data after transplantation showed direction-consistent trend for an association between donor kidney rs7918972 and development of GF in recipients. Thus, the SNP in *CUBN* locus was associated with susceptibility to develop ESRD in two settings, namely ESRD in native kidneys and GF in transplanted kidneys.

Transplantation represents a unique setting, also from genetic point view: an organ with its own genotype functions in an organism with another genotype. We tested both donor and recipient genotype for association with the renal outcome to investigate whether it is the kidney genotype that determines its own fate or it is the recipient genotype that influences function and survival of the transplanted organ. This unique design is useful for genetic research in nephrology as it enables discrimination between the renal and extra-renal mechanisms [12].

In our study, it was donor rather than recipient *CUBN* genotype that was associated with GF, suggesting involvement of local, intra-renal pathways in processes of transplanted kidney survival which are independent of systemic influences.

Albuminuria is known as a predictor of cardiovascular and non-cardiovascular mortality [13]. However, in our study *CUBN* genotypes did not associate with cerebro- or cardiovascular accident as a cause of death in donors and cardiovascular and all-cause mortality after transplantation in recipients.

Table 2. *CUBN* SNPs in the case-control study of ESRD patients versus kidney donors.

CUBN SNPs		ESRD patients, n = 1141	Kidney donors, n = 1182	OR [95% CI] per copy of the minor allele[a]	*p* value[a]
rs7918972	Genotypes, count	21/301/819	12/246/924		
	MAF, %	**15.0%**	**11.4%**	**1.39 [1.16–1.65]**	**0.0004**
rs1801239	Genotypes, count	8/276/857	14/266/902		
	MAF, %	12.8%	12.4%	1.04 [0.87–1.24]	0.6686

OR, odds ratio; CI, confidence interval.
[a]Logistic regression model adjusted for age and sex, with adjustment for case-control relatedness (DFAM algorithm).

Table 3. Interaction between the SNPs in the *CUBN* locus in the case-control study of ESRD patients versus kidney donors.

CUBN SNPs		rs7918972	
	N of the minor allele copies	0	1 or 2
		Reference	OR 0.93 [0.75–1.15]
	0	OR 1.00	$p = 0.484$
rs1801239		$n = 1352$	$n = 407$
		OR 0.65 [0.52–0.81]	OR 3.15 [2.21–4.48]
	1 or 2	$p = 1.7 \times 10^{-4}$	$p = 1.8 \times 10^{-10}$
		$n = 391$	$n = 173$

Logistic regression model adjusted for age and sex. Odds ratios (OR) [95% confidence intervals] for risk of ESRD, *p*-values and patients number (n) are presented in relation to simultaneous presence of both minor alleles in genotype.

As no albuminuria data were available and urinary albumin levels are known to correlate with total protein, we tested association of the *CUBN* SNPs with 24-h total urinary protein excretion as a surrogate phenotype. Interestingly, we found donor rs7918972 to be associated with elevated proteinuria levels cross-sectionally at 1 year after transplantation. This is consistent with our results of association with the outcome, and also in line with the results of a recent study which revealed, using exome sequencing, a deleterious mutation in *CUBN* in a family of proteinuric patients, thus confirming the *CUBN* gene involvement in proteinuria [14].

In the original GWAS [4] the *CUBN* SNP rs1801239, associated with elevated urinary albumine-to-creatinine ratio and microalbuminuria. However, this SNP was not associated with CKD or estimated GFR. In agreement with this, our case-control study showed no association between this SNP and ESRD. Also, rs1801239 was not associated with GF in our longitudinal study

Instead, it was the other *CUBN* polymorphism, the tagSNP rs7918972, that was associated with ESRD in our study.

The *CUBN* locus is characterized by a high variability, with both common and rare mutations. Mutations in the *CUBN* locus are known to be the cause of Imerslund-Gräsbeck syndrome (OMIM #261100, Finnish type) which is a rare (the estimated prevalence is <6:1,000,000) autosomal recessive disorder characterized by vitamin B12 deficiency commonly resulting in megaloblastic anemia, and also neurological damage and mild proteinuria [15]. However, we did not aim to address previously clinically-associated Mendelian mutations in the *CUBN* in our study. We aimed to investigate whether *common* variation, as opposed to rare mutations in Imerslund-Gräsbeck syndrome, in the *CUBN* associates with kidney disease. In the same time, we targeted a lower part of the common variability range, with MAFs between 10 and 15%, aiming to reveal allegedly stronger genetic effects. We selected two SNPs in the *CUBN* locus for the present study: first, the one previously published to be associated with

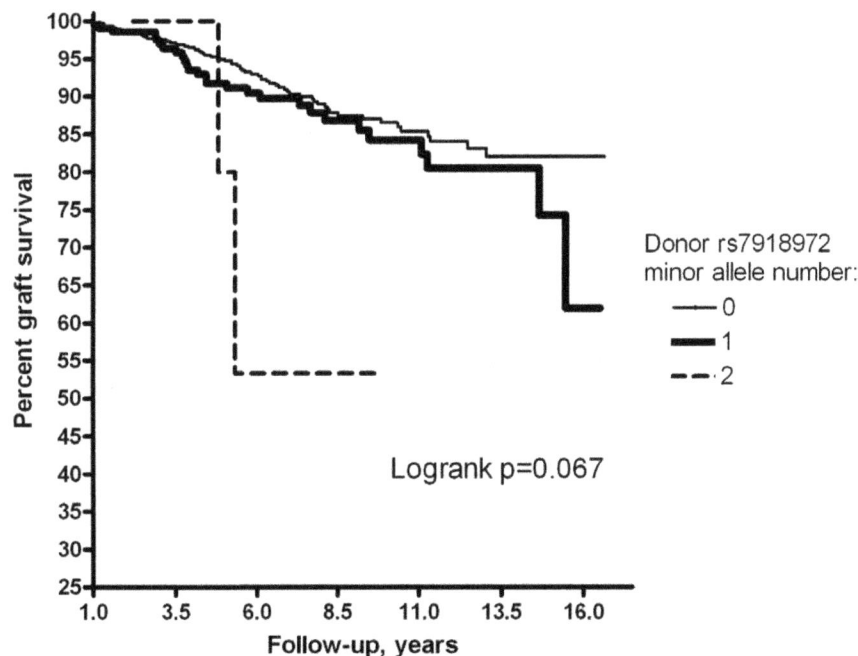

Figure 2. Curves of long-term renal graft survival by donor rs7918972 genotype. Numbers 0 to 2 designate corresponding number of the minor allele copies per genotype. The logrank test showed borderline statistical significance of the differences between the respective curves.

Table 4. CUBN SNPs in the longitudinal study with follow-up for graft failure.

Genotype	CUBN SNPs		Graft failure, n=92	Functioning graft, n=870	HR [95% CI] per copy of the minor allele[a]	p value[a]	HR [95% CI] per copy of the minor allele[b]	p value[b]
Donor	rs7918972	Genotypes, count	2/26/64	8/171/691				
		MAF, %	16.3%	10.7%	1.50 [0.99–2.26]	0.056	1.53 [0.99–2.37]	0.055
	rs1801239	Genotypes, count	2/15/75	11/201/658				
		MAF, %	10.3%	12.8%	0.80 [0.49–1.30]	0.363	0.75 [0.43–1.31]	0.311
Recipient	rs7918972	Genotypes, count	3/22/67	15/234/621				
		MAF, %	15.2%	15.2%	0.94 [0.62–1.43]	0.773	1.00 [0.64–1.56]	0.992
	rs1801239	Genotypes, count	0/20/72	6/212/651				
		MAF, %	10.9%	12.9%	0.78 [0.48–1.26]	0.308	0.70 [0.40–1.25]	0.229

HR, hazard ratio; CI, confidence interval.
[a] univariate Cox regression.
[b] multivariate Cox regression model adjusted for donor and recipient age and sex, donor type (living or deceased), ischemia times, immunosuppressive medication use, and history of acute rejection episodes.

albuminuria levels in the general population, i.e. the missense variant (Ile2984Val) rs1801239, and second the tagSNP in the CUBN intron, rs7918972. The latter is in high linkage disequilibrium ($r^2 = 0.831$) with another missense variant rs1801232 (Asn3552Lys) in CUBN, which might be responsible for the biological impact of the polymorphism on the protein level. The minor allele of rs1801232 leads to an asparagine-to-lysine amino acid substitution in the C-terminal CUB27 domain of cubilin. Despite the amino acids differ in chemical properties (isoelectric points: Asn 5.4, Lys 9.8), the substitution was predicted to be benign by bioinformatics algorithms. However, the mutation is close to sites of N-glycosylation (amino acid 3533) and di-sulfide bond (between amino acids 3564 and 3586) and therefore might potentially interfere with secondary protein structure and, consequently, function. The Imerslund-Gräsbeck syndrome mutations, for which functionality was proven, affect the IF-cobalamin-binding region in the CUB8 domain of cubilin (rs121434430 Pro1297Leu), CUB6 domain (CUBN IVS6 C-G in-frame insertion) or CUB23 domain (CUBN IVS23 G-T transversion at the conserved donor splice site of exon 23). The SNPs that we studied were spatially distant from these variants and located to the CUB22 domain (rs1801239) and CUB27 domain (rs1801232 tagged by rs7918972).

The rs7918972 CUBN SNP, associated with ESRD and GF in our study, is localized in high proximity to the neighboring gene, RSU1. Although the nine SNPs tagged by rs7918972 are all located in the CUBN locus, linkage disequilibrium with and involvement of the RSU1 is theoretically possible and cannot be entirely ruled out (Suppl. Fig. S1). The RSU1 gene encodes Ras suppressor protein 1, which participates in the Ras signal transduction pathway, growth inhibition and nerve-growth factor induced differentiation processes. Its mRNA is expressed in the kidney (according to the NCBI GEO profiles), in a low-to-moderate quantity (51 transcripts per million, according to the NCBI EST profiles). However, functional proof is beyond the scope of the present study, and further research will be needed to discriminate between the effects of these neighboring genes.

Interestingly, we found an interaction between the two SNPs studied. According to our data, the rs7918972 minor allele requires a copy of the rs1801239 minor allele to express its risk phenotype, whereas the minor allele of rs1801239 displays protective effect in the absence of rs7918972 minor allele. This pattern was observed in the case-control study and warrants further investigation to determine whether found statistical interaction has biological implications.

Our study was conducted in kidney transplant recipients, and thus reflects a population that developed ESRD in their native kidneys and was eligible to receive a transplantation. As such, renal transplant recipients represent a relatively healthy subset of the ESRD population, a selection bias inherent to any study in renal transplantation. This should be considered a limitation to our study. In chronic renal disease, both in native kidney disease and in transplantation, mortality is high, and for analyses on ESRD the competing risks of mortality, in particular cardiovascular, are therefore relevant to consider. In the current population, mortality with functioning graft was 15.8 percent, and no association with either of the CUBN SNPs was observed.

Our longitudinal study of graft failure may have been underpowered to detect a significant SNP effect. Insufficient power might thus be an explanation of the fact that convincing statistical significance was not reached in the graft survival analysis for association with rs7918972. Studies in larger populations are warranted to confirm an association between the CUBN SNP and GF.

Table 5. *CUBN* SNPs association with urinary total protein excretion cross-sectionally at 1 year after transplantation.

Genotype	SNP	Univariate Tobit regression			Multivariate Tobit regression[a]		
		Coefficient	SE	*p* value	Coefficient	SE	*p* value
Donor	rs7918972	0.223	0.083	0.007	0.201	0.082	0.015
	rs1801239	−0.039	0.078	0.617	−0.021	0.077	0.784
Recipient	rs7918972	−0.072	0.071	0.313	−0.049	0.070	0.488
	rs1801239	−0.028	0.081	0.726	−0.023	0.080	0.779

[a]Model adjusted for donor and recipient age and sex, donor type (living or deceased), systolic and diastolic blood pressure. Coefficients are given per copy of the minor allele.

Conclusion

Our study confirms association of the *CUBN* with renal phenotypes of progressive renal function loss and urine protein loss. We first identified *CUBN* SNP rs7918972 as a novel genetic variant of susceptibility for ESRD in a case-control design. In a separate proof-of-principle longitudinal study, which served as an internal replication, we reproduced the association. Thus, rs7918972 was associated with susceptibility to develop progressive renal function loss in two settings, namely ESRD in native kidneys and GF in transplanted kidneys. It was kidney genotype that associated with increased risk, supporting impact of intra-renal pathways on organ damage. Our study set-up – analyzing both donor and recipient genotypes – provides a powerful design for hypothesis-driven studies on risk loci for renal damage enabling differentiation between local, intra-renal, and systemic, extra-renal, influences.

Supporting Information

Figure S1 ***CUBN* regional LD plot.** The figure was generated using HapMap data (release 22, CEU population). The horizontal blue line represents an arbitrarily chosen LD threshold ($r^2 = 0.8$). SNPs are shown as diamonds. The color gradient between the diamonds reflects the pairwise LD between the SNPs, with color intensity of each diamond being directly proportional to the r^2 value. Boundaries of the gene coding regions are shown as green horizontal lines. The largest size diamonds represent the present study SNPs. The shaded area designates a span of the gene region tagged by rs7918972.

Author Contributions

Conceived and designed the experiments: AR HS MS GN. Analyzed the data: AR HS GN. Contributed reagents/materials/analysis tools: JvdB MHdB JD MCRFvD HvG BGH J-LH HGDL JN SJLB. Wrote the paper: AR HS GN.

References

1. Hunter DJ, Lange M, Snieder H, MacGregor AJ, Swaminathan R, et al. (2002) Genetic contribution to renal function and electrolyte balance: A twin study. Clin Sci (Lond) 103(3): 259–65.
2. Kottgen A (2010) Genome-wide association studies in nephrology research. Am J Kidney Dis 56(4): 743–58.
3. Boger CA, Heid IM (2011) Chronic kidney disease: Novel insights from genome-wide association studies. Kidney Blood Press Res 34(4): 225–34.
4. Boger CA, Chen MH, Tin A, Olden M, Kottgen A, et al. (2011) CUBN is a gene locus for albuminuria. J Am Soc Nephrol 22(3): 555–70.
5. Meguid El Nahas A, Bello AK (2005) Chronic kidney disease: The global challenge. Lancet 22–28;365(9456): 331–40.
6. Carlson CS, Eberle MA, Rieder MJ, Yi Q, Kruglyak L, et al. (2004) Selecting a maximally informative set of single-nucleotide polymorphisms for association analyses using linkage disequilibrium. Am J Hum Genet 74(1): 106–20.
7. Purcell S, Neale B, Todd-Brown K, Thomas L, Ferreira MA, et al. (2007) PLINK: A tool set for whole-genome association and population-based linkage analyses. Am J Hum Genet 81(3): 559–75.
8. Adzhubei IA, Schmidt S, Peshkin L, Ramensky VE, Gerasimova A, et al. (2010) A method and server for predicting damaging missense mutations. Nat Methods 7(4): 248–9.
9. Johnson AD, Handsaker RE, Pulit SL, Nizzari MM, O'Donnell CJ, et al. (2008) SNAP: A web-based tool for identification and annotation of proxy SNPs using HapMap. Bioinformatics 15;24(24): 2938–9.
10. Lubin JH, Colt JS, Camann D, Davis S, Cerhan JR, et al. (2004) Epidemiologic evaluation of measurement data in the presence of detection limits. Environ Health Perspect 112(17): 1691–6.
11. Tobin J (1958) Estimation of relationships for limited dependent variables. Econometrica 26: 24–36.
12. Broekroelofs J, Stegeman CA, Navis G, Tegzess AM, De Zeeuw D, et al. (1998) Risk factors for long-term renal survival after renal transplantation: A role for angiotensin-converting enzyme (insertion/deletion) polymorphism? J Am Soc Nephrol 9(11): 2075–81.
13. Hollenberg NK (2003) Urinary albumin excretion predicts cardiovascular and non-cardiovascular mortality in general population. Curr Hypertens Rep 5(5): 356–7.
14. Ovunc B, Otto EA, Vega-Warner V, Saisawat P, Ashraf S, et al. (2011) Exome sequencing reveals cubilin mutation as a single-gene cause of proteinuria. J Am Soc Nephrol 22(10): 1815–20.
15. Grasbeck R (2006) Imerslund-grasbeck syndrome (selective vitamin B(12) malabsorption with proteinuria). Orphanet J Rare Dis 19;1: 17.

4

Sex Differences in the Development of Malignancies among End-Stage Renal Disease Patients

Chi-Jung Chung[1,2], Chao-Yuan Huang[3], Hung-Bin Tsai[4], Chih-Hsin Muo[5,6], Mu-Chi Chung[7], Chao-Hsiang Chang[8,9], Chiu-Ching Huang[9,10]*

1 Department of Medical Research, China Medical University and Hospital, Taichung, Taiwan, 2 Department of Health Risk Management, College of Public Health, China Medical University, Taichung, Taiwan, 3 Department of Urology, National Taiwan University Hospital, College of Medicine National Taiwan University, Taipei, Taiwan, 4 Department of Traumatology, National Taiwan University Hospital, Taipei, Taiwan, 5 Department of Public Health, China Medical University, Taichung, Taiwan, 6 Management Office for Health Data, China Medical University and Hospital, Taichung, Taiwan, 7 Division of Nephrology, Department of Internal Medicine, Taichung Veterans General Hospital, Taichung, Taiwan, 8 Department of Urology, China Medical University and Hospital, Taichung, Taiwan, 9 Department of Medicine, College of Medicine, China Medical University and Hospital, Taichung, Taiwan, 10 Division of Nephrology and Kidney Institute, China Medical University and Hospital, Taichung, Taiwan

Abstract

Increasing evidence indicates that end-stage renal disease (ESRD) is associated with the morbidity of cancer. However, whether different dialysis modality and sex effect modify the cancer risks in ESRD patients remains unclear. A total of 3,570 newly diagnosed ESRD patients and 14,280 controls matched for age, sex, index month, and index year were recruited from the National Health Insurance Research Database in Taiwan. The ESRD status was ascertained from the registry of catastrophic illness patients. The incidence of cancer was identified through cross-referencing with the National Cancer Registry System. The Cox proportional hazards model and the Kaplan–Meier method were used for analyses. A similar twofold increase in cancer risk was observed among ESRD patients undergoing hemodialysis (HD) or peritoneal dialysis (PD) after adjusting for other potential risk factors. Patients with the highest cancer risk, approximately fourfold increased risk, were those received renal transplants. Urothelial carcinoma (UC) had the highest incidence in HD and PD patients. However, renal cell carcinoma (RCC) had the highest incidence in the renal transplantation (RT) group. In addition, female patients undergoing RT or PD had a higher incidence of RCC and UC, respectively. Male patients under HD had both higher incidence of RCC and UC. In conclusion, different dialysis modality could modify the cancer risks in ESRD patients. We also found sex effect on genitourinary malignancy when they are under different dialysis modality.

Editor: Emmanuel A. Burdmann, University of Sao Paulo Medical School, Brazil

Funding: The study was supported in part by grants from the Department of Health, Taiwan (DOH 97-HP-1101, 2008–2010), the Clinical Trial and Research Center of Excellence (DOH100-TD-B-111-004), the Cancer Research Center of Excellence (DOH99-TD-C-111-001, 2010–2011, DOH100-TD-C-111-005), the National Science Council (NSC 99-2621-M-039-001), and the China Medical University Hospital. The funders had no role in study design, data collection and analysis, decision to publish, or preparation of the manuscript.

Competing Interests: The authors have declared that no competing interests exist.

* E-mail: cch@mail.cmuh.org.tw

Introduction

End-stage renal disease (ESRD), as the fifth stage of chronic kidney disease (CKD), exemplifies progressive kidney damage. In Taiwan, chronic kidney disease was the tenth leading causes of death in 2010. From 1990 to 2007, the mortality rate increased from 11.4 to 22.2 per 100,000 persons (Department of Health, Executive Yuan, R.O.C.). Based on the United States Renal Data System (USRDS) Annual Data Report, Taiwan ranks first in the world in the incidence and prevalence of ESRD at 415 and 2288 per million population in 2007, respectively. Regular renal replacement therapy (RRT) with hemodialysis (HD), peritoneal dialysis (PD) or renal transplantation (RT) enhances the survival of patients with ESRD, but other complications might occur, including cardiovascular disease (CVD) [1–3]. These issues indicate that ESRD is a substantial burden to global health care and it reduces the quality of life of patients.

Until now, increasing evidence has indicated that CKD and ESRD are associated with the morbidity and mortality of cancer, including renal cell carcinoma (RCC), urothelial carcinoma (UC), and thyroid and lung cancer [4–6]. RCC and UC are the major malignancies among dialysis patients in Western countries and Taiwan, respectively [7,8]. The choice of RRT or dialysis duration might modify the risk of cancer [9,10]. Patients undergoing hemodialysis (HD) longer than ten years have greatly increased risk of developing RCC with a sarcomatoid component than those with shorter than ten years [11]. Moreover, the different histologic spectrum of RCC occurs according to the duration of dialysis [12]. Renal transplant recipients are known to have a higher cancer incidence compared with the general population [13,14]. According to the USRDS, renal transplantation is related to the incidence of renal cell carcinoma[15]. However, the mechanism through which renal transplantation increases the incidence of cancer has not yet been fully described.

In one study on ESRD patients, the top three of the most common cancer sites among males and females were the liver, the colon, and the urinary tract, in descending order, followed by thyroid and lung [6]. In general, the progression of renal failure in patients with CKD is more rapid in men than in women [6,16]. However, a recent study in Taiwan revealed that female ESRD patients have a higher risk of malignancy than male patients [17]. Furthermore, the gender effect on the relationship between dialysis modality and the renal outcome of patients with cancer remains unexamined.

The types of malignancies may occur differently because of distinct geographic regions and ethnic populations. Whether the comparison of dialysis modality or choice of transplantation also modifies the cancer outcomes in patients with ESRD remains unclear. Therefore, through a nationwide database, the effect of dialysis modality and renal transplantation on incident cancer morbidity was investigated and the interaction of gender effect and dialysis modality on survival among a cohort of patients with ESRD in Taiwan was assessed.

Materials and Methods

The present study was constructed as a retrospective cohort study through an encrypted database from the Bureau of National Health Insurance (BNHI); therefore the Institutional Review Board (IRB) waved the need for informed consent for this study.

Data source

The study used the Longitudinal Health Insurance Database (LHID) of the Taiwan National Health Research Institute (NHRI). The NHRI constructed insurant claims, which were released by the BNHI. The BNHI provided the medical claims data after scrambling the identification and this study was exempted by the IRB. The LHID included all medical records from 1996 to 2009, from which one million people were randomly selected from all insurant. There were no significant differences in the sex and age distributions between LHID and all insurant in the NHRI. The program was set up on March 1, 1995, with coverage of over 99.6% in 2009. The International Classification of Disease Revision 9th Clinical Modification (ICD-9-CM) was used for the diagnosis codes. Information about the databases has been detailed in a previous paper [18].

Study sample

Total 4,032 patients that were initially diagnosed with ESRD (ICD-9-CM 585) were selected from the registry of catastrophic illness patients, and the index date was the date of ESRD registration. Patients with a history of malignant cancer (ICD-9-CM 140–208) before the index date ($N = 246$), with incomplete age or sex information ($N = 34$), or did not undergo dialysis ($N = 253$) were excluded. Finally, all 3,570 ESRD patients were included as the ESRD group. All subjects without a history of ESRD were randomly selected from all NHI beneficiaries. Four controls for each case were frequency matched for age 5 years each, sex, index month, and index year as the control group. All controls were screened using the same exclusion criteria used for the ESRD cases. We used the method of 1:m matching to screen the control subjects, which can increase the statistical power and control the potential confounding. Even if $m > 4$, the statistical efficiency did not considerably increase. Therefore, we constructed a 1:4 matched study design. The ESRD group was divided into three subgroups according to RRT modality: the HD, PD and RT groups; those with a higher frequency of HD treatments were assigned to the HD group, and those with a higher frequency of

PD treatments were assigned to the PD group. All ESRD subjects were followed-up until the date at which they were diagnosed with malignant cancer. The incidence of kidney transplantation (ICD-9-CM V420) was ascertained before the said date.

Patient variables

Sociodemographic variables, such as age, sex, and level of urbanization, as well as comorbidities, such as hypertension (ICD-9-CM 401-405), diabetes (ICD-9-CM 250), and hyperlipidemia (ICD-9-CM 272) were analyzed. The level of urbanization of the patient residences was divided into two groups based on the NHRI report. All comorbidities were determined before the index date. Hypertension and hyperlipidemia were confirmed with at least three medical visits and diabetes by two visits within the first year of diagnosis.

Statistical analysis

All statistical analyses were performed using the SAS statistical software (version 9.1 for Windows; SAS Institute, Inc., Cary, NC, USA). We described and compared the distributions of age, sex, Urbanization level (high and low), and co-morbidities (%) between controls and patients with various RRT modalities by χ^2 tests. Person-year was calculated as the interval from the index date to the date of malignant cancer diagnosis, loss to follow-up, death, or the end of 2009. The incidence density (per 1,000 person-years) was assessed for each subgroup. Cox proportional hazard regression was used to estimate the hazard ratio (HR) of developing malignant cancer. The cumulative incidence of malignancy among the control group, HD group, and the PD group were assessed using the Kaplan–Meier method and the differences were estimated with a log-rank test.

Results

Baseline characteristics of the study subjects

The 3,570 ESRD patients consisted of 3,065 HD patients, 317 PD patients and 188 RT patients as well as 14,280 controls were recruited. Information on the demographic characteristics and co-morbidities of the ESRD patients by treatment status is provided in Table 1. The mean age of the ESRD patients was similar to the age of the normal control group. The PD group was younger than the HD group ($p < 0.0001$). Gender distribution was well balanced in both controls and cases as well as in all study groups. Compared with the control group, the ESRD group has more percentage of hypertension, diabetes, and hyperlipidemia ($p < 0.0001$).

Incidence and HR of all-site cancer according to treatment status

The mean duration of follow-up was 3.18 years in ESRD patients (3.13 years in HD patients, 2.96 years in PD patients and 4.3 years in RT patients) compared with 4.45 years in controls (Table 2). The incidence of malignancy among ESRD patients is higher by 1.74-fold than the control group. The highest incidence of malignancy was shown in RT patients. The adjusted hazard risk of malignancy was 1.92 among ESRD patients and the subgroups were 1.81, 2.07, and 3.83 in HD, PD, and RT patients, respectively (all $p < 0.05$). Further stratification by follow-up duration revealed that the patients with the highest risk of malignancy among the different-duration groups from the shortest to the longest period were RT, RT, and PD patients, respectively.

Table 1. Demographic characteristics and co-morbidities of patients with end-stage renal disease by treatment status.

Variables	End-stage renal disease										p-value
	Controls N = 14,280		Total N = 3,570		HD N = 3,065		PD N = 317		RT N = 188		
	n	%	N	%	n	%	n	%	n	%	
Age, years											1.00
<40	1,164	8.2	291	8.2	172	5.6	62	19.6	57	30.3	
40–49	1,988	13.9	497	13.9	387	12.6	62	19.6	48	25.5	
50–59	3,096	21.7	774	21.7	638	20.8	81	25.6	55	29.3	
60–69	3,528	24.7	881	24.7	803	26.2	55	17.4	24	12.8	
≥70	4,504	31.5	1,126	31.5	1,065	34.8	57	18.0	4	2.1	
mean (SD)	60.9	(15.0)	61.3	(14.9)	63.0	(14.0)	53.5	(16.6)	46.4	(12.8)	0.13
Sex											1.00
Women	7,248	50.8	1,812	50.8	1,548	50.5	172	54.3	92	48.9	
Men	7,032	49.2	1,758	49.2	1,517	49.5	145	45.7	96	51.1	
Urbanization level											0.42
High	7,860	55.0	1,992	50.8	1,684	54.9	198	62.5	110	58.5	
Low	6,419	45.0	1,578	44.2	1,381	45.1	119	37.5	78	41.5	
Co-morbidities											
Hypertension	5,977	41.9	3,215	90.1	2,784	90.8	272	85.8	159	84.6	<0.0001
Diabetes	1,998	14.0	1,836	51.4	1,699	55.4	111	35.0	26	13.8	<0.0001
Hyperlipidima	3,357	23.5	1,699	47.6	1,511	49.3	132	41.6	56	29.8	<0.0001

p-values were evaluated through chi-square tests.

Cause-specific cancer associated with ESRD patients receiving different RRT modalities

The HRs of cause-specific cancer associated with various ESRD treatments are shown in Table 3. Compared with the control group, the HR significantly increased among the ESRD and HD group patients for UC, followed by RCC, and thyroid cancer. In the PD group, the significant HRs were for UC. In the RT group, the highest risk was in RCC, followed UC.

The gender effect on the risk of all-site cancer, UC, and RCC

The highest incidence of overall cancers was noted in RT patients, followed by PD and HD patients after adjusted for potential risk factors (Figure 1). After stratification by sex, higher risk of cancer was noted in female patients in all RRT subgroups than in male patients. After considering the different RRT effects on the risks of UC or RCC, we found that the RT and PD groups had the highest incidence of RCC and UC among all the RRT subgroups, respectively, in the female group (data not shown). In

Table 2. Incidence rate and hazard ratios of overall cancer according to treatment status for patients with end-stage renal disease.

	Controls	Total	HD	PD	RT
Mean duration of follow-up (yr)	4.45	3.18	3.13	2.96	4.30
Person-years at risk	63,583	11,341	9,595	934	808
Overall cancer					
No. of events	655	203	172	13	18
Incidence*	10.3	17.9	17.9	13.9	22.3
Model 1	1.00 (reference)	2.01 (1.71–2.36)	1.90 (1.61–2.25)	2.17 (1.25–3.77)	4.04 (2.51–6.50)
Model 2	1.00 (reference)	1.92 (1.61–2.30)	1.81 (1.50–2.19)	2.07 (1.19–3.62)	3.83 (2.36–6.20)
Follow-up duration					
<2.5	1.00 (reference)	1.52 (1.17–1.96)	1.51 (1.15–1.97)	1.09 (0.45–2.66)	2.71 (1.18–6.23)
2.5–5.4	1.00 (reference)	1.91 (1.40–2.61)	1.61 (1.14–2.26)	3.28 (1.33–8.08)	6.31 (3.26–12.2)
≥5.5	1.00 (reference)	3.53 (2.36–5.28)	3.52 (2.32–5.35)	5.46 (1.69–17.6)	2.31 (0.56–9.56)

*Per 1000 person-years.
Models were adjusted for the following variables: Model 1, age and sex; Model 2, age, sex, and medical history of hypertension, hyperlipidima, diabetes.

Table 3. Hazard ratios and 95% confidence interval of cancer risks associated with end-stage renal disease in Cox's regression analysis in different cancers.

Cancer Type (ICD-9-CM)	Controls	Total		HD		PD		RT	
	Case	Case	HR (95% CI)	Case	HR (95% CI)	Case	HR (95% CI)	Case	HR (95% CI)
Overall cancer (140-208)	655	203	1.92 (1.61–2.30)	172	1.81 (1.50–2.19)	13	2.07 (1.19–3.62)	18	3.83 (2.36–6.20)
Oral cavity cancer (140–149)	32	5	1.03 (0.37–2.86)	4	0.99 (0.33–3.00)	0	–	1	2.27 (0.28–18.2)
Digestive									
All (150–159)	271	61	1.41 (1.04–1.92)	53	1.35 (0.98–1.87)	4	1.73 (0.64–4.69)	4	2.44 (0.89–6.67)
Colorectal cancer (153–154)	93	21	1.54 (0.92–2.59)	19	1.52 (0.89–2.60)	1	1.45 (0.20–10.6)	1	2.21 (0.30–16.3)
Liver cancer (155)	104	21	1.14 (0.67–1.92)	17	1.01 90.58–1.78)	2	2.04 (0.49–8.44)	2	2.64 (0.63–11.1)
Respiratory									
All (160–165)	126	14	0.75 (0.42–1.36)	11	0.65 (0.34–1.24)	2	2.02 (0.49–8.33)	1	1.59 (0.22–11.6)
Bone, skin and breast									
All (170–175)	70	16	1.24 (0.67–2.27)	13	1.16 (0.60–2.22)	1	0.99 (0.13–7.60)	2	2.86 (0.67–12.2)
Genitourinary									
All (179–189)	113	92	4.93 (3.56–6.84)	77	4.70 (3.35–6.60)	6	4.93 (2.12–11.5)	9	8.75 (4.24–18.0)
UC (188, 189.1–189.9)	35	53	13.3 (7.95–22.2)	44	12.5 (7.42–21.3)	5	19.0 (7.04–51.1)	4	17.9 (5.97–53.9)
RCC (189.0)	17	28	8.45 (4.16–17.2)	22	7.77 (3.73–16.2)	1	4.18 (0.53–32.9)	5	24.4 (7.87–75.6)
Other and unspecified									
All (190–199)	13	9	5.57 (2.02–15.3)	8	5.84 (2.06–16.5)	0	–	1	9.17 (1.06–79.4)
Thyroid cancer (193)	7	5	5.60 (1.42–22.1)	4	5.45 (1.28–23.2)	0	–	1	115.2 (1.51–153)
Haemopoietic									
All (200–208)	25	6	0.93 (0.35–2.44)	6	1.02 (0.39–2.70)	0	–	0	–

Models were adjusted for age, sex, and medical history of hypertension, hyperlipidima, and diabetes.

the male group, those patients who underwent HD had both the relatively higher risk of kidney cancer and UC than the other subgroups (data not shown). After adjusting for age, hypertension, hyperlipidemia, and diabetes, similar results were obtained (Figure 2).

Discussion

Thus far, the present study is the first to compare the effect of gender on susceptibility to malignancies in ESRD patients, as well as the effects of different RRT on cancer risks through national health database linkages in Taiwan. An approximately fourfold risk of cancer was observe among RT patients compared with the

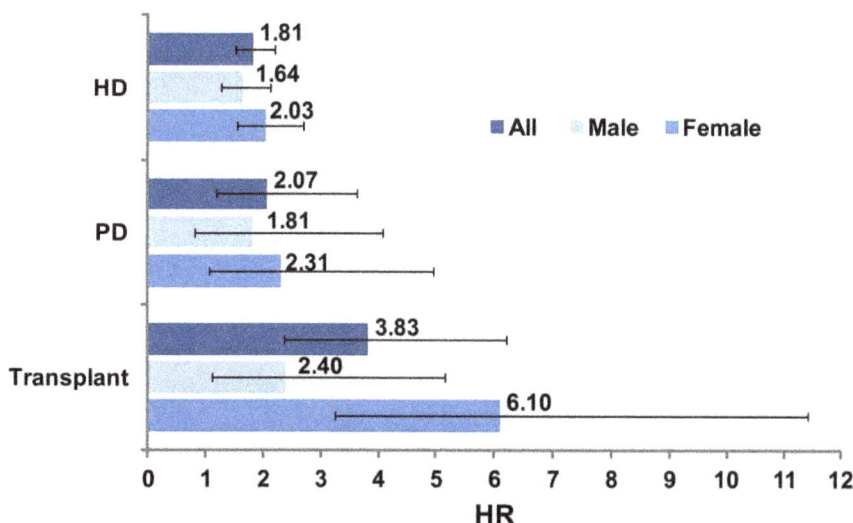

Figure 1. Hazard ratio and 95% confidence interval of overall cancer associated with end-stage renal disease in Cox's regression analysis by adjusted for age, sex, and medical history of hypertension, hyperlipidima, and diabetes.

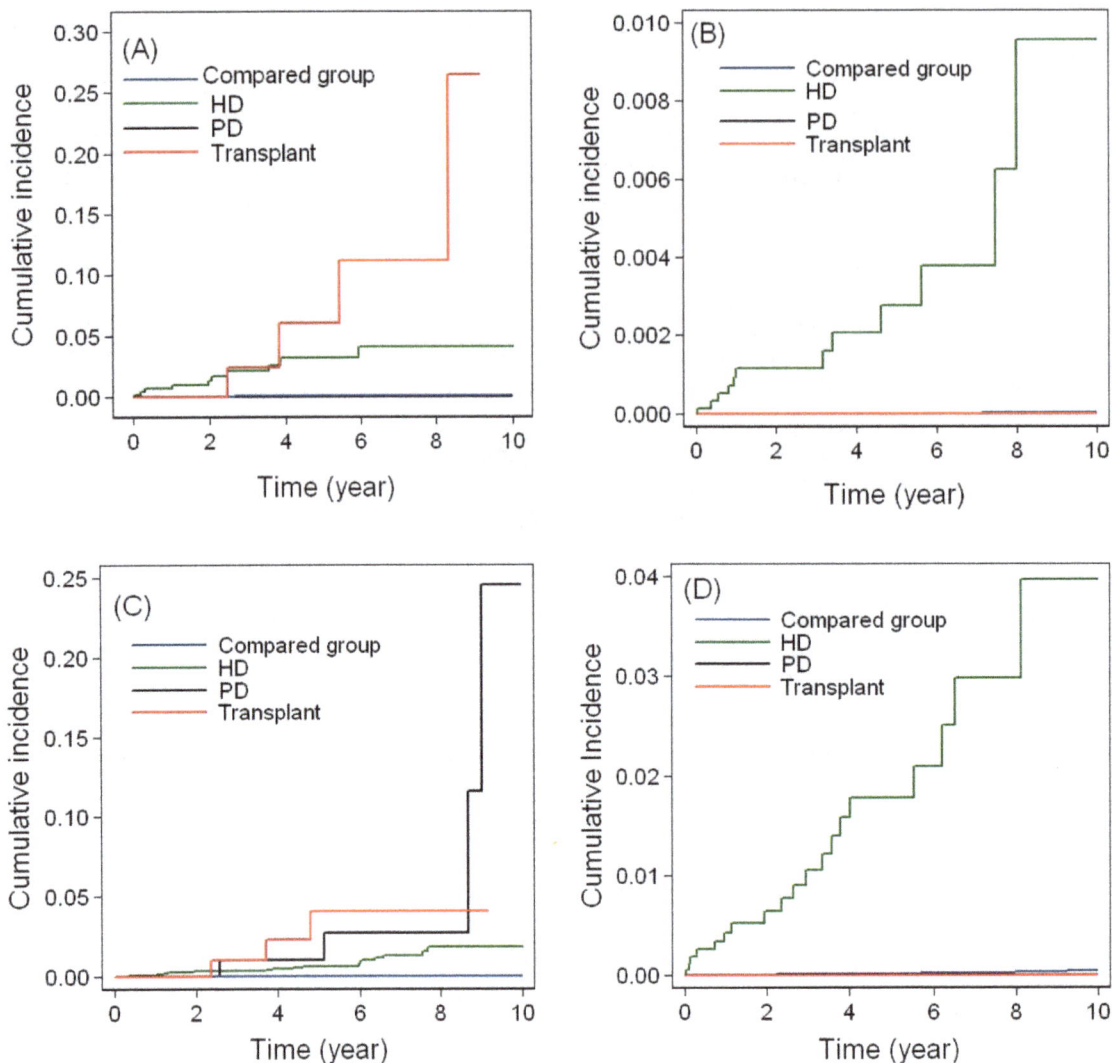

Figure 2. Cumulative incidence of cancer by sex after adjusting for age, hypertension, hyperlipidemia, and diabetes. (A) RCC in female, (B) RCC in male, (C) UC in female, (D) UC in male.

control group. Next, a similar twofold risk of all-site cancer was observed among ESRD patients undergoing HD or PD treatment. In addition, we also observed the gender effect in RRT-related malignancy. In female patients, those who have RT had higher risk of RCC and those having PD had higher risk of UC than those under other RRT. However, in male patients, those having HD had both higher risks of RCC and UC than those in other subgroups.

The cancer morbidity and mortality among patients with ESRD are reportedly higher compared with the general population even though they are receiving dialysis or renal transplantation [5,9]. The exact pathogenesis is not yet fully understood. However, several reasons were proposed, including viral infection, a weakened immune system, chronic inflammation, immunosuppressive treatment, and impairment of DNA repair [19,20]. An increased risk of morbidity of overall cancer is associated with longer dialysis duration in accordance with previous studies [5,21–23]. However, above studies had not compared the effect of different RRT on cancer risk. It might be mostly because of a low percentage of PD treatments. Recently, a Korean study analyzed a cohort of 4,562 ESRD patients from hospital-based database, and

indicated that among the 106 ESRD patients with cancer, 63 (59%) received HD and 43 received PD (41%) [6]. A recent study on another group in Taiwan indicated the significantly increase risk of post-transplantation malignancies using a standardized incidence ratio (SIR) based on the national health database [24]. The incidence rates of post-transplantation malignancies in our analysis were similar with the results of Li et al and the most common malignancies occurred in the urinary tract, which represent about 50% of the cancers diagnosed [24]. This suggests that urinary tract malignancies (RCC) are most common among the ESRD patients that received kidney transplants in the Taiwan area.

"Generally, male CKD or ESRD patients had worse progression of renal outcomes than women [6,16,25]. A total of 4,562 ESRD patients from Korea showed that male patients (73/2760) had more developed malignancies than female (33/1802) (ratio = 1.44) [6]. However, Kummer et al. recently suggested that both male and female CKD patients have the same poor survival once dialysis therapy has been initiated [26]. They proposed that the increased progression of renal outcomes for females may be due to genetic factors and gender hormones. Advanced analysis of the interaction of gender effect and dialysis modality on ESRD-related malignancies is rarely proposed in literature. Therefore, we want to explore the effect of sex difference and the interaction of sex and dialysis modality on the incidence of the risk of ESRD-related malignancies. In the present analysis, a higher risk of overall cancer morbidity was seen among female ESRD patients than among males. The results were in accordance with previous findings obtained by other investigators [22,24]. According to former literatures, a higher percentage of females than males preferred alternative therapies, including Chinese herbs containing aristolochic acid. In a Taiwan cohort with 6,548 Chinese herbalists, female herbalists were at higher risk for urologic cancers than males (standardized mortality ratio (SMR) = 3.10; 95% CI = 1.41–5.87) [27]. Another large prospective cohort study in Taiwan demonstrated a significantly increased risk of CKD among regular users of Chinese herbal medicines [28]. This hypothesis was in accordance with that of a Belgian cohort [29]. In a female rabbit model, chronic exposure to aristolochic acid, given as a single drug, casually induced renal hypocellular interstitial fibrosis, and even the development of urinary tract tumors [30]. Another Taiwanese study indicated that young women taking Mu-Tong and Fangchi (aristolochic acid–related herbal products) and over the counter drugs were more likely to develop transitional cell carcinoma, chronic tubulointerstitial nephritis [31], and renal failure, especially those less than 50 years old [32]. Further studies to verify the difference in cancer risk between males and female are needed. We also demonstrated that female patients undergoing RT or PD had higher risks of RCC and UC. The underlying mechanisms require further elucidation.

Another issue that warrants discussion is the possible gender difference in the competing risk mortality in the present study. The progression and mortality of ESRD may compete before the incidence of ESRD-related malignancies. In general, males have a higher mortality from cardiovascular disease than females [33]. However, according to the ANZDATA 2010 Annual Report, cancer is surpassing cardiovascular diseases as the leading cause of post-transplantation death [34]. Among our 17,850 study subjects, the average follow-up durations stratified by gender are 3.50 and 3.25 years in females and males with developed cancer, respectively, as well as 4.39 and 4.08 years in females and males without developed cancer (data not shown). The average follow-up from the date of recruitment through surrender stratified by gender are similar, i.e., 4.43 and 4.11 years in females and males,

respectively (data not shown). The similar follow-up periods of males and females may imply the low effect of competing risk mortality. Although the average follow-up period of recruitment to surrender may not represent the actual mortality rate, we believe that it is the approaching index in the present analysis. All ESRD patients who received any kind of dialysis modality should be recorded in the registry of catastrophic illness patients. Other than death, no other important reason to surrender is observed. However, further investigative studies are needed to confirm the links among the sex differences, mortality of competing risk, and incidences of ESRD-related malignancies.

A retrospective cohort study of the present study was used to evaluate cancer morbidity using population-based registries to avoid ascertainment bias during long-term follow-up. Morbidity rather than mortality was better for exploring the correlation between ESRD and all-site cancer because the mortality rate might be underestimated considering the risk can be improved by early screening and by increasing medical intervention. We also adopted frequency matching to balance the distributions of age, gender, and index date of ESRD diagnosis in the ESRD and non-ESRD groups to increase the comparability. The limitations of the current study are as follows: First, the limited sample size of people receiving PD or RT treatment resulted in a confidence interval too extensive to acquire meaningful conclusions or to execute stratified analyses. In addition, people receiving RT in foreign country could not recruit in the present analysis. Second, the related laboratory measurements or personal lifestyle risk factors were not included in the imbursement database. Therefore, the effects of potential covariates on the correlation between dialysis modality and cancer risk could not be evaluated.

In summary, ESRD is associated with an increased morbidity of all-site cancer regardless of different RRT modality, especially for female patients. Multicenter recruitment and measurements of laboratory data might be of benefit to have a sufficiently large sample size for stratification analysis and to explore further the possible mechanism of sex differences for ESRD-related cancer morbidity.

Author Contributions

Conceived and designed the experiments: CYH HBT MCC CHC CCH. Analyzed the data: CJC CHM. Wrote the paper: CJC.

References

1. Weiner DE, Tighiouart H, Stark PC, Amin MG, MacLeod B, et al. (2004) Kidney disease as a risk factor for recurrent cardiovascular disease and mortality. Am J Kidney Dis 44:198–206.
2. Parfrey PS, Foley RN, Rigatto C (1999) Risk issues in renal transplantation: cardiac aspects. Transplant Proc 31:291–293.
3. Parfrey PS, Foley RN (1999) The clinical epidemiology of cardiac disease in chronic renal failure. J Am Soc Nephrol 10:1606–1615.
4. Weng PH, Hung KY, Huang HL, Chen JH, Sung PK, et al. (2011) Cancer-specific mortality in chronic kidney disease: longitudinal follow-up of a large cohort. Clin J Am Soc Nephrol 6:1121–1128.
5. Maisonneuve P, Agodoa L, Gellert R, Stewart JH, Buccianti G, et al. (1999) Cancer in patients on dialysis for end-stage renal disease: an international collaborative study. Lancet 354:93–99.
6. Lee JE, Han SH, Cho BC, Park JT, Yoo TH, et al. (2009) Cancer in patients on chronic dialysis in Korea. J Korean Med Sci 24:S95–S101.
7. Chen KS, Lai MK, Huang CC, Chu SH, Leu ML (1995) Urologic cancers in uremic patients. Am J Kidney Dis 25:694–700.
8. Boon NA, Michael J (1984) Multiple neoplasia in a patient on dialysis presenting with haematuria. Br J Urol 56:96–97.
9. Stewart JH, Vajdic CM, van Leeuwen MT, Amin J, Webster AC, et al. (2009) The pattern of excess cancer in dialysis and transplantation. Nephrol Dial Transplant 24:3225–3231.
10. Birkeland SA, Lokkegaard H, Storm HH (2000) Cancer risk in patients on dialysis and after renal transplantation. Lancet 355:1886–1887.
11. Sassa N, Hattori R, Tsuzuki T, Watarai Y, Fukatsu A, et al. (2011) Renal cell carcinomas in haemodialysis patients: does haemodialysis duration influence pathological cell types and prognosis? Nephrol Dial Transplant 26:1677–1682.
12. Nouh MA, Kuroda N, Yamashita M, Hayashida Y, Yano T, et al. (2010) Renal cell carcinoma in patients with end-stage renal disease: relationship between histological type and duration of dialysis. BJU Int 105:620–627.
13. Suthanthiran M, Strom TB (1994) Renal transplantation. N Engl J Med 331:365–376.
14. Vajdic CM, McDonald SP, McCredie MR, van Leeuwen MT, Stewart JH, et al. (2006) Cancer incidence before and after kidney transplantation. JAMA 296:2823–2831.
15. Hurst FP, Jindal RM, Graham LJ, Falta EM, Elster EA, et al. (2010) Incidence, predictors, costs, and outcome of renal cell carcinoma after kidney transplantation: USRDS experience. Transplantation 90:898–904.
16. Silbiger SR, Neugarten J (1995) The impact of gender on the progression of chronic renal disease. Am J Kidney Dis 25:515–533.
17. Hung PH, Shen CH, Tsai HB, Hsiao CY, Chiang PC, et al. (2011) Gender effect on renal outcome in patients with urothelial carcinoma. World J Urol 29:511–516.
18. Lu JF, Hsiao WC (2003) Does universal health insurance make health care unaffordable? Lessons from Taiwan. Health Aff 22:77–88.
19. Vamvakas S, Bahner U, Heidland A (1998) Cancer in end-stage renal disease: potential factors involved -editorial-. Am J Nephrol 18:89-95.
20. Fischereder M (2008) Cancer in patients on dialysis and after renal

transplantation. Nephrol Dial Transplant 23:2457–2460.

21. Chen CH, Shun CT, Huang KH, Huang CY, Yu HJ, et al. (2008) Characteristics of female non-muscle-invasive bladder cancer in Taiwan: association with upper tract urothelial carcinoma and end-stage renal disease. Urology 71:1155–1160.

22. Liang JA, Sun LM, Yeh JJ, Sung FC, Chang SN, et al. (2011) The Association Between Malignancy and End-stage Renal Disease in Taiwan. Jpn J Clin Oncol 41:752–757.

23. Farivar-Mohseni H, Perlmutter AE, Wilson S, Shingleton WB, Bigler SA, et al. (2006) Renal cell carcinoma and end stage renal disease. J Urol 175:2018–2020.

24. Li WH, Chen YJ, Tseng WC, Lin MW, Chen TJ, et al. (2012) Malignancies after renal transplantation in Taiwan: a nationwide population-based study. Nephrol Dial Transplant 27:833–839.

25. Hurst FP, Jindal RM, Fletcher JJ, Dharnidharka V, Gorman G, et al. (2011) Incidence, predictors and associated outcomes of renal cell carcinoma in long-term dialysis patients. Urology 77: 1271–1276.

26. Kummer S, von GG, Kemper MJ, Oh J (2012) The influence of gender and sexual hormones on incidence and outcome of chronic kidney disease. Pediatr Nephrol 27: 1213–1219.

27. Yang HY, Wang JD, Lo TC, Chen PC (2009) Increased mortality risk for cancers of the kidney and other urinary organs among Chinese herbalists. J Epidemiol 19:17–23.

28. Wen CP, Cheng TY, Tsai MK, Chang YC, Chan HT, et al. (2008) All-cause mortality attributable to chronic kidney disease: a prospective cohort study based on 462 293 adults in Taiwan. Lancet 371:2173–2182.

29. Cosyns JP, Jadoul M, Squifflet JP, Wese FX, van Ypersele de SC (1999) Urothelial lesions in Chinese-herb nephropathy. Am J Kidney Dis 33:1011–1017.

30. Cosyns JP, Dehoux JP, Guiot Y, Goebbels RM, Robert A, et al. (2001) Chronic aristolochic acid toxicity in rabbits: a model of Chinese herbs nephropathy? Kidney Int 59:2164–2173.

31. Chang CH, Fang YW, Chen HS (2009) End-stage renal disease in both husband and wife in Taiwan. Clin Nephrol 72:298–302.

32. Lai MN, Lai JN, Chen PC, Tseng WL, Chen YY, et al. (2009) Increased risks of chronic kidney disease associated with prescribed Chinese herbal products suspected to contain aristolochic acid. Nephrology 14:227–234.

33. Orskov B, Sorensen VR, Feldt-Rasmussen B, Strandgaard S (2012) Changes in causes of death and risk of cancer in Danish patients with autosomal dominant polycystic kidney disease and end-stage renal disease. Nephrol Dial Transplant 27: 1607–1613.

34. Lindsay RM, Suri RS, Moist LM, Garg AX, Cuerden M, et al. (2011) International quotidian dialysis registry: Annual report 2010. Hemodial Int 15: 15–22.

5

Incidence and Predictors of End Stage Renal Disease among Low-Income Blacks and Whites

Loren Lipworth[1]*, Michael T. Mumma[2], Kerri L. Cavanaugh[3], Todd L. Edwards[1], T. Alp Ikizler[3], Robert E.Tarone[1,2], Joseph K. McLaughlin[1,2], William J. Blot[1,2]

1 Division of Epidemiology, Department of Medicine, Vanderbilt University Medical Center and Vanderbilt-Ingram Cancer Center, Nashville, Tennessee, United States of America, 2 International Epidemiology Institute, Rockville, Maryland, United States of America, 3 Division of Nephrology, Department of Medicine, Vanderbilt University Medical Center, Nashville, Tennessee, United States of America

Abstract

We evaluated whether black race is associated with higher incidence of End Stage Renal Disease (ESRD) among a cohort of blacks and whites of similar, generally low socioeconomic status, and whether risk factor patterns differ among blacks and whites and explain the poorly understood racial disparity in ESRD. Incident diagnoses of ESRD among 79,943 black and white participants in the Southern Community Cohort Study (SCCS) were ascertained by linkage with the United States Renal Data System (USRDS) from 2002 through 2009. Person-years of follow up were calculated from date of entry into the SCCS until date of ESRD diagnosis, date of death, or September 1, 2009, whichever occurred first. Cox proportional hazards models were used to estimate hazard ratios (HRs) and 95% confidence intervals (CI) for incident ESRD among black and white participants in relation to baseline characteristics. After 329,003 person-years of follow-up, 687 incident cases of ESRD were identified in the cohort. The age-adjusted ESRD incidence rate was 273 (per 100,000) among blacks, 3.5-fold higher than the rate of 78 among whites. Risk factors for ESRD included male sex (HR = 1.6; 95% CI 1.4–1.9), low income (HR = 1.5; 95% CI 1.2–1.8 for income below vs. above $15,000), smoking (HR = 1.2; 95% CI 1.02–1.4) and histories of diabetes (HRs increasing to 9.4 (95% CI 7.4–11.9) among those with ≥20 years diabetes duration) and hypertension (HR = 2.9; 95% CI 2.3–3.7). Patterns and magnitudes of association were virtually identical among blacks and whites. After adjustment for these risk factors, blacks continued to have a higher risk for ESRD (HR = 2.4; 95% CI = 1.9–3.0) relative to whites. The black-white disparity in risk of ESRD was attenuated but not eliminated after control for known risk factors in a closely socioeconomically matched cohort. Further research characterizing biomedical factors, including CKD progression, in ESRD occurrence in these two racial groups is needed.

Editor: Shree Ram Singh, National Cancer Institute, United States of America

Funding: The Southern Community Cohort Study (SCCS) is funded by grant R01 CA92447 from the National Cancer Institute (NCI), including American Recovery and Reinvestment Act funding (3R01 CA029447-08S1). Dr. Cavanaugh is funded by DK080952 and an American Society of Nephrology Carl W. Gottschalk Research Scholar Grant. Data on end stage renal disease diagnoses were provided by the United States Renal Data System (USRDS). The funders had no role in study design, data collection and analysis, decision to publish, or preparation of the manuscript.

Competing Interests: The authors have declared that no competing interests exist.

* E-mail: loren.lipworth@vanderbilt.edu

Introduction

In the last two decades, there has been a dramatic increase in the age-adjusted incidence of end stage renal disease (ESRD) in the United States, from 219 per million in 1991 to 355 per million in 2009 [1]. Since 2000, the rate of new ESRD cases has increased 7.2% among whites, while remaining stable among blacks [1], but in 2008 incidence for blacks was 3.5 times greater than for whites [1–3]. ESRD patients have a striking impact on national Medicare costs, which covers health care for incident ESRD in the United States regardless of age. At present, Medicare is the primary payer for 83% of hemodialysis patients, and total Medicare spending for treatment of ESRD in the United States is $29 billion, over 6% of the Medicare budget [1], and is expected to continue its rapid rise, in part due to the continued increasing prevalence of ESRD.

Although the higher rates of ESRD among blacks compared with whites are well-known, reasons for the increased ESRD risk among blacks and the extent to which differences in socioeconomic factors and other known determinants of ESRD may

account for the observed racial difference in incidence is more limited. A recent study conducted within the San Francisco Community Health Network, which serves an urban poor population, reported that among adults with non-dialysis dependent chronic kidney disease (CKD), 73% of whom had an annual income below $15,000, blacks had a substantially higher risk for progression to ESRD than whites after adjustment for socioeconomic variables and medical risk factors [4]. The Southern Community Cohort Study (SCCS) is a large, prospective cohort study examining health disparities among adults, over two-thirds black, residing in the southeastern United States where rates of ESRD are among the highest in the nation [1]. The SCCS provides unique advantages for examining differences in ESRD, since both black and white participants have similar (typically low) income and education levels, so that socioeconomic differences that sometimes confound racial comparisons are minimized. Thus, we have characterized and compared the incidence of ESRD among black and white participants in the SCCS, taking into account extensive well-defined data on socioeconomic factors, and we have examined race-specific associations between baseline demographic, lifestyle and medical factors and ESRD to enhance understanding of the independent determinants of ESRD among blacks versus whites.

Methods

Ethics statement

SCCS participants provided written informed consent, and protocols were approved by the Institutional Review Boards of Vanderbilt University Medical Center and Meharry Medical College.

Study population

The SCCS is an ongoing, prospective cohort study which enrolled nearly 86,000 adults, age 40–79, residing in 12 states in the southeastern United States during 2002–2009. Approximately 86% of participants were enrolled at participating community health centers (CHCs), institutions which provide primary health and preventive services in medically underserved areas and thus serve generally low-income populations [5], and the remaining 14% through mail-based general population sampling. The SCCS study design and methods have been described in detail previously [6].

Upon entry into the SCCS, participants were administered a baseline computer-assisted personal interview at the CHC while general population participants completed a self-administered mailed questionnaire. The questionnaire (available at www. southerncommunitystudy.org) ascertained information about demographic and socioeconomic characteristics, personal and family medical history, height, weight, tobacco and alcohol use history, and other factors. Many of the questions on the SCCS questionnaire were adapted from questionnaires used and validated in other settings, and a series of independent validation studies using biomarkers, repeat interviews or medical records have demonstrated the reliability of the questionnaire within the SCCS population for variables such as tobacco use status, self-reported diseases including diabetes, height and weight [6].

Outcome ascertainment

Incident diagnoses of ESRD among SCCS participants after entry into the cohort were ascertained by linkage, using Social Security number, date of birth, and first and last name, with the United States Renal Data System (USRDS) from January 1, 2002 through September 1, 2009 (the latest date for which data were available), providing virtually complete ascertainment of all persons in the United States receiving treatment for ESRD. Person-years of follow up for ascertainment of ESRD were calculated from date of entry into the SCCS until the date of diagnosis of ESRD, date of death, or September 1, 2009, whichever occurred first. Mortality (and date and cause of death) was ascertained by linkages with the Social Security Administration vital status service for epidemiologic researchers and the National Death Index through December 31, 2009. A total of 404 individuals with a diagnosis of ESRD recorded in the USRDS prior to enrollment in the SCCS (prevalent cases) were excluded from this analysis. Twenty-nine SCCS participants who did not have an incident diagnosis of ESRD identified through USRDS but had ESRD (ICD-10 N180, I120, I131, I132) listed as an underlying or contributing cause of death were not considered incident ESRD diagnoses, as misclassification of acute kidney injury could not be ruled out, and these 29 participants were excluded from the analysis.

Statistical analyses

Analyses were restricted to self-reported African American or black and non-Hispanic white SCCS participants who enrolled prior to September 1, 2009, since too few persons in other racial groups were available for stable statistical analysis. Percentage distributions of ESRD cases and age-adjusted (US 2000 standard population) incidence rates of ESRD were calculated in relation to demographic, socioeconomic, lifestyle, anthropometric and medical history characteristics reported at baseline, overall and by race and sex. Cox proportional hazards models, using age as the time scale, were used to estimate hazard ratios (HRs) and corresponding 95% confidence intervals (CI) for incident ESRD separately among black and white participants, and for both races combined, in relation to the following baseline characteristics: sex (male, female); recruitment source (CHC/general population); education (<12th grade, high/vocational school, some college or more); annual household income (<$15,000, ≥$15,000); cigarette smoking status (ever, never); history of diabetes (no/duration <10 years/duration 10–19 years/duration ≥20 years), hypertension, stroke, high cholesterol, and myocardial infarction (MI)/coronary artery bypass (CABG) (all yes/no). Tests for interaction of these variables with race were conducted by adding the corresponding cross-product terms to the models, and significance was based on two-sided tests with a nominal significance level of 0.05. Statistical analyses were conducted using SAS software, version 9.2 (SAS Institute Inc., Cary, NC).

Results

Among the 79,943 SCCS participants included in this analysis, 68% (N = 54,751) were black and 32% (N = 25,192) were white, and approximately 60% were women. Mean ages at the beginning of follow-up were 51.3 and 53.9 years among blacks and whites, respectively. Overall, 55% of participants had a household income below $15,000, and 29% reported an education level below high school. A diagnosis of diabetes, hypertension or MI/CABG was reported by 21%, 56% and 7% of participants, respectively.

After 329,003 person-years of follow-up, 687 incident cases of ESRD were identified in the cohort, yielding an overall age-adjusted incidence rate (IR) of 214 (per 100,000 person-years). The distribution and age-adjusted incidence rates of ESRD in relation to baseline characteristics are reported in Table 1. Six hundred and six (88.2%) of the ESRD cases were among blacks, yielding an incidence rate of 273, higher than the incidence rate of 78 among whites. Approximately 47% of the cases occurred among men, although the incidence of ESRD was higher among men (IR = 242) than women (IR = 194). Further, the substantially higher rate of ESRD among blacks than whites was apparent in both men and women, with rates (per 100,000) of 308, 248, 90 and 70 among black men, black women, white men and white women, respectively (data not shown).

A total of 258 cases of ESRD were observed among those aged 40–49 years at enrollment, yielding an IR of 244, which increased to an IR greater than 335 for those aged 60–69 at enrollment, but then dropped off to an IR of 242 at the oldest ages, likely reflecting a survivor effect (Table 1). The incidence of ESRD was inversely related to educational level and income. The IR of ESRD was approximately two-fold higher among those with less than 12 years of education (IR = 272) compared with those who had attended college (IR = 139), and among those with annual household income less than $15,000 (IR = 280) compared with higher income levels (IR = 128).

The association between BMI at enrollment and ESRD incidence varied by race. Black men and women who reported

Table 1. Distribution and age-adjusted (US 2000 standard) incidence rates (per 100,000) of end-stage renal disease (ESRD) in relation to baseline characteristics of 79,943 black and white SCCS participants, 2002–2009 (excluding those with prevalent ESRD at baseline).

Characteristic	Overall		African American		White	
	N (%)	IR	N (%)	IR	N (%)	IR
Total	687 (100)	214	606 (100)	273	81 (100)	78
Recruitment						
CHC Population	635 (92)	230	569 (94)	279	66 (81)	89
General Population	52 (8)	126	37 (6)	216	15 (19)	59
Age at enrollment (years)						
40–49	258 (38)	244	240 (40)	288	18 (22)	41
50–59	249 (36)	223	214 (35)	273	35 (43)	89
60–69	138 (20)	335	113 (19)	432	25 (31)	120
70–79	42 (6)	242	39 (6)	349	3 (4)	52
Sex						
Female	367 (53)	194	324 (53)	247	43 (53)	69
Male	320 (47)	242	282 (47)	308	38 (47)	90
Marital status						
Married	213 (31)	190	177 (29)	276	36 (44)	68
Separated/Divorced	222 (32)	203	194 (32)	224	28 (35)	134
Widowed	100 (15)	251	90 (15)	314	10 (12)	69
Single Never Married	149 (22)	315	142 (24)	368	7 (9)	87
Education						
Less than 12th grade	268 (39)	272	244 (40)	322	24 (30)	102
High/Vocational School	268 (39)	200	239 (39)	261	29 (36)	66
Some college or more	151 (22)	139	123 (20)	176	28 (35)	72
Annual household income ($)						
less than $15,000/year	482 (71)	280	429 (72)	328	53 (65)	123
$15,000/year or more	195 (29)	128	167 (28)	179	28 (35)	43
Health insurance						
No Insurance	224 (33)	140	201 (33)	171	23 (29)	56
Any Private/CHAMPUS/Other	127 (19)	122	107 (18)	173	20 (25)	47
Medicaid/Medicare Only	332 (49)	332	295 (49)	392	37 (46)	136
BMI at Enrollment (kg/m²)						
Underweight (<18.5)	7 (1)	201	6 (1)	260	1 (1)	73
Normal (18.5–24.9)	154 (23)	224	139 (23)	315	15 (19)	72
Overweight (25–29.9)	180 (27)	174	164 (28)	233	16 (20)	44
Obese (30+)	332 (49)	237	284 (48)	284	48 (60)	106
BMI at Age 21 (kg/m²)						
Underweight (<18.5)	57 (9)	206	53 (10)	290	4 (5)	43
Normal (18.5–24.9)	312 (49)	164	277 (50)	215	35 (45)	56
Overweight (25–29.9)	143 (23)	234	126 (23)	284	17 (22)	102
Obese (30+)	120 (19)	605	98 (18)	687	22 (28)	303
Smoking						
Ever	452 (66)	219	396 (65)	284	56 (69)	83
Never	234 (34)	202	209 (35)	252	25 (31)	68
Alcohol drinking						
None	405 (60)	252	342 (58)	311	63 (80)	113
Moderate (1–3/day)	195 (29)	147	182 (31)	202	13 (16)	31
Heavy (>3/day)	70 (10)	197	67 (11)	277	3 (4)	32
MI/CABG						

Table 1. Cont.

Characteristic	Overall		African American		White	
	N (%)	IR	N (%)	IR	N (%)	IR
No	580 (85)	194	521 (87)	249	59 (73)	61
Yes	103 (15)	452	81 (13)	614	22 (27)	200
Hypertension						
No	91 (13)	67	76 (13)	90	15 (19)	31
Yes	596 (87)	320	530 (87)	385	66 (81)	123
Diabetes						
No	245 (36)	103	219 (36)	136	26 (32)	29
Yes	442 (64)	611	387 (64)	716	55 (68)	283
Hypertension and Diabetes						
Both HTN and Diabetes	402 (59)	707	353 (58)	814	49 (60)	341
Diabetes Only	40 (6)	277	34 (6)	369	6 (7)	103
HTN Only	194 (28)	160	177 (29)	203	17 (21)	39
Neither HTN or Diabetes	51 (7)	39	42 (7)	44	9 (11)	25
Stroke						
No	592 (86)	199	525 (87)	255	67 (83)	68
Yes	95 (14)	447	81 (13)	556	14 (17)	228
High cholesterol						
No	343 (50)	162	314 (52)	205	29 (36)	41
Yes	343 (50)	306	292 (48)	404	51 (64)	128

being overweight or obese at enrollment had similar or lower rates of ESRD compared with those with normal BMI; among whites, rates were higher among men and women who were obese at enrollment compared with those of normal BMI, but remained substantially lower than for blacks across all categories of BMI. Self-reported BMI at age 21, however, was strongly and positively associated with ESRD in both races, with a greater than three-fold overall increase from a rate of 164 among those with normal BMI up to 605 among those who were obese at age 21. The association between BMI at age 21 and ESRD was more pronounced among whites, but the ESRD rate rose as high as 687 among blacks who reported having been obese at age 21, and as high as 1139 for black women when they were considered separately (data not shown).

Finally, the incidence of ESRD was strongly associated with history of MI/CABG, hypertension, diabetes, stroke and high cholesterol, overall and in each race stratum. In particular, the incidence of ESRD among those with hypertension or diabetes was five-fold and six-fold higher, respectively, than among those without, and was eighteen times higher among those with both hypertension and diabetes compared with those who had neither. Among blacks with both hypertension and diabetes, the incidence rate of ESRD reached 814.

Table 2 presents HRs and 95% CIs for the association between ESRD and selected baseline characteristics for the study population. Men and women were combined for these analyses as there were no material differences among estimates by sex. After adjustment for age, sex, education, income, smoking, and history of hypertension, diabetes and other medical conditions, blacks continued to have a higher risk for ESRD, with a HR of 2.4 (95% CI = 1.9–3.0) relative to whites. Women were at lower risk of ESRD than men (HR = 0.6; 95% CI 0.5–0.7), and smokers had a

modestly increased risk for ESRD compared with non-smokers (HR = 1.2; 95% CI 1.02–1.4). Income was inversely associated with ESRD, with a HR of 1.5 (95% CI 1.2–1.8) for those with income below $15,000, while level of education was no longer associated with ESRD in the adjusted model. For all of these variables, patterns and magnitudes of association were virtually identical among blacks and whites (Table 2). In this multivariate analysis, the inclusion of BMI, either at time of enrollment or at age 21, had no material effect on the HR estimates for the other examined covariates.

History of diabetes was the strongest predictor of ESRD in our study population, both overall and separately by race. Compared with those who had never been diagnosed with diabetes, HRs increased from 2.6 (95% CI 2.1–3.3) to 8.7 (95% CI 7.1–10.7) to 9.4 (95% CI 7.4–11.9) among those with a duration of diabetes of less than 10, 10–19, and 20 or more years, respectively (Table 2). Hypertension was also strongly associated with ESRD, with a nearly three-fold increased risk (HR = 2.9; 95% CI 2.3–3.7) among those who reported a diagnosis of hypertension at baseline. History of MI/CABG, stroke and high cholesterol were also modestly associated with ESRD overall, with HRs of 1.3 (95% CI 1.00–1.6), 1.3 (95% CI 1.1–1.7) and 1.2 (95% CI 1.01–1.4). For no risk factor was the formal test for interaction by race statistically significant, indicating that the ESRD HRs associated with the factors were similar between blacks and whites.

Discussion

In this population of socioeconomically similar black and white SCCS participants, the age-adjusted incidence of ESRD was more than 3.5 times higher among black than whites. Even after controlling for well-defined socioeconomic factors and extensive demographic, medical and lifestyle information collected at study

Table 2. Cox proportional hazard ratios (HR) and 95% confidence interval (CI) for end-stage renal disease (ESRD) in relation to baseline characteristics of black and white SCCS participants, 2002–2009 (excluding those with prevalent ESRD at baseline).

Characteristic	Overall			Black			White		
	ESRD events	HR	95% CI	ESRD events	HR	95% CI	ESRD events	HR	95% CI
Recruitment									
CHC Population	616	1.2	0.8–1.6	551	1.2	0.8–1.7	65	1.1	0.6–2.1
General Population	46	Ref		31	Ref		15	Ref	
Sex									
Female	357	0.6	0.5–0.7	314	0.6	0.5–0.7	43	0.7	0.4–1.02
Male	305	Ref		268	Ref		37	Ref	
Race									
Black	582	2.4	1.9–3.0						
White	80	Ref							
Education									
Less than 12th grade	256	0.9	0.8–1.1	232	0.9	0.8–1.1	24	0.9	0.5–1.6
High/Vocational School	259	Ref		230	Ref		29	Ref	
Some college or more	147	0.9	0.7–1.1	120	0.8	0.7–1.03	27	1.0	0.6–1.8
Annual Household Income									
less than $15,000/year	472	1.5	1.2–1.8	420	1.4	1.2–1.7	52	1.6	0.97–2.8
$15,000/year or more	190	Ref		162	Ref		28	Ref	
Smoking									
Ever	437	1.2	1.02–1.4	382	1.2	1.02–1.5	55	1.2	0.7–1.9
Never	225	Ref		200	Ref		25	Ref	
Hypertension Dx									
No	90	Ref		75	Ref		15	Ref	
Yes	572	2.9	2.3–3.7	507	3.0	2.3–3.9	65	2.1	1.1–3.8
Time Since Diabetes Dx									
Never Diagnosed	240	Ref		214	Ref		26	Ref	
less than 10 years	134	2.6	2.1–3.3	118	2.6	2.1–3.3	16	2.9	1.5–5.5
10–19 years	176	8.7	7.1–10.7	153	8.4	6.7–10.5	23	10.9	6.0–19.9
20 or more years	112	9.4	7.4–11.9	97	8.9	6.9–11.6	15	13.2	6.7–26.1
MI/CABG									
No	563	Ref		504	Ref		59	Ref	
Yes	99	1.3	1.00–1.6	78	1.3	0.97–1.6	21	1.2	0.7–2.1
Stroke									
No	569	Ref		503	Ref		66	Ref	
Yes	93	1.3	1.1–1.7	79	1.3	1.1–1.7	14	1.3	0.7–2.3
High cholesterol									
No	334	Ref		305	Ref		29	Ref	
Yes	328	1.2	1.01–1.4	277	1.2	1.01–1.4	51	1.2	0.7–1.9

entry, including comorbidities such as diabetes and hypertension, blacks continued to have a 2.4-fold greater risk of ESRD relative to whites. It is noteworthy that the strengths of the associations of the various factors with risk of ESRD tended to be the same for blacks and whites. Thus, although residual confounding cannot be ruled out entirely, the examined socioeconomic and other risk factors for ESRD do not explain the observed substantially higher incidence of ESRD observed among blacks.

Our data are consistent with national statistics [1] and observations of higher rates of ESRD observed among blacks in other study populations [7–9]. A small number of prospective studies have had sufficient sample size and length of follow up to directly compare risk factors for incident ESRD among blacks and whites. In the Atherosclerosis Risk in Communities (ARIC) study [7] of 3,954 blacks and 11,370 whites, older age, smoking, male sex, diabetes and hypertension were positively associated with incident ESRD, and African American race remained a strong predictor even after controlling for these factors, with a HR of 2.5. These results are very similar to what we found in the SCCS, and to results of the Multiple Risk Factor Intervention Trial (MRFIT) and a study among Medicare beneficiaries aged 66 years or older with hypertension or diabetes. [10]. Similarly, in. In a large population of veterans [8], including 311,790 blacks and 1,704,101 whites, the incidence of ESRD was consistently higher among blacks than whites at all levels of baseline kidney function, after adjustment for socioeconomic variables and comorbidities. Although that study included a larger number of ESRD cases (N = 4,379 cases among blacks, 10,769 among whites) than our study population, it did not report associations of ESRD with characteristics of the study participants other than estimated glomerular filtration rate (eGFR). Most recently, in the Reasons for Geographic and Racial Differences in Stroke (REGARDS) study, a total of 133 incident cases of ESRD were observed over a median of 3.6 years of follow-up among 27,911 participants [9]. ESRD rates among blacks and whites were comparable to those observed in the current study, but the fourfold greater risk of developing ESRD among blacks compared with whites decreased to 1.4 after adjustment for hypertension, diabetes, income, and education, as well as eGFR and albumin-to-creatinine ratio.

A striking pattern of racial differences exists also for CKD, and provides evidence that the observed disparity in ESRD incidence between blacks and whites may be due, at least in part, to racial differences in the rate of progression of CKD to ESRD. In the San Francisco Community Health Network study population, most similar to the SCCS population in terms of socioeconomic distribution, blacks with CKD stages 3 to 5 had a four-fold higher risk of progression to ESRD than whites after adjustment for socioeconomic status [4]. The prevalence of early stage CKD is higher among whites compared with blacks [11–14], with detailed analyses based on eGFR measurements showing that the white excess for mild CKD gives way to an excess for moderate to severe CKD in blacks [14–16]. It has been hypothesized that this "crossover" pattern may be due to lower mortality at higher GFR levels among blacks. Empirical evidence, however, demonstrates that death rates are higher among blacks than whites at all levels of CKD prior to ESRD [8,10], and rates of ESRD incidence are nearly five times higher than rates of cardiovascular death among blacks with hypertension [17], and thus does not lend support to this explanation. More intense surveillance among whites than blacks could contribute to elevated prevalence among whites of early stage CKD, for whom symptoms are less marked, or, on the contrary, whites may become symptomatic at higher GFR levels and thus have CKD diagnosed earlier. Shorter sojourn times in early stage disease by blacks than whites may also be involved, but explanations for speculated faster transitions to moderate and advanced CKD and potentially to ESRD for blacks remain clear.

We did not routinely measure baseline serum creatinine for estimation of GFR among SCCS participants, but blood samples were collected from over half of those who enrolled in CHCs. As part of ongoing nested case-control studies for breast, lung, colorectal and prostate cancer, independent of the current ESRD analysis, prediagnostic blood from 1,593 cases and age- and race-matched controls was assayed for several biomarkers, including serum creatinine. Wwe found that the mean creatinine levels were about 3% higher among black (1.10 mg/dl) than white men (1.07 mg/dl) and 14% higher among black (0.90 mg/dl) than white women (0.79 mg/dl), consistent with reports in other populations of blacks and whites [18,19]. Using the CKD-EPI equation to estimate GFR [20], the percentages in the SCCS sample of participants with eGFR of >90 ("normal"), 90–61 and ≤60ml/min/1.73 m^2 were 56.9%, 34.5% and 8.6% among black men, 39.5%, 51.3% and 9.2% among white men, 58.7%, 32.5% and 8.8% among black women and 47.7%, 39.5% and 12.8% among white women. These figures suggest that the overall prevalence of CKD at entry into the SCCS may be lower among blacks than whites. For severe CKD, defined by eGFR <30 ml/

min/1.73 m^2, a modest excess among blacks became apparent, with prevalences of 1.9%, 1.8%, 1.7% and 0.4% among black men, black women, white men, and white women, respectively, although based on very small numbers of study subjects. However, the observed excess in the incidence of ESRD among blacks in our study population was much greater than the excess in estimated severe CKD. Twenty-four of the incident ESRD cases in this study were among those who had existing baseline serum creatinine measurements; for these eGFR at study entry was below 90 ml/min/1.73 m^2 for 21 (88%) and below 60 ml/min/1.73 m^2 for 16 (67%). Further assessment of CKD is beyond the scope of this analysis, but additional research is needed using serum and urinary biomarkers collected at baseline, in conjunction with repeat blood collections to measure progression rates and times by race among SCCS participants with CKD.

While awareness and treatment of hypertension has improved among blacks over time, a substantially higher prevalence of hypertension among blacks compared with whites has been reported to persist, as well as the difference between blacks and whites in the proportion of patients with hypertension who are receiving treatment [21,22]. In the overall SCCS population, the prevalence of self-reported hypertension at baseline was 59% among blacks, significantly higher than the 50% among whites, but approximately 80% of both blacks and whites with hypertension reported use of anti-hypertensive medications. It has been suggested that a lower blood pressure level may be necessary to slow the decline of renal function among blacks with CKD and hypertension compared with whites [23,24], but racial differences in the susceptibility to renal damage from elevated blood pressure have been reported to persist even after adjustment for differences between blacks and whites in hypertension and hypertension-control [25]. In our study, the HR estimate associated with hypertension was somewhat (but not significantly) higher among blacks than whites (HR = 3.0 versus 2.1), which lends some support to the view that the higher incidence of ESRD in blacks may be attributable in part to a greater sensitivity to the effects of elevated blood pressure among blacks. With respect to diabetes, the onset of albuminuria, hypothesized to be an etiologic factor rather than simply a biomarker [26], appears to present earlier in the course of diabetes in blacks compared with whites, which may suggest more aggressive disease progression [27,28], but this is unlikely to explain the similar HR estimate observed between diabetes and ESRD among whites and blacks in our study population.

The SCCS is a unique cohort in which to study health effects in blacks compared with whites both because of the large number of blacks and the comparability of socioeconomic status between the racial groups. In addition, the collection of extensive baseline information for the entire SCCS cohort and the unbiased and virtually complete follow up for ascertainment of ESRD [29] are major strengths of our study. Over 85% of our study population was drawn from CHCs, which are expected to provide race-neutral care for diabetes, hypertension and other chronic illnesses. Limitations include the lack of data on baseline kidney function or proteinuria for the ESRD cases, the self-reported nature of the questionnaire data, and the lack of time-dependent covariates. However, we conducted internally valid comparisons of HRs for ESRD between blacks and whites, and our findings support the existing literature on this subject and warrant further etiologic research in future prospective studies of ESRD in blacks.

While race appears to be an independent predictor of ESRD, and possibly of more rapid loss of kidney function among those with moderate and advanced CKD [30], longitudinal studies with repeated measures of kidney function are critically needed to evaluate whether stage-specific kidney disease may progress more rapidly in blacks than in whites and to identify genetic, environmental or behavioral factors that may explain these differences in progression rate and incidence of ESRD among blacks in the United States. A recent study [31] showed that, among those of recent African ancestry, focal segmental glomerulosclerosis and hypertension-attributed ESRD are strongly associated with two coding sequence variants in the APOL1 gene on chromosome 22. The APOL1 genotype has also been shown to associate with microalbuminuria among nondiabetics [32], and with younger age at initiation of hemodialysis among nondiabetic blacks with ESRD [33]. The APOL1 risk alleles for renal disease occur in more than 30% of those with recent African ancestry, but to date have not been observed in European Americans [31,34]. Thus, these emerging data support the existence of a relatively common, high-risk genotype that confers susceptibility to nondiabetic kidney disease in African Americans [34].

Our study has demonstrated that, after taking into account traditional risk factors strongly associated with ESRD among both blacks and whites, blacks continue to have a substantially increased risk for ESRD compared with whites. Further research characterizing CKD progression and ESRD occurrence by race may help greatly in clarifying the natural history and etiologic events leading to ESRD in these two populations.

Author Contributions

Conceived and designed the experiments: LL MTM KC TLE TAI RET JKM WJB. Performed the experiments: LL MTM KC JKM WJB. Analyzed the data: LL MTM KC RET JKM WJB. Wrote the paper: LL MTM KC WJB. Interpretation of data: LL MTM KC TLE TAI RET JKM WJB. Critical revision of manuscript for important intellectual content: TLE TAI RET.

References

1. U.S. Renal Data System (2011) USRDS 2011 Annual Data Report: Atlas of End-Stage Renal Disease in the United States. In: National Institutes of Health NIoDaDaKD, editor. Bethesda, MD.
2. Klein JB, Nguyen CT, Saffore L, Modlin C 3rd, Modlin CS Jr. (2010) Racial disparities in urologic health care. J Natl Med Assoc 102: 108–117.
3. Martins D, Tareen N, Norris KC (2002) The epidemiology of end-stage renal disease among African Americans. Am J Med Sci 323: 65–71.
4. Hall YN, Choi AI, Chertow GM, Bindman AB (2010) Chronic kidney disease in the urban poor. Clin J Am Soc Nephrol 5: 828–835.
5. Hargreaves MK, Arnold CW, Blot WJ (2006) Community health centers: Their role in the treatment of minorities and in health disparities research. In: Satcher D, Pamies R, editors. Multicultural Medicine and Health Disparities. New York: McGraw-Hill. pp. 485–494.
6. Signorello LB, Hargreaves MK, Blot WJ (2010) The Southern Community Cohort Study: investigating health disparities. J Health Care Poor Underserved 21: 26–37.
7. Bash LD, Astor BC, Coresh J (2010) Risk of incident ESRD: a comprehensive look at cardiovascular risk factors and 17 years of follow-up in the Atherosclerosis Risk in Communities (ARIC) Study. Am J Kidney Dis 55: 31–41.
8. Choi AI, Rodriguez RA, Bacchetti P, Bertenthal D, Hernandez GT, et al. (2009) White/black racial differences in risk of end-stage renal disease and death. Am J Med 122: 672–678.
9. McClellan WM, Warnock DG, Judd S, Muntner P, Kewalramani R, et al. (2011) Albuminuria and racial disparities in the risk for ESRD. J Am Soc Nephrol 22: 1721–1728.
10. Xue JL, Eggers PW, Agodoa LY, Foley RN, Collins AJ (2007) Longitudinal study of racial and ethnic differences in developing end-stage renal disease among aged medicare beneficiaries. J Am Soc Nephrol 18: 1299–1306.
11. Clase CM, Garg AX, Kiberd BA (2002) Prevalence of low glomerular filtration rate in nondiabetic Americans: Third National Health and Nutrition Examination Survey (NHANES III). J Am Soc Nephrol 13: 1338–1349.
12. Coresh J, Astor BC, Greene T, Eknoyan G, Levey AS (2003) Prevalence of chronic kidney disease and decreased kidney function in the adult US population: Third National Health and Nutrition Examination Survey. Am J Kidney Dis 41: 1–12.
13. McClellan W, Warnock DG, McClure L, Campbell RC, Newsome BB, et al. (2006) Racial differences in the prevalence of chronic kidney disease among participants in the Reasons for Geographic and Racial Differences in Stroke (REGARDS) Cohort Study. J Am Soc Nephrol 17: 1710–1715.
14. U.S. Renal Data System (2011) USRDS 2011 Annual Data Report: Atlas of Chronic Kidney Disease in the United States. In: National Institutes of Health NIoDaDaKD, editor. Bethesda, MD.
15. Prevention CfDCa (2007) Prevalence of chronic kidney disease and associated risk factors–United States, 1999–2004. MMWR Morb Mortal Wkly Rep 56: 161–165.
16. McClellan WM, Newsome BB, McClure LA, Howard G, Volkova N, et al. (2010) Poverty and racial disparities in kidney disease: the REGARDS study. Am J Nephrol 32: 38–46.
17. Alves TP, Wang X, Wright JT Jr., Appel LJ, Greene T, et al. (2010) Rate of ESRD exceeds mortality among African Americans with hypertensive nephrosclerosis. J Am Soc Nephrol 21: 1361–1369.
18. Agamah ES, Webber LS, Lawrence M, Wattigney W, Berenson GS (1990) Serum creatinine and its relation to cardiovascular disease risk variables in children and young adults from a biracial community. The Bogalusa Heart Study. J Lab Clin Med 116: 327–334.
19. Jones CA, McQuillan GM, Kusek JW, Eberhardt MS, Herman WH, et al. (1998) Serum creatinine levels in the US population: third National Health and Nutrition Examination Survey. Am J Kidney Dis 32: 992–999.
20. Levey AS, Stevens LA, Schmid CH, Zhang YL, Castro AF 3rd, et al. (2009) A new equation to estimate glomerular filtration rate. Ann Intern Med 150: 604–612.
21. Egan BM, Zhao Y, Axon RN (2010) US trends in prevalence, awareness, treatment, and control of hypertension, 1988–2008. JAMA 303: 2043–2050.
22. Klag MJ, Whelton PK, Randall BL, Neaton JD, Brancati FL, et al. (1997) End-stage renal disease in African-American and white men. 16-year MRFIT findings. JAMA 277: 1293–1298.
23. Hebert LA, Kusek JW, Greene T, Agodoa LY, Jones CA, et al. (1997) Effects of blood pressure control on progressive renal disease in blacks and whites. Modification of Diet in Renal Disease Study Group. Hypertension 30: 428–435.
24. Walker WG, Neaton JD, Cutler JA, Neuwirth R, Cohen JD (1992) Renal function change in hypertensive members of the Multiple Risk Factor Intervention Trial. Racial and treatment effects. The MRFIT Research Group. JAMA 268: 3085–3091.
25. McClellan W, Tuttle E, Issa A (1988) Racial differences in the incidence of hypertensive end-stage renal disease (ESRD) are not entirely explained by differences in the prevalence of hypertension. Am J Kidney Dis 12: 285–290.
26. Burton C, Harris KP (1996) The role of proteinuria in the progression of chronic renal failure. Am J Kidney Dis 27: 765–775.
27. Goldschmid MG, Domin WS, Ziemer DC, Gallina DL, Phillips LS (1995) Diabetes in urban African-Americans. II. High prevalence of microalbuminuria and nephropathy in African-Americans with diabetes. Diabetes Care 18: 955–961.
28. Thaler LM, El-Kebbi IM, Ziemer DC, Gallina DL, Dunbar VG, et al. (1998) High prevalence of albuminuria among African-Americans with short duration of diabetes. Diabetes Care 21: 1576–1577.
29. Eggers PW (2010) CMS 2728: what good is it? Clin J Am Soc Nephrol 5: 1908–1909.
30. Hunsicker LG, Adler S, Caggiula A, England BK, Greene T, et al. (1997) Predictors of the progression of renal disease in the Modification of Diet in Renal Disease Study. Kidney Int 51: 1908–1919.
31. Genovese G, Friedman DJ, Ross MD, Lecordier L, Uzureau P, et al. (2010) Association of trypanolytic ApoL1 variants with kidney disease in African Americans. Science 329: 841–845.
32. Friedman DJ, Kozlitina J, Genovese G, Jog P, Pollak MR (2011) Population-based risk assessment of APOL1 on renal disease. J Am Soc Nephrol 22: 2098–2105.
33. Kanji Z, Powe CE, Wenger JB, Huang C, Ankers E, et al. (2011) Genetic variation in APOL1 associates with younger age at hemodialysis initiation. J Am Soc Nephrol 22: 2091–2097.
34. Pollak MR, Genovese G, Friedman DJ (2012) APOL1 and kidney disease. Curr Opin Nephrol Hypertens 21: 179–182.

6

CCR5Δ32 Genotype Leads to a Th2 Type Directed Immune Response in ESRD Patients

Friso L. H. Muntinghe[1]*, **Wayel H. Abdulahad**[2], **Minke G. Huitema**[2], **Jeffrey Damman**[3], **Marc A. Seelen**[3], **Simon P. M. Lems**[4], **Bouke G. Hepkema**[4], **Gerjan Navis**[3], **Johanna Westra**[2]

1 Internal Medicine, Vasculair Medicine, University Medical Center Groningen, Groningen, The Netherlands, 2 Rheumatology and Clinical Immunology, University Medical Center Groningen, Groningen, The Netherlands, 3 Internal Medicine, Nephrology, University Medical Center Groningen, Groningen, The Netherlands, 4 Laboratory Medicine, Transplantation Immunology, University Medical Center Groningen, Groningen, The Netherlands

Abstract

Background: In patients with end stage renal disease (ESRD) we observed protection from inflammation-associated mortality in CCR5Δ32 carriers, leading to CCR5 deficiency, suggesting impact of CCR5Δ32 on inflammatory processes. Animal studies have shown that CCR5 deficiency is associated with a more pronounced Th2 type immune response, suggesting that in human CCR5Δ32 carriers the immune response may be more Th2 type directed. So, in the present study we determined the Th1-Th2 type directed immune response in ESRD patients carrying and not carrying the CCR5Δ32 genetic variant after stimulation.

Methodology/Principal Findings: We tested this hypothesis by determining the levels of IFN-γ and IL-4 and the distribution of Th1, Th2 and Th17 directed circulating CD4+ and CD8+ T cells and regulatory T cells (Tregs) after stimulation in ESRD patients with (n = 10) and without (n = 9) the CCR5Δ32 genotype. The extracellular levels of IFN-γ and IL-4 did not differ between CCR5Δ32 carriers and non carriers. However, based on their intracellular cytokine profile the percentages IL-4 secreting CD4+ and CD8+ T cells carrying the CCR5Δ32 genotype were significantly increased (p = 0.02, respectively p = 0.02) compared to non carriers, indicating a more Th2 type directed response. Based on their intracellular cytokine profile the percentages IFN-γ and IL-17 secreting T cells did not differ between carriers and non-carriers nor did the percentage Tregs, indicating that the Th1, Th17 and T regulatory response was not affected by the CCR5Δ32 genotype.

Conclusions/Significance: This first, functional human study shows a more pronounced Th2 type immune response in CCR5Δ32 carriers compared to non carriers. These differences may be involved in the previously observed protection from inflammation-associated mortality in ESRD patients carrying CCR5Δ32.

Editor: Michael P. Bachmann, Carl-Gustav Carus Technical University-Dresden, Germany

Funding: The authors have no support or funding to report.

Competing Interests: The authors have declared that no competing interests exist.

* E-mail: f.l.h.muntinghe@umcg.nl

Introduction

Genetic variability in the chemokine cascades could potentially influence disease outcomes by modifying inflammatory processes. CC-chemokine receptor 5 (CCR5) is one of the chemokine receptors. It is expressed on T cells and monocytes and it is important for recruitment [1,2]. Several polymorphisms have been described for CCR5. The CCR5Δ32 genetic variant is located on the chromosome 3p21 and consists of a 32-basepair deletion in the open reading frame. It effectively results in functional CCR5 deficiency by absence of CCR5 membrane expression [3]. We observed protection from inflammation-associated mortality in carriers of the deletion 32 allele in end stage renal disease (ESRD), suggesting impact of CCR5Δ32 on the inflammatory process of atherosclerosis [4]. Also in other human populations, characterized by high cardiovascular risk, the presence of the CCR5Δ32 genotype has been associated with better outcome [5–8].

In chronic inflammatory processes like atherosclerosis T cells play an important role. Both CD4+ T cells and to a lesser extent CD8+ T cells are present in atherosclerotic lesions [9–12]. CD4+ T helper cells can differentiate into three effector lineages based on their cytokine expression: IFN-γ/TNF-α producers (Th1), IL-4 producers (Th2) and IL-17 producers (Th17) [12,13]. In addition, a small fraction of CD4+ T cells can develop into cells with a regulatory function (Tregs) that are defined by their co-expression of high levels of surface CD25 and intracellular transcription factor forkhead box P3 (FoxP3). These Tregs have the remarkable ability to suppress the proliferation and effector function of other T cells [9,12]. As with CD4+ T cells, CD8+ T cells can differentiate to T cytotoxic (Tc)1 or Tc2 cell subsets, secreting predominantly Th1 or Th2 cytokines respectively [13].

Atherosclerotic inflammation is regarded as a (partly) Th1 driven condition [12]. The CCR5 receptor is highly expressed T-lymphocytes, on both CD4+ T and CD8+ T cells [2,11]. In atherosclerotic mice CCR5 deficiency is associated with a more pronounced Th2 type immune response and less TNF-α and IFN-γ production hereby counteracting the Th1 directed Th1/Th2 disequilibrium of atherosclerotic inflammation [14–17].

These data fuel the hypothesis that the immune response in carriers of the CCR5Δ32 genotype is more Th2 type directed. Such differences in response might play a role in the protection against inflammation-associated mortality in ESRD in carriers of the CCR5Δ32 genotype. To test this hypothesis we studied the cell mediated immune responses in peripheral mononuclear cells (PBMCs) in ESRD patients. We first determined the extracellular levels of IFN-γ and IL-4 after stimulation of PBMCs, and second the distribution of Th1, Th2 and Th17 directed circulating CD4+ and CD8+ T cells, based on their intracellular cytokine profile after stimulation, and the percentage of Tregs in ESRD patients with and without the CCR5Δ32 genotype.

Methods

Objectives

The objective of the present study was to determine possible differences in cell mediated immune response between ESRD carriers and non carriers of the CCR5Δ32 genotype. To test this hypothesis we first determined the IFN-γ and IL-4 levels after stimulation of peripheral mononuclear cells (PBMCs) and secondly the distribution of Type-1, Type-2 and Type-17 directed circulating CD4+ and CD8+ T cells, based on their intracellular cytokine profile, as well as the frequency of FoxP3+ regulatory T cells.

Participants

Biosamples and data from twenty patients with ESRD were included in this study. These patients were part of an ESRD cohort from a single kidney transplant centre in the Netherlands (University Medical Center Groningen), in whom data and biosamples were collected prior to kidney transplantation. As part of a larger genotyping project, all patients were genotyped as described below. For the current project we randomly selected five homo- and five heterozygous carriers from the cohort. Ten wild type patients were matched with carriers according to time of inclusion, hereby creating similar preservation conditions.

Genotyping

The genotypes were determined with a PCR-based allelic discrimination assay using primers (Life Technologies) and allele-specific probes (PE Biosystems) as described previously [18]. Patients were grouped by CCR5 genotype, namely those homozygous for the major allele (non-carriers) and those with 1 or 2 deletion alleles (carriers). Patients with one or two deletion alleles were grouped together, as it has been demonstrated that presence of one deletion allele is sufficient to compromise CCR5 function [3].

Sample preparation and thawing

Heparinized venous blood was obtained from ESRD-patients who gave their informed consent. PBMCs were separated by conventional Ficoll gradient and frozen in 10% DMSO in FCS and stored in liquid nitrogen. PBMCs were thawed and washed twice with RPMI 1640 media (Cambrex Bio Science, Verviers, Belgium), supplemented with 10% heat inactivated fetal calf serum and 50 µg/mL gentamycin (Gibco, Scotland, UK).

Determination of extracellular cytokine by ELISA

Thawed PBMCs were cultured in a 5 mL polypropylene tubes (BD Biosciences) at $2,5 \times 10^6$ cells/mL per tube, and stimulated with 40 nM phorbol myristate acetate (PMA; Sigma-Aldrich, Steinheim, Germany) and 2 nM calcium ionophore (Sigma-Aldrich). Culture supernatants were collected over a period of 24 hours to determine the extracellular levels of IFN-γ, and IL-4 cytokines.

Cytokine levels of IFN-γ and IL-4 were measured by commercial sandwich enzyme linked immunoassay (ELISA) kits (Pelikine Compact, Sanquin, Amsterdam, The Netherlands), according to the instructions of the manufacturer.

Determination of intracellular cytokine by flow cytometry

The following conjugated antibodies were used in flow cytometry: allophycocyanin (APC)–Cy7–conjugated anti-CD69, peridin-chlorophyll protein (PerCP)–conjugated anti-CD8, phyco-erythrin (PE)– Cy7–conjugated anti-IL-4, and Alexa Fluor 700–conjugated anti-IFN-γ (all from Becton & Dickinson, Amsterdam, The Netherlands). Alexa Fluor 488–conjugated anti–IL-17, Alexa Fluor 647-conjugated anti-TNF-α, and eFluor605™–conjugated anti-CD3 were obtained from eBioscience (San Diego, CA). To determine the frequency of T cell subsets by measuring intracellular cytokine production, cells were stimulated for 4 hours with 40 nM PMA and 2 nM calcium ionophore. Brefeldin A (10 µg/mL) was added to inhibit cytokine release. After stimulation, cells were washed in wash buffer (phosphate buffered saline, 5% fetal bovine serum, 0.1% sodium azide; Merck, Darmstadt, Germany) and stained with eFluor 605-conjugated anti-CD3, PerCP–conjugated anti-CD8 and APC-Cy7–conjugated anti-CD69 for 15 minutes at room temperature. Cells were fixed with 100 µl Reagent A (Caltag, An Der Grab, Austria) for 15 minutes. After washing, the pellet was resuspended in 100 µl permeabiliza-tion Reagent B (Caltag) and labeled with PE-Cy7–conjugated anti-IL-4, Alexa Fluor 700–conjugated anti-IFN-γ, Alexa Fluor 647-conjugated anti-TNF-α, Alexa Fluor 488–conjugated anti–IL-17, and APC-Cy7–conjugated anti-CD69 for 30 minutes in the dark. After staining, the cells were washed and immediately analyzed on a FACS-LSRII flow cytometer (Becton Dickinson). Seven-color flow cytometric acquisition was performed using FACSDiva software (Becton Dickinson). For all flow cytometry analyses, data were collected for 2×10^5 cells and plotted using the Win-List software package (Verity Software House, Topsham, ME). Because stimulation reduces surface expression of CD4 on T cells, CD4 T cells were identified indirectly by gating on CD3+ and CD8– lymphocytes, whereas CD8+ T cells were identified by directly gating on CD3+ and CD8+ lymphocytes. Subsets of activated CD4+ and CD8+ T cells in response to mitogenic stimulation were evaluated by double expression of activation marker CD69 and intracellular cytokine production of IFN-γ (for type-1) or IL-17 (for type-17) or IL-4 (for type-2). The unstimulated samples were used as a guide for setting the linear gates to delineate positive and negative populations.

Determination of regulatory T cell frequencies

PBMCs were washed with cold PBS (pH 7.2) and incubated with appropriate concentrations of PerCP-conjugated anti-CD4, FITC-conjugated anti-CD3 and PE-conjugated anti-CD25 (all purchased from BD) for 30 min at 4°C in the dark. Cells were then washed with cold PBS, followed by fixation and permeabi-lization in Fix/Perm buffer (FoxP3 staining kit, eBioscience, Uithoorn, The Netherlands) for 45 min at 4°C. Subsequently, cells were washed with cold permeabilization buffer (FoxP3 staining kit, eBioscience, Uithoorn, The Netherlands). To block nonspecific binding, normal rat serum was added for 10 min, followed by the addition of APC-conjugated rat anti-human FoxP3 (eBioscience, Uithoorn, The Netherlands). After incubation for 30 min at 4°C, the cell suspension was washed twice with cold permeabilization buffer, and immediately analyzed on FACS-Calibur (BD). Data were collected for 2×10^5 cells and plotted using the Win-List software package (Verity Software House, Topsham, ME). Positively and negatively stained populations were calculated by quadrant dot-plot analysis, determined by the isotype matched control antibodies of irrelevant specificity (obtained from BD and eBioscience).

Ethics

All patients gave written informed consent and the local medical ethics committee from the University Medical Center Groningen (METc UMC Groningen), the Netherlands, gave their approval.

Statistical methods

Patients were grouped by CCR5 genotype, namely those homozygous for the major allele (non-carriers) and those with 1 or 2 deletion alleles (carriers). The latter were grouped together, as it has been demonstrated that presence of one deletion allele is sufficient to compromise CCR5 function [3]. Data are presented as the median. The nonparametric Mann-Whitney U test was used to compare data from patients with and without the CCR5Δ32 genotype. Differences were considered statistically significant at 2-sided p values less than 0.05.

Results

Patients

From the 20 patients who were included in this study 1 stimulation test failed due to the fact that the T cells could not be stimulated. Further statistical analyses were performed on the remaining 19 patients. Baseline characteristics are shown in Table 1. There were no statistically significant differences in baseline characteristics between the 2 genotype groups.

Extracellular cytokines of type-1 and type-2 T cells

To assess the functional capacity of the responding PBMCs the total amount of IFN-γ and IL-4 after stimulation was determined. As shown in Figure 1, the levels of extracellular IFN-γ and IL-4

were not statistically significant different between carriers and non carriers of the CCR5Δ32 genotype.

Intracellular cytokines of type-1, type-2, and type-17 T cells

To elucidate the functional phenotype of the CD4+ and CD8+ T cells responding to stimulation, activated T cells were gated and evaluated for expression of the activation marker CD69 versus intracellular expression of the cytokines IFN-γ, IL-17 and IL-4. The results are shown in Figure 2 and 3. The percentages IL-4 secreting CD4+ and CD8+ T cells from patients with the CCR5Δ32 genotype was significantly (p = 0.02, respectively p = 0.02) increased compared to patients not carrying the CCR5Δ32 genotype, indicating a more Th2 type directed response. The percentages IFN-γ secreting CD4+ and CD8+ T cells did not significantly differ between carriers and non carriers of CCR5Δ32, meaning the Th1 and Th17 response did not differ between these 2 groups. Comparing the CCR5Δ32 homozygous and heterozygous CD4+ and CD8+ T cells showed no significant differences.

Frequencies of regulatory T cells

To address the question whether differences in Tregs frequencies influence the distribution of T cell subsets between CCR5Δ32 carriers and non carriers, FoxP3+CD25^{High}CD4$^+$ T cells were analyzed in both groups. No significant differences were found between the 2 genotype groups (Figure 4). It seems, therefore, that

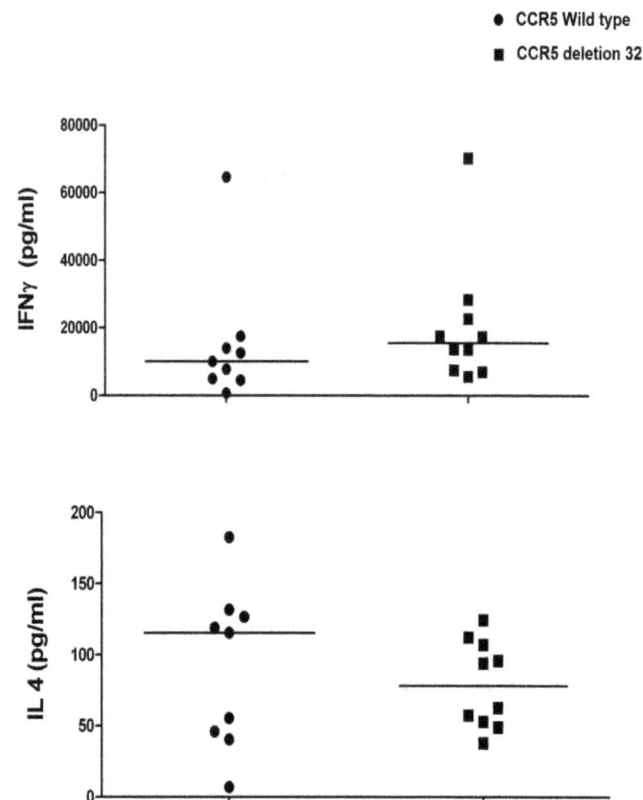

Figure 1. IFN-γ and IL-4 ELISA per 2,5×10⁶ PBMCs in carriers and non carriers of the CCR5Δ32 genotype. Levels of IFN-γ and IL-4 after stimulation from carriers (n = 10) and non carriers (n = 9) are shown. Horizontal lines represent the medians.

Table 1. Baseline characteristics.

	CCR5 wild type (n = 9)	CCR5 deletion 32 (n = 10)
Gender; male	4 (44.4)	7 (70.0)
Age (year)	51 (14)	51 (13)
Primary kidney disease		
Renal vascular disease and hypertension	3	3
Diabetes mellitus	1	0
Cystic kidney disease	1	3
Pyelonephritis	1	1
Primary oxalosis	1	0
Unknown	2	3
Dialysis duration (days)	1570 (880)	1005 (734)
Hemodialysis	5 (55.6)	4 (44.4)
Body Mass Index	26 (4.94)	25 (3.21)
Systolic bloodpressure (mmHg)	147 (19)	138 (10)
Diastolic bloodpressure (mmHg)	86 (8)	86 (9)

Data are presented as number (percentage), mean (SD).

CCR5 Wild type

CCR5 deletion 32

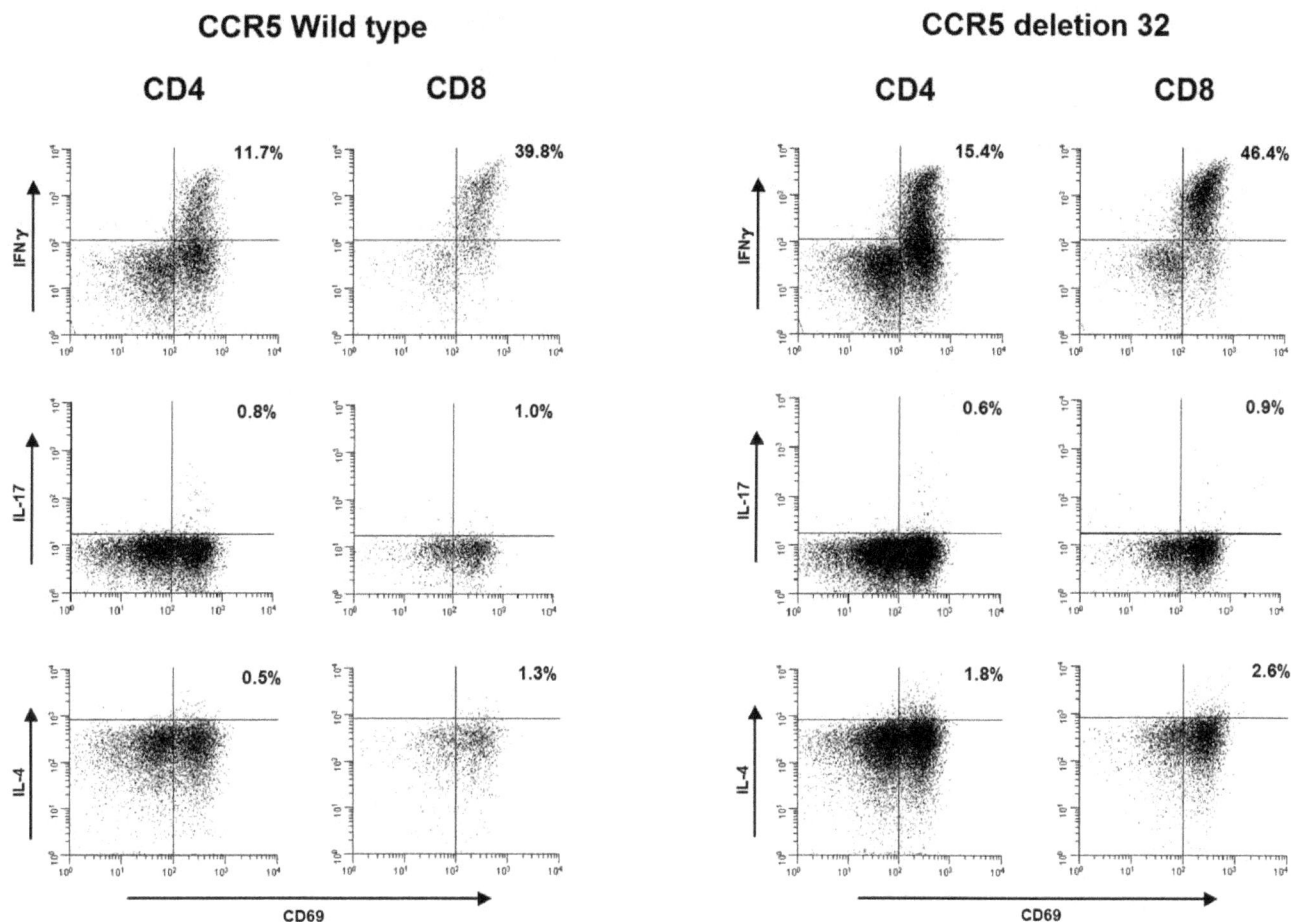

Figure 2. Flow cytometric characterization of CD4 and CD8 T cell subsets from CCR5 wild type (left panel) and CCR5 deletion 32 (right panel). PBMCs were stimulated *in vitro* with PMA and Ca-ionophore for 4 hours in the presence of BFA. The CD4 and CD8 T cell subsets were then assessed for the expression of activation marker CD69 versus intracellular cytokine (IFN-γ, IL-17, and IL-4). The percentage in the upper right corner of each plot represents the net percentage of positive cells.

Tregs are not responsible for the differences in Th2 response between CCR5Δ32 carriers and non carriers.

Discussion

In the present study we demonstrate a skewing of circulating CD4+ and CD8+ T cells towards the Th2 phenotype based on their intracellular cytokine profile after stimulation in ESRD patients carrying the CCR5Δ32 genotype. These data are in line with animal data showing that genetic deficiency of CCR5 results in a shift in immune response towards a Th2 type response, and support the assumption that genetic differences in immune response are involved in the protection against inflammation-associated mortality in ESRD patients reported previously [4].

In ESRD patients cardiovascular disease is a main cause of premature deaths [19]. Chronic inflammation is a major contributing factor [20,21]. The inflammatory nature of the process of atherosclerosis is nowadays well recognized [22]. In this process T cells play an important role [9–12]. Th1 cells, which produce IFN-γ as the principal cytokine, are thought to be pro-inflammatory and pro-atherogenic and are the most prevalent subtype in atherosclerotic lesions; Th2 cells, with IL-4 as the major cytokine, have the ability to inhibit Th1 differentiation and could therefore be anti-atherogenic. The role of Th17 cells, producing

IL-17, in atherosclerosis is not yet clear [23]. So, until now atherosclerotic inflammation is regarded as a Th1 directed Th1/Th2 disequilibrium [12].

To our knowledge, this is the first functional study investigating the Th1/Th2 directed immune response in relation to the CCR5Δ32 genetic variant in human. Animal studies consistently show a more pronounced Th2 immune response during genetic deficiency of CCR5 or pharmacological CCR5 blockade in atherosclerotic and other inflammatory conditions. In diet induced atherosclerotic inflammation in mice, genetic deletion of CCR5 was associated with a more stable plaque phenotype and reduced Th1 type immune response of stimulated splenocytes and an increased Th2 type response in splenocytes and lymph node cells [14]. After wire injury in mice with CCR5 deficiency a more atheroprotective immune response was seen, i.e. low IFN-γ and elevated IL-10 in CD4+ splenocytes compaired to CCR5 wild type mice [15]. Also in genetically CCR5 deficient mice with diet induced atherosclerosis, reduced lesion size, increased IL-10 and decreased TNF-α production by CD4+ and CD8+ T cells [16], and reduced macrophage accumulation in plaques and lowered circulating IL-6 levels was seen [17]. In CCR5 deficient mice a more CD4+ Th2 cell activation pattern was seen in colitis in contrast to CCR5 wild type mice [24]. Interestingly, in CCR5 genetically deficient mice who received a renal allograft less Th1

● **CCR5 Wild type**

■ **CCR5 deletion 32**

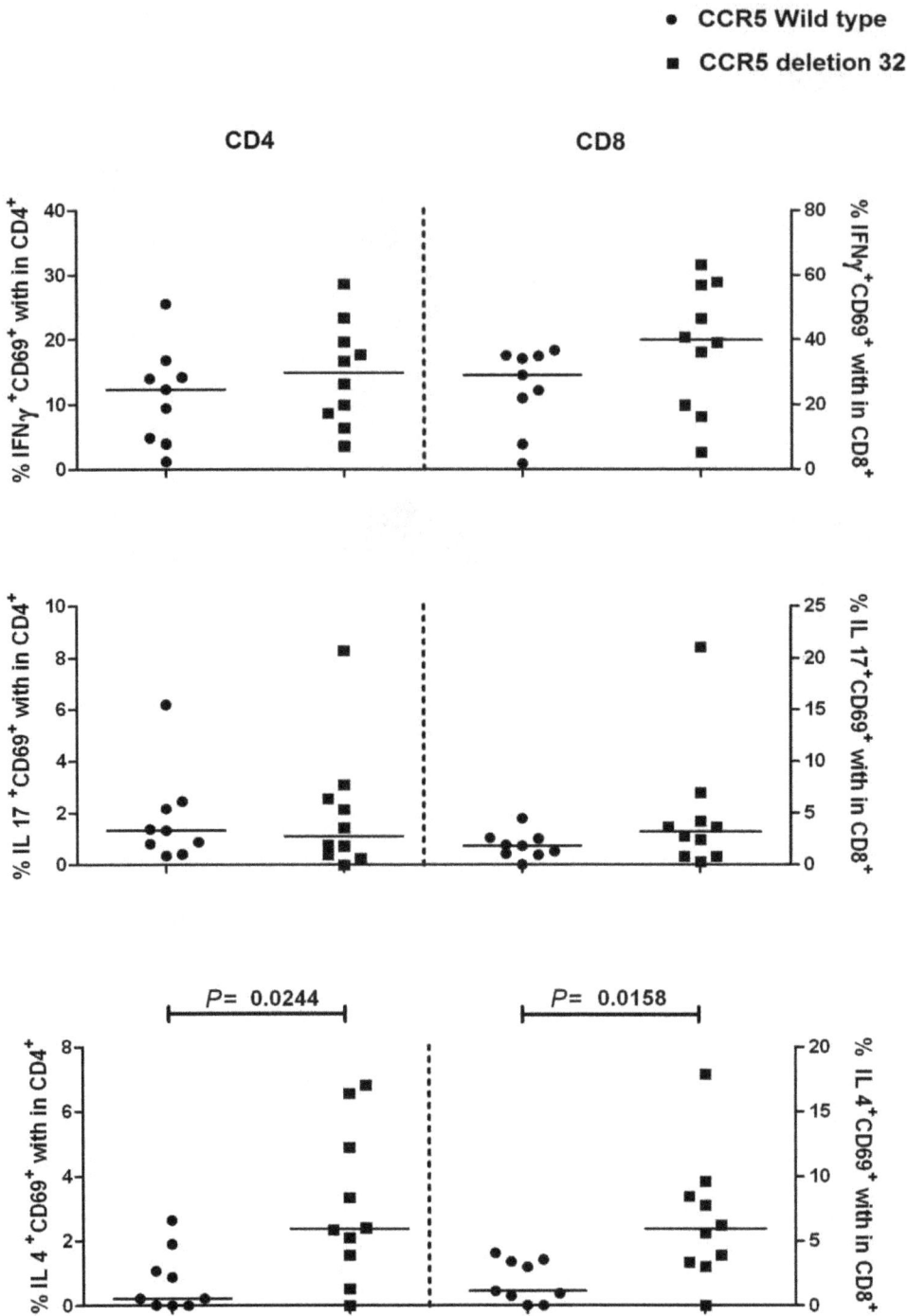

Figure 3. Percentages of IL-4, IL-17 and IFN-γ secreting CD4 and CD8+ T cells in carriers and non carriers of the CCR5Δ32 polymorphism. In the left panel the frequencies of IL-4, IL-17 and IFN-γ secreting cells among CD69+, CD4+ T cells from non carriers (n = 9) and carriers (n = 10) of the CCR5Δ32 genotype are shown. In the right panel the frequencies of IL-4, IL-17 and IFN-γ secreting cells among CD69+, CD8+ T cells from non carriers (n = 9) and carriers (n = 10) of the CCR5Δ32 polymorphism are shown. Horizontal lines represent the median percentage.

associated markers and increased Th2 associated markers were found during chronic intragraft immune response [25]. In an islet transplantation model it was shown that in genetically CCR5 deficient mice not only in the intragraft immune response but also in the periphery a Th2 shift occurred [26]. In mice with diet-induced atherosclerosis treatment with a RANTES chemokine antagonist, hereby blocking CCR5, reduced atherosclerotic plaque formation, associated with reduced proliferation and secretion of

Th1 cytokines IFN-γ and TNF-α, without difference in Th2 cytokine profile [27]. In rats pharmacological CCR5 blockade in stimulated endothelial cells inhibited selective transmigration of CD4+ Th1 cells [28].

Our results extend these animal data on functional differences in immune response for the first time to a human setting and support our previous human cross-sectional association study, showing absence of association between serum CRP and TNF-α

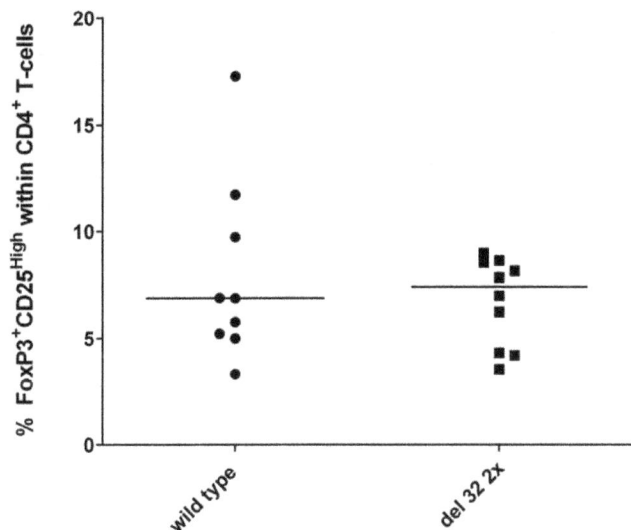

Figure 4. Percentages of Tregs (FoxP3$^+$CD25^{High} CD4$^+$ T cells) in carriers and non carriers of the CCR5Δ32 polymorphism. Horizontal lines represent the median percentage.

levels in ESRD patients carrying the CCR5Δ32 genotype, in contrast to patients without this genetic variant, supporting a reduced Th1 immune response in CCR5Δ32 [29]. It should be emphasized that ELISA and flowcytometry methods give different types of results and that measuring the intracellular cytokine production by FACS is more accurate than ELISA. The measured cytokines by ELISA can be released from several cells, whereas FACS-method identifies the intracellular cytokines produced on a single-cell level. In addition, difference in T cell numbers between the study samples may influence the results obtained from ELISA but not from FACS method hereby probably explaining why we did not find a difference in extracellular cytokine levels between CCR5Δ32 carriers and non carriers. Since Tregs are responsible for regulation and suppression of T cell responses [9,12], one may argue that differences in Tregs could underlie the increase in IL-4 expression in CCR5Δ32 carriers. However, no significant differences were observed in the percentages of Tregs between CCR5Δ32 carriers and non carriers. Thus, the increased Type 2

response in CCR5Δ32 carriers cannot be related to different frequencies of Tregs.

Together, these findings provide an explanation for the previously observed protection from inflammation-related mortality in ESRD in CCR5Δ32 carriers, as they support a less pro-inflammatory, pro-atherogenic immune response in carriers of the deletion [4]. Our results could also provide a mechanism underlying the protection against atherosclerosis by pharmacological blockade of the CCR5 pathway in animal studies [30–32]. Of note, CCR5 blockade has become feasible in humans, and is currently used for treatment of HIV-infection [33]. It has been proposed that CCR5 blockade may be a strategy for protection against inflammation driven cardiovascular disease in ESRD and/or transplantation [34,35]. Our current results contribute to understanding of mechanisms that could be affected by CCR5 blocking agents in ESRD.

Limitations

Acknowledged limitation in this study is the relatively small sample size. Besides this one blood sample failed to be stimulated. However, as mentioned above, the results are in accordance with animal data and extend the findings of a correlation study in ESRD patients, supporting the robustness of our findings. Another limitation is that we studied ESRD patients only. ESRD as such affects T-cell properties [36]. Whereas the effects of CCR5 deficiency appear to be remarkably consistent across different species and inflammatory conditions, nevertheless generalization of our results to other populations would require a separate study.

In conclusion, we present the first human data on a difference in Th1/Th2 balance dependent on the CCR5Δ32 genotype in ESRD patients. Stimulated CD4+ and CD8+ T cells of patients with one or two CCR5Δ32 alleles show an increased Th2 type phenotype base on their intracellular cytokine profile. Differences in immune response may be involved in the impact of CCR5Δ32 on outcome in ESRD, and possible other inflammatory conditions.

Author Contributions

Conceived and designed the experiments: FM WA MH JW . Performed the experiments: FM WA MH . Analyzed the data: FM WA JD GN JW. Contributed reagents/materials/analysis tools: FM WA MH JD MS SL BH GN JW. Wrote the paper: FM WA GN JW.

References

1. Raport CJ, Gosling J, Schweickart VL, Gray PW, Charo IF (1996) Molecular cloning and functional characterization of a novel human CC chemokine receptor (CCR5) for RANTES, MIP-1beta, and MIP-1alpha. J Biol Chem 271(0021-9258; 29): 17161–17166.

2. Wilcox JN, Nelken NA, Coughlin SR, Gordon D, Schall TJ (1994) Local expression of inflammatory cytokines in human atherosclerotic plaques. J Atheroscler Thromb 1 Suppl 1(1340-3478): S10–S13.

3. Benkirane M, Jin DY, Chun RF, Koup RA, Jeang KT (1997) Mechanism of transdominant inhibition of CCR5-mediated HIV-1 infection by ccr5delta32. J Biol Chem 272(0021-9258; 49): 30603–30606.

4. Muntinghe FL, Verduijn M, Zuurman MW, Grootendorst DC, Carrero JJ, et al. (2009) CCR5 deletion protects against inflammation-associated mortality in dialysis patients. J Am Soc Nephrol 20(1533-3450; 7): 1641–1649.

5. Gonzalez P, Alvarez R, Batalla A, Reguero JR, Alvarez V, et al. (2001) Genetic variation at the chemokine receptors CCR5/CCR2 in myocardial infarction. Genes Immun 2(1466-4879; 4): 191–195.

6. Pai JK, Kraft P, Cannuscio CC, Manson JE, Rexrode KM, et al. (2006) Polymorphisms in the CC-chemokine receptor-2 (CCR2) and -5 (CCR5) genes and risk of coronary heart disease among US women. Atherosclerosis 186(0021-9150; 1): 132–139.

7. Szalai C, Duba J, Prohaszka Z, Kalina A, Szabo T, et al. (2001) Involvement of polymorphisms in the chemokine system in the susceptibility for coronary artery disease (CAD). coincidence of elevated lp(a) and MCP-1 -2518 G/G genotype in CAD patients. Atherosclerosis 158(0021-9150; 1): 233–239.

8. Muntinghe FL, Gross S, Bakker SJ, Landman GW, van der Harst P, et al. (2009) CCR5Delta32 genotype is associated with outcome in type 2 diabetes mellitus. Diabetes Res Clin Pract 86(1872-8227; 2): 140–145.

9. Andersson J, Libby P, Hansson GK (2010) Adaptive immunity and atherosclerosis. Clin Immunol 134(1521-7035; 1521-6616; 1): 33–46.

10. Hansson GK (2005) Inflammation, atherosclerosis, and coronary artery disease. N Engl J Med 352(1533-4406; 16): 1685–1695.

11. Weber C, Zernecke A, Libby P (2008) The multifaceted contributions of leukocyte subsets to atherosclerosis: Lessons from mouse models. Nat Rev Immunol 8(1474-1741; 10): 802–815.

12. Robertson AK, Hansson GK (2006) T cells in atherogenesis: For better or for worse? Arterioscler Thromb Vasc Biol 26(1524-4636; 11): 2421–2432.

13. Carter LL, Dutton RW (1996) Type 1 and type 2: A fundamental dichotomy for all T-cell subsets. Curr Opin Immunol 8(0952-7915; 0952-7915; 3): 336–342.

14. Braunersreuther V, Zernecke A, Arnaud C, Liehn EA, Steffens S, et al. (2007) Ccr5 but not Ccr1 deficiency reduces development of diet-induced atherosclerosis in mice. Arterioscler Thromb Vasc Biol 27(1524-4636; 2): 373–379.

15. Zernecke A, Liehn EA, Gao JL, Kuziel WA, Murphy PM, et al. (2006) Deficiency in CCR5 but not CCR1 protects against neointima formation in atherosclerosis-prone mice: Involvement of IL-10. Blood 107(0006-4971; 11): 4240–4243.

16. Potteaux S, Combadiere C, Esposito B, Lecureuil C, it-Oufella H, et al. (2006) Role of bone marrow-derived CC-chemokine receptor 5 in the development of atherosclerosis of low-density lipoprotein receptor knockout mice. Arterioscler Thromb Vasc Biol 26(1524-4636; 8): 1858–1863.

17. Quinones MP, Martinez HG, Jimenez F, Estrada CA, Dudley M, et al. (2007) CC chemokine receptor 5 influences late-stage atherosclerosis. Atherosclerosis 195(1879-1484; 1): e92–103.

18. Clark VJ, Metheny N, Dean M, Peterson RJ (2001) Statistical estimation and pedigree analysis of CCR2-CCR5 haplotypes. Hum Genet 108(0340-6717; 6): 484–493.

19. Degoulet P, Legrain M, Reach I, Aime F, Devries C, et al. (1982) Mortality risk factors in patients treated by chronic hemodialysis. report of the diaphane collaborative study. Nephron 31(0028-2766; 0028-2766; 2): 103–110.

20. Stenvinkel P, Ketteler M, Johnson RJ, Lindholm B, Pecoits-Filho R, et al. (2005) IL-10, IL-6, and TNF-alpha: Central factors in the altered cytokine network of uremia–the good, the bad, and the ugly. Kidney Int 67(0085-2538; 4): 1216–1233.

21. Liu Y, Coresh J, Eustace JA, Longenecker JC, Jaar B, et al. (2004) Association between cholesterol level and mortality in dialysis patients: Role of inflammation and malnutrition. JAMA 291(1538-3598; 0098-7484; 4): 451–459.

22. Libby P (2002) Inflammation in atherosclerosis. Nature 420(0028-0836; 6917): 868–874.

23. Chen S, Crother TR, Arditi M (2010) Emerging role of IL-17 in atherosclerosis. J Innate Immun 2(1662-8128; 1662-811; 4): 325–333.

24. Andres PG, Beck PL, Mizoguchi E, Mizoguchi A, Bhan AK, et al. (2000) Mice with a selective deletion of the CC chemokine receptors 5 or 2 are protected from dextran sodium sulfate-mediated colitis: Lack of CC chemokine receptor 5 expression results in a NK1.1+ lymphocyte-associated Th2-type immune response in the intestine. J Immunol 164(0022-1767; 12): 6303–6312.

25. Dehmel S, Wang S, Schmidt C, Kiss E, Loewe RP, et al. (2010) Chemokine receptor Ccr5 deficiency induces alternative macrophage activation and improves long-term renal allograft outcome. Eur J Immunol 40(1521-4141; 0014-2980; 1): 267–278.

26. Abdi R, Smith RN, Makhlouf L, Najafian N, Luster AD, et al. (2002) The role of CC chemokine receptor 5 (CCR5) in islet allograft rejection. Diabetes 51(0012-1797; 0012-1797; 8): 2489–2495.

27. Braunersreuther V, Steffens S, Arnaud C, Pelli G, Burger F, et al. (2008) A novel RANTES antagonist prevents progression of established atherosclerotic lesions in mice. Arterioscler Thromb Vasc Biol 28(1524-4636; 1079-5642; 6): 1090–1096.

28. Kawai T, Seki M, Hiromatsu K, Eastcott JW, Watts GF, et al. (1999) Selective diapedesis of Th1 cells induced by endothelial cell RANTES. J Immunol 163(0022-1767; 6): 3269–3278.

29. Muntinghe FL, Carrero JJ, Navis G, Stenvinkel P (2011) TNF-alpha levels are not increased in inflamed patients carrying the CCR5 deletion 32. Cytokine 53(1096-0023; 1043-4666; 1): 16–18.

30. Schober A, Manka D, von Hundelshausen P, Huo Y, Hanrath P, et al. (2002) Deposition of platelet RANTES triggering monocyte recruitment requires P-selectin and is involved in neointima formation after arterial injury. Circulation 106(1524-4539; 12): 1523–1529.

31. van Wanrooij EJ, Happe H, Hauer AD, de Vos P, Imanishi T, et al. (2005) HIV entry inhibitor TAK-779 attenuates atherogenesis in low-density lipoprotein receptor-deficient mice. Arterioscler Thromb Vasc Biol 25(1524-4636; 12): 2642–2647.

32. Veillard NR, Kwak B, Pelli G, Mulhaupt F, James RW, et al. (2004) Antagonism of RANTES receptors reduces atherosclerotic plaque formation in mice. Circ Res 94(1524-4571; 2): 253–261.

33. Fatkenheuer G, Pozniak AL, Johnson MA, Plettenberg A, Staszewski S, et al. (2005) Efficacy of short-term monotherapy with maraviroc, a new CCR5 antagonist, in patients infected with HIV-1. Nat Med 11(1078-8956; 11): 1170–1172.

34. Kovesdy CP, Kalantar-Zadeh K (2009) Do genes allow inflammation to kill or not to kill? J Am Soc Nephrol 20(1533-3450; 1533-3450; 7): 1429–1431.

35. Muntinghe FL, Vegter S, Verduijn M, Boeschoten EW, Dekker FW, et al. (2011) Using a genetic, observational study as a strategy to estimate the potential cost-effectiveness of pharmacological CCR5 blockade in dialysis patients. Pharmacogenet Genomics 21(7): 417–425.

36. Hendrikx TK, van Gurp EA, Mol WM, Schoordijk W, Sewgobind VD, et al. (2009) End-stage renal failure and regulatory activities of CD4+CD25bright+ FoxP3+ T-cells. Nephrol Dial Transplant 24(1460-2385; 0931-0509; 6): 1969–1978.

7

Incidence of End-Stage Renal Disease in the Turkish-Cypriot Population of Northern Cyprus

Thomas M. F. Connor[1]*, D. Deren Oygar[2], Daniel P. Gale[1], Retha Steenkamp[3], Dorothea Nitsch[4], Guy H. Neild[1], Patrick H. Maxwell[1]

1 UCL Division of Medicine and Centre for Nephrology, University College London, London, United Kingdom, 2 Nicosia State Hospital, Burhan Nalbantoglu General Hospital, Nicosia, North Cyprus, 3 UK Renal Registry, Southmead Hospital, Bristol, United Kingdom, 4 London School of Hygiene and Tropical Medicine, London, United Kingdom

Abstract

Background: This is the first report of the incidence and causes of end-stage renal disease (ESRD) of the Turkish-Cypriot population in Northern Cyprus.

Methods: Data were collected over eight consecutive years (2004–2011) from all those starting renal replacement therapy (RRT) in this population. Crude and age-standardised incidence at 90 days was calculated and comparisons made with other national registries. We collected DNA from the entire prevalent population. As an initial experiment we looked for two genetic causes of ESRD that have been reported in Greek Cypriots.

Results: Crude and age-standardised incidence at 90 days was 234 and 327 per million population (pmp) per year, respectively. The mean age was 63, and 62% were male. The age-adjusted prevalence of RRT in Turkish-Cypriots was 1543 pmp on 01/01/2011. The incidence of RRT is higher than other countries reporting to the European Renal Association – European Dialysis and Transplant Association, with the exception of Turkey. Diabetes is a major cause of ESRD in those under 65, accounting for 36% of incident cases followed by 30% with uncertain aetiology. 18% of the incident population had a family history of ESRD. We identified two families with thin basement membrane nephropathy caused by a mutation in *COL4A3*, but no new cases of CFHR5 nephropathy.

Conclusions: This study provides the first estimate of RRT incidence in the Turkish-Cypriot population, describes the contribution of different underlying diagnoses to ESRD, and provides a basis for healthcare policy planning.

Editor: Leighton R. James, University of Florida, United States of America

Funding: This work was supported by a Clinical Research Training Fellowship to TMFC from the Medical Research Council (http://www.mrc.ac.uk/index.htm) and a grant from the St Peter's Trust for Kidney, Bladder and Prostate Research (http://www.stpeterstrust.org.uk/). The funders had no role in study design, data collection and analysis, decision to publish, or preparation of the manuscript.

Competing Interests: The authors have declared that no competing interests exist.

* E-mail: t.connor@ucl.ac.uk

Introduction

In recent years end-stage renal disease (ESRD) has become an increasing public health challenge for high and middle income countries, with an associated escalation of the cost of providing renal replacement therapy (RRT) [1–4]. The collection of accurate epidemiological data is of great importance for healthcare policy planning [1–3]. This is especially true for places where the infrastructure delivering RRT is improving, such as the island of Cyprus.

There are considerable differences in the incidence and prevalence of RRT within Europe. Registry data demonstrate a North-South gradient, with higher incidence of RRT and lower mortality around the Mediterranean [2,5]. Several factors have been suggested to contribute to this variation [6,7]. In order to understand the aetiology of ESRD and chronic kidney disease, which affects many more people, it is important to determine the primary renal diagnosis [8]. ESRD attributed to type 2 diabetes and hypertension continues to rise throughout the world, and this is increasingly true for countries such as Cyprus [2,9–11].

Cyprus is an island in the eastern Mediterranean that has been occupied by a series of historical powers, in particular the Greeks and Ottoman Turks. The Cypriot population is genetically distinct from mainland populations of either Greece or Turkey, although environmental factors, such as diet and lifestyle are broadly similar [12,13].

Turkish-Cypriots form a distinct ethno-linguistic community centered on Turkish administered Northern Cyprus (TRNC). The aim of this study was to describe the incidence and prevalence of RRT in this ethnically-defined Mediterranean population by type of primary renal disease. To put these data into context we compared these data with reported RRT incidence from Greece, Turkey, and the white population of England. An important, and probably unique, aspect of our registry is that every RRT patient has provided a DNA sample for research. Because the Greek and Turkish communities share many genetic characteristics [14,15], we initially undertook genetic testing for two conditions that have been identified in Greek Cypriots, CFHR5 nephropathy and thin basement membrane nephropathy [16,17].

Materials and Methods

Ethics Statement

This study was approved by the ethics committee of Lefkosa Burhan Nalbantoğlu State Hospital. All participants provided informed consent in writing, in accordance with the Declaration of Helsinki.

Study Population

The study was conducted at Nicosia State Hospital in Northern Cyprus. Nicosia State Hospital is a multi-specialty tertiary care hospital, and provides renal services to the whole of Turkish administered Northern Cyprus (TRNC). All citizens of TRNC are entitled to free RRT, regardless of ethnicity. All patients with symptomatic chronic kidney disease (CKD) from within this population present either through the village practitioners, private hospitals or directly to Nicosia State Hospital. Details of every individual admitted with acute or chronic renal failure in the last decade were collected with a unique identifier number, thus preventing any duplication of records or redundancy of referrals. ESRD was defined as chronic renal disease with an eGFR of <10 ml/min/1.73 m^2; but patients with diabetic nephropathy often started RRT with eGFR<15 ml/min/1.73 m^2.

The most recent census of the TRNC population in 2006 showed that of 178,031 *de jure* citizens, 120,007 were born to parents who were both themselves born in Cyprus, providing an effective measure of the size of the ethnic Turkish-Cypriot population that has been applied throughout this paper [18].

Variables

Basic demographic data (age at ESRD, sex, ethnic group, and probable diagnosis) were recorded for all patients receiving RRT at day 1, and again after 90 days on the renal replacement programme. Diabetic nephropathy was defined as ESRD in the presence of diabetes without evidence of an alternative diagnosis. Family history of ESRD was defined as a first or second degree relative with ESRD.

Data Sources for International Comparisons

European data was taken from the European Renal Association – European Dialysis and Transplant Association (ERA-EDTA) Registry report for 2008 [2]. Additional data for Greece, Turkey, and England were taken from the Hellenic Renal Registry (Dr GA Ioannidis personal communication), the National Haemodialysis, Transplantation and Nephrology Registry report of Turkey 2008 [19], and the 2008 Renal Registry Report [1]. The denominator population for international comparisons was calculated from the relevant national statistics [20,21].

Statistical Analysis

The incidence of RRT in this population was averaged over eight consecutive calendar years (2004–2011). Age-standardised incidence rates were calculated using the Eurostat EU27 population figures [22]. All comparisons with other populations were made using data for chronic RRT; that is those still on RRT at 90 days. The emphasis of this report will be on age-specific comparisons as these are not affected by age-referral biases. We

calculated 95% confidence intervals assuming a Poisson distribution for incidence rates. Statistical analysis was carried out using Stata version 11.

Genetic Testing of All Adult Patients on RRT in North Cyprus

After informed consent for this study, blood was taken from all patients on renal replacement therapy on 01/01/2011. Genetic analysis was performed at University College London, UK. DNA was extracted from peripheral blood using the QIAamp DNA Blood Mini Kit (Qiagen, Stanford, CA, USA). We designed primers to screen for the G1334E and 3854delG mutation in *COL4A4* and the G871C mutation in *COL4A3* [23]. Screening PCR was also performed to amplify both wild-type and mutant *CFHR5* alleles in a single reaction as described previously [16].

Results

A total of 225 Turkish-Cypriot patients were maintained on renal replacement therapy beyond 90 days during the study period (01/01/04–31/12/11). More males than females started RRT (139 vs 86), but the age distribution was similar between the sexes (Table 1). 18.2% of the incident population had a first or second degree relative with ESRD, and this rose to 27% in those with ESRD due to uncertain aetiology. The average crude and age-standardised incidence rates at day 1 for this period were 311.4 and 456.9 per million population, respectively. The Turkish-Cypriot case mix at 90 days included 36.0% with ESRD due to diabetic nephropathy, 29.8% with unknown diagnosis, and 3.6% with polycystic kidney disease (Table 2). Tetra primer PCR identified two individuals on RRT with the G871C mutation in COL4A3 previously reported in Greek-Cypriot pedigrees [17]. We did not detect the other previously cited mutations in *COL4A3* and *COL4A4* or the *CFHR5* duplication in the RRT population [16,17].

The majority (91.1%) of Turkish-Cypriot patients started RRT on haemodialysis; only a few started peritoneal dialysis (4.4%) or had pre-emptive renal transplantation (3.5%) (Table 1). The crude and age-standardised prevalence of RRT in Turkish-Cypriots was 1216 and 1543 pmp, respectively. The median age of the Turkish-Cypriot prevalent population was 60 for both men and women, and the mean duration on RRT was 5.0 years. The majority of patients on RRT in Northern Cyprus are treated with hemodialysis, which is carried out in two centers, Nicosia and Famagusta. The proportion of prevalent patients on peritoneal dialysis (14%) is similar to other countries [24]. Renal transplantation is performed in either Turkey or the Republic of Cyprus (Greek Cypriot), and benefits a high proportion of patients (prevalence 376 pmp).

We carried out international comparisons. Turkey, Greece, and Tunisia have an age-adjusted incidence rate at day 90 of 349.1, 159.5, and 238.7 pmp respectively [2]. In comparison the crude and age-adjusted incidence rates of chronic RRT for Turkish-Cypriots were 234.4 and 327.2 per million population, respectively. Figure 1 shows that the incidence of RRT in each age group in Turkish-Cypriots is comparable to that seen in Turkey. Despite the small number of cases, the incidence of RRT in the 45–64 age group in Turkish-Cypriots (412.0 pmp) is significantly higher than that seen in the white population of England (123.2 pmp).

There is a high rate of RRT for ESRD attributed to diabetic nephropathy in all eastern Mediterranean countries (84.4 pmp in Turkish-Cypriots, 53.5 pmp in Greece, and 61.6 pmp in Turkey) (Table 2). Table 2 also shows that the code 'uncertain aetiology' is more common in the Turkish-Cypriot registry (69.8 pmp) than in other populations. However there were lower levels of hyperten-

Table 1. Baseline characteristics of the incident Turkish-Cypriot renal replacement therapy (RRT) population at 90 days.

Characteristic	Category	Number	Percentage
Gender	Male	139	61.7%
	Female	86	38.3%
Median age of adult population at ESRF in years (lower and upper quartile)	Male	63 (54,69)	
	Female	64 (52,74)	
Modality of RRT at presentation	Haemodialysis	205	91.1%
	Peritoneal dialysis	10	4.4%
	Renal transplant	8	3.5%
Co-morbidities	Diabetes	93	41.3%
	Hypertension	145	64.4%
	Family History	41	18.2%
Mutation Analysis	COL4A3 (G871C)	2	0.9%
	COL4A3 (G1334E)	0	0%
	COL4A4 (3856delC)	0	0%
	CFHR5 duplication	0	0%

sive nephropathy in Turkish-Cypriots than in Greece or Turkey (1.0 pmp vs 19.1 pmp and 53.4 pmp respectively). The incidence of polycystic kidney disease was broadly similar across all registries (range 6.7–10.1 pmp).

The incidence of RRT in the minority Turkish population of Northern Cyprus is broadly in line with the rate seen in Turkish-Cypriots. An additional 76 Turkish patients were maintained on renal replacement therapy beyond 90 days during the study period, giving an overall incidence of 211.3 pmp in the *de jure* population of Northern Cyprus. However data on this population is less accurate due to significant migration to and from the mainland of Turkey [18].

Discussion

High Incidence of RRT

This study presents the first population-based RRT incidence figure from Cyprus, and reveals a high incidence of RRT that is RRT is higher than other countries reporting to the ERA-EDTA, with the exception of Turkey [2]. Diabetes is a major cause of ESRD overall and specifically in those under 65, with rates comparable to those seen in the USA [3]. We found that the high incidence of RRT in Turkish-Cypriots is not due to the specific mutations in *COL4A3*, *COL4A4*, and *CFHR5* assessed in this study [16,17]. Finally, a third of Turkish-Cypriot patients start RRT with unknown primary diagnosis. This highlights both the need for earlier detection of these cases and the possibility that there may be other uncharacterised conditions causing ESRD in this population.

Table 2. Provisional renal diagnosis in the Turkish-Cypriot renal replacement therapy (RRT) population at 90 days, by incidence per million population and percentage, in comparison with 2008 registry data for Greece, Turkey, and the UK.

Diagnosis	Turkish-Cypriots pmp	Turkish-Cypriots %	Greece pmp	Greece %	Turkey pmp	Turkey %	England whites pmp	England whites %
Diabetes	84.4	36.0%	53.5	30.3%	61.6	29.9%	24.5	19.5%
Glomerulonephritis	29.2*	12.4%*	14.8	8.4%	16.4	7.9%	13.5	10.7%
Hypertension	1.0	0.4%	19.1	10.8%	53.4	25.9%	6.8	5.4%
Renal Vascular Disease	12.5	5.3%	3.0	1.7%	2.8	1.3%	7.8	6.2%
Data not available	0.0	0.0%	0.0	0.0%	3.1	1.5%	9.8	7.8%
Other identified Category	12.5	5.3%	15.7	8.9%	21.0	10.2%	18.2	14.5%
Pyelonephritis	16.7	7.1%	9.9	5.6%	7.6	3.7%	9.7	7.7%
Polycystic Kidney	8.3	3.6%	6.7	3.8%	7.8	3.8%	10.1	8.0%
Uncertain aetiology	69.8	29.8%	53.9	30.5%	32.5	15.7%	25.5	20.3%
Total incidence at day 91	234.4	100.0%	176.7	100.0%	206.2	100.0%	125.9	100.0%

*Includes presumed glomerulonephritis not biopsy proven.

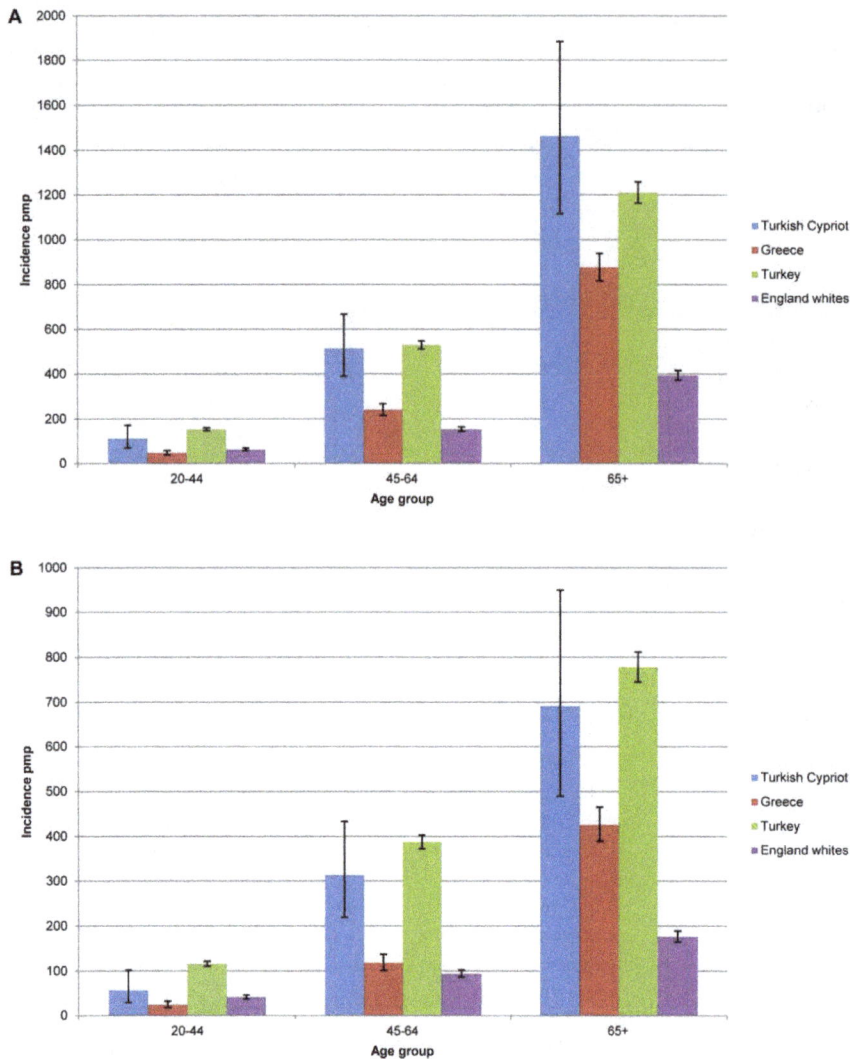

Figure 1. Incidence of renal replacement therapy (RRT) at 90 days by age and gender. Incidence of RRT at 90 days in Turkish Cypriots compared with 2008 registry data for Greece, Turkey, and English whites in males (A), and females (B). Error bars indicate 95% confidence intervals.

Diabetic Nephropathy

The Turkish-Cypriot case-mix, with a high incidence of RRT for ESRD due to diabetic nephropathy, is similar to that seen in Turkey and Greece (Table 2). Diabetes is also a common cause of ESRD in developing countries around the Eastern Mediterranean, such as Egypt, Kuwait, Lebanon and Saudi Arabia [11]. The incidence of RRT for ESRD attributed to diabetic nephropathy seen in Turkish-Cypriot less than 65 years old is striking (Figure 2). Currently data concerning the incidence of diabetes in Turkish-Cypriots is lacking. Diabetes is common in Greek-Cypriots and mainland Turkish patients [25–27], but not to the extent seen in some other populations with high levels of diabetic nephropathy, such as the Pima Indians of Arizona [28,29]. Moreover, childhood levels of obesity in Cyprus are much closer to those seen in other European countries than in the US [30,31]. It is therefore possible that, in common with other registries, some of these cases reflect a co-occurrence of Type 2 diabetes with ESRD due to an alternative aetiology [32].

Genetic Renal Disease in the Turkish-Cypriot Population

Congenital factors may also be important in the aetiology of ESRD in this population [33]. Previous estimates of the prevalence of family history of ESRD amongst incident dialysis patients, suggest that 7–15% Caucasians have a first or second-degree relative with ESRD [34,35]. This proportion is highest in young adults, non-Caucasians, and for those where ESRD is caused by diabetes or hypertension [34]. We observed a similar rate of familial ESRD in Turkish-Cypriot patients on RRT, which was even higher (27%) in the group with unknown diagnosis, suggesting the existence of conditions that are not yet char-acterised in this population. For comparison, the rate of RRT for ESRD due to polycystic kidney disease was similar across all registries.

In order to assess the contribution of inherited renal disease we collected DNA from the entire Turkish-Cypriot population on RRT. Previous work has demonstrated a number of important founder mutations and significant geographic clustering for several monogenetic diseases affecting the Greek-Cypriot population of Cyprus, including mutations of *COL4A3*, *COL4A4*, *PKD2*, and *MEFV* [17,36,37]. Although the *CFHR5* duplication is common in

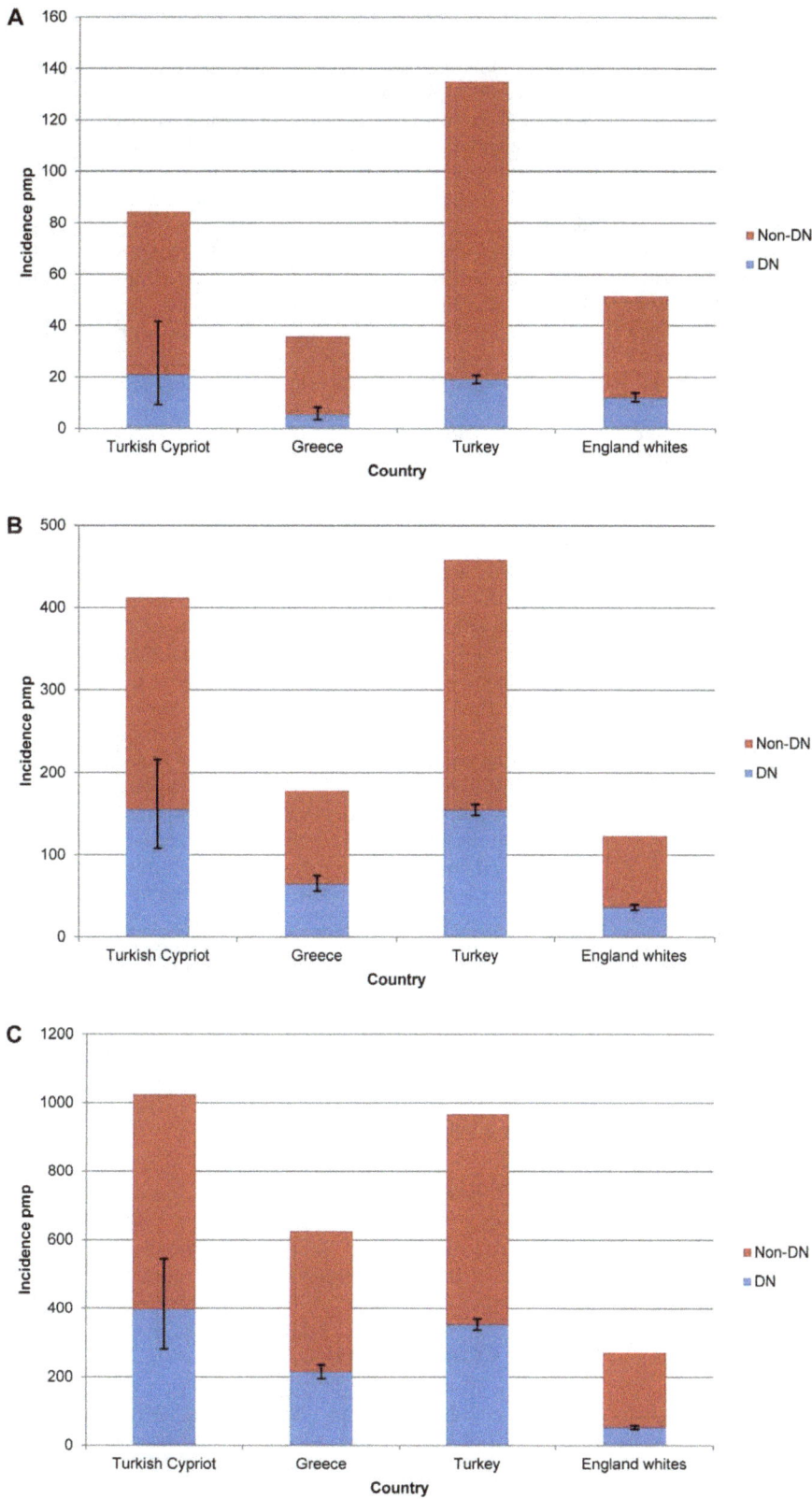

Figure 2. Incidence of renal replacement therapy (RRT) for end stage renal disease (ESRD) due to diabetic nephropathy. Incidence of RRT for ESRD due to diabetic nephropathy (DN) and all other causes (Non-DN) at 90 days in Turkish Cypriots compared with 2008 registry data for Greece, Turkey, and English whites in 20–44 year olds (A), 45–64 year-olds (B), and those over 65 years (C). Error bars indicate 95% confidence intervals.

Greek-Cypriots originating from the southern half of the island [38], we did not detect it in our sample of prevalent patients. However, due to the small size of our sample the allelic frequency may still lie within that observed for Greek Cypriots [39]. The familial clustering and high incidence of RRT in Turkish-Cypriots is therefore due to other monogenetic or polygenic diseases in this population.

Coding 'Uncertain Aetiology'

There is a significant group in the Turkish-Cypriot RRT population with unknown diagnosis (69.8 pmp). This group partly reflects late presentation and limited diagnostic investigations. Comparative data from the Eastern Mediterranean is difficult to obtain, and information on primary renal disease is less robust [8,32] but there is evidence for a reciprocal relationship with coding for hypertension in many registries [8,32,40]. The incidence of hypertensive nephropathy is conspicuously lower in Turkish-Cypriots than in neighbouring countries. In the absence of clear diagnostic criteria for hypertensive nephropathy, it may be appropriate to combine 'hypertension' with 'uncertain aetiology' in Table 2, which would imply that there is no established primary renal diagnosis in 40% of patients on RRT in the Greek, Turkish, and Turkish-Cypriot registries.

The majority of patients with an unknown diagnosis present clinically with minimal proteinuria (<1 g protein/day) and asymptomatic disease, consistent with a pathological process primarily affecting the renal tubules [8] and similar to the features of medullary cystic kidney disease type 1. A number of families presenting this way in the Greek Cypriot population have shown linkage to the region 1q21, but the gene responsible has not yet been identified [41]. It is possible that the medullary cystic phenotype reflects the final common pathway of a number of genetic and environmental factors that are common in this population.

Alternative Explanations for the Incidence of RRT in Turkish-Cypriots

Regional variations in RRT incidence may reflect both genetic and environmental factors [7,28,42]. Macroeconomic factors that influence regional variations in RRT incidence include per capita GDP and health-care expenditure [7]. Northern Cyprus has a developing economy, with per-capita GDP that is 76% of that in the Republic of Cyprus, and it is dependent on aid from the Turkish government [43]. RRT has only recently become widely available in TRNC and there is no long-term provision of private dialysis. Economic factors also influence the management of CKD and co-morbidities, as well as the competing risk of mortality, in the general population [7]. The high incidence of RRT in the Turkish-Cypriot population may therefore reflect suboptimal management of diabetes, hypertension, and associated complications. This has significance for healthcare planning on the island, and underlines the importance of prospective assessment of kidney function in this population.

Wider Relevance of these Findings

Our findings have several implications. First, these data highlight the need to examine the care of diabetics who are at risk of renal disease in the Turkish-Cypriot population, particularly in young people, to prevent rising rates of RRT. To this end, we are examining case records of patients who were diagnosed with diabetic nephropathy and reached ESRD at a young age. Second, there is a large diaspora of Turkish-Cypriots who may carry with them an increased risk of ESRD. Third, this study provides a template for other adult registries across the Middle-East, and highlights the proportion of patients with unknown diagnosis [8]. It is hoped that with greater access to diagnostic investigations this number will be reduced further.

The strength of this study is that we have a complete dataset from the study period, including DNA samples from the entire prevalent RRT population. Many countries with new RRT programs, such as Bangladesh or Malaysia, show increasing take-up of services with time [24]. However the incidence rate, mean age, and sex-ratio of patients on RRT at 90 days shown in Table 1 are broadly in line with other European populations [2]. Moreover, by examining incidence at 90-days in those aged <65 years we have sought to avoid misclassification and bias due to referral patterns, availability of RRT, and prevalence of co-morbidities.

The main limitations of this study are factors affecting the calculation of incidence rates. This study used the same definition of ethnicity as the 2006 census, and the size of the population remained stable over the study period. Referral bias is unlikely as RRT is freely available to all citizens, and because all ERSD is managed through one centre we were able to achieve a remarkably complete dataset.

In conclusion, this study provides a complete dataset of RRT in the Turkish-Cypriot population and shows that incidence and prevalence of RRT are high. Diabetes is a major cause of ESRD overall and specifically in those under 65. With the prevalence of diabetes and hypertension projected to rise further, facilities to target the earlier stages of diabetes and CKD need to be developed further in this population. Earlier identification of CKD together with long-term follow-up will enable more accurate determination of renal diagnosis before the onset of ESRD. Familial renal disease is common in this population, and this study represents the first complete collection of DNA from an ethnically-defined population on RRT. This population therefore provides an opportunity to look for genetic factors associated with an increased risk of ESRD in Cyprus. The high prevalence of RRT in Turkish-Cypriots has implications for healthcare policy planning.

Acknowledgments

We thank Meral Yükseliş for assistance with data collection, Dr G.A. Ioannidis for data from the Hellenic Renal Registry, and Professor Constantinos Deltas and Dr Konstantinos Voskarides for provision of DNA samples.

Author Contributions

Conceived and designed the experiments: TMFC DPG DN GHN PHM. Performed the experiments: TMFC DDO RS. Analyzed the data: TMFC DN GHN PHM. Contributed reagents/materials/analysis tools: DDO DPG RS DN. Wrote the paper: TMFC DN GHN PHM.

References

1. Byrne C, Ford D, Gilg J, Ansell D, Feehally J (2010) UK Renal Registry 12th Annual Report (December 2009): chapter 3: UK ESRD incident rates in 2008: national and centre-specific analyses. Nephron Clin Pract 115 Suppl 1: c9–39.
2. ERA (2008) ERA-EDTA Registry Annual Report 2008. Amsterdam, The Netherlands.
3. USRDS (2008) U.S. Renal Data System, USRDS 2011 Annual Data Report: Atlas of End-Stage Renal Disease in the United States, National Institutes of Health, National Institute of Diabetes and Digestive and Kidney Diseases, Bethesda, MD, 2011.

4. Meguid El Nahas A, Bello AK (2005) Chronic kidney disease: the global challenge. Lancet 365: 331–340.

5. van Dijk PC, Zwinderman AH, Dekker FW, Schon S, Stel VS, et al. (2007) Effect of general population mortality on the north-south mortality gradient in patients on replacement therapy in Europe. Kidney Int 71: 53–59.

6. Rosansky SJ, Clark WF, Eggers P, Glassock RJ (2009) Initiation of dialysis at higher GFRs: is the apparent rising tide of early dialysis harmful or helpful? Kidney Int 76: 257–261.

7. Caskey FJ, Kramer A, Elliott RF, Stel VS, Covic A, et al. (2011) Global variation in renal replacement therapy for end-stage renal disease. Nephrol Dial Transplant 26: 2604–2610.

8. Neild GH, Oygar DD, Hmida MB (2011) Can we improve the diagnosis of renal failure? A revised coding system for the Middle East and North Africa. Saudi J Kidney Dis Transpl 22: 651–661.

9. Stewart JH, McCredie MR, Williams SM, Jager KJ, Trpeski L, et al. (2007) Trends in incidence of treated end-stage renal disease, overall and by primary renal disease, in persons aged 20–64 years in Europe, Canada and the Asia-Pacific region, 1998–2002. Nephrology (Carlton) 12: 520–527.

10. White SL, Chadban SJ, Jan S, Chapman JR, Cass A (2008) How can we achieve global equity in provision of renal replacement therapy? Bull World Health Organ 86: 229–237.

11. Shaheen FA, Al-Khader AA (2005) Preventive strategies of renal failure in the Arab world. Kidney Int Suppl: S37–40.

12. Novembre J, Johnson T, Bryc K, Kutalik Z, Boyko AR, et al. (2008) Genes mirror geography within Europe. Nature 456: 98–101.

13. Irwin J, Saunier J, Strouss K, Paintner C, Diegoli T, et al. (2008) Mitochondrial control region sequences from northern Greece and Greek Cypriots. Int J Legal Med 122: 87–89.

14. Baysal E, Indrak K, Bozkurt G, Berkalp A, Aritkan E, et al. (1992) The beta-thalassaemia mutations in the population of Cyprus. Br J Haematol 81: 607–609.

15. Baysal E, Kleanthous M, Bozkurt G, Kyrri A, Kalogirou E, et al. (1995) alpha-Thalassaemia in the population of Cyprus. Br J Haematol 89: 496–499.

16. Gale DP, de Jorge EG, Cook HT, Martinez-Barricarte R, Hadjisavvas A, et al. (2010) Identification of a mutation in complement factor H-related protein 5 in patients of Cypriot origin with glomerulonephritis. Lancet 376: 794–801.

17. Voskarides K, Damianou L, Neocleous V, Zouvani I, Christodoulidou S, et al. (2007) COL4A3/COL4A4 mutations producing focal segmental glomeruloscle-rosis and renal failure in thin basement membrane nephropathy. J Am Soc Nephrol 18: 3004–3016.

18. Census (2006) The Final results of TRNC General Population and Housing Unit Census.

19. Nephrology TSo (2008) Registry of the Nephrology, Dialysis and Transplantation in Turkey. Annual Report Books. Istanbul.

20. ONS (2011) Mid Year population estimates 2008: 13/05/10. In: Statistics Ofn, editor.

21. Institute TS (2008) Midyear Population Projections by Age Groups and Sex. TurkStat.

22. Eurostat (2010) European Comission Population Statistics.

23. Ye S, Dhillon S, Ke X, Collins AR, Day IN (2001) An efficient procedure for genotyping single nucleotide polymorphisms. Nucleic Acids Res 29: E88–88.

24. Boddana P, Caskey F, Casula A, Ansell D (2009) UK Renal Registry 11th Annual Report (December 2008): Chapter 14 UK Renal Registry and international comparisons. Nephron Clin Pract 111 Suppl 1: c269–276.

25. Loizou T, Pouloukas S, Tountas C, Thanopoulou A, Karamanos V (2006) An epidemiologic study on the prevalence of diabetes, glucose intolerance, and metabolic syndrome in the adult population of the Republic of Cyprus. Diabetes Care 29: 1714–1715.

26. Suleymanlar G, Utas C, Arinsoy T, Ates K, Altun B, et al. (2011) A population-based survey of Chronic REnal Disease In Turkey–the CREDIT study. Nephrol Dial Transplant 26: 1862–1871.

27. NHANES (2010) National Health and Nutrition Examination Survey. In: Prevention CfDCa, editor. Chronic Disease Prevention and Health Promotion.

28. Agodoa L, Eggers P (2007) Racial and ethnic disparities in end-stage kidney failure-survival paradoxes in African-Americans. Semin Dial 20: 577–585.

29. Lemley KV (2008) Diabetes and chronic kidney disease: lessons from the Pima Indians. Pediatr Nephrol 23: 1933–1940.

30. Savva SC, Tornaritis MJ, Chadjigeorgiou C, Kourides YA, Siamounki M, et al. (2008) Prevalence of overweight and obesity among 11-year-old children in Cyprus, 1997–2003. Int J Pediatr Obes 3: 186–192.

31. Olds T, Maher C, Zumin S, Peneau S, Lioret S, et al. (2011) Evidence that the prevalence of childhood overweight is plateauing: data from nine countries. Int J Pediatr Obes 6: 342–360.

32. Suleymanlar G, Serdengecti K, Altiparmak MR, Jager K, Seyahi N, et al. (2011) Trends in renal replacement therapy in Turkey, 1996–2008. Am J Kidney Dis 57: 456–465.

33. Neild GH (2009) What do we know about chronic renal failure in young adults? I. Primary renal disease. Pediatr Nephrol 24: 1913–1919.

34. Freedman BI, Volkova NV, Satko SG, Krisher J, Jurkovitz C, et al. (2005) Population-based screening for family history of end-stage renal disease among incident dialysis patients. Am J Nephrol 25: 529–535.

35. Lubensky IA, Schmidt L, Zhuang Z, Weirich G, Pack S, et al. (1999) Hereditary and sporadic papillary renal carcinomas with c-met mutations share a distinct morphological phenotype. Am J Pathol 155: 517–526.

36. Deltas CC, Mean R, Rossou E, Costi C, Koupepidou P, et al. (2002) Familial Mediterranean fever (FMF) mutations occur frequently in the Greek-Cypriot population of Cyprus. Genet Test 6: 15–21.

37. Mochizuki T, Wu G, Hayashi T, Xenophontos SL, Veldhuisen B, et al. (1996) PKD2, a gene for polycystic kidney disease that encodes an integral membrane protein. Science 272: 1339–1342.

38. Gale DP (2011) The identification of CFHR5 nephropathy. J R Soc Med 104: 186–190.

39. Hanley JA, Lippman-Hand A (1983) If nothing goes wrong, is everything all right? Interpreting zero numerators. JAMA 249: 1743–1745.

40. Perneger TV, Whelton PK, Klag MJ, Rossiter KA (1995) Diagnosis of hypertensive end-stage renal disease: effect of patient's race. Am J Epidemiol 141: 10–15.

41. Stavrou C, Koptides M, Tombazos C, Psara E, Patsias C, et al. (2002) Autosomal-dominant medullary cystic kidney disease type 1: clinical and molecular findings in six large Cypriot families. Kidney Int 62: 1385–1394.

42. Palmer Alves T, Lewis J (2010) Racial differences in chronic kidney disease (CKD) and end-stage renal disease (ESRD) in the United States: a social and economic dilemma. Clin Nephrol 74 Suppl 1: S72–77.

43. Wikipedia editor (2011) Northern Cyprus.

8

Inflammation Disrupts the LDL Receptor Pathway and Accelerates the Progression of Vascular Calcification in ESRD Patients

Jing Liu[1], Kun Ling Ma[1]*, Min Gao[1], Chang Xian Wang[2], Jie Ni[1], Yang Zhang[1], Xiao Liang Zhang[1], Hong Liu[1], Yan Li Wang[1], Bi Cheng Liu[1]

1 Institute of Nephrology, Zhong Da Hospital, Southeast University School of Medicine, Nanjing City, Jiangsu Province, People's Republic of China, 2 Department of Infection Management, Zhong Da Hospital, Southeast University School of Medicine, Nanjing City, Jiangsu Province, People's Republic of China

Abstract

Background: Chronic inflammation plays a crucial role in the progression of vascular calcification (VC). This study was designed to investigate whether the low-density lipoprotein receptor (LDLr) pathway is involved in the progression of VC in patients with end-stage renal disease (ESRD) during inflammation.

Methods and Results: Twenty-eight ESRD patients were divided into control and inflamed groups according to plasma C-reactive protein (CRP) level. Surgically removed tissues from the radial arteries of patients receiving arteriovenostomy were used in the experiments. The expression of tumour necrosis factor-α (TNF-α) and monocyte chemotactic protein-1 (MCP-1) of the radial artery were increased in the inflamed group. Hematoxylin-eosin and alizarin red S staining revealed parallel increases in foam cell formation and calcium deposit formation in continuous cross-sections of radial arteries in the inflamed group compared to the control, which were closely correlated with increased LDLr, sterol regulatory element binding protein-2 (SREBP-2), bone morphogenetic proteins-2 (BMP-2), and collagen I protein expression, as shown by immunohistochemical and immunofluorescent staining. Confocal microscopy confirmed that inflammation enhanced the translocation of the SREBP cleavage-activating protein (SCAP)/SREBP-2 complex from the endoplasmic reticulum to the Golgi, thereby activating LDLr gene transcription. Inflammation increased alkaline phosphatase protein expression and reduced α-smooth muscle actin protein expression, contributing to the conversion of the vascular smooth muscle cells in calcified vessels from the fibroblastic to the osteogenic phenotype; osteogenic cells are the main cellular components involved in VC. Further analysis showed that the inflammation-induced disruption of the LDLr pathway was significantly associated with enhanced BMP-2 and collagen I expression.

Conclusions: Inflammation accelerated the progression of VC in ESRD patients by disrupting the LDLr pathway, which may represent a novel mechanism involved in the progression of both VC and atherosclerosis.

Editor: Alberico Catapano, University of Milan, Italy

Funding: This work was supported by the Natural Science Foundation of Jiangsu Province (BK2009279) and the National Natural Science Foundation of China (Grants 81170792 and 81070571). The funding agencies had no role in the study design, data collection and analysis, decision to publish, or preparation of the manuscript.

Competing Interests: The authors have declared that no competing interests exist.

* E-mail: mmkkll@hotmail.com

Introduction

Cardiovascular disease (CVD) is the leading cause of morbidity among patients with end-stage renal disease (ESRD), accounting for approximately 50% of deaths and 30% of hospitalisations in this population [1]. Annual CVD mortality is 10–20 fold higher in ESRD patients than in the general population, and this difference is not completely explained by traditional risk factors [2]. Recently, more attention has been paid to vascular calcification (VC), which induces arterial stiffness, high pulse pressure, and cardiac valve dysfunction, contributing to ventricular hypertrophy and heart failure [3,4]. Thus, VC results in an increased risk of CVD mortality, especially in ESRD patients, regardless of maintenance hemodialysis (HD) treatment status.

Vascular calcification is a complicated pathological process that develops primarily within the intimal and medial layers of the artery. Arterial intimal calcification (AIC) is an advanced form of atherosclerosis (AS), driven by cellular necrosis, inflammation, and lipid deposition manifested in a patchy, discontinuous course along the artery. Specific risk factors for AIC in uraemia patients include hyperphosphatemia, hypoalbuminemia, excessive calcium intake, and HD duration. Arterial medial calcification (AMC) is observed in the elastic lamella of the medial layer of the arteries. AMC is closely associated with HD duration even in patients with no CVD history at HD therapy onset. AMC is an active process that involves the transformation of medial vascular smooth muscle cells (VSMCs) from a fibroblastic to an osteogenic phenotype. Normally, VSMCs have a contractile phenotype and constitutively express proteins that inhibit mineralisation. In response to various stimuli, however, VSMCs express and/or release several key regulators of bone formation and bone structural associated proteins, such as bone morphogenetic protein-2 (BMP-2), alkaline phosphatase (ALP), and collagen I. In contrast, the expression of proteins such as α-smooth muscle cell (α-SMA) and collagen IV is reduced, ultimately transforming VSMCs into osteoblast-like cells [5,6]. However, the precise mechanisms that cause the osteogenic phenotype of VSMCs in calcified vessels are not completely clear.

Chronic systemic inflammation is a common feature in ESRD patients [7], and it may be correlated with the accumulation of pro-inflammatory compounds caused by a markedly decreased glomerular filtration rate (GFR) [8]. Other causes, including malnutrition, metabolic acidosis, hyperparathyroidism, the accumulation of advanced oxidation protein products and asymmetric dimethyl arginine, contribute to the release of inflammatory cytokines [9]. Inflammation accelerates the progression of AS and VC [10,11], which has been identified as an independent risk factor for the morbidity and mortality of CVD in ESRD patients [12].

It is well known that the low-density lipoprotein receptor (LDLr) pathway is a feedback system with important roles in regulating plasma and intracellular cholesterol homeostasis, and it is mainly modulated by the concentration of intracellular cholesterol and the interaction between sterol regulatory element binding protein (SREBP) and SREBP cleavage-activating protein (SCAP). Cholesterol deficiency enhances the translocation of SCAP from the endoplasmic reticulum (ER) to the Golgi, where it cleaves SREBP, thus increasing LDLr gene expression.

Our previous studies demonstrated that inflammation accelerated the progression of AS by disrupting LDLr feedback regulation [13,14]. The present study was performed to evaluate whether the inflammation exacerbates the progression of VC in ESRD patients and explore the underlying mechanisms.

Materials and Methods

Ethics Statement

All studies were approved by the Ethical Committee of Southeast University. Each patient provided written informed consent to the use of their tissues for research purposes.

Patient Selection and Clinical Data

We studied 28 ESRD patients from Zhong Da Hospital, Southeast University between January 2010 and May 2011. Patients with ESRD who were to undergo arteriovenostomy before hemodialysis were included in the study. Patients with acute infection, cancer, and/or chronic active hepatitis were excluded. The included patients were divided into two groups based on plasma C-reactive protein (CRP) levels: control (CRP<3.0 mg/l, n = 14) and inflamed (CRP>= 3.0 mg/l, n = 14) group. Inflamed group was defined as the patients with persistent increased plasma levels of CRP checked at the start and the second week after hospitalization. The patients were comprehensively monitored by the symptoms, signs, and serum indexes, in order to detect timely any confounding condition which may potentially affect serum CRP level.

Clinical Biochemical Tests

Blood samples were assayed to determine erythrocyte sedimentation rate (ESR), CRP, red blood cells (RBC), haemoglobin (Hb), total protein (TP), albumin (ALB), glucose (GLU), triglyceride (TG), total cholesterol (TC), low density lipoprotein (LDL), high density lipoprotein (HDL), apolipoprotein A1 (Apo A1), Apo B, lipoprotein (a), calcium (Ca), phosphate (P), and intact parathyroid hormone (iPTH) using an automatic biochemistry analyser at the clinical chemistry centre of the hospital.

Tissue Processing

Tissues from the radial artery were taken during radial-cephalic anastomosis surgery. The tissue sections were rinsed with saline and placed in 10% buffered formalin. After treatment, representative sections of the grafts were obtained and embedded in O.C.T. medium or paraffin.

Hematoxylin-eosin (HE) Staining

The paraffin embedded tissues were sliced and dewaxed. The slices were dyed for 15 minutes with hematoxylin, dipped in 1% hydrochloric alcohol, and then stained with 1% eosin for 3 minutes. The slices were sealed with resinene after they were dehydrated to transparency. The results were observed under light microscope (×200).

Alizarin red S Staining

The paraffin-embedded tissues were dewaxed and hydrated in 70% alcohol. After rinsing rapidly in distilled water, the slices were dyed with alizarin red S solution for one minute. Positive results were shown in an orange-red colour in light microscope (×200).

Immunohistochemical Staining

Paraffin-embedded sections (4 μm) were subjected to immunohistochemical staining. After deparaffinisation, sections were placed in citrate-buffered solution (pH 6.0) and then heated for antigen retrieval. Endogenous peroxidase was blocked with 3% hydrogen peroxide, and nonspecific antibody binding was blocked with 10% goat serum. Subsequently, sections were incubated with goat, rabbit or mouse anti-human primary antibodies against TNF-α (Santa Cruz, USA), MCP-1 (Santa Cruz, USA), LDLr (Abcam, UK), BMP-2 (Santa Cruz, USA), and collagen I (Abcam, UK) overnight at 4°C, followed by incubation with biotinylated secondary antibodies. Finally, a diaminobenzidine tetrahydrochloride substrate was used to develop the reaction. The results were observed under a light microscope (×200). Semiquantitative analysis was performed by the software of Image-Pro Plus version 5.0.

Immunofluorescent Staining

The frozen sections were fixed with 4% formalin solution and then blocked with 5% bovine serum albumin (BSA). Subsequently, the sections were incubated with rabbit, mouse, or goat anti-human primary antibodies against SCAP (Abcam, UK), α-SMA (Abcam, UK), Golgi (Invitrogen, USA), and ALP (Santa Cruz, USA), followed by goat anti-rabbit Fluor 488, donkey anti-rabbit Fluor 594, goat anti-mouse Fluor 594, and donkey anti-goat Fluor 488 secondary uorescent antibodies (Invitrogen, USA), respectively. After washing, the slides were examined by laser confocal microscopy (×100). Semi-quantitative analysis was performed by the software of Image-Pro Plus version 5.0.

Statistical Analysis

All the data were expressed as the mean ± standard deviation (SD) and were analysed with SPSS 13.0. Continuous variables were compared between the two groups with the independent-sample t test (where appropriate), and correlations between variables were analysed by Spearman's R coefficient. A difference was considered significant if the P value was less than 0.05.

7

Results

Basic Clinical Data of the Patients in the Two Groups

As shown in Table 1, there were no differences in age, body weight, ESR, RBC, Hb, TP, ALB, lipid profiles, Ca, P, Ca×P, or iPTH (P>0.05) between the inflamed group and the control group.

Local Upregulation of Inflammation in the Artery was Consistent with Plasma CRP Level

Using immunohistochemical staining, we demonstrated that the expression of TNF-α and MCP-1 were increased in the radial artery in the inflamed group, which indicated that the local inflammation in the artery was upregulated, consistent with the observation of systemic inflammation stress (Fig. 1A, Fig. 1B).

Inflammation Induced Foam Cell Formation and Calcified Plaque Deposition of Radial Arteries

HE staining showed that there was significant foam cell formation in the radial arteries of the inflamed group compared to the control (Fig. 2A, Fig. 2B). Interestingly, there was a parallel increase in calcified plaque deposition in the radial arteries of the inflamed group compared to controls, as evaluated by alizarin red S staining, suggesting that a common mechanism could be involved in both AS and VC (Fig. 2C, Fig. 2D).

Inflammation Disrupted the Feedback Regulation of the LDL Receptor

To explore the potential mechanisms underlying this phenomenon, we evaluated the effects of inflammation on the protein expression of LDLr and SREBP-2 by immunohistochemical staining in radial arteries. Inflammation significantly increased LDLr and SREBP-2 protein expression (Fig. 3A I–VI, Fig. 3B).

Table 1. Basic clinical and biochemical data for the patients.

Parameters	control (n=14)	inflamed group (n=14)
Weight(Kg)	63.71±9.82	63.54±12.47
Age (ys)	49.07±16.34	57.71±17.32
RBC(10¹²/L)	2.57±0.57	2.72±0.63
Hb(g/L)	76.89±17.39	78.67±18.29
TP(g/L)	57.07±10.51	57.36±9.6
ALB(g/L)	28.14±6.20	28.36±4.89
GLU (mmol/L)	5.34±2.46	5.52±1.92
TG (mmol/L)	1.33±1.06	1.18±0.64
T-CHO (mmol/L)	4.81±1.26	4.51±1.00
LDL (mmol/L)	3.09±1.09	2.83±0.87
HDL(mmol/L)	1.21±0.28	1.08±0.37
ApoA1 (mmol/L)	1.11±0.23	0.97±0.29
ApoB (mmol/L)	0.89±0.30	0.81±0.21
LP(a) (mmol/L)	395.43±204.79	366.43±203.45
Ca (mmol/L)	2.00±0.24	2.01±0.27
P (mmol/L)	1.89±0.31	1.83±0.47
Ca*P (mmol/L)²	3.75±0.55	3.57±0.54
iPTH (pg/mL)	255.84±168.57	205.05±133.97

There was no difference compared every index in the inflamed group with that in the control, P>0.05.

Moreover, the plasma CRP level was positively correlated with the expression of the LDLr protein (Fig. 3C). Therefore, we further investigated the effect of inflammation on the translocation of SCAP escorting SREBP-2 from the ER to the Golgi in the radial arteries. Confocal microscopy showed that inflammation significantly increased SCAP translocation from the ER to the Golgi, thereby activating LDLr gene transcription (Fig. 3D, Fig. 3E.).

Inflammation Accelerated VC by Contributing to VSMC Conversion from the Fibroblastic to the Osteogenic Phenotype

To investigate the possible mechanisms of VC in the context of inflammation, we evaluated the effects of inflammation on the expression of the bone formation biomarkers BMP-2 and collagen I in the radial arteries during VC progression. As shown by immunohistochemical staining, BMP-2 and collagen I protein expression were significantly increased in the inflamed group compared to the control group (Fig. 4A I–VI, Fig. 4B). It is well known that VSMC is one of the major cellular components involved in the progression of AMC. Therefore, we evaluated the protein expressions of ALP and α-SMA. As shown by immunofluorescent staining, inflammation significantly increased ALP expression and decreased α-SMA expression (Fig. 4C, Fig. 4D). This suggests that inflammation induces VSMC conversion from the fibroblastic to the osteogenic phenotype, thereby accelerating the progression of AMC.

The Disruption of the LDLr Pathway was Closely Associated with AS and VC of the Radial Arteries

Correlation analysis demonstrated that LDLr protein expression was positively associated with BMP-2 and collagen I protein expression (Fig. 5A and Fig. 5B). These findings, in combination with those of our previous studies, suggest that the disruption of the LDLr pathway under inflammatory stress may be closely associated with the progression of AS and VC.

Discussion

Dyslipidemia and chronic inflammation are common complications in chronic kidney disease (CKD), especially ESRD. It has been reported that dyslipidemia and inflammation act together as "partners in crime" to accelerate the progression of AS and vascular calcification in HD patients. Our previous in vivo and in vitro studies showed that inflammation induced intracellular lipid accumulation and foam cell formation by disrupting LDLr feedback regulation, exacerbating the progression of AS [13–15]. The present study was designed to investigate whether the LDLr pathway was involved in the progression of VC in HD patients under inflammatory stress.

Using immunohistochemical staining, we found that TNF-α and MCP-1 protein expression were increased in the arteries of the inflamed group compared to controls, suggesting that local arterial inflammation was also upregulated in the inflamed group.

By evaluating continuous cross-sections, we demonstrated that there was a significant increase in foam cell formation and calcium deposition in the inflamed group, as shown by hematoxylin eosin and alizarin red S staining, respectively. The parallel pathological changes in AS and VC appeared in the same area of the radial artery, suggesting that a common pathway mediated by inflammation and dyslipidemia may be involved in the progression of both AS and VC.

We found that LDLr protein expression in the radial artery tissues was increased in the inflamed group compared to the control group and that this increase was positively associated with

A

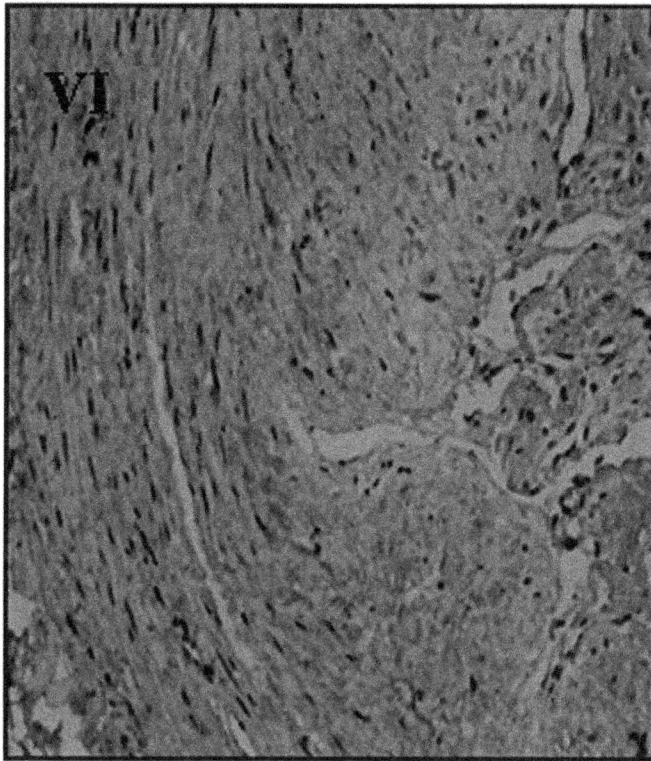

B

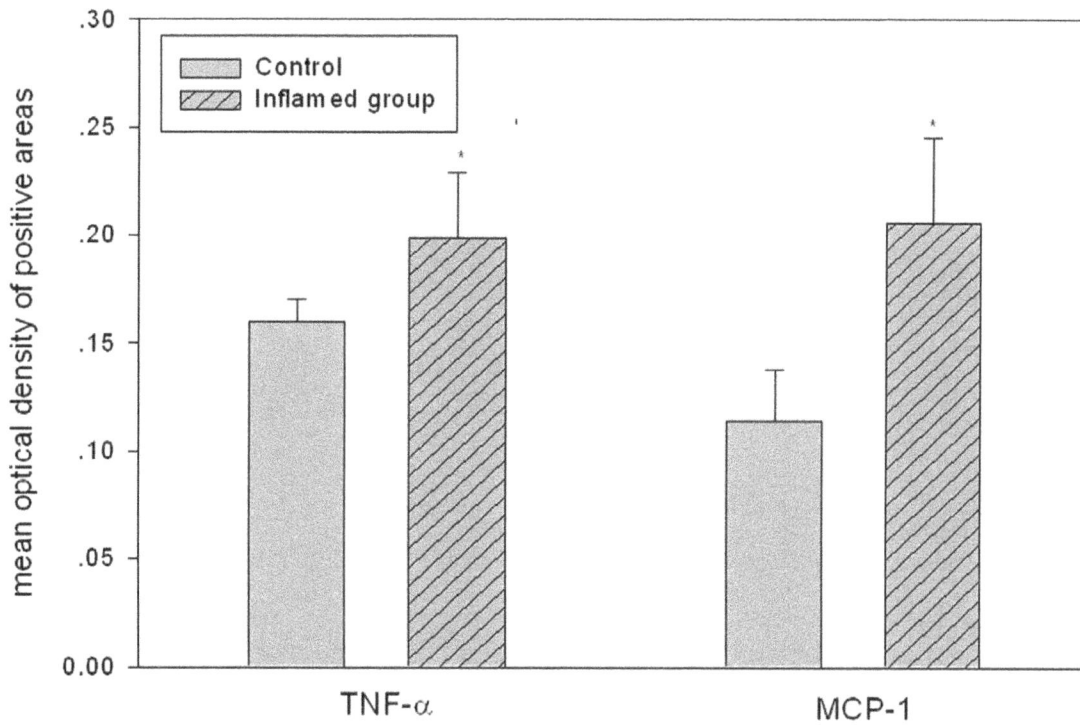

Figure 1. Locally upregulated inflammation in the artery was consistent with the plasma CRP level. The local inflammation status in the radial artery was examined by immunohistochemical staining. The positive areas were stained brown in cross-sections of radial arteries (Fig. 1, I–VI, original magnification ×200). The values of semiquantitative analysis for the positive areas were expressed as the mean ±SD from five patients in each group (n = 14). * $P < 0.05$ vs control (Fig. 1B).

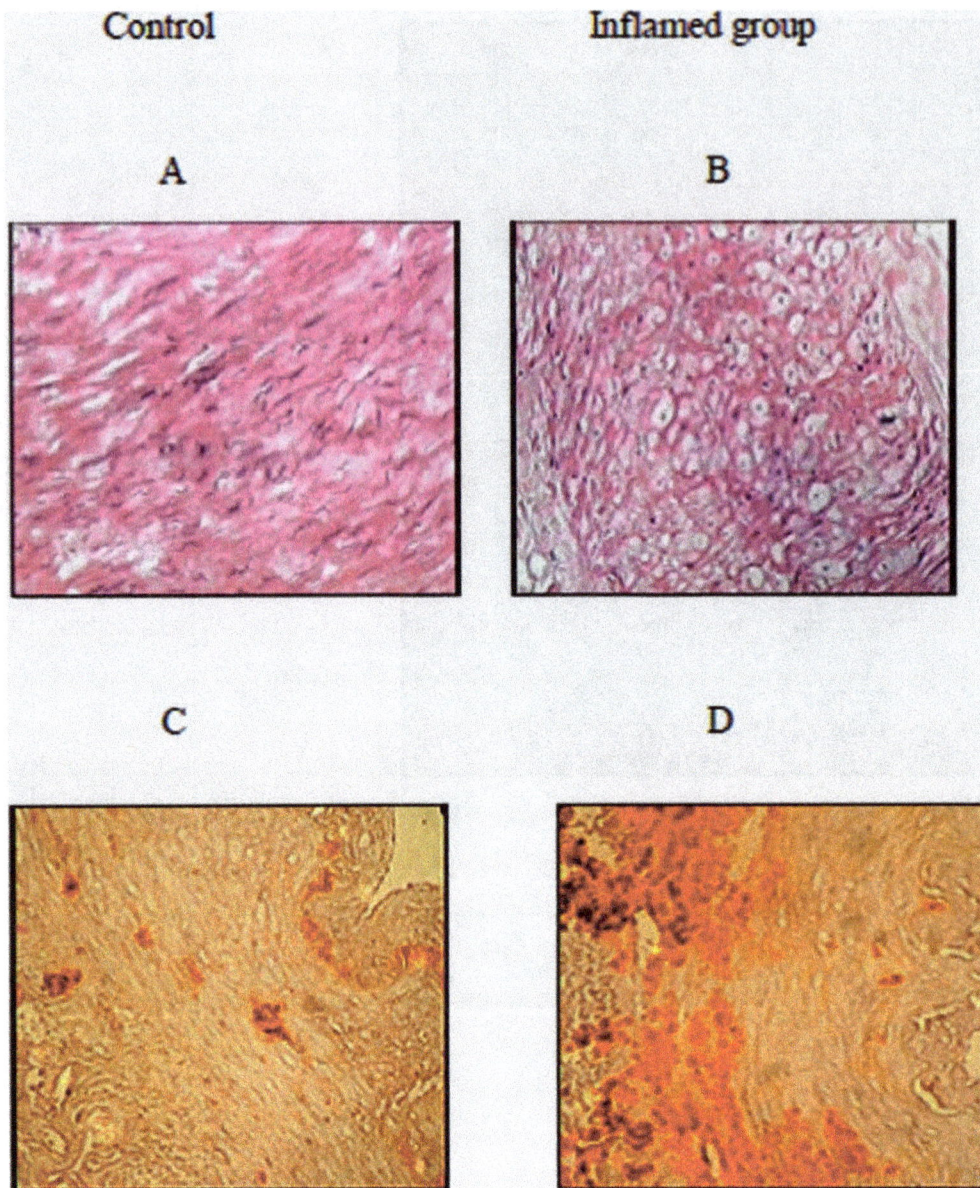

Figure 2. Inflammation induced foam cell formation and calcified plaque deposition in the radial arteries. The lipid accumulation in the radial arteries was checked by hematoxylin-eosin staining (Fig. 2A and Fig. 2B, original magnification ×200) Calcification was examined by alizarin red S staining, and calcium deposits were stained orange-red (Fig. 2C and Fig. 2D, original magnification ×200).

plasma CRP level. Further analysis showed that upregulated LDLr protein expression was mediated by increased SREBP-2 protein expression and enhanced SCAP/SREBP-2 complex translocation. These clinical findings were consistent with our previous *in vivo* and *in vitro* studies, showing that the disruption of the LDLr pathway played crucial roles in the progression of AS.

It is accepted that AMC, the main calcification mechanism in CKD patients, is closely associated with the conversion of VSMCs from fibroblastic to osteogenic phenotypes and the upregulation of osteogenic programs [16]. Although Proudfoot *et al* reported that acetylated LDL stimulates human VSMC calcification by promoting osteoblastic differentiation, little is known about the roles of LDLr feedback regulation in modulating the phenotype conversion of VSMCs in calcified vessels in the context of inflammation. To investigate the possible link between the disruption of the LDLr pathway and VC, we further evaluated the effects of inflammation on AMC in the tissues of the radial artery. Using tissues removed from the radial arteries of HD patients, we demonstrated that inflammation significantly increased the expression of the bone formation biomarker proteins BMP-2 and collagen I during VC progression. Immunofluorescent staining showed that inflammation significantly increased ALP expression and decreased α-SMA expression. The correlation analysis further showed that LDLr protein expression was positively associated with BMP-2 and collagen I protein expression. These observations suggest that inflammation accelerates the progression of AMC by disrupting the LDLr pathway, which is closely associated with the induction of VSMC phenotype conversion. Recently, using LDL receptor deficient mice, Geng Y *et al* [17] demonstrated that up-regulation of cholesterol

A

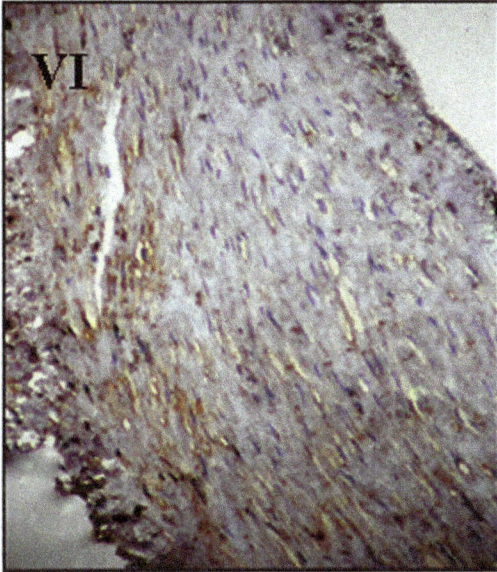

B

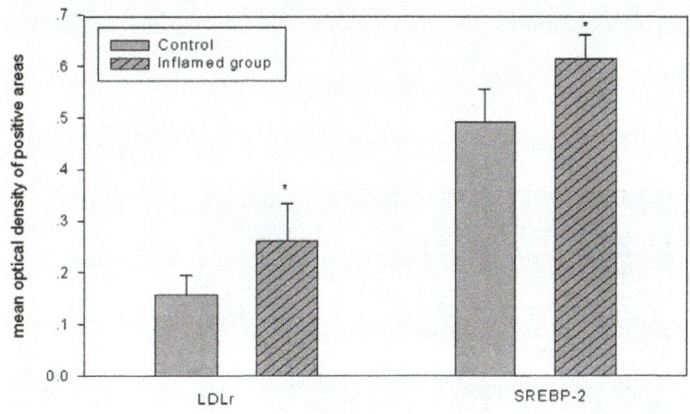

C

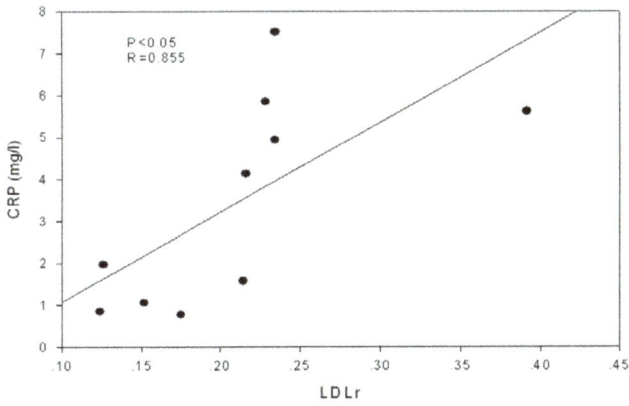

D

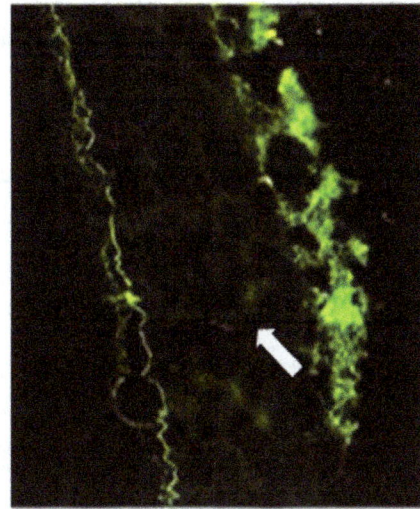

E

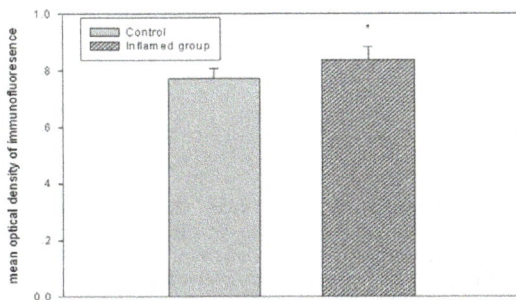

Figure 3. Inflammation disrupted the feedback regulation of the LDL receptor. LDLr and SREBP-2 protein expression were measured by immunohistochemical staining. The positive areas were stained brown in radial artery cross sections (Fig. 3A I–VI, original magnification ×200). The

values of semiquantitative analysis for the positive areas are expressed as the mean ±SD from five patients at each group (n = 14). * P<0.05 vs control (Fig. 3B). Correlation analysis of plasma CRP level with LDLr expression (Fig. 3C). The translocation of SCAP from the ER to Golgi was evaluated by immunofluorescent staining. SCAP and Golgi are stained in green and red, respectively. The colocalisation of SCAP with Golgi was evaluated by laser confocal microscopy (Fig. 3D, arrow indicates colocalisation, original magnification ×100). Overlay areas were quantified and expressed as the mean ± SD from five patients at each group (n = 14). * P<0.05 vs control (Fig. 3E).

A

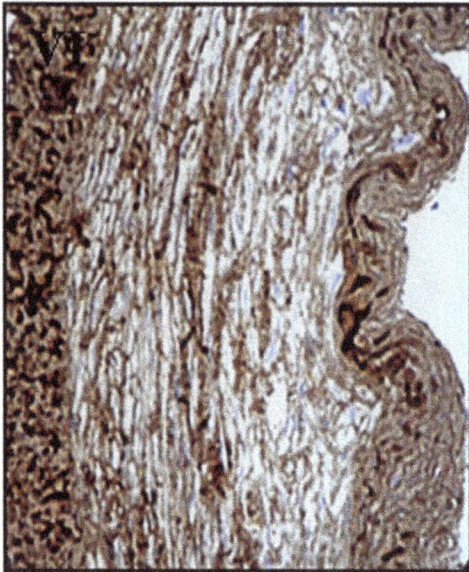

B

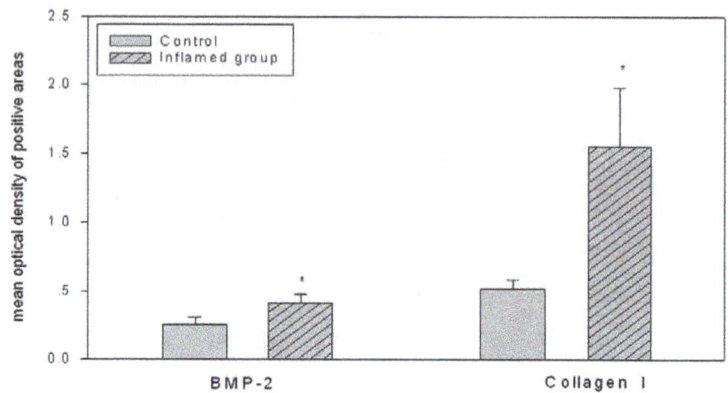

C

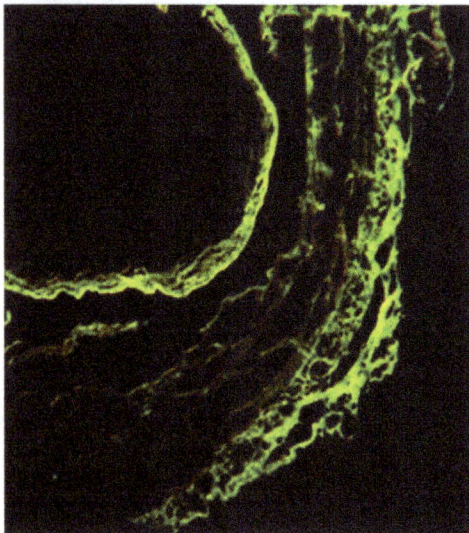

D

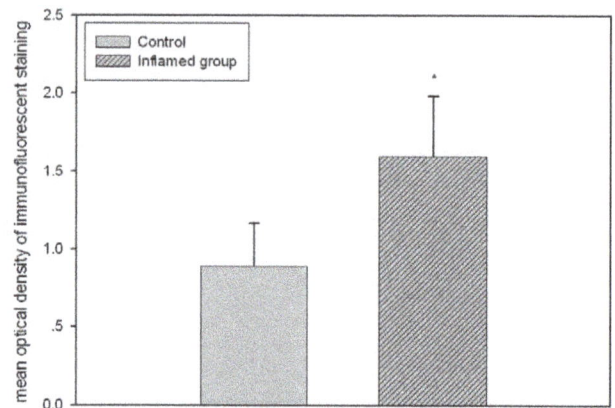

Figure 4. Inflammation accelerated the VC by contributing to the phenotype conversion of VSMC from the fibroblastic to the osteogenic. The protein expressions of BMP-2 and Collagen I were checked by immunohistochemical staining. The positive areas were stained as brown in cross-sections of radial arteries (Fig. 4A I–VI, original magnification ×200). The values of semiquantitative analysis for the positive areas were expressed as the mean ±SD from five patients at each group (n = 14). * P<0.05 vs control (Fig. 4B). The co-expression of the ALP and α-SMA proteins was checked by immunofluorescent double staining. ALP and α-SMA are stained with green and red fluorescence, respectively (Fig. 4C, original magnification ×100). The ratio of green to red in the overlay areas were quantified and expressed as the mean±SD from five patients in each group (n = 14). * P<0.05 vs control (Fig. 4D).

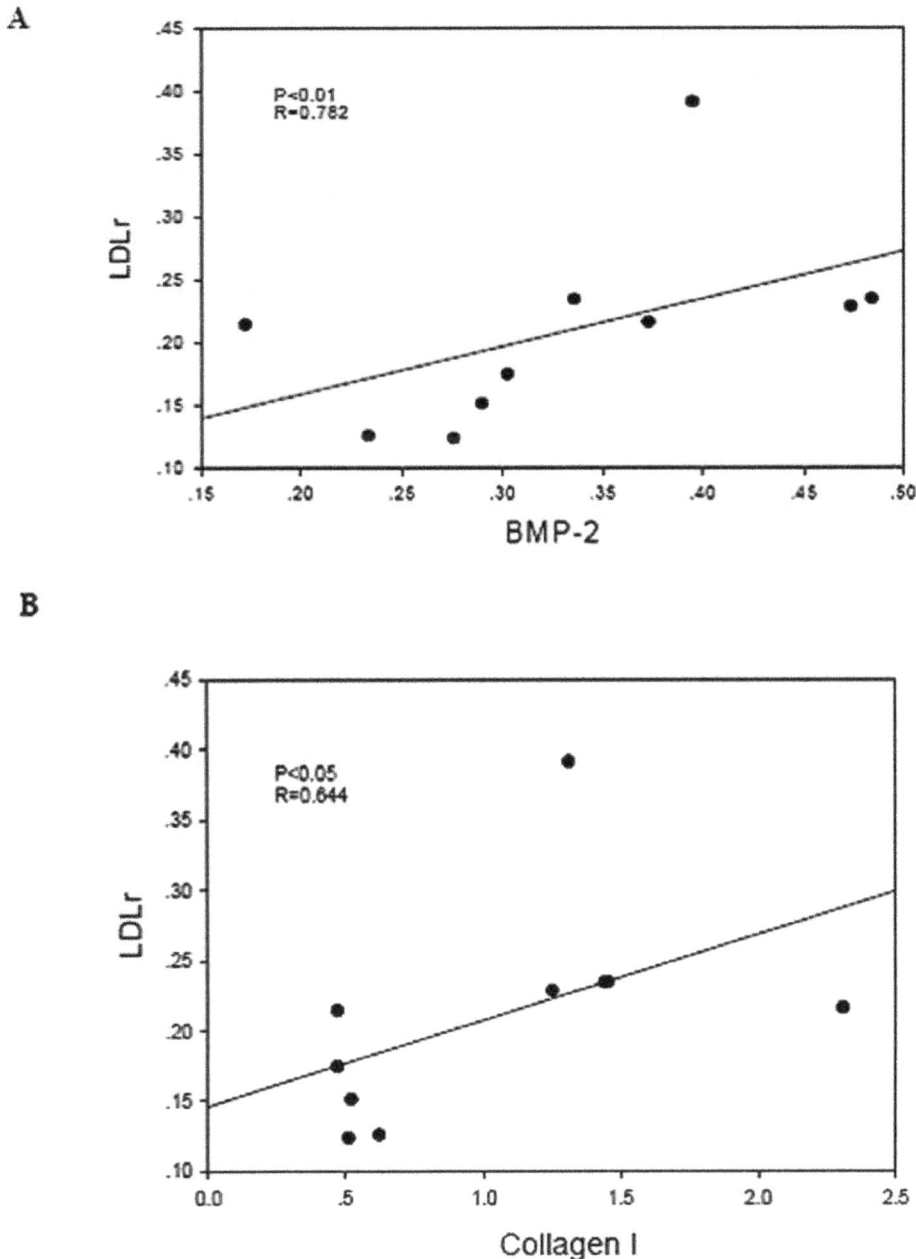

Figure 5. The disruption of the LDLr pathway was closely associated with VC of the radial arteries. Correlation analysis demonstrated that LDLr protein expression was positively associated with BMP-2 (Fig. 5A, R = 0.782, P<0.01) and collagen I (Fig. 5B, R = 0.644, P<0.05) expression.

metabolism is essential for matrix mineralization by vascular cells, which were further confirmed by our findings.

In summary, our findings demonstrate for the first time that inflammation accelerates the progression of VC in HD patients by disrupting the LDLr pathway. This may be a novel mechanism involved in the progression of both VC and AS.

Limitations

The main limitation was low number of patients and small size of samples acquired from radial arteries in two groups, which may limit providing more evidence with the evaluation of VC. CRP, as a biomarker in this study for the evaluation of inflammatory status in ESRD patients, should be understood objectively. Although it

has been widely accepted as a valuable and well recognized index of inflammation, some studies recently have reported that CRP partly depends upon commonly unmeasured factors (e. g. genetic traits) [18,19]. In addition, as each patient had different conditions, such as age, complications, treatments, serum levels of phosphate, calcium, and intact parathyroid hormone, the data could be not well-controlled.

Author Contributions

Conceived and designed the experiments: KLM. Performed the experiments: JN J. Liu Y. Zhang. Analyzed the data: KLM C.X. Wang B.C. Liu. Contributed reagents/materials/analysis tools: KLM J. Liu. Wrote the paper: MG H. Liu X.L. Zhang Y.L. Wang.

References

1. Locatelli F, Pisoni RL, Combe C, Bommer J, Andreucci VE, et al (2004) Anaemia in haemodialysis patients of five European countries: association with morbidity and mortality in the Dialysis Outcomes and Practice Patterns Study (DOPPS). Nephrol Dial Transplant 19: 121–132.
2. Foley RN, Parfrey PS, Sarnak MJ (1998) Clinical epidemiology of cardiovascular disease in chronic renal disease. Am J Kidney Dis 32: S112–S119.
3. London GM, Guerin AP, Marchais SJ, Metivier F, Pannier B, et al (2003) Arterial media calcification in end-stage renal disease: impact on all-cause and cardiovascular mortality. Nephrol Dial Transplant 18: 1731–1740.
4. London GM (2003) Cardiovascular calcifications in uremic patients: clinical impact on cardiovascular function. J Am Soc Nephrol 14: S305–S309.
5. Giachelli CM (2004) Vascular calcification mechanisms. J Am Soc Nephrol 15: 2959–2964.
6. Shanahan CM, Crouthamel MH, Kapustin A, Giachelli CM (2011) Arterial calcification in chronic kidney disease: key roles for calcium and phosphate. Circ Res 109: 697–711.
7. Kaysen GA (2001) The microinflammatory state in uremia: causes and potential consequences. J Am Soc Nephrol 12: 1549–1557.
8. Akahoshi T, Kobayashi N, Hosaka S, Sekiyama N, Wada C, et al (1995) In-vivo induction of monocyte chemotactic and activating factor in patients with chronic renal failure. Nephrol Dial Transplant 10: 2244–2249.
9. Silverstein DM (2009) Inflammation in chronic kidney disease: role in the progression of renal and cardiovascular disease. Pediatr Nephrol 24: 1445–1452.
10. Hansson GK, Robertson AK, Soderberg-Naucler C (2006) Inflammation and atherosclerosis. Annu Rev Pathol 1: 297–329.
11. Moe SM, Chen NX (2005) Inflammation and vascular calcification. Blood Purif 23: 64–71.
12. Zimmermann J, Herrlinger S, Pruy A, Metzger T, Wanner C (1999) Inflammation enhances cardiovascular risk and mortality in hemodialysis patients. Kidney Int 55: 648–658.
13. Ma KL, Ruan XZ, Powis SH, Moorhead JF, Varghese Z (2007) Anti-atherosclerotic effects of sirolimus on human vascular smooth muscle cells. Am J Physiol Heart Circ Physiol 292: H2721–H2728.
14. Ruan XZ, Moorhead JF, Tao JL, Ma KL, Wheeler DC, et al (2006) Mechanisms of Dysregulation of Low-Density Lipoprotein Receptor Expression in Vascular Smooth Muscle Cells by Inflammatory Cytokines. Arterioscler Thromb Vasc Biol 26(5): 1150–5.
15. Ma KL, Ruan XZ, Powis SH, Chen Y, Moorhead JF, et al (2008) Inflammatory stress exacerbates lipid accumulation in hepatic cells and fatty livers of apolipoprotein E knockout mice. Hepatology 48: 770–781.
16. Amann K (2008) Media calcification and intima calcification are distinct entities in chronic kidney disease. Clin J Am Soc Nephrol 3: 1599–1605.
17. Geng Y, Hsu JJ, Lu J, Ting TC, Miyazaki M, et al (2011) Role of cellular cholesterol metabolism in vascular cell calcification. J Biol Chem 286: 33701–33706.
18. Crawford DC, Sanders CL, Qin X, Smith JD, Shephard C, et al (2006) Genetic variation is associated with C-reactive protein levels in the Third National Health and Nutrition Examination Survey. Circulation 114: 2458–2465.
19. Thalmaier D, Dambacher J, Seiderer J, Konrad A, Schachinger V, et al (2006) The +1059G/C polymorphism in the C-reactive protein (CRP) gene is associated with involvement of the terminal ileum and decreased serum CRP levels in patients with Crohn's disease. Aliment Pharmacol Ther 24: 1105–1115.

9

Early Referral to a Nephrologist Improved Patient Survival: Prospective Cohort Study for End-Stage Renal Disease in Korea

Do Hyoung Kim[1,9], Myounghee Kim[2,9], Ho Kim[3,9], Yong-Lim Kim[4,9], Shin-Wook Kang[5,9], Chul Woo Yang[6,9], Nam-Ho Kim[7,9], Yon Su Kim[1,9], Jung Pyo Lee[8,9]*

1 Department of Internal Medicine, Seoul National University College of Medicine, Seoul, Korea, 2 Department of Dental Hygiene, College of Health Science, Eulji University, Seongnam, Korea, 3 Department of Epidemiology and Biostatistics, School of Public Health, Seoul National University, Seoul, Korea, 4 Department of Internal Medicine, Kyungpook National University School of Medicine, Daegu, Korea, 5 Department of Internal Medicine, Yonsei University College of Medicine, Seoul, Korea, 6 Department of Internal Medicine, The Catholic University of Korea College of Medicine, Seoul, Korea, 7 Department of Internal Medicine, Chonnam National University Medical School, Gwangju, Korea, 8 Department of Internal Medicine, Seoul National University Boramae Medical Center, Seoul, Korea, 9 Clinical Research Center for End Stage Renal Disease in Korea, Daegu, Korea

Abstract

The timing of referral to a nephrologist may influence the outcome of chronic kidney disease patients, but its impact has not been evaluated thoroughly. The results of a recent study showing an association between early referral and patient survival are still being debated. A total of 1028 patients newly diagnosed as end-stage renal disease (ESRD) from July 2008 to October 2011 were enrolled. Early referral (ER) was defined as patients meeting with a nephrologist more than a year before dialysis and dialysis education were provided, and all others were considered late referral (LR). The relationship of referral pattern with mortality in ESRD patients was explored using a Cox proportional hazards regression models. Time from referral to dialysis was significantly longer in 599 ER patients than in 429 LR patients (62.3 ± 58.9 versus 2.9 ± 3.4 months, $P<0.001$). Emergency HD using a temporary vascular catheter was required in 485 (47.2%) out of all patients and in 262 (43.7%) of ER compared with 223 (52.0%) of LR ($P=0.009$). After 2 years of follow-up, the survival rate in ER was better than that in LR (hazard ratio [HR] 2.38, 95% confidence interval [CI] 1.27–4.45, $P=0.007$). In patients with diabetes nephropathy, patient survival was also significantly higher in ER than in LR (HR 4.74, 95% CI 1.73–13.00, $P=0.002$). With increasing age, HR also increased. Timely referral to a nephrologist in the predialytic stage is associated with reduced mortality.

Editor: Jung Eun Lee, Sookmyung Women's University, Republic of Korea

Funding: This study was supported by a grant from the Korea Healthcare Technology R&D Project, Ministry for Health and Welfare, Republic of Korea (A102065). The funders had no role in study design, data collection and analysis, decision to publish, or preparation of the manuscript.

Competing Interests: The authors have declared that no competing interests exist.

* E-mail: nephrolee@gmail.com

Introduction

Patients with end-stage renal disease (ESRD) have an exceedingly high morbidity and mortality compared to the general population [1]. The number of ESRD patients is growing at a much faster rate than the total population. The increasing prevalence of ESRD has led to its recognition as a significant clinical and public health problem, in terms of its use of medical resources and public health expenditure. According to data from the National Health Insurance Corporation, chronic kidney disease (CKD) ranked first in public health expenditure [2]. Also, it was the single most expensive disease.

Over the past several years, interest has evolved in evaluating the timing of nephrology referral in the predialytic stage of CKD. The potential benefits of timely nephrology referral include identification of reversible causes of CKD, provision of treatments that may slow the progression of CKD, management of the metabolic complications of advanced CKD, coordination of education regarding ESRD treatment options, and optimal preparation for the chosen dialysis modality or kidney transplantation [3]. Therefore, delayed nephrology care could be associated with several unfavorable outcomes, including reduced access to peritoneal dialysis (PD) [4,5] and kidney transplantation [6,7], higher rates of dialysis initiation through a temporary venous catheter, and an higher mortality rate after starting maintenance dialysis, especially during the first few months [8–10].

To date, most referral studies have had a retrospective design [4,5,11–13] and there have been few prospective multi-center studies examining referral practices [14,15]. The results of a recent study showing an association between early referral and patient survival are still being debated [16]. Additionally, late referral was defined as the first encounter with a nephrologist occurring within 1 to 3 months of the commencement of dialysis in most studies. This duration was too short to ensure effective education of the patients by the nephrologist [17]. Therefore, a large prospective study is required to investigate the relationship between early referral to a nephrologist and patient survival.

Table 1. Patient characteristics by referral pattern.[a]

	Total ESRD				DM ESRD			
	Total (N=1028)	Early referral (N=599)	Late referral (N=429)	P Value	Total (N=511)	Early referral (N=302)	Late referral (N=209)	P Value
Age at the time of dialysis (year)	57.0±13.9	57.4±13.5	56.5±14.4	0.329	59.1±11.5	59.9±11.4	57.8±11.5	0.044
Gender (male, %)	59.6	58.3	61.5	0.303	63.0	60.6	66.5	0.174
Length of follow-up (mo)	10.2±6.9	10.7±7.1	9.4±6.6	0.003	10.1±6.8	10.8±7.3	9.1±5.9	0.004
Drop out (N, %)	95 (9.2)	49 (8.2)	46 (10.7)	0.190	46 (9.0)	24 (7.9)	22 (10.5)	0.347
Findings at the time of referral to nephrologist								
Underlying kidney disease (%)				0.181				
Diabetes mellitus	49.7	50.4	48.7					
Hypertension	17.5	15.5	20.3					
Glomerulonephritis	15.3	18.0	11.4					
Polycystic kidney disease	2.0	2.8	0.9					
Others	7.8	8.0	7.5					
Unknown	7.7	5.2	11.2					
Systolic BP (mmHg)	147.1±27.6	143.3±26.8	151.0±28.0	<0.001	146.0±26.2	143.8±26.2	148.7±26.0	0.086
Diastolic BP (mmHg)	84.7±16.5	83.4±16.0	86.1±16.9	0.032	81.3±14.8	80.5±15.1	82.2±14.5	0.311
Serum creatinine (mg/dL)	4.8±4.1	2.6±1.5	7.2±4.6	<0.001	4.1±3.0	2.6±1.4	6.0±3.4	<0.001
eGFR (mL/min/1.73m^2)	24.5±33.9	36.1±42.7	11.4±8.0	<0.001	24.5±21.3	34.2±24.0	12.8±8.2	<0.001
Hemoglobin (g/dL)	10.0±5.0	11.2±6.4	8.8±1.8	<0.001	9.7±1.9	10.5±1.8	8.9±1.7	<0.001
Number of visits to nephrologist from referral to dialysis (%)				<0.001				<0.001
None	8.6	0	20.5		6.1	0	14.8	
1 time	7.4	1.8	15.2		6.7	2.3	12.9	
2 times or more	84.0	98.2	64.3		87.2	97.7	72.2	
Time from referral to dialysis (month)	37.7±53.8	62.3±58.9	2.9±3.4	<0.001	29.1±37.0	46.8±39.1	3.3±3.5	<0.001
Findings at the time of dialysis								
Modified Charlson co-morbidity index	5.1±2.5	5.2±2.5	5.0±2.5	0.218	6.1±2.2	6.2±2.3	6.0±2.1	0.189
Davies co-morbidity index	1.0±0.9	1.0±0.9	1.0±1.0	0.919	1.5±0.8	1.5±0.8	1.6±0.8	0.656
Serum creatinine (mg/dL)	8.4±3.9	8.3±3.6	8.5±4.2	0.147	7.8±3.1	7.8±3.1	7.7±3.2	0.642
eGFR (mL/min/1.73m^2)	7.6±3.4	7.5±3.2	7.7±3.7	0.288	8.1±3.4	7.9±3.2	8.4±3.6	0.115
Hemoglobin (g/dL)	9.0±3.5	8.9±1.6	8.8±1.7	0.468	9.1±3.8	8.9±1.5	8.9±1.6	0.854
Transferrin saturation (%)	33.3±51.8	33.0±46.2	33.8±58.6	0.825	32.4±62.3	30.9±44.6	34.5±81.2	0.553
Hemoglobin A1c (%)					6.9±2.5	6.9±1.7	6.6±1.3	0.039
Uric acid (mg/dL)	8.2±5.1	8.0±2.5	8.2±2.6	0.228	8.2±5.5	8.0±2.4	7.9±2.3	0.850

Table 1. Cont.

	Total ESRD				DM ESRD			
	Total (N=1028)	Early referral (N=599)	Late referral (N=429)	P Value	Total (N=511)	Early referral (N=302)	Late referral (N=209)	P Value
Calcium (mg/dL)	7.9±3.9	7.8±1.0	7.7±1.1	0.331	8.0±4.2	7.8±0.9	7.7±0.9	0.148
Phosphate (mg/dL)	5.5±3.0	5.3±1.8	5.6±2.0	0.042	5.5±2.8	5.3±1.7	5.5±1.8	0.437
iPTH (pg/mL)	256.0±239.9	267.2±258.0	240.0±210.9	0.105	219.0±189.5	218.1±174.8	220.4±210.4	0.905
Systolic BP (mmHg)	140.3±23.7	138.2±23.8	143.2±23.3	0.001	141.8±24.5	139.8±24.5	144.9±24.1	0.023
Diastolic BP (mmHg)	78.4±14.1	77.3±13.2	80.1±15.0	0.002	76.7±13.1	75.4±12.4	78.5±13.4	0.008
BMI (kg/m^2)	23.3±6.3	23.1±3.3	23.6±8.9	0.211	23.5±3.4	23.6±3.3	23.4±3.6	0.625
Total cholesterol (mg/dL)	159.2±50.7	156.2±48.5	163.4±53.2	0.030	157.7±55.7	153.5±51.1	163.9±61.4	0.053
Triglycerides (mg/dL)	129.8±82.4	129.7±86.6	129.8±76.3	0.991	135.9±86.4	134.0±85.2	138.5±88.3	0.593
LDL cholesterol (mg/dL)	93.6±55.1	90.0±53.7	98.5±56.6	0.038	93.7±66.9	89.1±66.0	100.0±67.8	0.117
HDL cholesterol (mg/dL)	39.7±14.3	39.7±14.6	39.8±13.9	0.902	38.3±13.2	37.6±12.3	39.5±14.3	0.149

a Values for continuous variables are means ± standard deviation; values for categorical variables expressed as proportion. BP, blood pressure; eGFR, estimated glomerular filtration rate; iPTH, intact parathyroid hormone; BMI, body mass index; LDL, low-density lipoprotein; HDL, high-density lipoprotein.

The purpose of this study was to explore the impact of early nephrology referral and frequent attendance at nephrology clinics before ESRD treatment initiation on patient survival in a subset of patients from the Comprehensive Prospective Study of the Clinical Research Center for End Stage Renal Disease (CRC ESRD) in Korea.

Subjects and Methods

Study Design and Definition

This study was a multi-center, prospective cohort study of patients with ESRD in Korea who were initiated on dialysis therapy. Patients were divided into two groups according to timing of referral to a nephrologist.

Patients were classified as early referral (ER) if their first encounter with a nephrologist occurred more than 1 year prior to initiation of dialysis and education about dialysis (from a nurse or nephrologist), and all others were considered late referral (LR), as described previously by Di Napoli et al. [18].

Estimated glomerular filtration rate (eGFR) was calculated by the modified Modification of Diet in Renal Disease equation as follows: eGFR (mL/min/1.73 m^2) = 186.3× (serum creatinine)$^{-1.154}$× (age)$^{-0.203}$ (×0.742 for females) where serum creatinine is measured in milligrams per deciliter and age is measured in years [19].

Study Population

Patients aged 20 years or more with ESRD who were initiated on dialysis were enrolled in the CRC ESRD. It was a nationwide web-based multi-center joint network prospective cohort of patients with ESRD in Korea designed to improve survival rates and quality of life in patients with ESRD and to create effective treatment guidelines (clinicaltrial.gov NCT00931970). Thirty-one hospitals and clinics in Korea participated in the CRC ESRD and shared the clinical data of 1,211 newly diagnosed adult ESRD patients from July 2008 to October 2011. In the present study 1,028 patients were enrolled among them. Of the 183 patients who were excluded, data regarding visits to a nephrologist were unknown in 133 patients and data regarding the type of initial dialysis were unknown in 50 patients. All patients provided their

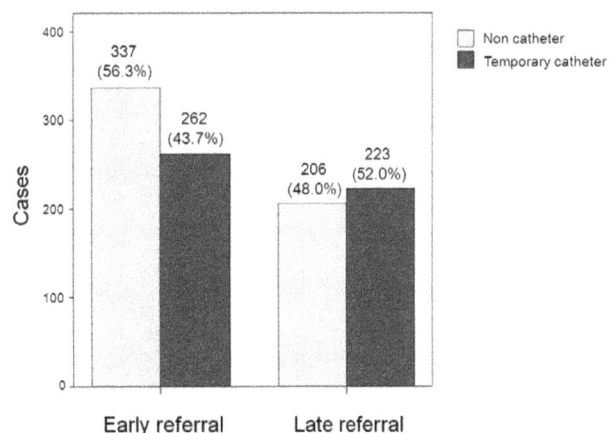

Figure 1. Pattern of emergency dialysis using a temporary vascular catheter according to the timing of referral. Early referral were defined as the patient's first encounter with a nephrologist occurring more than 1 year before first dialysis, with education about dialysis prior to initiation of dialysis, and all others were considered late referral (P = 0.009).

Table 2. Univariate analysis of predictors associated with mortality.[a]

Variable	Total ESRD (N=1028)			DM ESRD (N=511)		
	HR	95% CI	P Value	HR	95% CI	P Value
Age at the time of dialysis (per year increase)	1.07	1.04–1.09	<0.001	1.08	1.05–1.12	<0.001
Gender (female)	0.95	0.58–1.57	0.851	1.23	0.65–2.35	0.523
Underlying kidney disease						
Diabetes mellitus	Ref					
Hypertension	0.56	0.25–1.25	0.154			
Glomerulonephritis	0.63	0.30–1.30	0.207			
Polycystic kidney disease	0.59	0.08–4.27	0.598			
Others	0.70	0.25–1.96	0.497			
Unknown	1.17	0.49–2.77	0.727			
Number of visits to nephrologist from referral to dialysis						
None	Ref			Ref		
1 time	0.79	0.28–2.27	0.668	0.71	0.14–3.52	0.675
2 times or more	0.52	0.23–1.15	0.104	0.43	0.13–1.41	0.163
Late referral (ref = Early referral)	2.16	1.32–3.53	0.002	2.42	1.26–4.64	0.008
Emergency HD (ref = no)	1.63	1.00–2.67	0.053	1.08	0.57–2.04	0.812
Hospitalization (ref = no)	2.75	1.66–4.56	<0.001	2.07	1.05–4.07	0.035
Findings at the time of dialysis						
Modified Charlson co-morbidity index	1.33	1.22–1.46	<0.001	1.26	1.10–1.43	0.001
Davies co-morbidity index	1.65	1.32–2.06	<0.001	1.44	1.00–2.07	0.052
eGFR (mL/min/1.73m^2)	1.13	1.06–1.20	<0.001	1.08	0.99–1.17	0.090
Hemoglobin (g/dL)	1.02	0.88–1.18	0.775	0.93	0.75–1.15	0.505
Transferrin saturation (%)	1.00	0.99–1.01	0.692	1.00	0.99–1.01	0.865
Hemoglobin A1c (%)				0.99	0.77–1.27	0.922
Uric acid (mg/dL)	0.95	0.86–1.06	0.365	1.01	0.88–1.15	0.891
Calcium (mg/dL)	1.11	0.88–1.40	0.392	0.91	0.65–1.27	0.571
Phosphate (mg/dL)	0.82	0.71–0.95	0.007	0.82	0.67–1.01	0.060
iPTH (pg/mL)	1.00	0.99–1.00	0.020	1.00	0.99–1.00	0.883
Systolic BP (mmHg)	1.00	0.99–1.01	0.958	1.00	0.98–1.01	0.620
Diastolic BP (mmHg)	0.98	0.97–1.00	0.082	1.00	0.97–1.02	0.915
BMI (kg/m^2)	0.92	0.85–1.00	0.046	0.84	0.75–0.95	0.004
Total cholesterol (mg/dL)	1.00	0.99–1.00	0.192	1.00	0.99–1.00	0.386
Triglycerides (mg/dL)	1.00	0.99–1.00	0.568	1.00	0.99–1.00	0.456
LDL cholesterol (mg/dL)	0.99	0.99–1.00	0.146	0.99	0.98–1.00	0.231
HDL cholesterol (mg/dL)	0.99	0.97–1.01	0.438	0.99	0.97–1.02	0.684

[a]HR, hazard ratio; CI, confidence interval; BP, blood pressure; HD, hemodialysis; eGFR, estimated glomerular filtration rate; iPTH, intact parathyroid hormone; BMI, body mass index; LDL, low-density lipoprotein; HDL, high-density lipoprotein.

written consent to participate in this study. All traceable identifiers were removed before analysis to protect patient confidentiality. The study was approved by the institutional review board at each center [The Catholic University of Korea, Bucheon St. Mary's Hospital; The Catholic University of Korea, Incheon St. Mary's Hospital; The Catholic University of Korea, Seoul St. Mary's Hospital; The Catholic University of Korea, St. Mary's Hospital; The Catholic University of Korea, St. Vincent's Hospital; The Catholic University of Korea, Uijeongbu St. Mary's Hospital; Cheju Halla General Hospital; Chonbuk National University Hospital; Chonnam National University Hospital; Chung-Ang University Medical Center; Chungbuk National University Hospital; Chungnam National University Hospital; Dong-A University Medical Center; Ehwa Womens University Medical Center; Fatima Hospital, Daegu; Gachon University Gil Medical Center; Inje University Pusan Paik Hospital; Kyungpook National University Hospital; Kwandong University College of Medicine, Myongji Hospital; National Health Insurance Corporation Ilsan Hospital; National Medical Center; Pusan National University Hospital; Samsung Medical Center, Seoul; Seoul Metropolitan Government, Seoul National University, Boramae Medical Center; Seoul National University Hospital; Seoul National University, Bundang Hospital; Yeungnam University Medical Center; Yonsei University, Severance Hospital; Yonsei University, Gangnam Severance Hospital; Ulsan University Hospital; Wonju Christian Hospital (in alphabetical order)]. All clinical investiga-

Table 3. Multivariate Cox proportional hazard models of independent factors of survival.[a]

Total patients (N= 1028)	Model 1		Model 2		Model 3	
	HR (95% CI)	P Value	HR (95% CI)	P Value	HR (95% CI)	P Value
Type of referral						
Early referral	Ref		Ref		Ref	
Late referral	2.16 (1.32–3.53)	0.002	2.28 (1.39–3.74)	0.001	2.38 (1.27–4.45)	0.007
Age (years)			3.73 (2.43–5.73)	<0.001	1.06 (1.03–1.09)	<0.001
Gender (female)			0.87 (0.53–1.44)	0.599	1.11 (0.56–2.21)	0.760
BMI					0.95 (0.86–1.05)	0.342
Calcium					1.00 (0.93–1.08)	0.964
Modified Charlson co-morbidity Index					1.09 (0.93–1.28)	0.268
HDL cholesterol					1.00 (0.97–1.03)	0.887
Triglycerides					1.00 (1.00–1.01)	0.822
Total cholesterol					1.00 (1.00–1.01)	0.326
Hemoglobin					0.90 (0.73–1.10)	0.302
eGFR					1.03 (0.94–1.13)	0.504
iPTH					1.00 (1.00–1.00)	0.163
Uric acid					1.02 (0.91–1.14)	0.794
SBP at the time of dialysis					1.00 (0.98–1.01)	0.744

DM ESRD patients (N= 511)	Model 1		Model 2		Model 3	
	HR (95% CI)	P Value	HR (95% CI)	P Value	HR (95% CI)	P Value
Type of referral						
Early referral	Ref		Ref		Ref	
Late referral	2.42 (1.26–4.64)	0.008	2.88 (1.49–5.59)	0.002	4.74 (1.73–13.00)	0.002
Age (years)			3.71 (2.17–6.34)	<0.001	1.08 (1.03–1.13)	0.002
Gender (female)			1.30 (0.67–2.52)	0.437	1.90 (0.67–5.38)	0.230
BMI					0.83 (0.70–0.99)	0.042
Calcium					1.00 (0.81–1.22)	0.989
Modified Charlson co-morbidity Index					1.10 (0.87–1.39)	0.440
HDL cholesterol					1.00 (0.95–1.04)	0.843
Triglycerides					1.00 (0.99–1.01)	0.640
Total cholesterol					1.01 (0.99–1.02)	0.331
Hemoglobin					0.67 (0.50–0.91)	0.010
eGFR					1.03 (0.89–1.18)	0.713
iPTH					1.00 (1.00–1.00)	0.162
Uric acid					1.03 (0.87–1.22)	0.727
SBP at the time of dialysis					0.99 (0.98–1.01)	0.341

[a]HR, hazard ratio; CI, confidence interval; BMI, body mass index; HDL, high-density lipoprotein; eGFR, estimated glomerular filtration rate; iPTH, intact parathyroid hormone; SBP, systolic blood pressure.

tions were conducted in accordance with the guidelines of the 2008 Declaration of Helsinki.

Outcomes

The primary outcome of interest was all-cause mortality after initiation of dialysis in the LR versus ER patients. The secondary outcomes consisted of various clinical and laboratory parameters in the LR versus ER group: emergency hemodialysis (HD), cardiovascular death, cause of death, hospitalization.

Data Sources

CRC ESRD served as the primary source of data for these analyses. Clinical and laboratory data were collected by web-based medical and patient questionnaires [20].

Each centers collected the information of several outcomes including cause of death with the clinical and laboratory data in this study. Then, they reported to CRC-ESRD web-based registry about the outcomes. Research coordinators from central center carried out a regular sample survey on enrolled patients to confirm the medical records twice a year. They had checked all the

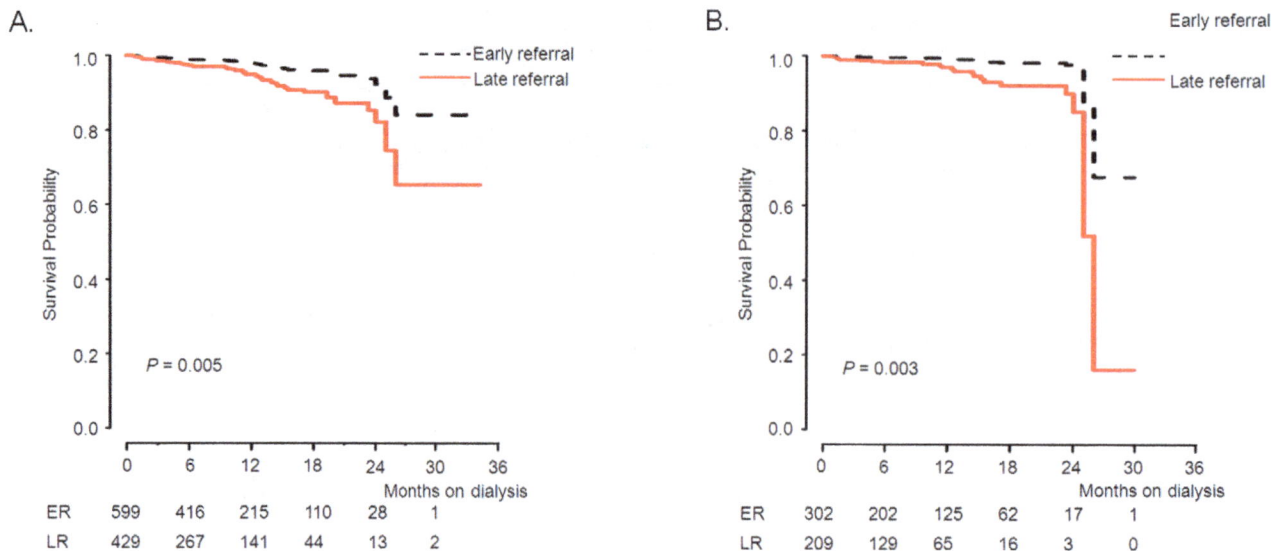

Figure 2. Kaplan-Meier survival curve by timing of referral. (A) Total patients, adjusted for age, gender, modified CCI, BMI, eGFR, serum hemoglobin, calcium, iPTH, uric acid, triglycerides, total cholesterol, and HDL cholesterol. (B) DM ESRD patients, adjusted for age, gender, modified CCI, BMI, eGFR, serum hemoglobin, calcium, iPTH, uric acid, triglycerides, total cholesterol, and HDL cholesterol.

medical records of patients who died in hospital registered in CRC-ESRD to confirm the cause-specific death and the mortality date. In the case of patient death in other hospitals, information of cause-specific death was extracted from the Korean National Statistical Office data as of December 31, 2010.

A medical questionnaire was completed by data coordinators, who were trained in each center to collect patient data by a combination of chart reviews and informal interviews using a standardized form. The questionnaires included data on demographics, previous medical history, laboratory results, dialysis modality and prescription, presence and type of permanent access used for the first dialysis, and medications including erythropoietin use. eGFR, modified Charlson co-morbidity index (CCI), and Davies co-morbidity index (DCI) at the initiation of dialysis were recorded for each patient.

The modified CCI and DCI values were calculated using the method described in a previous study [21–23]. The modified CCI includes age (weight 1 for every 10 years starting from 50 years of age) and contains 19 categories of comorbidities including congestive heart failure (weight 1), myocardial infarction (weight 1), chronic pulmonary disease (weight 1), cerebrovascular disease (weight 1), hemiplegia or paraplegia (weight 2), dementia (weight 1), diabetes (weight 1), diabetes with complications (weight 2), leukemia (weight 2), lymphoma (weight 2), malignancy (weight 2), metastatic solid tumor (weight 6), mild liver disease (weight 1), moderate or severe liver disease (weight 3), peptic ulcer disease (weight 1), peripheral vascular disease (weight 1), rheumatologic disease (weight 1), renal disease (weight 2) and acquired immune deficiency syndrome (weight 6) [21,22]. The DCI includes malignancy (1 point), ischemic heart disease (1 point), peripheral vascular disease (1 point), left ventricular dysfunction (1 point), diabetes mellitus (1 point), systemic collagen vascular disease (1 point), and other significant pathology (1 point). These data were obtained from a systematic review of all available records [23].

Patients who responded to the questionnaire were asked when they first received medical attention from a kidney specialist before starting dialysis. In a similar fashion, respondents to the questionnaire were asked about the number of visits they had

with a nephrologist during the year and about education concerning dialysis and diet before the start of ESRD.

Statistical Analysis

Univariate analyses of the differences in the clinical and laboratory variables between ER and LR were performed using the t test for continuous variables and the chi-square or Fisher exact test for discrete variables. The multivariate Cox proportional hazards regression models were used to explore the relationships of each of the independent factors with mortality risk in ESRD patients. A stepwise selection process was used to develop the multivariate Cox proportional hazards regression model. Model 1 was built to explore the relationship of timing of referral with mortality risk without the use of any explanatory variables. Model 2 was only controlled for age and gender. Model 3 was adjusted for body mass index (BMI), modified CCI, serum calcium, high-density lipoprotein cholesterol, triglycerides, total cholesterol, hemoglobin, intact parathyroid hormone, uric acid, and eGFR. The effects of the multivariate Cox proportional hazards regression models are shown as hazard ratio (HR) and 95% confidence index (CI). The Kaplan-Meier method was used to compare survival curves, and differences were assessed by means of the log rank test. The statistical analysis was performed using SAS version 9.2 (SAS Institute Inc., Cary, NC, USA) and R 2.14.1. Significant differences were defined as P less than 0.05.

Results

Patient Characteristics by Referral Pattern

Of 1028 patients enrolled in the CRC ESRD, 599 were referred early and 429 were referred late. Patients' clinical and laboratory characteristics are listed in Table 1. Time from referral to dialysis was significantly longer in the ER group compared to the LR group (62.3±58.9 months versus 2.9±3.4 months, P<0.001). The most common etiology of kidney failure was diabetic nephropathy in both groups. At the time of referral to a nephrologist, blood pressure (BP) was lower, renal function was better, and hemoglobin level was higher in the ER group compared to the LR group.

Table 4. Cause of death in patients.

		Total			DM ESRD		
		Early referral (N)	Late referral (N)	Sum (N)	Early referral (N)	Late referral (N)	Sum (N)
Cardiovascular disease	Myocardial infarction	0	2	2	0	2	2
	Cardiomyopathy	0	1	1	0	0	0
	Cardiac arrest, cause unknown	4	6	10	2	3	5
	Pulmonary edema	0	2	2	0	1	1
	Pulmonary embolus	0	1	1	0	0	0
	Cerebrovascular accident including intracranial hemorrhage	1	0	1	1	0	1
	Hemorrhage from ruptured vascular aneurysm	1	1	2	0	0	0
	Other hemorrhage	0	1	1	0	1	1
	Mesenteric infarction/ischemic bowel	0	1	1	0	1	1
Infection	Peritoneal access infectious complication, bacterial	0	1	1	0	0	0
	Peritoneal access infectious complication, fungal	0	1	1	0	1	1
	Peritonitis (complication of peritoneal dialysis)	0	1	1	0	0	0
	Septicemia, other	4	2	6	1	2	3
	Cardiac infection (endocarditis)	0	1	1	0	1	1
	Pulmonary infection (pneumonia, influenza)	4	6	10	2	4	6
Liver disease	Liver failure, cause unknown or other	0	1	1	0	0	0
Gastro-intestinal disease	Perforation of bowel	1	0	1	0	0	0
Other	Cachexia/failure to thrive	1	0	1	1	0	1
	Malignant disease, patient on immunosuppressive therapy	2	0	2	1	0	1
	Malignant disease	0	3	3	0	1	1
	Hyperkalemia	1	0	1	1	0	1
	Suicide	0	1	1	0	1	1
	Other cause of death	2	2	4	2	1	3
	Unknown	5	6	11	3	4	7
Sum		26	40	66	14	23	37

However, at the time of dialysis, most findings including co-morbidity index were similar in both groups, except for BP, serum phosphate, total cholesterol, and low-density lipoprotein (LDL) cholesterol. Hemoglobin level or iron status was the same for the two groups. BP was well controlled in the ER group. Serum phosphate, total cholesterol, and LDL cholesterol levels in the ER group were significantly lower than for the LR group.

There were no significant differences in clinical and laboratory characteristics at the time of dialysis between the ER group and the LR group with diabetes nephropathy as a cause of ESRD (DM ESRD), except in terms of BP and hemoglobin A1c.

Emergency HD using a temporary vascular catheter was required in 262 of 599 ER patients compared to 223 of 429 LR patients. The rate of emergency HD in ER patients was significantly lower than in LR patients (Figure 1, 43.7% versus 52.0%, P = 0.009).

Improved Survival in Early Referral Patients with End-stage Renal Disease

In the univariate analysis, late referral was significantly associated with patient mortality (HR 2.16, 95% CI 1.32–3.53, P = 0.002). Age (HR 1.07, 95% CI 1.04–1.09, P<0.001), hospitalization (HR 2.75, 95% CI 1.66–4.56, P<0.001), modified CCI (HR 1.33, 95% CI 1.22–1.46, P<0.001), DCI (HR 1.65, 95% CI 1.32–2.06, P<0.001), and eGFR (HR 1.13, 95% CI 1.06–1.20, P<0.001) were also significant risk factors associated with increased risk of death (Table 2). Variables that proved significant in the univariate analysis and referral pattern were included in the multivariate Cox proportional hazards model to determine factors associated with mortality. In the multivariate Cox analysis, late referral (HR 2.38, 95% CI 1.27–4.45, P = 0.007) and age (HR

A.

B.

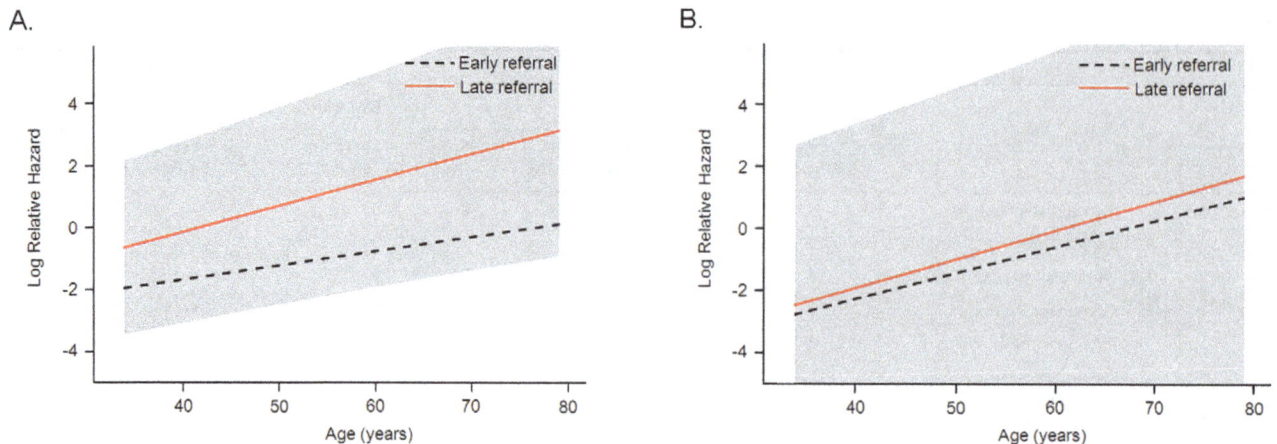

Figure 3. Relationship between log relative hazard for mortality and age according to timing of referral. (A) Total patients, adjusted for age, gender, modified CCI, BMI, eGFR, serum hemoglobin, calcium, iPTH, uric acid, triglycerides, total cholesterol, and HDL cholesterol. (B) DM ESRD patients, adjusted for age, gender, modified CCI, BMI, eGFR, serum hemoglobin, calcium, iPTH, uric acid, triglycerides, total cholesterol, and HDL cholesterol.

1.06, 95% CI 1.03–1.09, P<0.001) had an adverse association with survival (Table 3).

In the Kaplan-Meier analysis, the survival rate in ER patients was significantly better than that in LR patients after adjusting for several risk factors of model 3 (Figure 2A, P = 0.005). The 1-year and 2-year survival rates in ER patients were 97.2% and 95.7%, respectively, compared to 93.9%, and 91.3% in LR patients.

Next, we performed a subgroup analysis in the DM ESRD patients. In DM ESRD patients, age (HR 1.08, 95% CI 1.05–1.12, P<0.001), late referral (HR 2.42, 95% CI 1.26–4.64, P = 0.008), hospitalization (HR 2.07, 95% CI 1.05–4.07, P = 0.035), and modified CCI (HR 1.26, 95% CI 1.10–1.43, P = 0.001) were the univariate factors associated with increased risk of death. In the multivariate Cox analysis, late referral (HR 4.74, 95% CI 1.73–13.00, P = 0.002) and age (HR 1.08, 95% CI 1.03–1.13, P = 0.002) had an adverse association with survival (Table 3). The survival rate in ER patients was significantly higher than that in LR patients (Figure 2B, P = 0.003).

During follow-up, 66 patients (6%) died overall. Causes of death are listed in Table 4. Cardiovascular death represented the most common cause of death (32%), followed by infection (30%), unknown cause (17%), and neoplasm (8%). The remaining deaths (13%) were due to other causes (Table 4). In LR, cardiovascular death was the most common cause of death. However, infection was the most common cause of death in ER. In the Kaplan-Meier analysis, the cardiovascular death free survival rate was significantly worse in LR patients compared with ER patients in total (P = 0.004) and DM ESRD (P = 0.008). In the multivariate Cox analysis, LR (Table S1, HR 4.99, 95% CI 1.48–16.82, P = 0.009) was significant risk factors associated with cardiovascular death. Among patients with DM ESRD, LR was still significant factor associated with increased risk of cardiovascular death (Table S1, HR 26.71, 95% CI 1.49–478.99, P = 0.026).

Hospitalization-free survival rate and cardiovascular event-free survival rates were not different between ER and LR patients (data not shown).

Relationship between Mortality and Age at the Time of Referral

The relationship between age and mortality was evaluated. As the age of patients increased, the hazard ratio for death also

increased (Figure 3A). In particular, in older patients the hazard ratios for ER and LR patients were quite different, with survival rates for ER patients increasing against LR patients. This trend was observed in DM ESRD patients (Figure 3B).

Discussion

The present nationwide multi-center prospective cohort study showed that early nephrology referral in the predialytic stage of CKD improves survival rate in ESRD. Late referral remains an important predictor of mortality even after adjusting for age, gender, co-morbidity, BMI, and biochemical variables.

Previous studies on the association of the timing of referral to a nephrologist with mortality have demonstrated conflicting results. Kazmi et al. studied 2,195 patients between 1996 and 1997 and found that, compared with ER patients, LR (<4 months) patients had a 44% higher risk of death at 1 year after initiation of dialysis, which remained significant after adjusting for the quintile of the propensity score [11]. Dogan et al studied 101 patients between 1998 and 2002 and found that ER (>12 weeks) and/or early diagnosis of ESRD resulted in better biochemical variables, shorter length of first hospitalization, a higher percentage of elective construction of arteriovenous fistula, and the availability to start with an alternative dialysis modality [12]. In contrast, two studies have shown no difference in mortality between ER and LR patients. Schmidt et al showed that there was no statistically significant difference in long-term survival when ER (>1 month) patients were compared with LR patients at 4 months among 238 patients [13]. Roubicek et al showed that the referral pattern (LR <4 months) was not associated with mortality rate among 270 patients [24].

Many previous studies incorporated an observational retrospective design, and the definition of the timing of ER was different in each study. In addition, some prospective studies were of small size and/or single-center design. Furthermore, the referral timing of 3 months or more in most previous studies was too short to assess and educate patients.

In a recent study, Di Napoli et al reported that late referral patients had a lower frequency of hepatitis B virus vaccination, arteriovenous fistula and information about renal replacement therapy modalities, and they more often started chronic dialysis in an emergency [18]. They defined LR patients as those who had not been regularly referred to a nephrologist in the one year before chronic dialysis began. And, they considered a period of 12 months as adequate to describe the role of individual and health service characteristics in early access to renal services for ESRD care. In addition, de Jager DJ *et al* classified referral (time between first pre-dialysis visit to a nephrologist and dialysis initiation) as: late (<3 months), early (3–12 months) or very early (≥12 months). They reported that early and late referrals were associated with increased mortality compared with very early referral [25]. Quaglia M *et al* also mentioned that predialysis nephrology care had a much wider concept than providing the patient with a dialysis access and consequently demanded a longer time (ie, several years) to produce results, and that 3-month period before dialysis was inadequate to assess any impacts on hard end points [17].

This study is a prospective nationwide multi-center cohort study. ER was defined as a group undergoing follow-up for 12 months or longer prior to the initiation of dialysis. And, a 1-year period before dialysis was enough to control a BP, metabolic condition of patients, and provided the predialysis care for patients. Thus, this study design provides for a proper evaluation of the association between referral pattern and mortality in ESRD patients.

Our study showed that the mortality rate increased by 2.4 times during overall follow-up and this risk remained after adjusting for age, gender, and other covariates. Furthermore, we analyzed the cause of death in ESRD patients according to referral pattern. There were few researches studied about association between referral pattern and causes of death in dialysis patients. Lorenzo *et al* reported that referral pattern was no significant association with causes of death in dialysis patients [15]. However, Herget-Rosenthal *et al* showed that cardiovascular death was increased in LR versus ER (patient number, 4 versus 1) [26]. In this study, we showed the data that cardiovascular death was increased in LR versus ER, and the cardiovascular death free survival rate in ER was significantly better than that in LR. Blood pressure was well controlled in the early referral (ER) group. However, ER significantly lowered all-cause mortality and cardiovascular mortality after adjusting for systolic blood pressure in the multivariate analysis. Recently, Winkelmayer *et al* reported that estimated annual reductions in 1-year mortality rates were 0.9% (95% CI, 0.7%–1.1%) in ER (>90 days), and there was no material improvement in 1-year survival rates after dialysis initiation among 323,977 patients [5]. But, considering the duration of patients' referrals to a nephrologist, the timing of early referral (>90 days) was a short period in which to evaluate and educate ESRD patients. In the present study, with increasing age, the risk for mortality due to late referral increased in the total patient population. In particular, in older patients there was a big difference in the hazard ratio between ER and LR (<1 year) patients.

It has been reported that patient education by nephrologists before initiation of dialysis decreases the likelihood of the need for urgent dialysis, resulting in a reduction in the need for the creation of a temporary vascular access [27]. Schmidt *et al* showed that the need for emergency HD was significantly less among ER patients compared with LR patients (22% versus 90%) [13]. Our analysis also found that the likelihood of patients referred early receiving emergency HD using a temporary vascular catheter was significantly reduced. A previous study has shown that reduced use of a temporary vascular catheter is associated with decreased patient morbidity and mortality through reduced systemic infection rates [28].

Patients who are referred earlier are prepared for dialysis initiation, resulting in fewer emergent hospitalizations. Smart *et al* showed a reduction of 8.8 days (95% CI, -10.7 to -7.0 days, P<0.00001) in those referred earlier to a nephrologist [29]. However, the hospitalization-free survival rate was no different for ER and LR patients in our study.

In this study, ER patients were well educated about dialysis by a nurse or nephrologist. Furthermore, BP, serum phosphate, total cholesterol, and LDL cholesterol were well controlled in the ER group. This could reduce the cardiovascular mortality rate and all-cause mortality in ER patients. Thus, timely referral to a nephrologist at least 1 year before dialysis initiation is important to reduce mortality even in older patients. Predialysis nephrology care is a much wider concept than providing the patient with dialysis access. It is important for the nephrologist to give patients information about CKD and offer personal education about dialysis or lifestyle modification. ER provides identification and correction of reversible causes of CKD, and preparation of dialysis. Timely referral is expected to influence long-term survival in ESRD patients.

Our results are informative, but this study has a limitation. This study had a relatively short follow-up period, with a maximum of 36 months. This was a short period in which to analyze the survival in ESRD patients.

In conclusion, timely referral to a nephrologist in the predialytic stage is associated with reduced mortality.

Author Contributions

Conceived and designed the experiments: DHK JPL. Performed the experiments: YLK SWK CWY NHK YSK. Analyzed the data: MK HK. Wrote the paper: DHK YSK JPL.

References

1. Collins AJ, Foley RN, Herzog C, Chavers BM, Gilbertson D, et al. (2010) Excerpts from the US Renal Data System 2009 Annual Data Report. Am J Kidney Dis 55: S1–420, A426–427.
2. NHIC (2004) 2003 National Health Insurance Statistical Yearbook. Seoul, Korea. National Health Insurance Corporation (NHIC).
3. Jones C, Roderick P, Harris S, Rogerson M (2006) Decline in kidney function before and after nephrology referral and the effect on survival in moderate to advanced chronic kidney disease. Nephrol Dial Transplant 21: 2133–2143.
4. Stack AG (2002) Determinants of modality selection among incident US dialysis patients: results from a national study. J Am Soc Nephrol 13: 1279–1287.
5. Winkelmayer WC, Glynn RJ, Levin R, Owen W Jr, Avorn J (2001) Late referral and modality choice in end-stage renal disease. Kidney Int 60: 1547–1554.
6. Cass A, Cunningham J, Snelling P, Ayanian JZ (2003) Late referral to a nephrologist reduces access to renal transplantation. Am J Kidney Dis 42: 1043–1049.
7. Winkelmayer WC, Mehta J, Chandraker A, Owen WF Jr, Avorn J (2007) Predialysis nephrologist care and access to kidney transplantation in the United States. Am J Transplant 7: 872–879.
8. Stehman-Breen CO, Sherrard DJ, Gillen D, Caps M (2000) Determinants of type and timing of initial permanent hemodialysis vascular access. Kidney Int 57: 639–645.
9. Astor BC, Eustace JA, Powe NR, Klag MJ, Sadler JH, et al. (2001) Timing of nephrologist referral and arteriovenous access use: the CHOICE Study. Am J Kidney Dis 38: 494–501.

10. Avorn J, Winkelmayer WC, Bohn RL, Levin R, Glynn RJ, et al. (2002) Delayed nephrologist referral and inadequate vascular access in patients with advanced chronic kidney failure. J Clin Epidemiol 55: 711–716.

11. Kazmi WH, Obrador GT, Khan SS, Pereira BJ, Kausz AT (2004) Late nephrology referral and mortality among patients with end-stage renal disease: a propensity score analysis. Nephrol Dial Transplant 19: 1808–1814.

12. Dogan E, Erkoc R, Sayarlioglu H, Durmus A, Topal C (2005) Effects of late referral to a nephrologist in patients with chronic renal failure. Nephrology (Carlton) 10: 516–519.

13. Schmidt RJ, Domico JR, Sorkin MI, Hobbs G (1998) Early referral and its impact on emergent first dialyses, health care costs, and outcome. Am J Kidney Dis 32: 278–283.

14. Curtis BM, Barret BJ, Jindal K, Djurdjev O, Levin A, et al. (2002) Canadian survey of clinical status at dialysis initiation 1998–1999: a multicenter prospective survey. Clin Nephrol 58: 282–288.

15. Lorenzo V, Martn M, Rufino M, Hernandez D, Torres A, et al. (2004) Predialysis nephrologic care and a functioning arteriovenous fistula at entry are associated with better survival in incident hemodialysis patients: an observational cohort study. Am J Kidney Dis 43: 999–1007.

16. Winkelmayer WC, Liu J, Chertow GM, Tamura MK (2011) Predialysis nephrology care of older patients approaching end-stage renal disease. Arch Intern Med 171: 1371–1378.

17. Quaglia M, Canavese C, Stratta P (2011) Early nephrology referral: how early is early enough? Arch Intern Med 171: 2065–2066; author reply 2067.

18. Di Napoli A, Valle S, d'Adamo G, Pezzotti P, Chicca S, et al. (2010) Survey of determinants and effects of timing of referral to a nephrologist: the patient's point of view. J Nephrol 23: 603–613.

19. Levey AS, Bosch JP, Lewis JB, Greene T, Rogers N, et al. (1999) A more accurate method to estimate glomerular filtration rate from serum creatinine: a new prediction equation. Modification of Diet in Renal Disease Study Group. Ann Intern Med 130: 461–470.

20. (2012) Comprehensive Prospective Study of Clinical Research Center for End Stage Renal Disease (CRC ESRD). Available: http://webdb.crc-esrd.or.kr. Accessed July.

21. Charlson ME, Pompei P, Ales KL, MacKenzie CR (1987) A new method of classifying prognostic comorbidity in longitudinal studies: development and validation. J Chronic Dis 40: 373–383.

22. Chae JW, Song CS, Kim H, Lee KB, Seo BS, et al. (2011) Prediction of mortality in patients undergoing maintenance hemodialysis by Charlson Comorbidity Index using ICD-10 database. Nephron Clin Pract 117: c379–384.

23. Davies SJ, Russell L, Bryan J, Phillips L, Russell GI (1995) Comorbidity, urea kinetics, and appetite in continuous ambulatory peritoneal dialysis patients: their interrelationship and prediction of survival. Am J Kidney Dis 26: 353–361.

24. Roubicek C, Brunet P, Huiart L, Thirion X, Leonetti F, et al. (2000) Timing of nephrology referral: influence on mortality and morbidity. Am J Kidney Dis 36: 35–41.

25. de Jager DJ, Voormolen N, Krediet RT, Dekker FW, Boeschoten EW, et al. (2011) Association between time of referral and survival in the first year of dialysis in diabetics and the elderly. Nephrol Dial Transplant 26: 652–658.

26. Herget-Rosenthal S, Quellmann T, Linden C, Hollenbeck M, Jankowski V, et al. (2010) How does late nephrological co-management impact chronic kidney disease? – an observational study. Int J Clin Pract 64: 1784–1792.

27. Inaguma D, Tatematsu M, Shinjo H, Suzuki S, Mishima T, et al. (2006) Effect of an educational program on the predialysis period for patients with chronic renal failure. Clin Exp Nephrol 10: 274–278.

28. Lemaire X, Morena M, Leray-Moragues H, Henriet-Viprey D, Chenine L, et al. (2009) Analysis of risk factors for catheter-related bacteremia in 2000 permanent dual catheters for hemodialysis. Blood Purif 28: 21–28.

29. Smart NA, Titus TT (2011) Outcomes of early versus late nephrology referral in chronic kidney disease: a systematic review. Am J Med 124: 1073–1080 e1072.

10

Predicting Progression of IgA Nephropathy: New Clinical Progression Risk Score

Jingyuan Xie[1,2,9], Krzysztof Kiryluk[2,9], Weiming Wang[1], Zhaohui Wang[1], Shanmai Guo[1], Pingyan Shen[1], Hong Ren[1], Xiaoxia Pan[1], Xiaonong Chen[1], Wen Zhang[1], Xiao Li[1], Hao Shi[1], Yifu Li[2], Ali G. Gharavi[2]*, Nan Chen[1]*

1 Nephrology Department, Ruijin Hospital, Shanghai Jiao Tong University School of Medicine, Shanghai, China, 2 Division of Nephrology, Department of Medicine, College of Physicians and Surgeons, Columbia University, New York, New York, United States of America

Abstract

IgA nephropathy (IgAN) is a common cause of end-stage renal disease (ESRD) in Asia. In this study, based on a large cohort of Chinese patients with IgAN, we aim to identify independent predictive factors associated with disease progression to ESRD. We collected retrospective clinical data and renal outcomes on 619 biopsy-diagnosed IgAN patients with a mean follow-up time of 41.3 months. In total, 67 individuals reached the study endpoint defined by occurrence of ESRD necessitating renal replacement therapy. In the fully adjusted Cox proportional hazards model, there were four baseline variables with a significant independent effect on the risk of ESRD. These included: eGFR [HR = 0.96(0.95–0.97)], serum albumin [HR = 0.47(0.32–0.68)], hemoglobin [HR = 0.79(0.72–0.88)], and SBP [HR = 1.02(1.00–1.03)]. Based on these observations, we developed a 4-variable equation of a clinical risk score for disease progression. Our risk score explained nearly 22% of the total variance in the primary outcome. Survival ROC curves revealed that the risk score provided improved prediction of ESRD at 24th, 60th and 120th month of follow-up compared to the three previously proposed risk scores. In summary, our data indicate that IgAN patients with higher systolic blood pressure, lower eGFR, hemoglobin, and albumin levels at baseline are at a greatest risk of progression to ESRD. The new progression risk score calculated based on these four baseline variables offers a simple clinical tool for risk stratification.

Editor: Ivan Cruz Moura, Institut national de la santé et de la recherche médicale (INSERM), France

Funding: This work was supported by the National Basic Research Program of China 973 Program No.2012CB517600 (No.2012CB517604), the National Natural Science Foundation of China (No. 81000295). XJ is supported by the Schrier Family Fellowship from the International Society of Nephrology (ISN). KK is supported by the National Institutes of Health grant K23DK090207 (NIDDK). This work was also supported by the Leading Academic Discipline Project of Shanghai Health Bureau (05III 001 and 2003ZD002) and Shanghai Leading Academic Discipline Project (T0201). The funders had no role in study design, data collection and analysis, decision to publish, or preparation of the manuscript.

Competing Interests: The authors have declared that no competing interests exist.

* E-mail: ag2239@columbia.edu (AG); cnrj100@126.com (NC)

9 These authors contributed equally to this work.

Introduction

IgA nephropathy (IgAN) is the most common form of primary glomerulonephritis (GN) worldwide [1]. The disease is characterized by a highly variable clinical course ranging from a benign condition to a rapidly progressive irreversible kidney failure. About 15 to 40 percent of IgAN patients will develop worsening renal dysfunction and eventually end stage renal disease (ESRD) within 10–20 years of diagnosis [2,3,4]. A major challenge in the field is the identification of individuals at highest risk of progression to ESRD. Notably, IgAN is most prevalent in Asia, and studies suggest that the disease may have a more severe course in individuals of Asian ancestry [5,6]. Thus, studies based on Asian populations may be more effective in identifying risk factors for progression.

Numerous prior studies identified several potential clinical predictors of progression, including degree of renal impairment at diagnosis [2,7,8,9], histologic grading [2,7,8,9,10] and proteinuria [10,11,12]_ENREF_8. These factors appear to contribute independently to the risk of progression in multivariate models. Moreover, some studies suggest an independent prognostic value of high blood pressure at presentation [6,7,10] ?r during follow-up [12], hematuria [9], family history of hypertension [7] or chronic renal failure [9], serum albumin level [9,13], age [9], and male gender [9].

One of the problems in the field is that several of the above predictors reflect the degree of disease severity on presentation and are thus strongly inter-correlated. Their individual contribution to the overall risk of progression is difficult to assess without powerful and well-characterized patient cohorts. In addition, the overall predictive value of these variables is relatively low. The development of a risk score that reflects cumulative effects of individual predictors may be helpful to identify individuals that are most likely to progress to ESRD. This approach has been successfully utilized in the RENAAL study of 1,513 type 2 diabetics with nephropathy [14]. Based on the longitudinal data from this study, a relatively simple risk score was proposed that incorporates serum creatinine, albumin, hemoglobin, and urine albumin-to-creatinine ratio into an equation that accurately determines the risk of progression to ESRD. Another powerful example of this approach is provided by a large-scale progression study of all-cause chronic kidney disease (CKD) [15]. Here, the most accurate model that predicted ESRD included age, sex,

Table 1. Baseline characteristics of IgAN patients.

Variable	IgAN Patients, N = 619
Follow-up mean (scope), [month]	41.3 (3.03–248.1)
Age at biopsy (±s.d.), [years]	36.0±12.3
Gender (Male: Female)	1.03:1.00
Family history of chronic kidney disease (%)	78 (12.6)
Body mass index mean (±s.d.), [kg/m^2]	23.0±3.5
Serum creatinine mean (±s.d.), [mg/dL]	1.5±1.1
GFR mean (±s.d.), [mL/min/1.73 m^2]	87.9±44.4
CKD stage 1 (%)	289 (46.7)
CKD stage 2 (%)	135 (21.8)
CKD stage 3 (%)	145 (23.4)
CKD stage 4 (%)	38 (6.1)
CKD stage 5 (%)	12 (1.9)
SBP mean (±s.d.), [mm Hg]	128.2±18.9
DBP mean (±s.d.), [mm Hg]	82.5±13.0
MAP mean (±s.d.), [mm Hg]	97.7±14.1
Pulse pressure mean (±s.d.), [mm Hg]	45.7±12.1
Hypertension (%)	290 (46.9)
Urine protein median (scope), [g/24 h]	1.42 (0–13.9)
Urine protein groups	
Mild (<1 g/24 h) (%)	237 (38.3)
Moderate (1~3 g/24 h) (%)	254 (41)
Severe (>=3 g/24 h) (%)	128 (20.7)
Gross hematuria (%)	125 (20.2)
Serum UA mean (±s.d.), [mg/dl]	6.5±1.7
Hyperuricemia (%)	256 (41.4)
Serum albumin mean (±s.d.), [g/dL]	3.4±0.8
Hypoalbuminemia (%)	128 (20.7)
Serum triglycerides median (scope), [mg/dL]	175.7(42.5–1033.6)
Serum cholesterol median (scope), [mg/dL]	198.1(32.1–469.1)
Hemoglobin mean (±s.d.), [g/dl]	13.0±2.2
Anemia (%)	261 (42.2)
WBC mean (±s.d.), [10^3/mm^3]	7.7±2.7
Serum IgA mean (±s.d.), [mg/L]	3238.5±1422.9
Haas classification	
Grade I (%)	16(2.6)
Grade II (%)	136(22)
Grade III (%)	251(40.5)
Grade IV (%)	130(21)
Grade V (%)	86(13.9)
ACEI or ARB treatment (%)	368(67.8%)
Glucocorticoid treatment (%)	293(54.7)

SBP: systolic blood pressure;
DBP: diastolic blood pressure;
MAP: mean arterial pressure;
UA: uric acid;
WBC: white blood cell count.

Table 2. Univariate analysis of baseline variables with renal end points for ESRD.

Predictor	IgAN Patients, N = 619		
	HR	95% CI	P value
Age at biopsy [year]	1.02[#]	1.01–1.04	4*10^{-2}
Female Gender	0.69	0.42–1.13	0.14
Family history	0.75	0.37–1.52	0.42
Body mass index [kg/m^2]	0.94	0.82–1.09	0.41
Serum creatinine [mg/dL]	2.30[#]	2.03–2.61	<2.0*10^{-16}
eGFR [mL/min/1.73 m^2]	0.95[#]	0.94–0.96	<2.0*10^{-16}
eGFR [<60 to >=60 mL/min/1.73 m^2]	7.91[#]	4.60–13.6	7.6*10^{-14}
SBP [mm Hg]	1.03[#]	1.02–1.04	1.2*10^{-7}
SBP [>=140 to <140 mmHg]	2.85[#]	1.76–4.63	2.3*10^{-5}
DBP [mm Hg]	1.04[#]	1.02–1.06	7.5*10^{-6}
DBP [>=90 to <90 mmHg]	2.90[#]	1.76–4.77	2.9*10^{-5}
MAP [mm Hg]	1.04[#]	1.03–1.06	3.6*10^{-7}
Pulse pressure [mm Hg]	1.03[#]	1.01–1.05	5.5*10^{-4}
Hypertension	3.59[#]	2.07–6.23	5.7*10^{-6}
Urine protein [g/24 h]	1.12[#]	1.03–1.21	6.9*10^{-3}
Degree of proteinuria [per group]	2.28[#]	1.64–3.18	1.0*10^{-6}
Gross hematuria	0.57	0.31–1.06	0.07
Serum UA [mg/dl]	1.40[#]	1.23–1.60	6.1*10^{-7}
Hyperuricemia	2.11[#]	1.29–3.45	2.9*10^{-3}
Serum albumin [g/dL]	0.60[#]	0.45–0.79	2.3*10^{-4}
Hypoalbuminemia	2.45[#]	1.48–4.07	5.0*10^{-4}
Serum triglycerides [mg/dL]	1.00	0.99–1.00	0.64
Serum cholesterol [mg/dL]	1.00	0.99–1.01	0.15
Hemoglobin [g/dl]	0.75[#]	0.69–0.82	2.0*10^{-11}
Anemia	4.98[#]	2.80–8.85	4.8*10^{-8}
WBC [10^3/mm^3]	0.90	0.72–1.13	0.38
Serum IgA [mg/L]	1.00	0.99–1.00	0.99
Haas classification	2.71[#]	2.05–3.57	2.1*10^{-12}
ACEI or ARB treatment (%)	0.71	0.42–1.20	0.21
Glucocorticoid treatment	1.52	0.95–2.40	0.10

SBP: systolic blood pressure;
DBP: diastolic blood pressure;
MAP: mean arterial pressure;
UA: uric acid;
WBC: white blood cell count.
# p<0.05.

eGFR, albuminuria, as well as basic serum measurements of calcium, phosphate, bicarbonate, and albumin. This model was further validated in an independent cohort of 4,942 patients with an estimated C-statistic of 0.84 (95%CI 0.83–0.86).

To date, there have been two studies that applied a similar approach to the prediction of ESRD in patients with newly diagnosed IgAN: the study by Berthoux et al. of 332 French patients followed for a median of 136 months [10] and the study by Goto et al. of 2,283 Japanese patients followed for a median of 87 months [9]. The French study derived a 3-variable risk score (based on hypertension, proteinuria, and a histology score), while the Japanese study derived an 8-variable score (based on age, gender, hypertension, proteinuria, hematuria, hypoalbuminacmia, eGFR, and histological grade). The performance of these risk scores, however, has not yet been validated in independent cohorts.

In this study, we systematically evaluate the predictive value of a complete set of baseline clinical and laboratory factors in the

Table 3. Multivariate Cox Regression with Stepwise Selection (n = 619).

Variable	Coefficient	HR (95%CI)	R² (%)	P-value
Model 1* (events = 67)				
eGFR [ml/min/1.73 m²]	−0.039	0.96 (0.95–0.97)	16.3	$1.3*10^{-14}$
Hemoglobin [g/dL]	−0.230	0.79 (0.72–0.88)	6.4	$1.2*10^{-5}$
Serum albumin [g/dL]	−0.762	0.47 (0.32–0.68)	1.9	$7.4*10^{-5}$
SBP [mmHg]	0.016	1.02 (1.00–1.03)	3.7	$5.4*10^{-3}$
Risk Score #		2.73 (2.27–3.28)	21.9	$<2*10^{-16}$
Model 2** (events = 85)				
eGFR [ml/min/1.73 m²]	−0.018	0.98 (0.98–0.99)	7.5	$1.6*10^{-8}$
Hemoglobin [g/dL]	−0.206	0.81 (0.75–0.89)	6.5	$1.5*10^{-6}$
Serum albumin [g/dL]	−0.769	0.46 (0.35–0.62)	3.2	$2.7*10^{-7}$
SBP [mmHg]	0.015	1.02 (1.00–1.03)	3.0	$6.4*10^{-3}$
Risk Score #		1.78 (1.56–2.02)	14.0	$<2*10^{-16}$

SBP: systolic blood pressure.
*Renal outcome defined as end-stage renal disease (ESRD).
**Renal outcome defined as 50% decline from baseline eGFR.
The risk score was calculated from the coefficients of independent risk factors in model 1.

progression of renal disease in a large cohort of IgAN patients from Shanghai, China. We formulate a new 4-variable risk score equation that best predicts renal disease progression in our cohort. We also compare the performance of our Risk Score to the French and the Japanese progression scores, as well as to the risk score based on the RENAAL study.

Methods

Ethics Statement

This study was approved by the Institutional Review Board of the Ruijin Hospital, Shanghai Jiao Tong University School of Medicine and was in accordance with the principle of the Helsinki Declaration II. The written informed consent was obtained from each participant.

Study Population and Clinical Data

To identify cases eligible to participate in the study, we reviewed all kidney biopsy reports of Shanghai Jiao Tong University Ruijin Hospital, a major referral center for Southern China, between years 1989 and 2010. All cases included in the study were defined by dominant and at least 2+ (on a scale from 0 to 3+) mesangial staining for IgA by immunoflorescence, in addition to compatible findings of mesangial expansion or proliferation on light microscopy. The patients with systemic diseases, such as systemic lupus erythematosus, Henoch-Schonlein purpura, and chronic liver disease were excluded from this analysis. We also recruited a large group of age and gender matched healthy controls from the Ruijin Hospital Health Care Center defined by the absence of abnormalities on a routine urinalysis and normal renal function (serum creatinine <1.1 mg/dL).

In total, 619 individuals fulfilled our diagnostic criteria for IgAN and had a minimum of 3 months of follow-up data available for analysis. Baseline demographic and clinical data were collected from all patients at the time of renal biopsy. These included: age, gender, body mass index (BMI), serum creatinine, serum uric acid (UA), triglyceride levels, cholesterol levels, hemoglobin (Hb), systolic blood pressure (SBP), diastolic blood pressure (DBP), family history of kidney disease, history of gross hematuria, serum

immunoglobulin A (IgA) levels, and 24-hour protein excretion. The diagnosis of hypertension was based on SBP≥140 mmHg, or DBP≥90 mmHg, or history of antihypertensive medication use. Hyperuricemia was defined by gender-specific criteria of serum UA >450 umol/L in males and >340 umol/L in females. Anemia was defined by gender-specific criteria of hemoglobin concentrations <13.5 g/dL in males and <12 g/dL in females. Hypoalbuminemia was defined by serum albumin <3 g/dL. Estimated glomerular filtration rate (eGFR) was evaluated by an abbreviated Modification of Diet in Renal Disease (MDRD) equation modified for Chinese: eGFR (ml/min/1.73 m²) = $186*Pcr^{-1.154}*age^{-0.203}*0.742$(if female)*1.233 [16]. Chronic kidney disease (CKD) was classified based to the Kidney Disease Outcomes Quality Initiative (K/DOQI) practice guidelines [17]. Most patients were treated according to the accepted standards at our center: IgAN patients with hypertension and/or proteinuria were treated with ACE inhibitors (ACEI) and/or angiotensin receptor blockers (ARB). Glucocortoids were added in individuals with a new onset of massive proteinuria, and proteinuric patients who did not respond to an ACEI or ARB therapy. Patients with crescentic disease and rapidly progressive glomerulonephritis were treated with combined immunosuppressive agents and glucocorticoids. The mean follow-up time after renal biopsy was 41.3 months (range 3.03–248.1 months).

Statistical Methods

The distributions of quantitative variables were assessed for normality and summarized as means and standard deviations (or medians and ranges for non-normally distributed variables). Statistical testing of continuous variables was performed using Student's t-test (or Mann-Whitney U-test if appropriate). All categorical variables were expressed as frequencies or percentages (%) and comparison of proportions was performed using a standard X^2 test. Baseline clinical variables included sex, age, family history, BMI, baseline serum creatinine, eGFR, SBP, DBP, mean arterial pressure, pulse pressure, urine protein, gross hematuria, serum UA, serum albumin, serum triglycerides, serum cholesterol, hemoglobin, platelets, WBC, serum IgA, Haas classification, and treatment type. All slides of kidney biopsies were reviewed by a single experienced

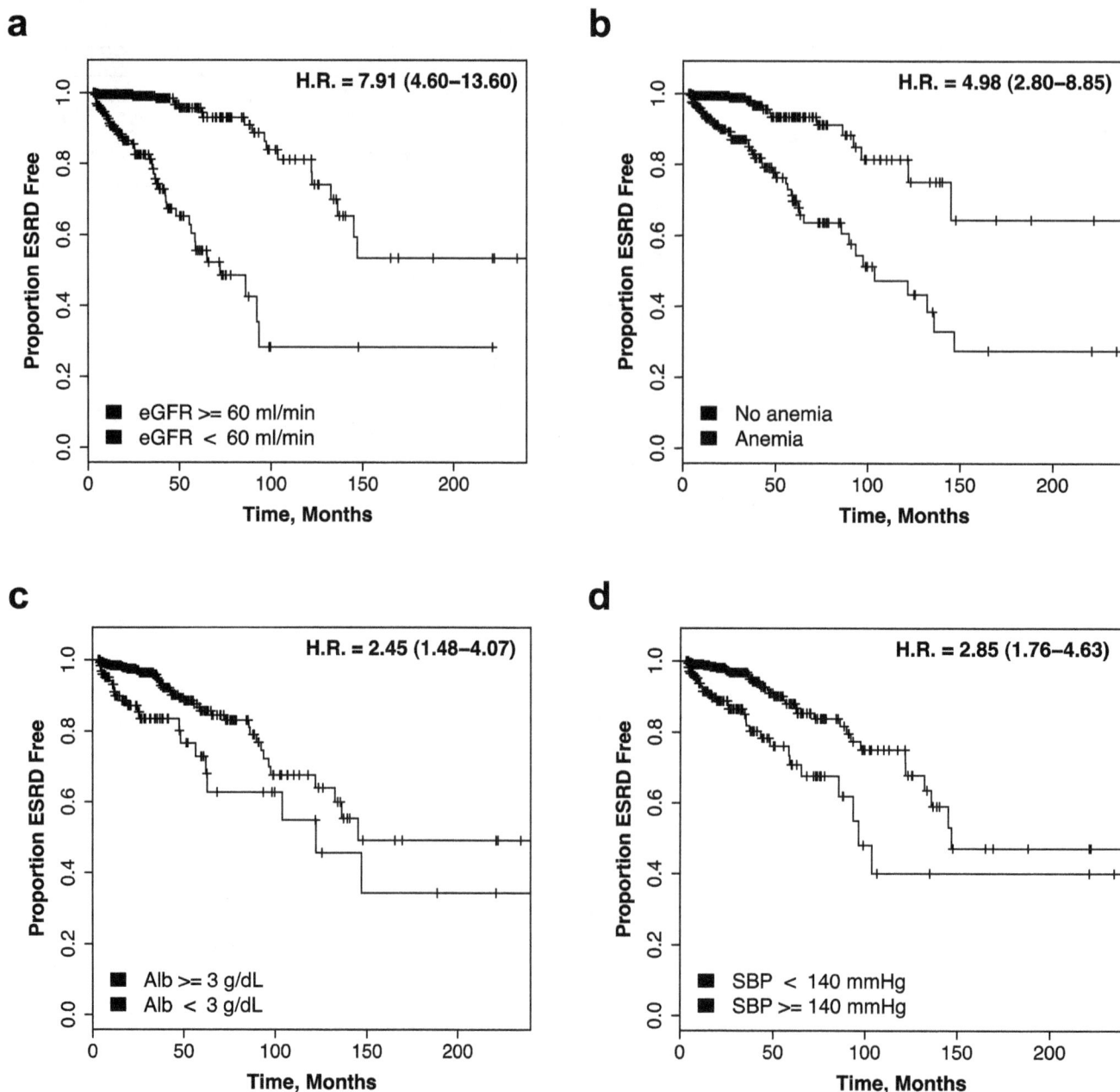

Figure 1. Kaplan-Meier Outcome-free Survival Curves. (a) low (red) versus high (black) baseline eGFR group; **(b)** patients with a baseline diagnosis of anemia (red) versus no anemia (black); **(c)** patients with hypoalbuminemia (red) versus normoalbuminemia (black); **(d)** patients with systolic hypertension (red) versus normotensives (black). Censor points are denoted by vertical tick lines.

renal pathologist. The primary outcome was defined as occurrence of ESRD defined by a need for renal replacement therapy (dialysis or renal transplantation). The association of baseline variables with the primary outcome was tested using Cox regression proportional hazards models. A two sided P<0.05 was considered statistically significant. To identify independent predictors of progression, we performed a multivariate Cox regression analysis with a stepwise selection of variables (entry and elimination P<0.05). Patients were censored at the time of death or loss to follow-up. The proportional hazards assumption was formally tested for each of the outcomes using the method proposed by Grambsch and Therneau [18] and implemented in the R survival package version 2.36 (R v.2.9). The independent predictors retained in the final model were used to

derive the Risk Score. The effects of each independent predictor, as well as their cumulative effect in the form of the Risk Score were next tested using the Kaplan-Meier approach. We also scored our patients using the Japanese [9], the French [10] and the RENAAL [14] risk scores. The R^2 (reflecting the fraction of variance in the primary outcome explained) was determined for each of the models [19]. In addition, survival areas under receiver operating characteristic (ROC) curves were also assessed for the 24th, 60th and 120th month time points. These analyses were performed using Survcomp [20] package version 1.1.6 (R v.2.9) and ROCR package version 1.0–2 (R v.2.9) [21]. Based on the size and median follow-up of our cohort, we estimate 80% power to detect hazard ratios greater than

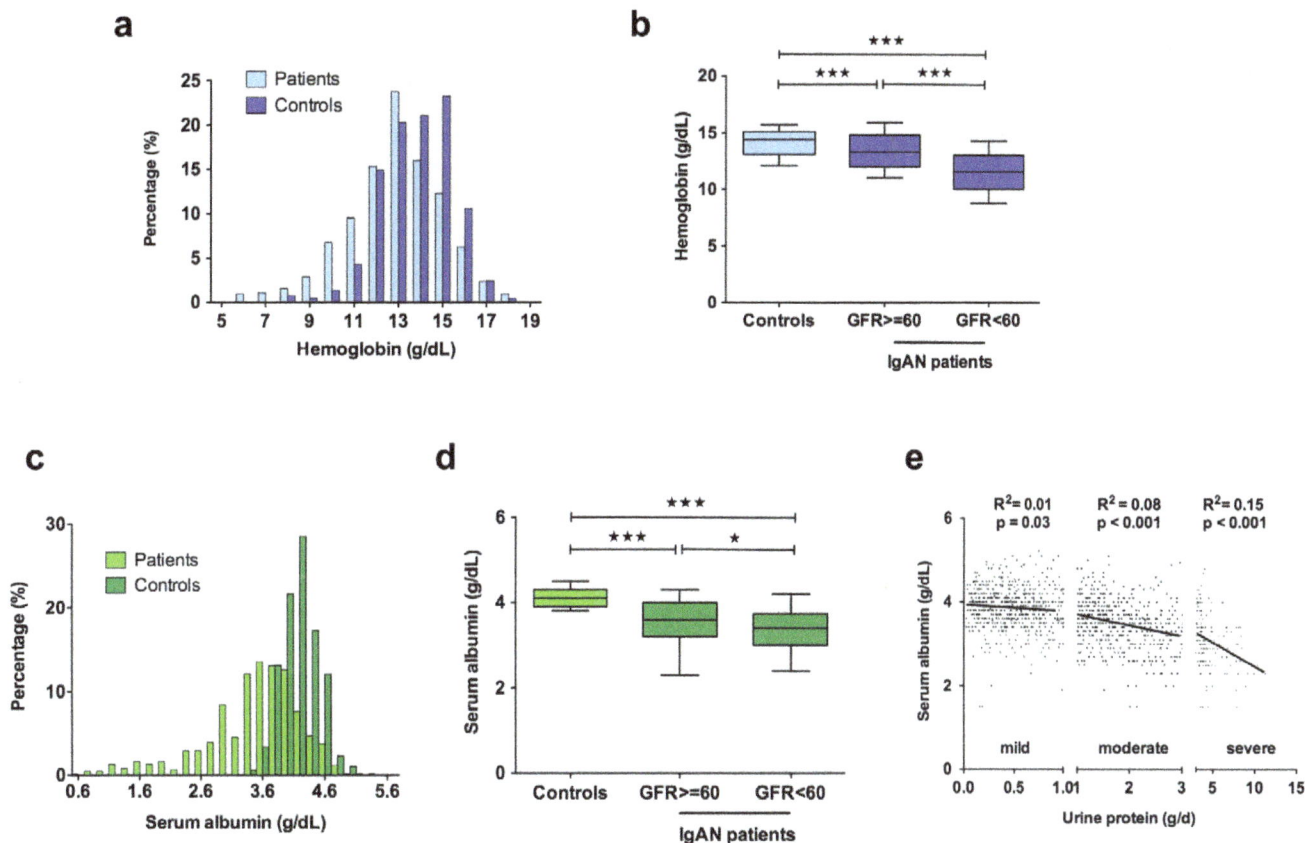

Figure 2. Detailed Analysis of Hemoglobin and Serum Albumin Levels. (a) the distributions of hemoglobin levels for IgAN patients and healthy controls; **(b)** hemoglobin levels by the degree of renal impairment; **(c)** serum albumin distributions in IgAN patients and healthy controls; **(d)** serum albumin levels by the degree of renal impairment; **(e)** correlation between serum albumin and urine protein excretion by three different groups of proteinuria. Significance code: * p<0.05, ** p<0.01, *** p<0.001.

1.4 in this study. Our power calculations were performed with the PS software version 3.0 [22].

Results

Baseline Demographic and Clinical Data

We analyzed clinical data from a total of 619 IgAN patients (Table 1). There were 314 males and 305 females in the study; the average age was 36±12 years. Of all the IgAN patients, 78 (12.6%) had positive family history of chronic kidney disease. Most IgAN patients had moderate to severe pathology grade at diagnosis (75.4% with Haas III-V). Moreover, 46.9% were hypertensive, 61.7% had urine protein higher than 1 g/24 h, and 20.2% reported history of gross hematuria (Table 1). We first explored the associations of clinical variables with baseline renal function (eGFR). In univariate analyses, 17 of 25 baseline clinical variables correlated with the degree of renal impairment at the time of biopsy (Table S1). In multivariate analysis, older age [beta = -1.06, p<$2.0*10^{-16}$], higher degree of proteinuria [beta = -5.18, p = $2*10^{-3}$], elevated UA [beta = -8.23, p<$2.0*10^{-16}$], higher Haas grade [beta = -11.3, p = <$2.0*10^{-16}$), lower hemoglobin, [beta = 2.90, p = $9*10^{-7}$] and increased SBP [beta = -0.37, p = $2*10^{-7}$] were independently associated with lower eGFR at the time of biopsy (Table S2).

Predictors of Progression in IgAN

In total, 67 individuals reached the study endpoint defined as occurrence of ESRD. In univariate analyses, 21 of 30 baseline variables were significantly associated with this outcome (Table 2). In the multivariate stepwise Cox proportional hazards models, only four baseline variables had a significant, independent effect on the risk of ESRD (Model 1): baseline eGFR [HR = 0.96, 95% CI 0.95–0.97, p = $1.3*10^{-14}$], serum albumin [HR = 0.47, 95% CI 0.32–0.68, p = $7.4*10^{-5}$], hemoglobin [HR = 0.79, 95% CI 0.72–0.88, p = $1.2*10^{-5}$], and SBP [HR = 1.02, 95% CI 1.00–1.03, p = $5.4*10^{-3}$] (Table 3). Similarly, the same four variables were also highly significant independent predictors of eGFR decline (defined as 50% reduction from the baseline eGFR) in our cohort (Model 2): baseline eGFR [HR = 0.98, 95% CI 0.98–0.99, p = $1.6*10^{-8}$], serum albumin [HR = 0.46, 95% CI 0.35–0.62, p = $2.7*10^{-7}$], hemoglobin [HR = 0.81, 95% CI 0.75–0.89, p = $1.5*10^{-6}$], and SBP [HR = 1.02, 95% CI 1.00–1.03, p = $6.4*10^{-3}$]. We also explored all pairwise interactions and considered quadratic terms in these models, but none these alternative analyses provided a better fit to the data.

As expected, eGFR at presentation was the strongest predictor of ESRD: each unit decrease in baseline eGFR was associated with 4% increase in the risk of ESRD during the follow-up period. Accordingly, individuals with baseline eGFR $\geq$60 ml/min/1.73 m^2 had considerably longer median outcome-free survival time when compared to those with eGFR <60 ml/min/1.73 m^2

a

b

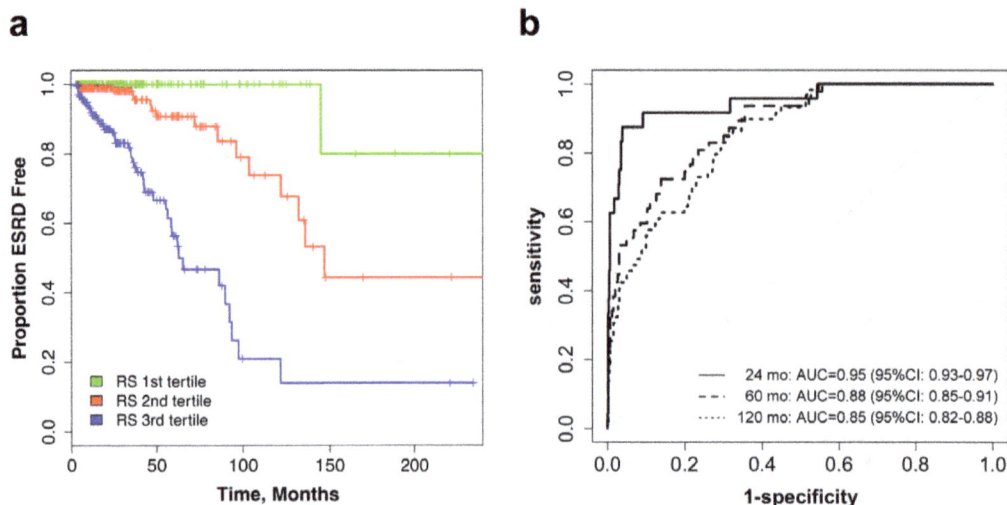

Figure 3. Survival and Survival ROC curves for the Risk Score. (a) Kaplan-Meier outcome-free survival curves by risk score tertiles; **(b)** the Risk Score's ROC curves for predicting ESRD at 24 months, 60 months and 120 months.

(242 months versus 72 months) [HR = 7.91, 95%CI: 4.60–13.60, Figure 1A].

On average, the cases were three times more likely to fulfill our diagnostic criteria for anemia compared to the healthy population controls (42.2% vs. 14.5%) (Table S3). Each unit drop in hemoglobin was associated with 20% increase in the risk of ESRD. Median outcome-free survival times were 104 and 247 months in individuals with and without the diagnosis of anemia, respectively [HR = 4.98, 95% CI 2.80–8.85, Figure 1B]. In addition to the risk of ESRD, anemia was associated with male sex, older age, lower eGFR, higher SBP, more severe proteinuria, higher uric acid level, lower albumin level, and more severe Haas class (Table S4). Individuals with low hemoglobin levels were also more frequently treated with glucocorticoids.

The patients with hypoalbuminemia had a shorter median ESRD-free survival of 122 months, compared to 145 months for those with normal albumin levels [HR = 2.45, 95% CI 1.48–4.07, Figure 1C]. Serum albumin was strongly correlated with daily protein excretion (Figure 2C-E, Table S4). Surprisingly, proteinuria did not independently contribute to the risk of ESRD in multivariate analysis. We formally explored if albumin and/or hemoglobin account for the effect of proteinuria in the final risk model (Table S5). The exclusion of albumin from the full model unmasked highly significant association of proteinuria with the risk of progression (HR 1.56, $p = 9.7 \times 10^{-3}$), but at the cost of overall reduction in the model's goodness of fit. This suggests that albumin is a superior predictor of outcome and captures most of the variance contributed by proteinuria.

Progression Risk Score

Next we developed a risk score for disease progression based on the regression coefficients for the four independent predictors retained in the best model (Table 3). The risk score equation is provided by the following formula:

$$RiskScore = 6.932 - 0.039 * (eGFR[ml/min/1.73m]) - 0.230 * (Hb[g/dL]) - 0.762 * (serumalbumin[g/dL]) + 0.016 * (SBP[mmHg]).$$

When considered in a stepwise multivariate analysis with all 21 other baseline variables at entry, the risk score was the only independent predictor of adverse renal outcome. It conveyed 2.7-fold increase in the risk of ESRD per one score unit [HR = 2.73, 95%CI: 2.27–3.28] and explained 21.9% of the total variance in the primary outcome. The median ESRD-free survival times for the lowest, middle, and highest tertiles of the Risk Score were 247, 147, and 65 months, respectively. Accordingly, when compared to the first tertile, individuals in the second Risk Score tertile had a 15-fold increase in the risk of ESRD [HR = 15.3, 95%CI: 2.0–115.0)], while individuals in the highest tertile had over 79-fold risk increase [HR = 79.8, 95%CI 11.0–580.3] (Figure 3A and Table S6).

Survival ROC analysis revealed that the risk score provided considerably improved discriminative power at 24, 60 and 120 months of follow-up compared to individual predictors. The area under the survival ROC curves was estimated at 0.95 (95%CI: 0.93–0.97) at 24 months, 0.88 (95% CI: 0.85–0.91) at 60 months, and 0.85 (95%CI: 0.82–0.88) at 120 months of follow-up. Impressively, at the cutoff point of 3.27, the Risk Score's sensitivity and specificity of predicting ESRD within 2 years of diagnosis were 87.5% and 96.0%, respectively (Figure 3B).

Next, we compared the performance of the three other published risk scores in predicting ESRD in our dataset (Figure 4). The Goto et al. Japanese progression score performed better compared to the Berthoux et al. and the RENAAL scores, with the AUC of 0.93, 0.87 and 0.82 at 24, 60, and 120 months of follow-up, respectively. This score explained 14.4%, 17.9% and 18.3% of variance in the primary outcome for each respective follow-up period. The performance of the Goto et al. score was only slightly worse compared to the Risk Score derived in our study (AUC of 0.95, 0.88, and 0.85; variance explained: 16.2%, 20.3% and 22.3%). The RENAAL risk score provided slightly less accurate prediction compared to the Goto et al. score, with respective AUCs of 0.92, 0.85, and 0.79. These differences in performance are likely due to the fact that this score was originally derived for patients with diabetic nephropathy. Finally, the risk score proposed by Berthoux et al. was considerably less accurate, with respective AUCs of 0.77, 0.75 and 0.73.

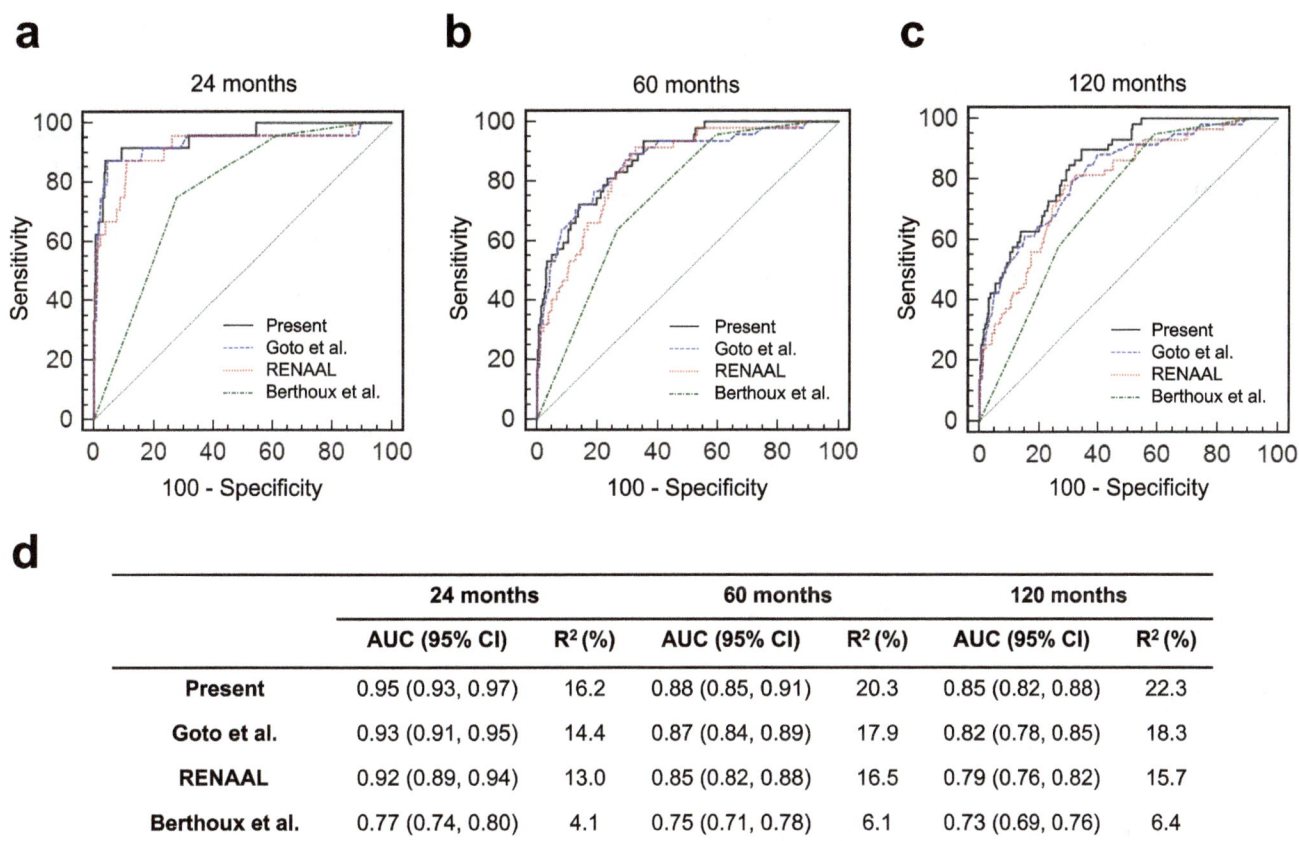

Figure 4. Performance of the Published ESRD Prediction Scores. The ROC curves for predicting renal outcomes within (a) 24 months, (b) 60 months, and (c) 120 months of follow-up. The Risk Score from this study (black) is contrasted against the Goto et al. score (blue), RENAAL score (red) and the Berthoux et al. score (green); (d) comparisons of AUCs (and their 95% CIs) and R^2 for the four risk score prediction models.

Discussion

IgAN is a progressive disease with high variability of clinical presentation and outcomes [23]. Presently, clinician's ability to identify patients at a highest risk of progression is limited. Such patients, however, are more likely to benefit from early or more aggressive therapy. In this study, we systematically test a complete set of over 28 baseline clinical parameters in multivariate models to detect independent predictors of renal disease progression. This is one of the largest observational studies of IgAN, involving over 600 patients. Accordingly, we are well powered to detect relatively small effect sizes. Other strengths of our study include: homogenous patient cohort, uniform histology scoring of renal biopsies, and application of a robust definition of progression (ESRD requiring renal replacement therapy).

To our knowledge, our study is the first to identify hemoglobin level as an independent risk factor for progression of IgAN. In the adjusted models, each 1 g/dL drop in hemoglobin was associated with 20% increase in the risk of renal progression. Additionally, hemoglobin levels explained nearly 6.4% of variance in renal outcome. Anemia is a common complication of CKD that has recently emerged as an important independent risk factor for kidney disease progression [24,25]. For example, in the RENNAL cohort, baseline hemoglobin concentration was inversely correlated with the risk of ESRD, with the average increase in the risk of 11% per each 1 g/dL decline in hemoglobin levels after adjustment for baseline renal function and other covariates. The exact mechanism that underlies these observations is not clear. It is possible that anemia has a direct causal effect on the deterioration of renal function. Alternatively, this association may reflect the severity of underlying systemic inflammation, or may mark additional kidney damage that is not yet reflected by a decline in eGFR.

In addition to hemoglobin levels, our study provides strong support for predictive value of serum albumin in the assessment of ESRD risk. Serum albumin is widely recognized as a biomarker of nutritional status and inflammation, but it is also closely correlated with age, proteinuria, and hemoglobin levels (Figure 3C-D, Table S4). Multiple prior studies have found independent associations of low serum albumin with disease progression outcomes among patients with diabetic nephropathy and CKD [14,15,25,26,27,28]. Thus, similar to hemoglobin levels, our study contributes to the growing evidence for hypoalbuminemia as a major risk factor for ESRD and validates its utility in patients with IgA nephropathy.

Our findings also confirm strong independent associations of decreased eGFR, and elevated SBP with accelerated renal disease progression. These clinical parameters are among the most consistently reported predictors of progression, with similar findings observed across multiple cohorts [29,30,31,32].

Interestingly, proteinuria was strongly associated with the risk of ESRD in univariate analysis, however, it did not independently contribute to the risk in multivariate models. Notably, urinary protein had strong inverse correlation with serum albumin. Accordingly, inclusion of albumin in the prediction model captured most of the variance in outcome contributed by proteinuria. Although albumin appears to be a superior predictor of progression in our cohort, it is also possible that additional predictive value of proteinuria would become more evident with larger cohort size or longer follow-up.

Based on our results, we formulated a new four-variable risk score model for predicting ESRD. Our Risk Score explained nearly 22% of the total variance in the outcome. In addition, when tested against the three previously proposed scores, our Risk Score provided improved prediction of ESRD at 24th, 60th and 120th month of follow-up.

Previously, the largest and most comprehensive IgAN progression study with a similar endpoint of ESRD was performed in Japanese individuals by Goto et al. [9] This nation-wide study followed 2,283 IgAN patients from 97 clinical units in Japan for a median of 87 months with the primary outcome of ESRD. The study formulated an 8-variable progression score that included age, gender, hypertension, proteinuria, hematuria, hypoalbuminaemia, eGFR, and histological grade. In our study, we provide the first independent validation of this risk score. However, our Risk Score had better discrimination power despite comprising of a smaller number of variables. It is noteworthy that the Japanese study did not consider hemoglobin levels and/or anemia diagnosis as potential predictors of ESRD. Based on our findings, the addition of anemia would significantly strengthen their model.

Other risk scoring systems, such as the Bethoux et al. [10] or the Bartosik et al. [33] are not directly comparable to our risk score because they did not examine hemoglobin, serum albumin, or other baseline laboratory measurements. The Bethoux's formula incorporates proteinuria, hypertension, and histology score, while the Bartosik's formula includes mean arterial pressure and proteinuria, but requires follow-up data of at least 2 years. Neither of these risk scores uses the generally accepted Haas or Oxford classification systems. Not surprisingly, the Berthoux risk score did not perform well in predicting ESRD in our dataset. Although the Bartosik formula was validated by another small cohort [34], it uses a less definitive clinical outcome (slope of eGFR decline) and the requirement of two year's follow-up has limited its routine implementation.

We also compared our risk score with the RENAAL progression score, which was based on a powerful and well-characterized cohort of patients with diabetic nephropathy. Similar to our study, RENAAL score included both baseline hemoglobin and serum albumin. The finding that we identify the same risk factors for progression as in the RENAAL study strongly suggests that the same factors affect nephropathy progression regardless of the original insult.

While our risk score is highly promising, it will require validation in independent cohorts. Moreover, our data is based on a retrospective chart reviews, and a prospective evaluation of this score would be useful, perhaps in more ethnically diverse patients. In addition, newer pathology classifications, as well as novel genetic and serologic markers are likely to enhance the predictive power of our risk score. For example, we have previously demonstrated that levels of galactose-deficient IgA1 are elevated in IgAN and may have a diagnostic value [35,36]?

Moreover, we have recently discovered five new genetic susceptibility loci for IgAN in a genome-wide association study (GWAS) [37]. The predictive value of both, galactose-deficient IgA1 as well as GWAS susceptibility alleles on disease progression has not yet been evaluated. Finally, the new Oxford classification of IgAN holds promise to improve risk prediction compared to the Haas grading [38]. Thus, inclusion of newer pathologic scores, and novel biomarkers may further improve the performance of the risk score and enable better risk stratification.

In summary, our new 4-variable Risk Score model is highly predictive of an individual risk of disease progression, explaining nearly 22% of the variance in outcome. In contrast with prior studies, there are three main advantages of this Risk Score: (1) the score equation is relatively simple, thus it is easy to implement in clinical practice, (2) the score has a superb sensitivity and specificity to predict ESRD when compared with other proposed scoring systems, and (3) our score is based entirely on the objective clinical variables that include routine laboratory measurements available for all newly diagnosed patients in clinical practice.

Supporting Information

Table S1 Unadjusted association of baseline parameters with eGFR at presentation (univariate analysis).

Table S2 Multivariate linear regression with stepwise selection for eGFR at the time of biopsy.

Table S3 Baseline characteristics of age and gender-matched healthy population controls.

Table S4 Patient characteristics by anemia and hypoalbuminemia diagnosis.

Table S5 Assessment of the predictive value of proteinuria in the risk of ESRD.

Table S6 Patient characteristics by risk score tertiles.

Acknowledgments

We are grateful to all patients for their participation in this study. This work is the result of a collaborative effort between the Nephrology Department of Ruijin Hospital, Shanghai Jiao Tong University, China and the Nephrology Division at Columbia University, New York.

Author Contributions

Conceived and designed the experiments: NC AG KK JX. Performed the experiments: JX KK WW ZW. Analyzed the data: JX KK AG YL. Contributed reagents/materials/analysis tools: NC JX WW ZW PS SG HR XP XC WZ XL HS. Wrote the paper: KK JX AG.

References

1. Levy M, Berger J (1988) Worldwide perspective of IgA nephropathy. Am J Kidney Dis 12: 340–347.
2. Radford MG Jr, Donadio JV Jr, Bergstralh EJ, Grande JP (1997) Predicting renal outcome in IgA nephropathy. J Am Soc Nephrol 8: 199–207.
3. D'Amico G, Colasanti G, Barbiano di Belgioioso G, Fellin G, Ragni A, et al. (1987) Long-term follow-up of IgA mesangial nephropathy: clinico-histological study in 374 patients. Semin Nephrol 7: 355–358.
4. Donadio JV, Grande JP (2002) IgA nephropathy. N Engl J Med 347: 738–748.
5. Li L (1996) End-stage renal disease in China. Kidney Int 49: 287–301.
6. Koyama A, Igarashi M, Kobayashi M (1997) Natural history and risk factors for immunoglobulin A nephropathy in Japan. Research Group on Progressive Renal Diseases. Am J Kidney Dis 29: 526–532.
7. Li PK, Ho KK, Szeto CC, Yu L, Lai FM (2002) Prognostic indicators of IgA nephropathy in the Chinese–clinical and pathological perspectives. Nephrol Dial Transplant 17: 64–69.
8. Lv J, Zhang H, Zhou Y, Li G, Zou W, et al. (2008) Natural history of immunoglobulin A nephropathy and predictive factors of prognosis: a long-term follow up of 204 cases in China. Nephrology 13: 242–246.

9. Goto M, Wakai K, Kawamura T, Ando M, Endoh M, et al. (2009) A scoring system to predict renal outcome in IgA nephropathy: a nationwide 10-year prospective cohort study. Nephrology, dialysis, transplantation : official publication of the European Dialysis and Transplant Association - European Renal Association 24: 3068–3074.

10. Berthoux F, Mohey H, Laurent B, Mariat C, Afiani A, et al. (2011) Predicting the risk for dialysis or death in IgA nephropathy. Journal of the American Society of Nephrology : JASN 22: 752–761.

11. Donadio JV, Bergstralh EJ, Grande JP, Rademcher DM (2002) Proteinuria patterns and their association with subsequent end-stage renal disease in IgA nephropathy. Nephrology, dialysis, transplantation : official publication of the European Dialysis and Transplant Association - European Renal Association 17: 1197–1203.

12. Reich HN, Troyanov S, Scholey JW, Cattran DC (2007) Remission of proteinuria improves prognosis in IgA nephropathy. Journal of the American Society of Nephrology : JASN 18: 3177–3183.

13. Kaartinen K, Syrjanen J, Porsti I, Hurme M, Harmoinen A, et al. (2008) Inflammatory markers and the progression of IgA glomerulonephritis. Nephrol Dial Transplant 23: 1285–1290.

14. Keane WF, Zhang Z, Lyle PA, Cooper ME, de Zeeuw D, et al. (2006) Risk scores for predicting outcomes in patients with type 2 diabetes and nephropathy: the RENAAL study. Clinical journal of the American Society of Nephrology : CJASN 1: 761–767.

15. Tangri N, Stevens LA, Griffith J, Tighiouart H, Djurdjev O, et al. (2011) A predictive model for progression of chronic kidney disease to kidney failure. JAMA : the journal of the American Medical Association 305: 1553–1559.

16. Ma YC, Zuo L, Chen JH, Luo Q, Yu XQ, et al. (2006) Modified glomerular filtration rate estimating equation for Chinese patients with chronic kidney disease. J Am Soc Nephrol 17: 2937–2944.

17. National Kidney Foundation (2002) K/DOQI clinical practice guidelines for chronic kidney disease: evaluation, classification, and stratification. American journal of kidney diseases : the official journal of the National Kidney Foundation 39: S1–266.

18. Therneau PGaT (1994) Proportional hazards tests and diagnostics based on weighted residuals. Biometrika 81: 11.

19. Nagelkerke NJD (1991) A note on a general definition of the coefficient of determination. Biometrika 78: 691–692.

20. Haibe-Kains B, Desmedt C, Sotiriou C, Bontempi G (2008) A comparative study of survival models for breast cancer prognostication based on microarray data: does a single gene beat them all? Bioinformatics 24: 2200–2208.

21. Sing T, Sander O, Beerenwinkel N, Lengauer T (2005) ROCR: visualizing classifier performance in R. Bioinformatics 21: 3940–3941.

22. Dupont WD, Plummer WD Jr (1990) Power and Sample Size Calculations: A Review and Computer Program. Controlled Clinical Trials 11: 116–128.

23. Kiryluk K, Julian BA, Wyatt RJ, Scolari F, Zhang H, et al. (2010) Genetic studies of IgA nephropathy: past, present, and future. Pediatric nephrology 25: 2257–2268.

24. Mohanram A, Zhang Z, Shahinfar S, Keane WF, Brenner BM, et al. (2004) Anemia and end-stage renal disease in patients with type 2 diabetes and nephropathy. Kidney Int 66: 1131–1138.

25. Staples AO, Greenbaum LA, Smith JM, Gipson DS, Filler G, et al. (2010) Association between clinical risk factors and progression of chronic kidney disease in children. Clinical journal of the American Society of Nephrology : CJASN 5: 2172–2179.

26. Yokoyama H, Tomonaga O, Hirayama M, Ishii A, Takeda M, et al. (1997) Predictors of the progression of diabetic nephropathy and the beneficial effect of angiotensin-converting enzyme inhibitors in NIDDM patients. Diabetologia 40: 405–411.

27. Keane WF, Brenner BM, de Zeeuw D, Grunfeld JP, McGill J, et al. (2003) The risk of developing end-stage renal disease in patients with type 2 diabetes and nephropathy: the RENAAL study. Kidney international 63: 1499–1507.

28. Leehey DJ, Kramer HJ, Daoud TM, Chatha MP, Isreb MA (2005) Progression of kidney disease in type 2 diabetes - beyond blood pressure control: an observational study. BMC Nephrol 6: 8.

29. Fox CS, Larson MG, Leip EP, Culleton B, Wilson PW, et al. (2004) Predictors of new-onset kidney disease in a community-based population. JAMA : the journal of the American Medical Association 291: 844–850.

30. Retnakaran R, Cull CA, Thorne KI, Adler AI, Holman RR (2006) Risk factors for renal dysfunction in type 2 diabetes: U.K. Prospective Diabetes Study 74. Diabetes 55: 1832–1839.

31. Hunsicker LG, Adler S, Caggiula A, England BK, Greene T, et al. (1997) Predictors of the progression of renal disease in the Modification of Diet in Renal Disease Study. Kidney Int 51: 1908–1919.

32. Klahr S, Levey AS, Beck GJ, Caggiula AW, Hunsicker L, et al. (1994) The effects of dietary protein restriction and blood-pressure control on the progression of chronic renal disease. Modification of Diet in Renal Disease Study Group. N Engl J Med 330: 877–884.

33. Bartosik LP, Lajoie G, Sugar L, Cattran DC (2001) Predicting progression in IgA nephropathy. American journal of kidney diseases : the official journal of the National Kidney Foundation 38: 728–735.

34. Mackinnon B, Fraser EP, Cattran DC, Fox JG, Geddes CC (2008) Validation of the Toronto formula to predict progression in IgA nephropathy. Nephron Clinical practice 109: c148–153.

35. Kiryluk K, Moldoveanu Z, Sanders JT, Eison TM, Suzuki H, et al. (2011) Aberrant glycosylation of IgA1 is inherited in both pediatric IgA nephropathy and Henoch-Schonlein purpura nephritis. Kidney international 80: 79–87.

36. Moldoveanu Z, Wyatt RJ, Lee JY, Tomana M, Julian BA, et al. (2007) Patients with IgA nephropathy have increased serum galactose-deficient IgA1 levels. Kidney international 71: 1148–1154.

37. Gharavi AG, Kiryluk K, Choi M, Li Y, Hou P, et al. (2011) Genome-wide association study identifies susceptibility loci for IgA nephropathy. Nature genetics 43: 321–327.

38. Cattran DC, Coppo R, Cook HT, Feehally J, Roberts IS, et al. (2009) The Oxford classification of IgA nephropathy: rationale, clinicopathological correlations, and classification. Kidney international 76: 534–545.

11

Serum Fatty Acid-Binding Protein 4 is a Predictor of Cardiovascular Events in End-Stage Renal Disease

Masato Furuhashi[1]*, Shutaro Ishimura[1], Hideki Ota[1], Manabu Hayashi[2], Takahiro Nishitani[3], Marenao Tanaka[1], Hideaki Yoshida[1], Kazuaki Shimamoto[4], Gökhan S. Hotamisligil[5], Tetsuji Miura[1]

1 Second Department of Internal Medicine, Sapporo Medical University School of Medicine, Sapporo, Japan, 2 Second Department of Internal Medicine, Obihiro Kosei Hospital, Obihiro, Japan, 3 Obihiro East Medical and Cardiovascular Clinic, Obihiro, Japan, 4 Sapporo Medical University, Sapporo, Japan, 5 Department of Genetics and Complex Diseases, Harvard School of Public Health, Boston, Massachusetts, United States of America

Abstract

Background: Fatty acid-binding protein 4 (FABP4/A-FABP/aP2), a lipid chaperone, is expressed in both adipocytes and macrophages. Recent studies have shown that FABP4 is secreted from adipocytes and that FABP4 level is associated with obesity, insulin resistance, and atherosclerosis. However, little is known about the impact of FABP4 concentrations on prognosis. We tested the hypothesis that FABP4 level predicts prognosis of patients with end-stage renal disease (ESRD), a group at high risk for atherosclerosis-associated morbidity and mortality.

Methods and Results: Biochemical markers including FABP4 were determined in 61 ESRD patients on chronic hemodialysis (HD). Serum FABP4 level in females (404.2±30.5 ng/ml) was significantly higher than that in males (315.8±30.0 ng/ml), and the levels in ESRD patients were about 20-times higher than those in age-, gender- and body mass index (BMI)-matched control subjects with normal renal function. FABP4 level was decreased by 57.2% after HD and was positively correlated with blood pressure, BMI, and levels of lipids and insulin. Multiple regression analysis indicated that HD duration, BMI, and triglycerides level were independent determinants for FABP4 level. ESRD patients with high FABP4 levels had higher cardiovascular mortality during the 7-year follow-up period. Cox proportional hazard regression analysis showed that logarithmically transformed FABP4 level was an independent predictor of cardiovascular death adjusted for age, gender, HD duration, BMI, and triglycerides level (hazard ratio, 7.75; 95% CI, 1.05–25.31).

Conclusion: These findings suggest that FABP4 level, being related to adiposity and metabolic disorders, is a novel predictor of cardiovascular mortality in ESRD.

Editor: Harald H. H. W. Schmidt, Maastricht University, The Netherlands

Funding: This work was supported by grants from Grant-in-Aid for Scientific Research for The Ministry of Education, Culture, Sports, Science and Technology, Uehara Memorial Foundation, Senshin Medical Research Foundation, Naito Foundation Natural Science Scholarship, Takeda Science Foundation, Mochida Memorial Foundation for Medical and Pharmaceutical Research, Kanae Foundation for the Promotion of Medical Science, Cardiovascular Research Foundation, Suzuken Memorial Foundation, Sumitomo Foundation, Tokyo Biochemical Research Foundation, Japan Diabetes Foundation, Ono Medical Research Foundation, Novartis Foundation (Japan) for the Promotion of Science, Japan Foundation for Applied Enzymology, and The Ichiro Kanehara Foundation (to M.F.). The funders had no role in study design, data collection and analysis, decision to publish, or preparation of the manuscript.

Competing Interests: The authors have declared that no competing interests exist.

* E-mail: furuhasi@sapmed.ac.jp

Introduction

Intracellular lipid chaperones known as fatty acid-binding proteins (FABPs) are a group of molecules that coordinate lipid responses in cells [1]. FABPs are abundantly expressed 14–15 kDa proteins that can reversibly bind to hydrophobic ligands, such as saturated and unsaturated long chain fatty acids, eicosanoids, and other lipids, with high affinity[1]. FABPs have been proposed to facilitate the transport of lipids to specific compartments in the cell, such as to the lipid droplet for storage, to the endoplasmic reticulum for signaling, trafficking, and membrane synthesis, to the mitochondria or peroxisome for oxidation, to cytosolic or other enzymes to regulate their activity, and to the nucleus for lipid-mediated transcriptional regulation. One of the FABPs, fatty acid-binding protein 4 (FABP4), known as adipocyte FABP (A-FABP) or aP2, is expressed in both adipocytes and macrophages and plays important roles in the

regulation of insulin sensitivity and the development of atherosclerosis [2–8]. Therefore, it is expected that modification of FABP4 function will provide a new class of therapeutic agents. In fact, we recently demonstrated that chemical inhibition of FABP4 could be a therapeutic strategy against insulin resistance, diabetes mellitus (DM), fatty liver disease, and atherosclerosis in experimental models[9].

In the present study, we hypothesized that serum FABP4 is a novel marker for risk stratification of end-stage renal disease (ESRD) patients on hemodialysis (HD). The rationale for this hypothesis is four-fold. First, it has been shown that FABP4 is secreted from adipocytes [10], although there is no typical sequence of secretory signal peptides. At least, we previously confirmed that FABP4 release from adipocytes was not an escape due to apoptosis or necrosis of adipocytes [7]. Second, recent studies have shown that elevation of serum FABP4 is associated with obesity and insulin resistance, risk factors of atherosclerosis, and carotid atherosclerosis [10–13]. Third, chronic kidney disease has been shown to be a risk factor of atherosclerosis [14]. Fourth, atherosclerotic vascular diseases are a major cause of death in ESRD patients [14].

Methods

Ethics statement

This study was performed with the approval of the institutional ethical committee of Sapporo Medical University, and written informed consent was received from all of the subjects.

Participants

Sixty-one HD patients (31 males and 30 females) aged 39–78 years (mean age: 61.6 ± 1.8 years, mean$\pm$SEM) were recruited. All of the patients had anuria or oliguria (urine volume <200 ml/day). None of the patients had a history of acute myocardial infarction within 6 months prior to the start of this study, chest pain at rest or in the peridialysis period, unstable hemodynamics during dialysis, critical illness, or a history of recent major vascular surgery. The mean duration of HD was 63.4 ± 7.1 months. The underlying renal diseases of the HD patients were diabetes mellitus (n = 21), glomerulonephritis (n = 22), nephrosclerosis (n = 6) and other diseases (n = 12). Diabetic patients treated with thiazolidinediones, PPARγ agonists, were excluded because the FABP4 gene is known as a target of PPARγ. All HD patients were dialyzed 2 or 3 times per week on Monday-Wednesday–Friday, Tuesday–Thursday–Saturday, or Tuesday–Satur day using high-flux membranes (dialysis filter surface area, 1.1– 2.1 m^2). Sixty-one age-, gender- and body mass index-matched control subjects (31 men and 30 women; mean age, 61.2 ± 2.0 years) who had been taking no medication were also enrolled to compare FABP4 levels between subjects with and without renal dysfunction. None of the control subjects had any evidence of complications such as endocrine or metabolic disturbances, cerebrovascular or cardiovascular disease, and renal disease.

Measurement of biochemical markers

Blood samples in HD patients were drawn before the start and at the end of a routine HD treatment on Monday or Tuesday. Assays of FABP4 (ng/ml) were per-formed using blood samples taken before and after HD. Other biochemical assays, such as assays of total protein, creatinine, blood urea nitrogen, lipid variables, glucose, insulin, and adiponectin, were performed using blood samples taken before hemodi-alysis. Serum FABP4 level was measured using a commercially available enzyme-linked immunosorbent assay kit (Biovendor R&D, Mordrice, Czech Republic). The accu-racy, precision and reproducibility of this kit have been described previously [10]. Plasma glucose was determined by the glucose oxidase method. Plasma insulin was measured by a radioimmunoassay method (Insulin RIA bead, Dianabot, Tokyo, Japan). Serum lipid profiles, including total cholesterol, high-density lipoprotein (HDL)-cholesterol and triglycerides, were estimated by enzymatic methods. Serum adiponectin level was measured using a commercially available sandwich enzyme-linked immunosorbent assay kit (Otsuka Pharmaceuticals Co., Ltd., Tokushima, Japan).

Statistical analysis

Numeric variables are expressed as means$\pm$SEM. The Mann-Whitney U test was used for comparisons between two unpaired variables. The difference between two paired variables was analyzed by the Wilcoxon signed rank test. Group statistical comparisons were assessed by the chi-square test. Before performing regression

analyses, the distribution of each parameter was tested for normality using the Shapiro-Wilk W test, and non-normally distributed parameters were logarithmically transformed. Simple linear regression analysis was used to determine the correlation between two variables. Multiple linear regression analysis was used to identify independent determinants of the FABP4 concentrations and the percentage of variance in the FABP4 concentrations that they explained (R^2). Receiver operating characteristic (ROC) analysis was performed to determine the inflection point at which the FABP4 level provided the most sensitive prediction of cardiovascular death as a result of sudden cardiac death/arrhythmia, heart failure, atherothrombotic events (myocardial infarction, stroke, mesenteric ischemia). For a given FABP4 level, the ordinate value shows the percentage of patients with that FABP4 level who died (true-positive rate or sensitivity), and the abscissa value shows the percentage of patients with that FABP4 level who did not die (false-positive rate or 1-specificty). Using the ROC-derived optimal cutoff value, patients were divided into two groups. Survival rate was analyzed by log-rank tests of Kaplan-Meier curves in the two groups. Cox regression analyses were performed for cardiovascular death as an end point. A p value of <0.05 was considered statistically significant. All data were analyzed by using JMP 8 for Macintosh (SAS Institute, Cary, NC).

Results

FABP4 levels in hemodialysis patients

The FABP4 level in HD males were significantly lower than that in HD females (Figure 1A; males vs. females: 315.8 ± 30.0 vs. 404.2 ± 30.5 ng/ml), and these levels were about 20-times higher than those in both male and female controls with normal renal function (Figure 1B; males vs. females: 16.0 ± 1.7 vs. 20.5 ± 1.6 ng/ml). After HD, the FABP4 level was significantly decreased by 57.2% (before vs. after: 359.3 ± 22.0 vs. 153.9 ± 10.5 ng/ml) but was still higher than that in control subjects (Figure 1C).

Simple and multiple regression analyses for FABP4

In all of the HD patients, FABP4 levels were positively correlated with HD duration, body mass index, waist circumference, blood pressures, and levels of total cholesterol, LDL-cholesterol, triglycerides, and insulin and were negatively correlated with levels of HDL-cholesterol and adiponectin (Table 1). Multiple regression analysis for predicting FABP4 level was performed using the correlated and nonconfounding parameters, such as age, gender, HD duration, body mass index as an index of adiposity, systolic blood pressure, and levels of triglycerides as a lipid profile, insulin, and adiponectin. The result revealed that HD duration, body mass index, and level of triglycerides were independent predictors for FABP4 level, explaining a total of 55% of the variance in this measure ($R^2=0.55$) (Table 2).

Predictor of cardiovascular mortality in ESRD

During the 7-year follow-up period, we confirmed 13 out of 61 patients who died of cardiovascular events. ROC analysis of the correlation between FABP4 levels in HD patients and the occurrence of cardiovascular death was performed. We chose the inflection point as the optimal cutoff value, 364.1 ng/ml (Figure 2A; sensitivity: 76.9%, specificity: 68.8%, area under the curve: 0.70). Using the cutoff point, HD patients were divided into two groups: Low-FABP4 (HD patients with FABP4 levels below the point) and High-FABP4 (HD patients with FABP4 levels above the cutoff) groups. During the 7-year follow-up period, 3 out of 36 Low-FABP4 patients and 10 out of 25 High-FABP4 patients died of cardiovascular events. Kaplan-Meier survival curves showed that

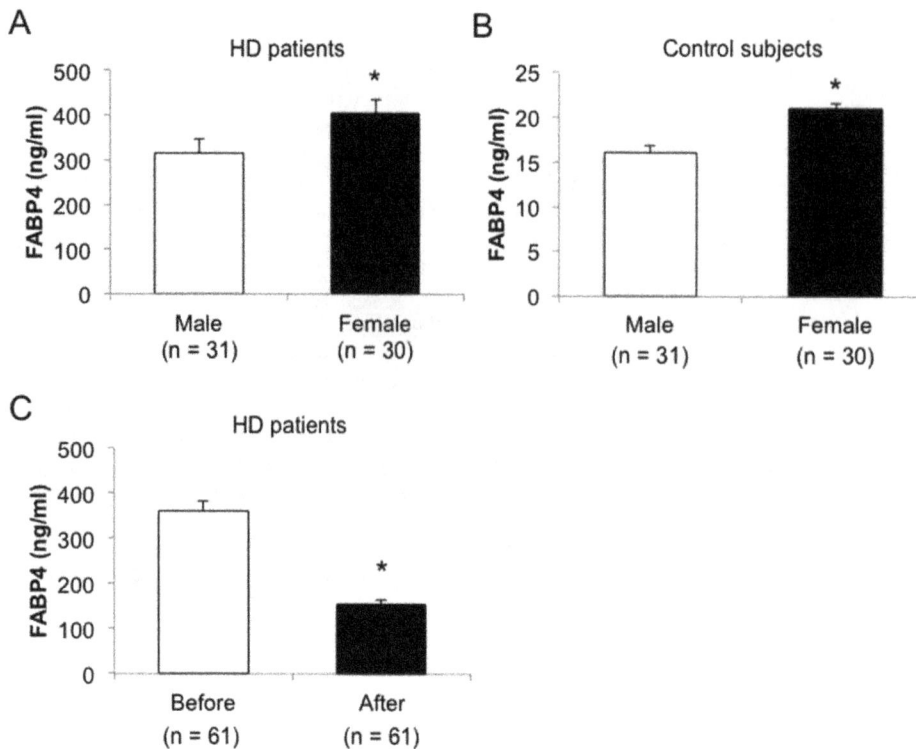

Figure 1. Concentrations of FABP4. FABP4 levels were investigated in the males and females of hemodialysis patients (A) and control subjects with normal renal function (B). FABP4 levels were determined before and after hemodialysis (C). Values are presented as means±SEM. *P <0.05.

the High-FABP4 patients had a significantly higher mortality than did the Low-FABP4 patients (Figure 2B).

Clinical characteristics of the HD patients split by the two groups are shown in Table 3. There were no significant inter-group differences in age, gender, presence of DM, blood pressure, and Kt/V as an index of dialysis adequacy. Drug therapies including administration of antihypertensive drugs and statins were comparable in the Low-FABP4 and High-FABP4 groups. Body mass index and waist circumference were significantly higher in the High-FABP4 patients than in the Low-FABP4 patients. The High-FABP4 patients had significantly higher levels of total cholesterol, triglycerides, and insulin

and lower levels of adiponectin than did the Low-FABP4 patients. No significant differences were found in other parameters, including serum total protein, blood urea nitrogen, creatinine, potassium, and C-reactive protein, between the Low-FABP4 and High-FABP4 groups.

Cox proportional hazard regression analysis for predicting cardiovascular death was performed including FABP4 level, age, gender, presence of DM, and the independent determinants of FABP4 level (HD duration, body mass index, and level of triglycerides) in the multiple regression analysis (Table 2) which also have a significant difference between the Low-FABP4 and High FABP4 groups (Table 3). The result demonstrated that FABP4 concentration was a significant explanatory variable after adjustment of the other parameters, suggesting that FABP4 level was an independent predictor of long-term cardiovascular mortality (Table 4).

Table 1. Simple regression analysis for log FABP4.

	r	p
Age	−0.175	0.178
HD duration	0.253	0.049
Body mass index	0.315	0.013
Waist circumference	0.345	0.012
Systolic blood pressure	0.259	0.043
Diastolic blood pressure	0.325	0.011
Total cholesterol	0.378	0.004
LDL cholesterol	0.291	0.024
HDL cholesterol	−0.256	0.046
Triglycerides	0.506	<0.001
Insulin	0.430	0.002
Adiponectin	−0.366	0.004

Table 2. Multiple regression analysis for log FABP4.

	t	p
Age	0.118	0.907
Gender (Male)	−1.280	0.207
HD duration	4.215	<0.001
Body mass index	2.320	0.025
Systolic blood pressure	0.192	0.849
Triglycerides	3.277	0.002
Insulin	0.563	0.576
Adiponectin	−1.651	0.106
$R^2 = 0.55$		

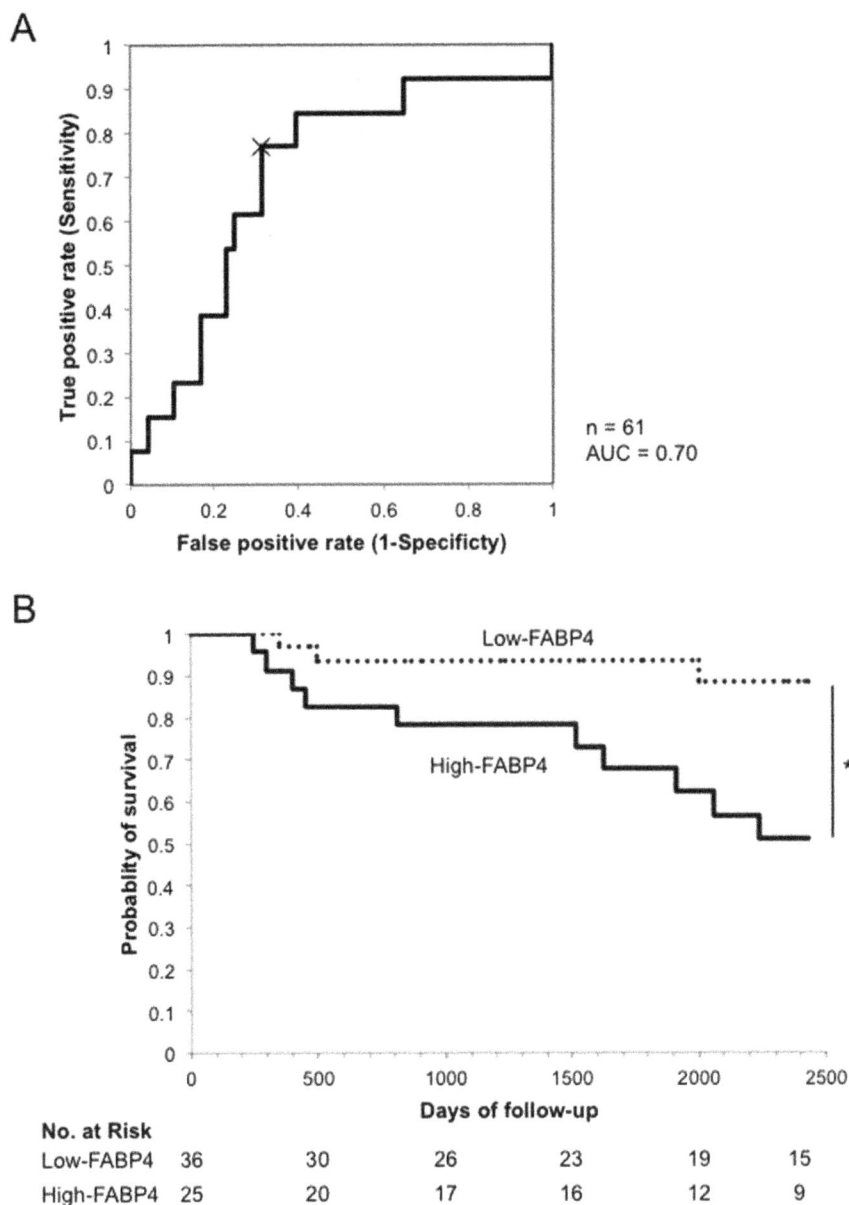

Figure 2. Receiver operating characteristic (ROC) analysis and Kaplan-Meier survival curve. (A) ROC analysis of the correlation between FABP4 levels in HD patients and the occurrence of cardiovascular death is shown. The ordinate values show the corresponding true-positive rate (fraction of patients with that FABP4 level who died) and the abscissa values show the corresponding false-positive rate (fraction of patients with that FABP4 level who did not die). The inflection point (indicated by X) was chosen as the optimal cutoff value, 364.1 ng/ml (sensitivity: 76.9%, specificity: 68.8%, area under the curve [AUC]: 0.70). (B) According to the cutoff point of FABP4 level, HD patients were divided into two groups: Low-FABP4 and High-FABP4 groups, and Kaplan-Meier curves for cardiovascular death are analyzed in the two groups. Broken lines (Low-FABP4 group), patients with FABP4 levels of <364.1 ng/ml (n = 36, 22 males and 14 females); Solid lines (High-FABP4 group), patients with FABP4 levels of ≥364.1 ng/ml (n = 25, 9 males and 16 females). Survival rates were compared by log-rank test. *P <0.05.

Discussion

To the best of our knowledge, this is the first report on the impact of elevation of circulating FABP4 concentrations on long-term prognosis of ESRD. Previous studies using animal models indicate that FABP4 plays a significant role in several aspects of metabolic syndrome, including insulin resistance, type 2 DM and atherosclerosis, through its action at the interface of metabolic and inflammatory pathways in adipocytes and macrophages [1–8]. In a human study, reduced expression of FABP4 in adipose tissue was suggested to have beneficial effects on cardiovascular and

metabolic health [15]. Subjects with a genetic variation of the FABP4 locus (T-87C) leading to decreased FABP4 expression in adipose tissue showed lower levels of triglycerides as well as a significantly reduced risk for cardiovascular disease. Taken together, these observations support the notion that measurement of FABP4 concentration is useful for risk stratification and for guiding treatment in observational or interventional studies. However, it is clearly necessary to prospectively evaluate whether a change in the FABP4 value indeed reflects conditions of metabolic syndrome and atherosclerosis and predicts long-term cardiovascular outcomes in patients regardless of ESRD.

Table 3. Basal and biochemical characteristics of 61 patients.

	Whole	Low-FABP4	High-FABP4
n	61	36	25
Male/Female	31/30	22/14	9/16
Age (years)	61.6±1.8	62.6±2.3	60.2±2.8
Diagnosis			
Diabetes mellitus	21	12	9
Glomerulonephritis	22	10	12
Nephrosclerosis	6	6	0
Others	12	8	4
HD duration (months)	63.4±7.1	51.4±9.0	80.6±10.8*
Body mass index (kg/m²)	21.4±0.5	20.7±0.6	22.4±0.4*
Waist circumference (cm)	78.0±1.5	75.3±2.0	81.4±2.3*
Systolic blood pressure (mmHg)	140.0±2.9	137.4±3.8	143.7±4.5
Diastolic blood pressure (mmHg)	77.0±1.8	74.0±2.3	80.4±2.7
Kt/V	1.44±0.05	1.42±0.06	1.45±0.08
Drug therapy			
ACE inhibitors	5 (8.2)	2 (5.6)	3 (12.0)
Angiotensin II receptor blockers	16 (26.2)	11 (30.5)	5 (20.0)
Calcium channel blockers	26 (42.6)	18 (50.0)	8 (32.0)
α blockers	4 (6.6)	4 (11.1)	0 (0)
β blockers	7 (11.5)	4 (11.1)	3 (12.0)
Diuretics	13 (21.3)	8 (22.2)	5 (20.0)
Statins	8 (13.1)	4 (11.1)	4 (16.0)
Total protein (g/l)	6.4±0.1	6.4±0.1	6.4±0.1
BUN (mg/dl)	63.4±2.4	62.4±3.1	64.9±3.8
Cr (mg/dl)	10.1±0.3	9.7±0.4	10.6±0.5
K (mEq/l)	5.3±0.1	5.2±0.1	5.5±0.2
Total cholesterol (mg/dl)	168.6±4.7	159.4±5.9	181.7±7.0*
HDL cholesterol (mg/dl)	40.9±1.7	43.5±2.2	37.2±2.6
LDL cholesterol (mg/dl)	101.5±3.6	96.2±4.6	109.4±5.6
Triglycerides (mg/dl)	112.5±7.2	90.2±8.2	142.7±9.7**
Blood glucose (mg/dl)	124.7±6.4	115.4±8.2	137.5±9.7
Insulin (μU/ml)	20.4±2.4	15.7±3.1	27.0±3.6*
HbA1c (%)	5.4±0.2	5.2±0.3	5.6±0.3
C-reactive protein (mg/dl)	0.45±0.08	0.44±0.10	0.47±0.12
Adiponectin (μg/ml)	17.7±1.0	19.5±1.3	15.0±1.6*

Variables are expressed as means±SEM or number (%).
*P <0.05 vs. Low-FABP4.
**P <0.01 vs. Low-FABP4.

Table 4. Cox proportional hazard model for prognosis at 7 year follow-up.

	HR	95% CI	p
Age	1.054	1.005 – 1.117	0.029
Gender (Male)	2.447	0.715 – 9.177	0.153
Diabetes mellitus	1.198	0.317 – 4.390	0.783
HD duration	0.993	0.978 – 1.006	0.293
Body mass index	0.866	0.678 – 1.079	0.209
log Triglycerides	0.881	0.135 – 6.511	0.898
log FABP4	7.751	1.052 – 25.316	0.044

previously measured concentrations of FABP3, which is another member of the FABP family known as heart-type FABP (H-FABP), in HD patients [19]. We found the concentration of FABP3 was increased 13.8-fold in HD patients compared to that in control subjects with normal renal function and was reduced by 40% after HD but was still higher than that in control subjects. Those results are similar to the results of the present study. The molecular weights of FABP3 and FABP4 are almost the same, about 15 kD. It is expected that the sieving effects of HD dialyzers on these two proteins are similar. These findings suggest that renal elimination is a major route by which physiological levels of FABPs are maintained. Interestingly, similar mechanisms of elimination have been proposed for other adipocyte-derived factors, such as leptin, adiponectin, and retinol-binding protein 4 [20–22]. Taking these into consideration, FABP4 appears to be accumulated in circulation due to diminished renal excretion in chronic kidney disease.

Recent studies have demonstrated an association between increased FABP4 levels and metabolic parameters even in HD patients [17,18]. In the present study, we confirmed that FABP4 levels were significantly correlated with adiposity, blood pressure, insulin resistance, and dyslipidemia in HD patients. Furthermore, body mass index and triglycerides were independent predictors for FABP4 concentration, and this relationship was independent of HD duration, suggesting that a high level of FABP4 is attributable to metabolic syndrome even in patients with ESRD. Strikingly, FABP4 level was an independent predictor of cardiovascular death after adjustment of metabolic parameters.

One limitation in this study is the small number of patients enrolled. As another limitation, we did not directly assess the extent of atherosclerosis in each patient. Thus, the relationship between FABP4 level and progression of atherosclerosis remains unclear. These issues warrant further investigation in a prospective study recruiting a larger number of patients.

In conclusion, concentration of serum FABP4 may be not only a marker of metabolic syndrome that can be used even for ESRD patients but also a novel predictor of cardiovascular mortality in patients at high risk of atherosclerotic cardiovascular events.

Acknowledgments

We are grateful to group members of our department, IZAYOI (Boston, MA), and G-PUC (Sapporo, Japan) for their scientific inputs, discussions, and contributions.

Author Contributions

Conceived and designed the experiments: MF KS. Performed the experiments: MF SI HO MH TN MT HY. Analyzed the data: MF MH TN. Wrote the paper: MF GSH TM.

In the present study, FABP4 concentrations were sex-related, being higher in females than in males as previously reported [10–13,16]. However, multiple regression analysis showed that gender was not a significant determinant of FABP4 concentration in HD patients. FABP4 level was significantly higher in HD patients than in the controls, which is consistent with previous findings in patients with renal dysfunction [16–18]. In the control subjects, FABP4 levels were negatively correlated with estimated glomerular filtration rate (data not shown), which is an index of renal function, as previously reported in DM patients with nephropathy [16]. We

References

1. Furuhashi M, Hotamisligil GS (2008) Fatty acid-binding proteins: role in metabolic diseases and potential as drug targets. Nat Rev Drug Discov 7: 489–503.
2. Hotamisligil GS, Johnson RS, Distel RJ, Ellis R, Papaioannou VE, et al. (1996) Uncoupling of obesity from insulin resistance through a targeted mutation in aP2, the adipocyte fatty acid binding protein. Science 274: 1377–1379.
3. Uysal KT, Scheja L, Wiesbrock SM, Bonner-Weir S, Hotamisligil GS (2000) Improved glucose and lipid metabolism in genetically obese mice lacking aP2. Endocrinology 141: 3388–3396.
4. Makowski L, Boord JB, Maeda K, Babaev VR, Uysal KT, et al. (2001) Lack of macrophage fatty-acid-binding protein aP2 protects mice deficient in apolipo-protein E against atherosclerosis. Nat Med 7: 699–705.
5. Maeda K, Cao H, Kono K, Görgün CZ, Furuhashi M, et al. (2005) Adipocyte/macrophage fatty acid binding proteins control integrated metabolic responses in obesity and diabetes. Cell Metab 1: 107–119.
6. Boord JB, Maeda K, Makowski L, Babaev VR, Fazio S, et al. (2004) Combined adipocyte-macrophage fatty acid-binding protein deficiency improves metabo-lism, atherosclerosis, and survival in apolipoprotein E-deficient mice. Circulation 110: 1492–1498.
7. Furuhashi M, Fucho R, Görgün CZ, Tuncman G, Cao H, et al. (2008) Adipocyte/macrophage fatty acid-binding proteins contribute to metabolic deterioration through actions in both macrophages and adipocytes in mice. J Clin Invest 118: 2640–2650.
8. Erbay E, Babaev VR, Mayers JR, Makowski L, Charles KN, et al. (2009) Reducing endoplasmic reticulum stress through a macrophage lipid chaperone alleviates atherosclerosis. Nat Med 15: 1383–1391.
9. Furuhashi M, Tuncman G, Görgün CZ, Makowski L, Atsumi G, et al. (2007) Treatment of diabetes and atherosclerosis by inhibiting fatty-acid-binding protein aP2. Nature 447: 959–965.
10. Xu A, Wang Y, Xu JY, Stejskal D, Tam S, et al. (2006) Adipocyte fatty acid-binding protein is a plasma biomarker closely associated with obesity and metabolic syndrome. Clin Chem 52: 405–413.
11. Yeung DC, Xu A, Cheung CW, Wat NM, Yau MH, et al. (2007) Serum adipocyte fatty acid-binding protein levels were independently associated with carotid atherosclerosis. Arterioscler Thromb Vasc Biol 27: 1796–1802.
12. Xu A, Tso AW, Cheung BM, Wang Y, Wat NM, et al. (2007) Circulating adipocyte-fatty acid binding protein levels predict the development of the metabolic syndrome: a 5-year prospective study. Circulation 115: 1537–1543.
13. Tso AW, Xu A, Sham PC, Wat NM, Wang Y, et al. (2007) Serum adipocyte fatty acid binding protein as a new biomarker predicting the development of type 2 diabetes: a 10-year prospective study in a Chinese cohort. Diabetes Care 30: 2667–2672.
14. El Nahas M (2010) Cardio-Kidney-Damage: a unifying concept. Kidney Int 78: 14–18.
15. Tuncman G, Erbay E, Hom X, De Vivo I, Campos H, et al. (2006) A genetic variant at the fatty acid-binding protein aP2 locus reduces the risk for hypertriglyceridemia, type 2 diabetes, and cardiovascular disease. Proc Natl Acad Sci USA 103: 6970–6975.
16. Yeung DC, Xu A, Tso AW, Chow WS, Wat NM, et al. (2009) Circulating levels of adipocyte and epidermal fatty acid-binding proteins in relation to nephropathy staging and macrovascular complications in type 2 diabetic patients. Diabetes Care 32: 132–134.
17. Sommer G, Ziegelmeier M, Bachmann A, Kralisch S, Lossner U, et al. (2008) Serum levels of adipocyte fatty acid-binding protein (AFABP) are increased in chronic haemodialysis (CD). Clin Endocrinol 69: 901–905.
18. Tsai JP, Liou HH, Liu HM, Lee CJ, Lee RP, et al. (2010) Fasting serum fatty acid-binding protein 4 level positively correlates with metabolic syndrome in hemodialysis patients. Arch Med Res 41: 536–540.
19. Furuhashi M, Ura N, Hasegawa K, Yoshida H, Tsuchihashi K, et al. (2003) Serum ratio of heart-type fatty acid-binding protein to myoglobin. A novel marker of cardiac damage and volume overload in hemodialysis patients. Nephron Clin Pract 93: C69–74.
20. Merabet E, Dagogo-Jack S, Coyne DW, Klein S, Santiago JV, et al. (1997) Increased plasma leptin concentration in end-stage renal disease. J Clin Endocrinol Metab 82: 847–850.
21. Zoccali C, Mallamaci F, Tripepi G, Benedetto FA, Cutrupi S, et al. (2002) Adiponectin, metabolic risk factors, and cardiovascular events among patients with end-stage renal disease. J Am Soc Nephrol 13: 134–141.
22. Ziegelmeier M, Bachmann A, Seeger J, Lossner U, Kratzsch J, et al. (2007) Serum levels of adipokine retinol-binding protein-4 in relation to renal function. Diabetes Care 30: 2588–2592.

12

Risk of ESRD and All Cause Mortality in Type 2 Diabetes According to Circulating Levels of FGF-23 and TNFR1

Jung Eun Lee[1,2,3], Tomohito Gohda[1,3,4], William H. Walker[1], Jan Skupien[1,3,5], Adam M. Smiles[1], Rita R. Holak[1], Jackson Jeong[1], Kevin P. McDonnell[1], Andrzej S. Krolewski[1,3], Monika A. Niewczas[1,3]*

1 Research Division, Joslin Diabetes Center, Boston, Massachusetts, United States of America, 2 Division of Nephrology, Samsung Medical Center, Sungkyunkwan University School of Medicine, Seoul, Korea, 3 Department of Medicine, Harvard Medical School, Boston, Massachusetts, United States of America, 4 Division of Nephrology, Department of Internal Medicine, Juntendo University School of Medicine, Tokyo, Japan, 5 Department of Metabolic Diseases, Jagiellonian University Medical College, Krakow, Poland

Abstract

Introduction: Recent studies demonstrated that circulating fibroblast growth factor (FGF)-23 was associated with risk of end stage renal disease (ESRD) and mortality. This study aims to examine whether the predictive effect of FGF-23 is independent from circulating levels of tumor necrosis factor receptor 1 (TNFR1), a strong predictor of ESRD in Type 2 diabetes (T2D).

Methods: We studied 380 patients with T2D who were followed for 8–12 years and were used previously to examine the effect of TNFR1. Baseline plasma FGF-23 was measured by immunoassay.

Results: During follow-up, 48 patients (13%) developed ESRD and 83 patients (22%) died without ESRD. In a univariate analysis, baseline circulating levels of FGF-23 and TNFR1 were significantly higher in subjects who subsequently developed ESRD or died without ESRD than in those who remained alive. In a Cox proportional hazard model, baseline concentration of FGF-23 was associated with increased risk of ESRD, however its effect was no longer significant after controlling for TNFR1 and other clinical characteristics (HR 1.3, p = 0.15). The strong effect of circulating level of TNFR1 on risk of ESRD was not changed by including circulating levels of FGF-23 (HR 8.7, p<0.001). In the Cox multivariate model, circulating levels of FGF-23 remained a significant independent predictor of all-cause mortality unrelated to ESRD (HR 1.5, p<0.001).

Conclusions: We demonstrated that the effect of circulating levels of FGF-23 on the risk of ESRD is accounted for by circulating levels of TNFR1. We confirmed that circulating levels of FGF-23 have an independent effect on all-cause mortality in T2D.

Editor: Paolo Fiorina, Children's Hospital Boston/Harvard Medical School, United States of America

Funding: This study was supported by grants from the National Institutes of Health DK041526 and DK067638 (ASK), DERC Joslin Diabetes Center Pilot and Feasibility grant (MAN) and a JDRF fellowship grant 3-2009-397 (JS). The funders had no role in study design, data collection and analysis, decision to publish, or preparation of the manuscript.

Competing Interests: ASK and MAN are co-inventors of the patent application on TNFRs Methods of Diagnosing and Predicting Renal Disease, ref JDP-131US01 that has been assigned to Joslin Diabetes Center/Harvard Medical School, and subsequently transferred to Argutus Medical. These authors declare this does alter their adherence to all PLOS ONE policies on sharing data and materials.

* E-mail: Monika.Niewczas@joslin.harvard.edu

Introduction

Diabetic nephropathy is one of the most devastating complications of diabetes. It remains the leading cause of end-stage renal disease (ESRD), accounting for 44% of ESRD incident cases in the United States [1]. Type 2 diabetes (T2D) also increases risk of mortality [2]. Increased urinary excretion of albumin has long been considered a major determinant of diabetic nephropathy progression. However, its value as an accurate marker of the progression to ESRD was recently challenged [3–5]. Thus, new markers that will better identify diabetes patients with at risk of ESRD or mortality unrelated to ESRD are needed.

Recently, results from the Joslin Kidney Study demonstrated that among several inflammatory markers measured, increased concentrations of circulating Tumor Necrosis Factor Receptor (TNFR) 1 and TNFR2 emerged as very strong predictors of

diabetic nephropathy progression to chronic kidney disease (CKD) stage 3 or ESRD [6,7]. TNFR1 and TNFR2 are cell membrane-bound receptors involved in apoptosis, inflammation and immune response [8]. They are released into the extracellular space by the action of a cleavage enzyme or by exocytosis within exosome-like vesicles [9]. It remains unclear how circulating levels of TNFRs impact risk of renal function decline in diabetes [6,7].

Fibroblast growth factor (FGF)-23 is an endocrine hormone secreted by bone cells [10]. The primary physiologic actions of FGF-23 levels are to induce phosphaturia by decreasing urinary reabsorption in proximal tubule, to reduce active vitamin D production and to inhibit PTH secretion [11,12]. Recent epidemiologic studies have focused on the prognostic values of plasma FGF-23 levels and demonstrated that the circulating level of FGF-23 is strongly associated with higher risk of ESRD and death in subjects with CKD [13–17]. Also, circulating levels of

FGF-23 are associated with serum levels of several inflammatory markers in non-diabetic subjects with CKD [18,19], and with circulating levels of TNFR1 in diabetic patients [20].

This study aims to evaluate the effect of circulating levels of FGF-23 on risk of ESRD and mortality unrelated to ESRD in a prospective study of T2D subjects. The question of great importance is whether the effect of TNFR1 can account for the effect of FGF-23, or are these two effects independent.

Materials and Methods

Study patients

The Joslin Kidney Study in T2D patients was previously described [7]. Briefly, a random sample of Joslin Clinic patients with T2D was recruited into the Joslin Study between 1991 and 1995. Eligibility criteria included residence in Massachusetts, T2D diagnosed between ages 35 and 64 years, and age at examination 40 to 69 years. The study protocol and informed written consent procedures were approved by the Joslin Diabetes Center Institutional Review Board. Trained recruiters performed a physical examination that included standardized measurements of blood pressure and collected samples of urine and blood biochemical determinations (stored at $-80°C$). Questionnaires were supplemented with data from medical records and clinical laboratory database. Of the 600 patients selected, 509 were examined and enrolled into the study. Patients with evidence of nephropathy unrelated to diabetes and patients in CKD stage 5 [defined as an estimated glomerular filtration rate (eGFR) <15 ml/min per 1.73 m^2 using the Modified Diet in Renal Disease formula] were excluded. This left 410 patients, with 85% defining themselves as Caucasian. Three hundred eighty patients with available plasma samples for FGF-23 measurements were included in this study.

Assessment of albuminuria status and estimated GFR at baseline

We determined the albumin to creatinine ratio (ACR, mg/g Cr) using the urine sample obtained at the baseline examination. The ACR value was converted to an albumin excretion rate (AER) according to a previously published formula [21]. This AER was used in the univariate and multivariate analyses.

In addition to the baseline urine, we retrieved the results of urinalysis performed on these patients' urine during the preceding two-year interval from the Joslin Clinical computer database, and converted it to an AER as previously described [21]. We determined geometric mean AER for the preceding two-year interval to assign an albuminuria status: normoalbuminuria (AER<30 μg/min), microalbuminuria (AER 30–300 μg/min) and macroalbuminuria/proteinuria (>300 μg/min).

Plasma creatinine was measured in stored baseline samples at the University of Minnesota with the Roche enzymatic assay (Prod No. 11775685) on a Roche/Hitachi Mod P analyzer. eGFR was obtained from plasma concentrations of creatinine using the IDMS-traceable Modified Diet in Renal Disease formula [5]. These measurements were performed in 2009.

Measurements of plasma markers

All plasma markers were measured in baseline specimens by immunoassays in 2009. Circulating TNFR1 levels were determined with ELISA (Cat# DRT100, R&D Systems, Minneapolis, MN) as previously described [7]. Plasma concentrations of C-terminal FGF-23 were determined with ELISA (Cat# 60-6100, Immutopics, San Clemente, CA). All measurements were performed according to the manufacturer's protocols.

Ascertainment of outcomes

The US Renal Data System (USRDS) maintains a roster of US patients receiving renal replacement therapy that includes dates of dialysis and transplantation [22]. The National Death Index (NDI) is a comprehensive roster of deaths in the United States, and includes date and causes of death [23]. All patients were queried against rosters of the USRDS and the NDI covering all events up to the end of 2004, as formerly reported [7].

Statistical Analysis

Analyses were performed in SAS software (SAS Institute, Cary, NC, version 9.2). Differences among the three outcome groups were tested using the chi-squared test for categorical variables, and ANOVA with post hoc Tukey's t-test for continuous variables. Bonferroni correction was applied for the number of group comparisons. Spearman rank correlation matrix was created to evaluate the relationships among clinical variables and plasma markers. AER and the levels of markers were transformed to their logarithms for statistical analysis. Incidence rates of ESRD and deaths were tested for trend across quartiles of marker distribution using SAS macro provided by the Mayo Clinic [24,25]. To evaluate the independent effects of markers for the prediction of outcome, we applied Cox proportional hazard models. $P<0.05$ was considered significant.

Results

Baseline characteristics of the study subjects according to outcomes

At study entry, the mean eGFR of the study group was 92 ± 31 mL/min per 1.73 m^2 and 325 subjects (86%) had preserved renal function (eGFR ≥60 mL/min per 1.73 m^2). One hundred ninety five subjects (51%) had normoalbuminuria, 114 (30%) had microalbuminuria and 71 (19%) had proteinuria.

At the end of follow-up, 249 of the 380 subjects (65%) remained alive. ESRD had developed in 48 (13%) patients. The remaining 83 patients (22%) died without ESRD. Baseline characteristics are summarized in Table 1 according to three outcomes: Alive, ESRD, and Deceased. Those categorized as ESRD or Deceased were older, had longer duration of diabetes, higher AER and lower eGFR than those who remained Alive. The three outcome groups did not differ significantly with regard to HbA1c.

Concentrations of two markers in baseline plasma are also summarized in Table 1. As we previously reported, the ESRD group showed higher baseline concentrations of TNFR1 compared with the Alive group [7]. The Deceased group had levels that, while elevated, were only half as high as the ESRD group. Differences in plasma concentrations of FGF-23 according to outcome groups mirrored the pattern of TNFR1. However, the differences were weaker in case of FGF-23. Interestingly, the plasma concentrations of FGF-23 and TNFR1 in the total study subjects were only moderately correlated (Spearman correlation coefficient = 0.49, p<0.001).

Results of Follow-up Study

To further evaluate the effects of plasma markers on the occurrence of ESRD and all-cause mortality, we used prospective analysis. During 8–12 years of follow-up the cohort of 380 patients with T2D had 3585 person-years of observation; 48 patients developed ESRD (incidence rate; 13/1000 person-years) and 83 died due to causes unrelated to ESRD (mortality rate; 23/1000 person-years). Incidence rate of ESRD increased from 3 to 6, 10 and 46 per 1000 person-years according to increasing quartiles of baseline FGF-23 (p<0.0001 for trend). An even more dramatic

Table 1. Baseline characteristics of subjects with T2D according to their outcome during 8–12 years of follow-up.

Baseline Characteristics	Outcome			P-value	
	Alive (n=249)	ESRD (n=48)	Deceased (n=83)	Alive vs ESRD	Alive vs Deceased
Clinical Characteristics					
Male (%)	54.6	43.8	65.1	0.1672	0.0959
Age (yr)	54±10	60±7	60±7	3.8×10^{-4}	7.9×10^{-7}
Duration of Diabetes (yr)	12±8	18±6	16±8	8.5×10^{-7}	5.9×10^{-5}
HbA1c (%)	8.3±1.7	8.9±1.5	8.6±1.6	0.0607	0.506
AER (μg/min)	20 (12–68)	657 (359–1544)	77 (20–217)	$<10^{-28}$	4.8×10^{-7}
eGFR (mL/min per 1.73 m²)	100±27	60±27	90±30	$<10^{-28}$	0.0093
Plasma Markers					
TNFR1 (pg/mL)	1188 (1006–1447)	2543 (2151–3771)	1597 (1171–2079)	$<10^{-28}$	5.8×10^{-12}
FGF-23 (RU/mL)	50 (36–75)	117 (65–238)	84 (53–133)	5.6×10^{-8}	2.9×10^{-6}

Data are mean ± SD, median (25th, 75th percentiles), or percentage. AER and plasma markers were transformed to base 10 logarithms for the statistical analyses. Bonferroni correction for a number of groups was applied.

increase was seen for incidence rate of ESRD (rates 0, 1, 3 and 72 per 1000 person-years, p<0.0001 for trend) according to quartiles of baseline TNFR1. Mortality rates increased from 10 to 18, 26 and 49 per 1000 person-years with increasing quartiles of baseline FGF-23 (p<0.0001 for trend). Mortality rate increase (rates 13, 14, 26 and 53 per 1000 person-years, p<0.0001 for trend) according to quartiles of baseline TNFR1 were very similar to that observed for quartiles of baseline FGF-23. More detailed data about incidence rates of ESRD and all cause mortality according to both

quartiles of baseline concentrations of FGF-23 and TNFR1 are shown in Table 2 and in Table S1, respectively.

Risk of ESRD according to both plasma markers

Incidence rates of ESRD by quartiles of baseline plasma concentrations of FGF-23 and TNFR1 are presented in Figure 1A. Darker bars represent higher concentrations of FGF-23. It was clear that although the rates increased with quartiles of FGF-23 in univariate analysis, the risk of ESRD was restricted almost exclusively to patients with the highest quartile of TNFR1. Among

Table 2. Incidence rate of ESRD in subjects with T2D stratified by quartiles of FGF-23 and TNFR1.

	FGF-23 Q1	FGF-23 Q2	FGF-23 Q3	FGF-23 Q4	Total
TNFR1 Q1					
Incidence rate (/1000 person-year)	0	0	0	0	0
No of Events/No of person-years	0/439	0/396	0/203	0/45	0/1083
No of subjects	37	36	18	4	95
TNFR1 Q2					
Incidence rate (/1000 person-year)	0	0	0	8.7	1.0
No of Events/No of person-years	0/355	0/246	0/302	1/115	1/1019
No of subjects	31	23	29	13	96
TNFR1 Q3					
Incidence rate (/1000 person-year)	4.8	0	0	10.4	3.4
No of Events/No of person-years	1/208	0/220	0/259	2/193	3/880
No of subjects	22	22	27	23	94
TNFR1 Q4					
Incidence rate (/1000 person-year)	52.8	55.9	55.4	91.3	72.9
No of Events/No of person-years	2/38	6/107	9/163	27/296	44/603
No of subjects	5	14	21	55	95
Total					
Incidence rate (/1000 person-year)	2.9	6.2	9.7	46.3	13.4
No of Events/No of person-years	3/1039	6/970	9/927	30/648	48/3585
No of subjects	95	95	95	95	380

Quartile cut-off values were 1049, 1302, and 1812 pg/mL for TNFR1 and 42, 60, and 96 RU/mL for FGF-23, respectively.

subjects with the highest quartile of TNFR1, the concentrations of FGF-23 did not discriminate the risk of ESRD (p = 0.13 for trend according to FGF-23 quartiles). Subjects who had plasma TNFR1 concentrations in quartiles 1-2 did not develop ESRD regardless of FGF-23 concentrations. To evaluate the effect of FGF-23 on the development of ESRD controlling for other clinical characteristics and plasma TNFR1, we used Cox proportional hazard models. The results are shown in Table 3. In a univariate analyses, clinical characteristics and both plasma markers were strongly associated with risk of ESRD. In multivariate analyses (model #1),when clinical characteristics were considered together with each marker, the hazard ratio (HR) for TNFR1 and FGF-23 declined significantly but still remained associated with risk of ESRD (HR 8.4, 95% C.I. 3.1–22.6 for one quartile increase of TNFR1 and HR 1.6, 95% C.I. 1.2–2.1 for one quartile increase of FGF-23). In model #2 when both markers were considered together with clinical characteristics, only the HR for TNFR1 was significant (HR 6.9, 95% C.I. 2.5–19.0 for one quartile increase). The effect of FGF-23 was not significant (HR 1.2, 95% C.I. 0.9–1.7 for one quartile increase).

Mortality according to plasma markers

Rates of all-cause mortality according to quartiles of baseline FGF-23 and TNFR1 are presented in Figure 1B. Darker bars represent higher concentrations of FGF-23. Mortality rates clearly increased with quartiles of FGF-23 and with quartiles of TNFR1. The two effects were additive. To evaluate the effect of FGF-23 on the mortality controlling for other clinical characteristics and plasma TNFR1, we used Cox proportional hazard models. The results are shown in Table 4. In univariate analyses only two clinical characteristics, age and AER, were significant together with baseline concentrations of FGF-23 and TNFR1. In multivariate analyses (model #1) when clinical characteristics were considered together with each marker, the HRs for TNFR1 and FGF-23 declined somewhat but remained strongly associated with mortality (for one quartile increase of TNFR1, HR 1.4, 95% C.I. 1.1–1.7 and for one quartile increase of FGF-23, HR 1.6, 95% C.I. 1.3–2.0). In model #2 when both markers were considered together with clinical characteristics, the HR for FGF-23 was

significant (for one quartile increase of TNFR1, HR 1.1, 95% C.I. 0.8–1.5 and for one quartile increase of FGF-23, HR 1.5, 95% C.I. 1.2–2.0).

When cardiovascular death risk (n = 47) was analyzed separately, FGF-23 levels remained independent predictors in the model, which included age, AER and TNFR1 (effect for one quartile FGF-23 increase HR 1.4, 95% C.I. 1.0–2.0). More detailed results are presented in Table S2.

Discussion

In our prospective study of subjects with T2D, we demonstrated that baseline plasma concentration of FGF-23 was associated with increased risk of ESRD. However its effect was no longer significant after controlling for plasma concentration of TNFR1. In other words, plasma concentration of TNFR1 accounted for the effect of FGF-23 on risk of ESRD. However, baseline level of FGF-23 was a significant independent predictor of all-cause as well as cardiovascular mortality unrelated to ESRD.

Recent epidemiologic studies reported association between plasma FGF-23 levels and clinical outcomes in patients with CKD [13–17]. Several cross-sectional studies demonstrated that FGF-23 levels were increased in patients with CKD [26]. Several reports show high levels of circulating FGF-23 as a predictor of progression to ESRD [13,14,17]. In the Chronic Renal Insufficiency Cohort Study during 3.5 years of follow-up elevated FGF-23 was an independent risk factor for ESRD [14]. In another follow-up study of 177 patients with non-diabetic CKD, higher levels of C-terminal FGF-23 and intact FGF-23 were independently associated with incident ESRD [17]. A small study of subjects with diabetes and impaired renal function at baseline reported that FGF-23 was a predictor of renal outcome independent of creatinine clearance, although its 12 ESRD events did not allow a fully adjusted Cox analysis [16].

The mechanisms are unclear as to which circulating FGF-23 may impact/be associated with impaired renal function and contributes to progression to ESRD. In non-diabetic subjects with impaired renal function, circulating levels of FGF-23 were correlated with serum concentrations of several markers of

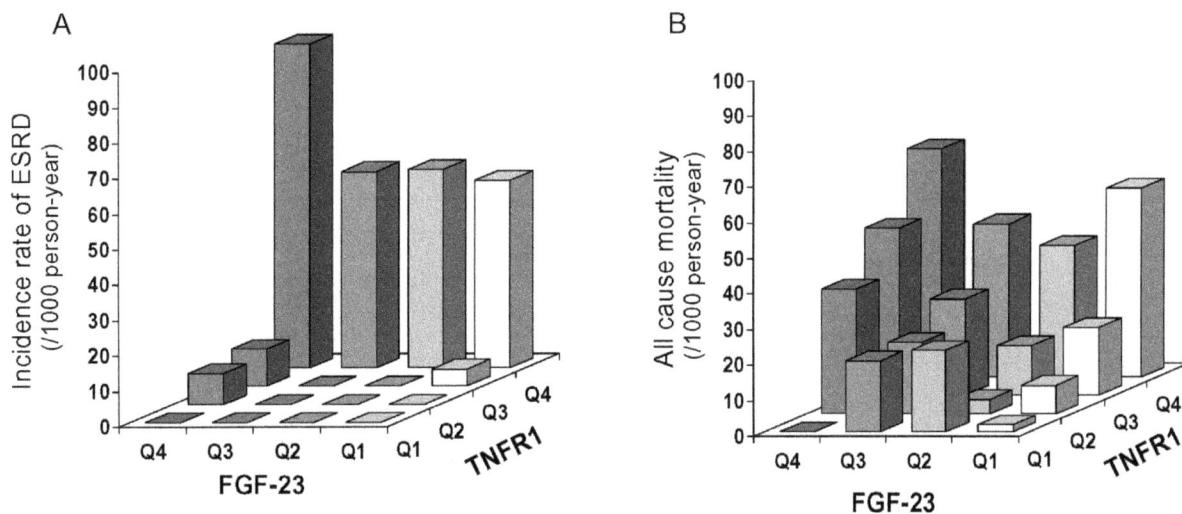

Figure 1. Incidence rate of ESRD and all-cause mortality stratified by quartiles of FGF-23 and TNFR1. Figure 1A demonstrates incidence rate of ESRD and Figure 1B shows incidence of all cause mortality. Q1–Q4 represents quartiles 1 to 4. Quartile cut-off values were 1049, 1302, and 1812 pg/mL for TNFR1 and 42, 60, and 96 RU/mL for FGF-23, respectively. Increasing color intensity of the columns corresponds to higher concentrations (quartiles) of FGF-23.

Table 3. Univariate and multivariate Cox proportional hazard models assessing risk of ESRD adjusting for relevant baseline clinical characteristics and plasma markers in subjects with T2D followed for 8–12 years.

| | Univariate analyses | | Multivariate analyses | | | |
| | | | Model #1 | | Model #2 | |
	HR* (95% CI)	P-value	HR* (95% CI)	P-value	HR* (95% CI)	P-value
Clinical Characteristics						
AER	4.3 (3.2–5.9)	<0.0001	2.4 (1.7–3.5)	<0.0001	2.5 (1.7–3.6)	<0.0001
eGFR	2.0 (1.7–2.3)	<0.0001	1.3 (1.1–1.6)	0.0106	1.3 (1.1–1.6)	0.01
HbA1c	1.3 (1.0–1.6)	0.027	1.3 (1.1–1.7)	0.0092	1.4 (1.1–1.7)	0.008
Plasma Markers						
TNFR1	35.5 (15.0–84.0)	<0.0001	8.4 (3.1–22.6)	<0.0001	6.9 (2.5–19.0)	0.0002
FGF-23	2.8 (2.0–3.9)	<0.0001	1.6 (1.2–2.1)	0.002	1.2 (0.9–1.7)	0.15

*Effect measures are expressed as the HR for a one-quartile increase in the distribution of each covariate except for eGFR, for which it is a one-quartile decrease.
Model #1 included relevant clinical characteristics and plasma TNFR1 and FGF-23 independently.
Model #2 included relevant clinical characteristics and plasma TNFR1 and FGF-23 together.

systemic inflammation such as IL-6, C-reactive protein and TNFα [18,19]. One study reported that elevated FGF-23 levels were associated with TNFR1 levels in subjects with diabetic nephropathy [20]. Interestingly these findings were confirmed in our study. Table S3 shows correlations between baseline plasma levels of FGF-23 and ACR, eGFR and plasma markers such as CRP, IL-6, free and total TNFα, TNFR1 and TNFR2. Although these correlations were statistically significant, they were only moderate. The correlations between these markers and plasma level of TNFR1, a marker that accounted for the initial effect of FGF-23 on risk of ESRD in T2D, were almost twice as strong. These patterns of associations may indicate that both FGF-23 and TNFR1 (TNF markers) cause progression to ESRD in the same pathway. TNFR1 appeared to be stronger predictor, either because it is more directly involved in progression to ESRD or because its features as a biomarker are potentially better (i.e. better stability over time). Another possibility is that FGF-23 is simply a correlate of circulating level of TNFRs and is not causally related to progression to ESRD.

The role of FGF-23 on the inflammatory pathway has not yet been studied in depth. The effect of FGF-23 may be mediated via expression of Klotho. Klotho is an essential cofactor of FGF-23, expressed highly in renal tubules [27]. Higher FGF-23 levels may be associated with low Klotho tissue expression [28,29]. Klotho expression is down-regulated in several kidney injury models and its over-expression attenuates renal damage in the experimental models of kidney injury [30]. Moreno et al. reported that TNF (TNFRs ligand) decreases Klotho expression [31]. The relation between expression of Klotho and plasma levels of TNFRs is unknown. On the other hand, exogenous administration of Klotho suppressed NF-kB activation and subsequent inflammatory cytokines production in in-vitro study [32]. A few studies examined the clinical implication of plasma Klotho levels in subjects with CKD, but failed to demonstrate consistent association of Klotho levels with renal function or poor outcome [33]. Additionally, increased FGF-23 levels reduce vitamin D activation, which has known anti-inflammatory properties [34,35]. Increase of vitamin D levels by dietary supplement resulted in decrease of systemic inflammatory markers such as CRP and TNFα in subjects with T2D [36].

In contrast to the lack of independent effect of circulating FGF-23 on progression to ESRD, our study demonstrated that FGF-23

Table 4. Univariate and multivariate Cox proportional hazard models assessing risk of all-cause mortality adjusting for relevant baseline clinical characteristics and plasma markers in subjects with T2D followed for 8–12 years.

| | Univariate analyses | | Multivariate analyses | | | |
| | | | Model #1 | | Model #2 | |
	HR* (95% CI)	P-value	HR* (95% CI)	P-value	HR* (95% CI)	P-value
Clinical Characteristics						
Age	1.6 (1.3–1.9)	<0.0001	1.4 (1.1–1.8)	<0.0001	1.4 (1.1–1.7)	0.0011
AER	1.4 (1.2–1.7)	<0.0001	1.2 (0.99–1.5)	0.059	1.3 (1.04–1.6)	0.0206
Plasma Markers						
TNFR1	1.9 (1.5–2.4)	<0.0001	1.4 (1.1–1.8)	0.012	1.1 (0.8–1.5)	0.42
FGF-23	1.8 (1.5–2.3)	<0.0001	1.6 (1.3–2.0)	<0.0001	1.5 (1.2–2.0)	0.0005

*Effect measures are expressed as the HR for a one-quartile increase in the distribution of each covariate except for eGFR, for which it is a one-quartile decrease.
Model #1 included relevant clinical characteristics and plasma TNFR1 and FGF-23 independently.
Model #2 included relevant clinical characteristics and plasma TNFR1 and FGF-23 together.

had an independent impact on risk of death unrelated to ESRD, including CVD deaths. Interestingly, in multivariate analyses, FGF-23 effect accounted for an effect of circulating TNFRs on mortality in T2D shown in our previous report [7]. The mechanism underlying the association between FGF-23 levels and mortality remains unclear. First, some investigators suggest that FGF-23 levels may be a sensitive surrogate marker for the toxicity of disturbance in phosphate and mineral metabolism in CKD patients [15]. However, the predictive effect of FGF-23 levels is not attenuated by serum phosphate, PTH, and vitamin D levels and FGF-23 levels are stronger predictors of mortality than other bone-related markers [13,16]. Alternatively, FGF-23 levels may be a surrogate marker of the severity of CKD and subsequent increased risk of mortality. However, this scenario is also unlikely given the observation that the association with mortality was independent of TNFR1 levels in this study, while the association with ESRD was not. The third possibility is that elevated FGF-23 levels may be a causal factor contributing to increased mortality. This possibility is indirectly supported by the observation that higher FGF-23 levels are associated with vascular calcification, endothelial dysfunction and left ventricular hypertrophy in CKD patients [15,37,38].

Finally, we should mention a few limitations of our study. First, we measured only C-terminal, and not the intact form of FGF-23. However, a recent study showed the following: both forms are highly correlated; biologically active FGF-23 is accurately measured by either form; and clinical associations are comparably strong between the two [39]. Second, it is not clear how stable plasma concentration of FGF-23 is over a period of several years. For example, we showed that plasma concentrations of TNFR1 are very stable in patients with T1D over several years [6]. Third,

our study was conducted in mostly Caucasian subjects with T2D so it is uncertain if our findings could be applied to Non-Caucasians and to the subjects with T1D.

Supporting Information

Table S1 All-cause mortality in subjects with T2D stratified by quartiles of FGF-23 and TNFR1.

Table S2 Univariate and multivariate Cox proportional hazard models assessing risk of cardiovascular mortality adjusting for relevant baseline clinical characteristics and plasma markers in subjects with T2D followed for 8–12 years.

Table S3 Spearman correlation coefficients among clinical variables and plasma markers at baseline.

Acknowledgments

The authors wish to thank for Harry Spaulding editorial assistance in the preparation of this article.

Author Contributions

Guarantor of this work, having full access to all the data in the study and taking responsibility for the integrity of the data and the accuracy of the data analyses: MAN. Conceived and designed the experiments: JL ASK MAN. Performed the experiments: JL TG WHW AMS RRH JJ KPM. Analyzed the data: JL TG JS AMS ASK MAN. Contributed reagents/materials/analysis tools: JS ASK MAN. Wrote the paper: JL ASK MAN.

References

1. Collins AJ, Foley RN, Chavers B, Gilbertson D, Herzog C, et al. (2012) United States Renal Data System 2011 Annual Data Report: Atlas of chronic kidney disease & end-stage renal disease in the United States. Am J Kidney Dis 59: A7, e1–A7,420.
2. McEwen LN, Karter AJ, Waitzfelder BE, Crosson JC, Marrero DG, et al. (2011) Predictors of Mortality Over 8 Years in Type 2 Diabetic Patients: Translating Research Into Action for Diabetes (TRIAD). Diabetes Care. dc11–2281.
3. Perkins BA, Ficociello LH, Silva KH, Finkelstein DM, Warram JH, et al. (2003) Regression of microalbuminuria in type 1 diabetes. N Engl J Med 348: 2285–2293.
4. MacIsaac RJ, Jerums G (2011) Diabetic kidney disease with and without albuminuria. Curr Opin Nephrol Hypertens 20: 246–257.
5. Levey AS, Coresh J, Greene T, Marsh J, Stevens LA, et al. (2007) Expressing the Modification of Diet in Renal Disease Study equation for estimating glomerular filtration rate with standardized serum creatinine values. Clin Chem 53: 766–772.
6. Gohda T, Niewczas MA, Ficociello LH, Walker WH, Skupien J, et al. (2012) Circulating TNF Receptors 1 and 2 Predict Stage 3 CKD in Type 1 Diabetes. J Am Soc Nephrol 23: 516–524.
7. Niewczas MA, Gohda T, Skupien J, Smiles AM, Walker WH, et al. (2012) Circulating TNF Receptors 1 and 2 Predict ESRD in Type 2 Diabetes. J Am Soc Nephrol 23: 507–515.
8. Aderka D (1996) The potential biological and clinical significance of the soluble tumor necrosis factor receptors. Cytokine Growth Factor Rev 7: 231–240.
9. Levine SJ (2008) Molecular mechanisms of soluble cytokine receptor generation. J Biol Chem 283: 14177–14181.
10. Prie D, Friedlander G (2010) Reciprocal control of 1,25-dihydroxyvitamin D and FGF23 formation involving the FGF23/Klotho system. Clin J Am Soc Nephrol 5: 1717–1722.
11. Saito H, Kusano K, Kinosaki M, Ito H, Hirata M, et al. (2003) Human fibroblast growth factor-23 mutants suppress Na+-dependent phosphate co-transport activity and 1alpha,25-dihydroxyvitamin D3 production. J Biol Chem 278: 2206–2211.
12. Baum M, Schiavi S, Dwarakanath V, Quigley R (2005) Effect of fibroblast growth factor-23 on phosphate transport in proximal tubules. Kidney Int 68: 1148–1153.
13. Kendrick J, Cheung AK, Kaufman JS, Greene T, Roberts WL, et al. (2011) FGF-23 associates with death, cardiovascular events, and initiation of chronic dialysis. J Am Soc Nephrol 22: 1913–1922.
14. Fliser D, Kollerits B, Neyer U, Ankerst DP, Lhotta K, et al. (2007) Fibroblast growth factor 23 (FGF23) predicts progression of chronic kidney disease: the Mild to Moderate Kidney Disease (MMKD) Study. J Am Soc Nephrol 18: 2600–2608.
15. Gutierrez OM, Mannstadt M, Isakova T, Rauh-Hain JA, Tamez H, et al. (2008) Fibroblast growth factor 23 and mortality among patients undergoing hemodialysis. N Engl J Med 359: 584–592.
16. Titan SM, Zatz R, Graciolli FG, dos Reis LM, Barros RT, et al. (2011) FGF-23 as a predictor of renal outcome in diabetic nephropathy. Clin J Am Soc Nephrol 6: 241–247.
17. Isakova T, Xie H, Yang W, Xie D, Anderson AH, et al. (2011) Fibroblast growth factor 23 and risks of mortality and end-stage renal disease in patients with chronic kidney disease. JAMA 305: 2432–2439.
18. Krieger NS, Culbertson CD, Kyker-Snowman K, Bushinsky DA (2012) Metabolic acidosis increases fibroblast growth factor 23 in neonatal mouse bone. Am J Physiol Renal Physiol 303: F431–F436.
19. Mendoza JM, Isakova T, Ricardo AC, Xie H, Navaneethan SD, et al. (2012) Fibroblast Growth Factor 23 and Inflammation in CKD. Clin J Am Soc Nephrol 7: 1155–1162.
20. Sharma K, Ix JH, Mathew AV, Cho M, Pflueger A, et al. (2011) Pirfenidone for diabetic nephropathy. J Am Soc Nephrol 22: 1144–1151.
21. Krolewski AS, Laffel LM, Krolewski M, Quinn M, Warram JH (1995) Glycosylated hemoglobin and the risk of microalbuminuria in patients with insulin-dependent diabetes mellitus. N Engl J Med 332: 1251–1255.
22. Agodoa LY, Eggers PW (1995) Renal replacement therapy in the United States: data from the United States Renal Data System. Am J Kidney Dis 25: 119–133.
23. Centers for Disease Control and Prevention, National Center for Health Statistics website. Avaiable: http://www.cdc.gov/nchs/ndi.htm. Accessed 2010 Oct 10.
24. Gooley TA, Leisenring W, Crowley J, Storer BE (1999) Estimation of failure probabilities in the presence of competing risks: new representations of old estimators. Stat Med 18: 695–706.
25. Bergstralh E: SAS Macro That Performs Cumulative Incidence in Presence of Completing Risks. Available: http://mayoresearch.mayo.edu/mayo/research/biostat/upload/comprisk.sas. Accessed 2010 Feb 3.
26. Larsson T, Nisbeth U, Ljunggren O, Juppner H, Jonsson KB (2003) Circulating concentration of FGF-23 increases as renal function declines in patients with chronic kidney disease, but does not change in response to variation in phosphate intake in healthy volunteers. Kidney Int 64: 2272–2279.

27. Li SA, Watanabe M, Yamada H, Nagai A, Kinuta M, et al. (2004) Immunohistochemical localization of Klotho protein in brain, kidney, and reproductive organs of mice. Cell Struct Funct 29: 91–99.

28. Kurosu H, Ogawa Y, Miyoshi M, Yamamoto M, Nandi A, et al. (2006) Regulation of fibroblast growth factor-23 signaling by klotho. J Biol Chem 281: 6120–6123.

29. Koh N, Fujimori T, Nishiguchi S, Tamori A, Shiomi S, et al. (2001) Severely reduced production of klotho in human chronic renal failure kidney. Biochem Biophys Res Commun 280: 1015–1020.

30. Bernheim J, Benchetrit S (2011) The potential roles of FGF23 and Klotho in the prognosis of renal and cardiovascular diseases. Nephrol Dial Transplant 26: 2433–2438.

31. Moreno JA, Izquierdo MC, Sanchez-Nino MD, Suarez-Alvarez B, Lopez-Larrea C, et al. (2011) The inflammatory cytokines TWEAK and TNFalpha reduce renal klotho expression through NFkappaB. J Am Soc Nephrol 22: 1315–1325.

32. Zhao Y, Banerjee S, Dey N, LeJeune WS, Sarkar PS, et al. (2011) Klotho depletion contributes to increased inflammation in kidney of the db/db mouse model of diabetes via RelA (serine)536 phosphorylation. Diabetes 60: 1907–1916.

33. Seiler S, Wen M, Roth HJ, Fehrenz M, Flugge F, et al. (2012) Plasma Klotho is not related to kidney function and does not predict adverse outcome in patients with chronic kidney disease. Kidney Int 10.1038/ki.2012.288 [doi].

34. Alborzi P, Patel NA, Peterson C, Bills JE, Bekele DM, et al. (2008) Paricalcitol reduces albuminuria and inflammation in chronic kidney disease: a randomized double-blind pilot trial. Hypertension 52: 249–255.

35. Shimada T, Hasegawa H, Yamazaki Y, Muto T, Hino R, et al. (2004) FGF-23 is a potent regulator of vitamin D metabolism and phosphate homeostasis. J Bone Miner Res 19: 429–435.

36. Shab-Bidar S, Neyestani TR, Djazayery A, Eshraghian MR, Houshiarrad A, et al. (2012) Improvement of vitamin D status resulted in amelioration of biomarkers of systemic inflammation in the subjects with type 2 diabetes. Diabetes Metab Res Rev 28: 424–430.

37. Yilmaz MI, Sonmez A, Saglam M, Yaman H, Kilic S, et al. (2010) FGF-23 and vascular dysfunction in patients with stage 3 and 4 chronic kidney disease. Kidney Int 78: 679–685.

38. Gutierrez OM, Januzzi JL, Isakova T, Laliberte K, Smith K, et al. (2009) Fibroblast growth factor 23 and left ventricular hypertrophy in chronic kidney disease. Circulation 119: 2545–2552.

39. Shimada T, Urakawa I, Isakova T, Yamazaki Y, Epstein M, et al. (2010) Circulating fibroblast growth factor 23 in patients with end-stage renal disease treated by peritoneal dialysis is intact and biologically active. J Clin Endocrinol Metab 95: 578–585.

13

Decreased Circulating C3 Levels and Mesangial C3 Deposition Predict Renal Outcome in Patients with IgA Nephropathy

Seung Jun Kim[1]◊, Hyang Mo Koo[1]◊, Beom Jin Lim[2], Hyung Jung Oh[1], Dong Eun Yoo[1], Dong Ho Shin[1], Mi Jung Lee[1], Fa Mee Doh[1], Jung Tak Park[1], Tae-Hyun Yoo[1], Shin-Wook Kang[1,3], Kyu Hun Choi[1], Hyeon Joo Jeong[3], Seung Hyeok Han[1]*

1 Department of Internal Medicine, Yonsei University College of Medicine, Seoul, Korea, **2** Department of Pathology, Yonsei University College of Medicine, Seoul, Korea, **3** Severance Biomedical Science Institute, Brain Korea 21, Yonsei University, Seoul, Korea

Abstract

Background and Aims: Mesangial C3 deposition is frequently observed in patients with IgA nephropathy (IgAN). However, the role of complement in the pathogenesis or progression of IgAN is uncertain. In this observational cohort study, we aimed to identify the clinical implications of circulating C3 levels and mesangial C3 deposition and to investigate their utility as predictors of renal outcomes in patients with IgAN.

Methods: A total of 343 patients with biopsy-proven IgAN were enrolled between January 2000 and December 2008. Decreased serum C3 level (hypoC3) was defined as C3 <90 mg/dl. The study endpoint was end-stage renal disease (ESRD) and a doubling of the baseline serum creatinine (D-SCr).

Results: Of the patients, there were 66 patients (19.2%) with hypoC3. During a mean follow-up of 53.7 months, ESRD occurred in 5 patients (7.6%) with hypoC3 compared with 9 patients (3.2%) with normal C3 levels (P = 0.11). However, 12 patients (18.2%) with hypoC3 reached D-SCr compared with 17 patients (6.1%) with normal C3 levels [Hazard ratio (HR), 3.59; 95% confidence interval (CI), 1.33–10.36; P = 0.018]. In a multivariable model in which serum C3 levels were treated as a continuous variable, hypoC3 significantly predicted renal outcome of D-SCr (per 1 mg/dl increase of C3; HR, 0.95; 95% CI, 0.92–0.99; P = 0.011). The risk of reaching renal outcome was significantly higher in patients with mesangial C3 deposition 2+ to 3+ than in patients without deposition (HR 9.37; 95% CI, 1.10–80.26; P = 0.04).

Conclusions: This study showed that hypoC3 and mesangial C3 deposition were independent risk factors for progression, suggesting that complement activation may play a pathogenic role in patients with IgAN.

Editor: Ivan Cruz Moura, Institut national de la santé et de la recherche médicale (INSERM), France

Funding: This work was supported by the Brain Korea 21 Project for Medical Science, Yonsei University, by the National Research Foundation of Korea (NRF) grant funded by the Korean government (MEST) (No. 2011-0030711), and by a grant from the Korea Healthcare Technology R&D Project, Ministry of Health and Welfare, Republic of Korea (A102065). The funders had no role in study design, data collection and analysis, decision to publish, or preparation of the manuscript.

Competing Interests: The authors have declared that no competing interests exist.

* E-mail: hansh@yuhs.ac

◊ These authors contributed equally to this work.

Introduction

IgA nephropathy (IgAN) is most common primary glomerulonephritis worldwide [1]. Patients with IgAN have a variable clinical course, ranging from a totally benign condition to progressive deterioration in kidney function over time. Approximately 20 to 30% of the patients with IgAN will eventually develop end stage renal disease (ESRD) within 20 to 25 years after disease onset [2]. Previous studies have identified clinical and pathologic features associated with adverse outcomes. These include heavy proteinuria, reduced renal function, hypertension at the time of diagnosis, interstitial fibrosis, and glomerular sclerosis [3–5]. However, there are no available serologic tests that can be employed to assess disease activity or to predict renal outcomes in these patients.

Although IgA deposits within the mesangium are a key diagnostic finding in IgAN, mesangial C3 deposition is also frequently observed. However, the role of complement activation in the pathogenesis or progression of IgAN is uncertain [6]. In previous studies, dimeric and polymeric IgA have been found to activate complement system in the glomeruli via the alternative or lectin pathway, thus leading to glomerular damage [7–12]. It was also reported that systemic complement activation occurs in patients with IgAN [13,14]. Specifically, Zwirner showed that activated C3 was associated with increased proteinuria and subsequent deterioration in kidney function in these patients, suggesting that systemic complement activation might play a role in renal injury in this glomerulopathy [14]. However, their findings have not yet been validated, thus whether hypocomplementemia may have prognostic value for predicting renal outcomes is currently unknown. Therefore, we undertook an observational cohort study to determine the clinical implications of decreased serum C3 levels (hypoC3) and to investigate its utility as a predictor of renal outcomes in patients with IgAN. We also examined clinical features and outcomes according to the pathologic findings, particularly mesangial C3 deposition in these patients.

Methods

Ethics statement

The study was carried out in accordance with the Declaration of Helsinki and approved by the Institutional Review Board of Yonsei University Health System Clinical Trial Center. We obtained informed written consent from all participants involved in our study.

Patients

Renal biopsy was performed in 1181 patients at Yonsei University Severance Hospital between January 2000 and December 2008. Among these patients, 436 were diagnosed with IgAN. Patients with Henoch-Schonlein purpura were considered ineligible. Our routine practice to assess glomerular disease encompasses the measurement of serum concentrations of complement. However, patients in whom serum complement levels were not available at the time of renal biopsy were excluded (n = 27). We also excluded patients who had features of IgA-dominant acute post-infectious glomerulonephritis exhibiting hypocomplementemia, diffuse glomerular endocapillary hypercellularity, and subepithelial humps on electron microscopy (n = 3)

[15], and patients who had features of lupus nephritis, such as the presence of typical autoantibodies and "full house" immunofluorescence pattern which was defined as the mesangial co-deposits of IgG, IgA, IgM, and/or C1q (n = 2) [16]. In addition, patients with age <20 years (n = 6) or >75 years (n = 3), inadequate biopsy sample with the number of glomeruli ≤7 (n = 7), and patients who initially presented with nephrotic syndrome (n = 38), crescentic glomerulonephritis (n = 2), and advanced chronic liver diseases (n = 5) were also excluded. Therefore, a total of 343 patients were included in this study (Figure 1).

Data collection

At the time of the renal biopsy, patients' demographic and clinical data such as age, gender, blood pressure, episode of gross hematuria, and presence of hypertension were recorded. Hypertension was defined as systolic blood pressure >140 mmHg or 90 mmHg and the need for antihypertensive medication to maintain pressures below these levels. In addition, laboratory parameters such as serum albumin, blood urea nitrogen, creatinine, uric acid, total cholesterol, triglycerides, C-reactive protein (CRP) and urinary protein-to-creatinine ratio (UPCR) were measured. Serum concentrations of immunoglobulins (Igs) A or G and C3 were measured by immunoturbidimetry (Cobas C501, Roche, Mannhein, Germany). Using this method, the normal reference range of C3 levels are 90–180 mg/dl. We calculated eGFR using the Modification of Diet in Renal Disease (MDRD) study equation [17].

Renal biopsy

All renal biopsy specimens were re-assessed blindly by a single pathologist using the Oxford classification [18]. The biopsy specimens were processed for light microscopy, immunofluorescence study, and electron microscopy. IgAN was diagnosed by the

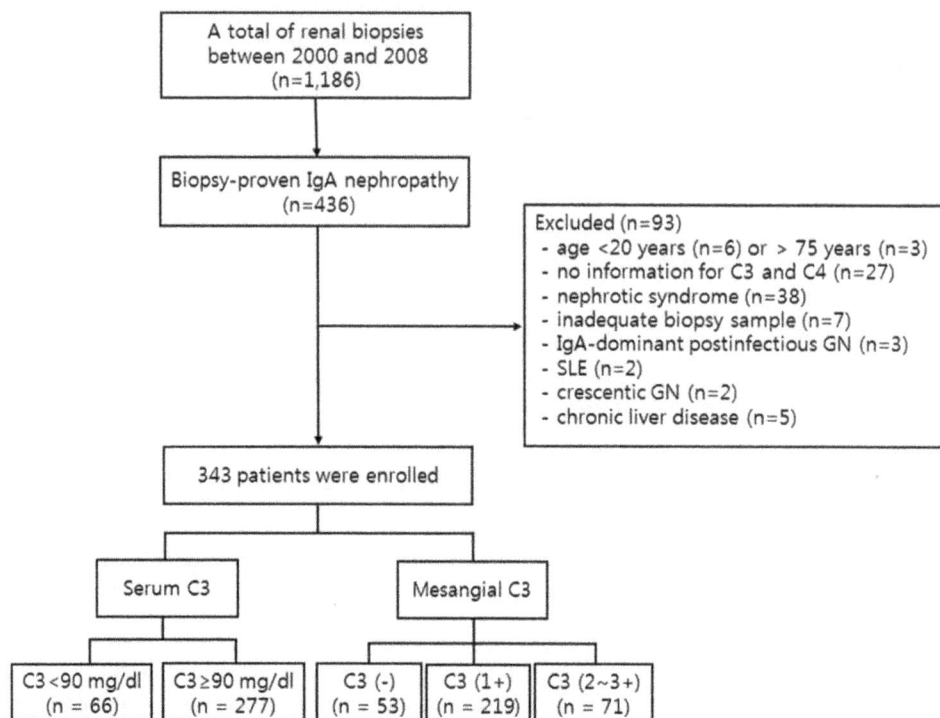

Figure 1. Flow diagram of the study. IgA nephropathy was diagnosed in 436 patients between January 2000 and December 2008. Excluding 93 patients, a total of 343 patients were enrolled. eGFR, estimated glomerular filtration rate; GN, glomerulonephritis; SLE, systemic lupus erythematosus.

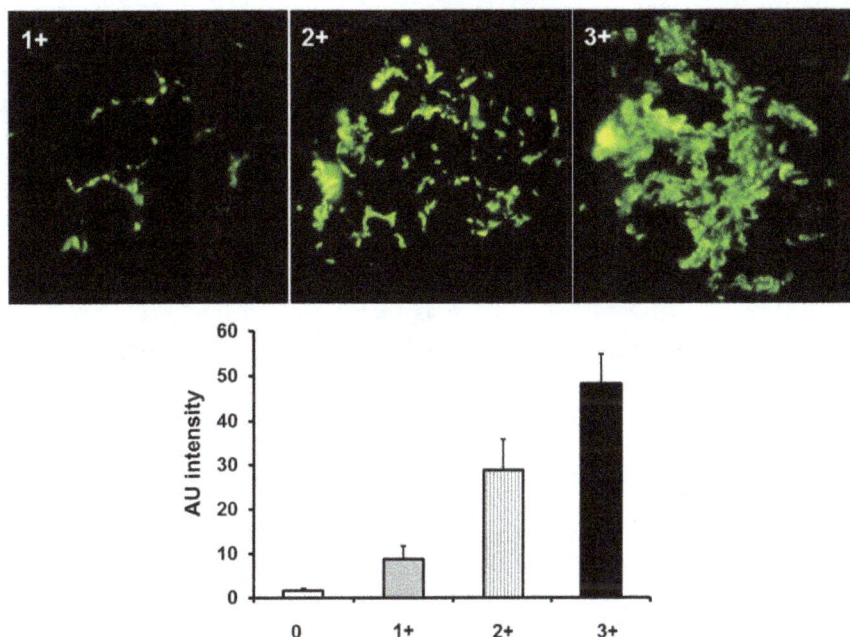

Figure 2. Representative pictures of immunofluorescence staining of mesangial C3 1+ to 3+. Immunofluorescence intensity was quantified by ImageJ software.

following findings: (1) the presence of predominant IgA deposits (at least 1+) mainly in the mesangium by immunofluorescence, (2) the presence of mesangial electron-dense deposits by electron microscopic examination, and (3) the absence of other systemic inflammatory diseases such as systemic lupus erythematosus. The mesangial hypercellularity score was preferred to the percentage of glomeruli showing severe mesangial hypercellularity. The cutoff for the mesangial hypercellularity score was 0.5. Segmental glomerulosclerosis and endocapillary hypercellularity were categorized as either present or absent. Tubular atrophy/interstitial fibrosis was classified as T0 (0–25% of cortical area), T1 (26–50% of cortical area), or T2 (>50% of cortical area) [18]. We quantified the immunofluorescence staining of C3 deposition in the mesangial area by ImageJ software v1.60 (NIH, Bethesda, Maryland, USA; online at http://rsbweb.nih.gov/ij). With the use of this method, quantification of immunofluorescence was expressed as arbitrary unit (AU), which was calculated as (mean pixel intensity X glomerular area)/100,000. Mesangial C3 deposits were classified into four groups: 0, AU level <5; 1+, 5≤ AU level <20; 2+, 20≤ AU level <40; and 3+, 40≤ AU level (Figure 2).

Study outcomes

The study endpoint was ESRD and a doubling of the baseline serum creatinine (D-SCr). ESRD was defined as initiation of renal replacement therapy including permanent hemodialysis, peritoneal dialysis, or renal transplantation. We also evaluated the decline rate of eGFR between patients with hypoC3 and patients with normal C3 levels.

Statistical analysis

Statistical analysis was performed using SPSS version 17.0 (SPSS Inc., Chicago, Illinois, USA). Continuous data were expressed as mean ± SD, and categorical data were expressed as a number (percentage). The two groups were compared using the t-test or chi-squared test. The Kolmogorov-Smirnov test was used to analyze the normality of the distribution of parameters. Nonparametric variables were expressed as median and interquartile range and compared using the Mann–Whitney test or Kruskal–Wallis test. Probability of renal survival curves were generated by the Kaplan-Meier method, and between-group survival was compared by the log-rank test. The independent prognostic values of clinical and pathological parameters for the study outcomes were analyzed by multiple Cox regression analyses. Hazard ratios (HRs) and 95% confidence intervals (CIs) were calculated with the use of the estimated regression coefficients and standard errors in the Cox regression analysis. The predictive value for renal outcome was also analyzed by receiver operating characteristic (ROC) curve analysis with calculated area under the ROC curve (AUC). Finally, to compare

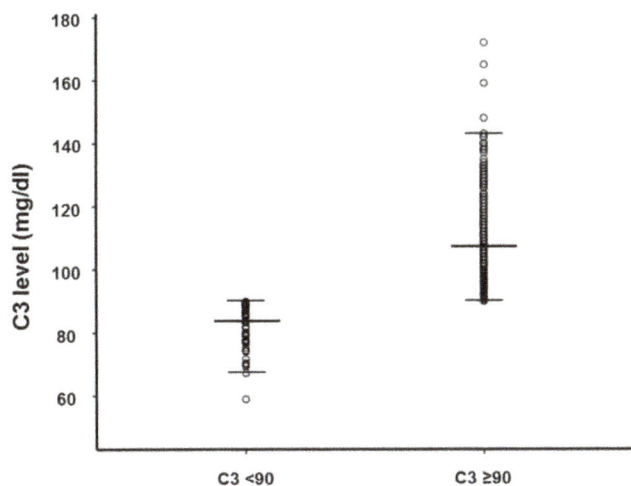

Figure 3. A scattered plot of each level of serum C3 between patients with C3 levels <90 mg/dl and patients with C3 levels ≥90 mg/dl.

Table 1. Demographic, clinical and biochemical characteristics.

	All (n = 343)	C3 <90 mg/dl (n = 66)	C3 ≥90 mg/dl (n = 277)	P-value
Age (years)	34.5±11.7	31.1±9.2	35.4±12.1	0.002
Male gender (n, %)	159 (46.4%)	30 (45.5%)	129 (46.6%)	0.87
Hypertension (n, %)	85 (24.8%)	8 (12.1%)	77 (27.8%)	0.008
Diabetes (n, %)	4 (1.2%)	1 (1.5%)	3 (1.1%)	0.77
Coronary artery disease (n, %)	8 (2.3%)	2 (3.0%)	6 (2.2%)	0.68
Hepatitis B antigen positivity (n, %)	15 (4.4%)	2 (3.2%)	13 (5.1%)	0.74
Hepatitis C antibody positivity (n, %)	1 (0.3%)	0 (0%)	1 (0.6%)	1.00
Episodes of gross hematuria (n, %)	93 (27.1%)	16 (24.2%)	77 (27.8%)	0.56
Body mass index (kg/m^2)	22.7±3.3	20.9±2.4	23.2±3.3	<0.001
Systolic blood pressure (mmHg)	125.7±15.3	121.5±11.1	126.8±16.0	0.002
141 to 160 mmHg (n, %)	34 (9.9%)	7 (10.6%)	27 (9.7%)	
161 to 180 mmHg (n, %)	2 (0.6%)	0 (0%)	2 (0.7%)	
>180 mmHg (n, %)	2 (0.6%)	0 (0%)	2 (0.7%)	
MAP (mmHg)	94.2±11.4	91.4±9.5	94.8±11.7	0.031
Blood urea nitrogen (mg/dl)	15.0±5.6	15.2±6.4	15.0±5.5	0.74
Creatinine (mg/dl)	1.1±0.4	1.1±0.4	1.1±0.4	0.34
eGFR (ml/min/1.73 m^2)	79.8±24.2	78.8±26.1	80.0±23.8	0.71
eGFR <30 (n, %)	9 (2.6%)	3 (4.5%)	6 (2.2%)	
30≤ eGFR <60 (n, %)	65 (19.0%)	15 (22.7%)	50 (18.1%)	
eGFR ≥60 (n, %)	269 (78.4%)	48 (72.7%)	221 (79.8%)	
Protein (g/dl)	6.8±0.6	6.6±0.6	6.8±0.6	0.10
Albumin (g/dl)	4.1±0.5	4.0±0.5	4.1±0.5	0.10
Uric acid (mg/dl)	5.7±1.6	5.6±1.7	5.8±1.6	0.45
Cholesterol (mg/dl)	181.8±38.5	170.8±39.9	184.4±37.8	0.01
Triglycerides (mg/dl)	132.3±91.0	106.1±50.1	139.2±97.9	0.002
Urine PCR (mg/mg)	1.3±1.4	1.2±1.4	1.4±1.4	0.34
IgG (mg/dl)	1238.7±301.2	1200.7±294.2	1247.9±302.9	0.30
IgA (mg/dl)	309.5±103.8	296.5±95.8	312.7±105.7	0.28
C3 (mg/dl)	104.2±17.1	82.0±6.8	109.5±14.3	<0.001
C-reactive protein (mg/l)*	1.0 (0.3–2.72)	1.0 (0.5–1.3)	1.1 (0.5–3.1)	0.53
Medications				
ACE inhibitors or ARBs	215 (62.7%)	39 (59.1%)	176 (63.5%)	0.50
Diuretics	60 (17.5%)	7 (10.6%)	53 (19.1%)	0.09
Other antihypertensive drugs	53 (15.5%)	6 (9.1%)	47 (17.0%)	0.11
More than 2 antihypertensive drugs	50 (14.6%)	6 (9.1%)	44 (15.9%)	0.16
More than 3 antihypertensive drugs	18 (5.2%)	1 (1.5%)	17 (6.1%)	0.22
HMG-CoA reductase inhibitors	49 (14.3%)	6 (9.1%)	43 (15.5%)	0.18
Corticosteroid	10 (2.9%)	2 (3.0%)	8 (2.9%)	0.95
Cyclosporine	3 (0.9%)	0 (0%)	3 (1.1%)	0.40
Time to renal biopsy (months)*	12 (3–36)	11 (3–30)	12 (3–36)	0.48

Data are presented as n (%) or mean ± SD or *median and interquartile range.
MAP, mean arterial pressure; eGFR, estimated glomerular filtration rate; PCR, protein to creatinine ratio; Ig, immunoglobulin; C, complement; ACE, angiotensin converting enzyme; ARB, angiotensin II receptor blocker.

the decline rate of eGFR between the two groups, multivariate linear regression analysis was conducted. All probabilities were two-tailed and the level of significance was set at 0.05.

Results

Baseline characteristics

The demographic, clinical, and biochemical characteristics of the study population are shown in Table 1. Of the 343 patients, 66 patients (19.2%) had C3 levels below the lower limit of the normal range (<90 mg/dl) and were considered to have hypoC3. A

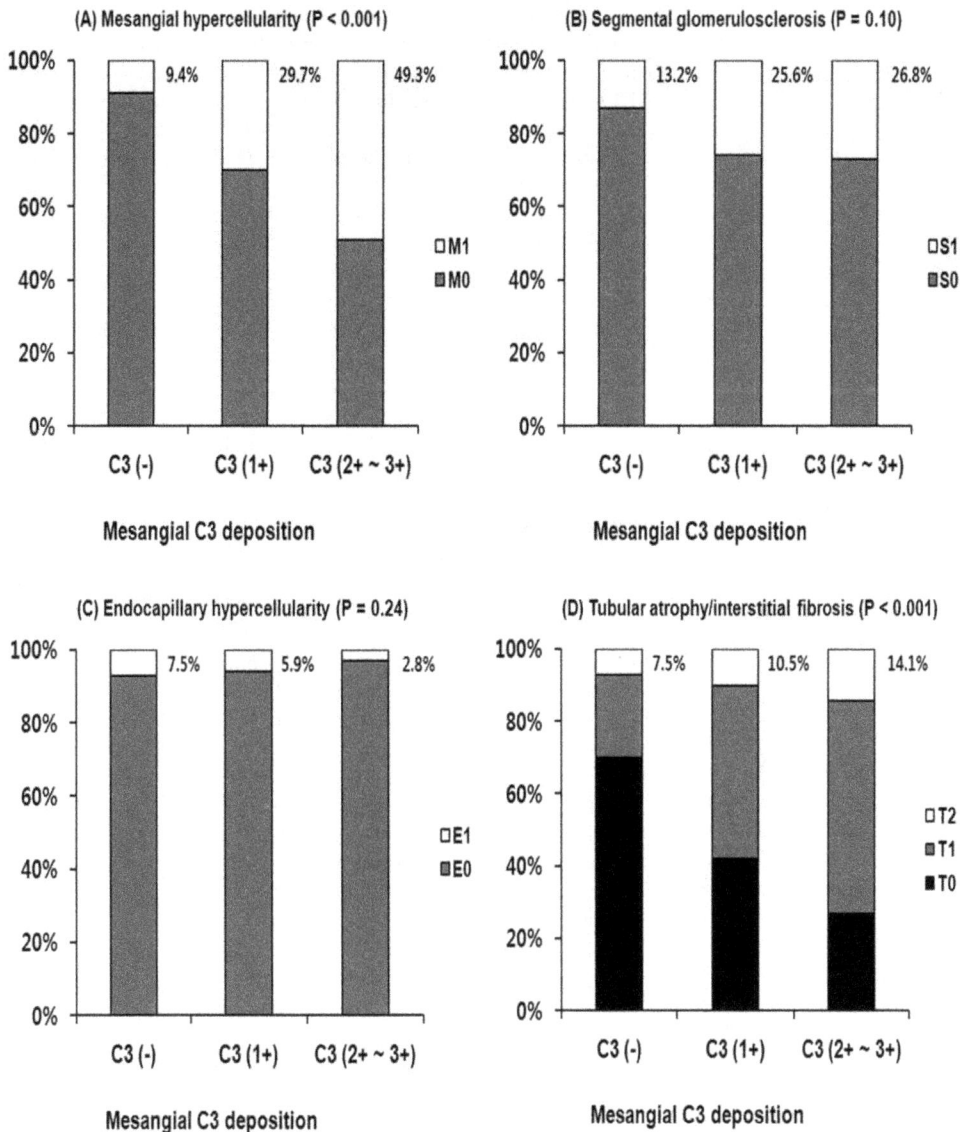

Figure 4. The histopathologic grades such as (A) mesangial hypercellularity, (B) segmental glomerulosclerosis, (C) endocapillary hypercellularity, and (D) tubular atrophy/interstitial fibrosis according to mesangial C3 deposition. Mesangial hypercellularity (C3 deposition 0, 9.4%; 1+, 29.7%; 2+~3+, 49.3%; P<0.001) and high-grade tubular atrophy/interstitial fibrosis (C3 deposition 0, 7.5%; 1+, 10.5%; 2+~3+, 14.1%; P<0.001) were more prominent as the mesangial area of C3 deposition increased.

scattered plot of each level of serum C3 was presented in Figure 3. Compared to patients with C3 ≥90 mg/dl, those with C3 <90 mg/dl were younger (31.1±9.2 vs. 35.4±12.1 years, P=0.002) and had lower mean arterial blood pressure (91.4±9.5 vs. 94.8±11.7 mmHg, P=0.031). Patients with uncontrolled hypertension were more common in patients with C3 ≥90 mg/dl. Of note, these patients had higher BMI, and cholesterol and triglyceride levels than patients with C3 levels <90 mg/dl (Table 1). Between the two groups, however there were no differences in eGFR, UPCR, Ig levels, CRP, comorbidities, or medications including immuno-suppressants and antihypertensive agents during follow-up. Meanwhile, no patients underwent tonsillectomy for the prevention of disease progression in our study.

In patients with nephrotic syndrome, serum C3 levels were 97.8±14.7 mg/dl and 6 (15.8%), 25 (65.7%), and 7 (18.4%) patients had mesangial C3 deposits of 0, 1+, and 2+ or more,

respectively. Whether complement activation is involved in the development of nephrotic syndrome in IgA nephropathy is currently unknown. We recently demonstrated that IgAN patients with nephrotic syndrome exhibited different features and had worse prognosis compared with patients with typical IgA nephropathy [19]. In addition, they are usually more likely to be treated with immunosuppressive drugs. These may lead to a biased result, thus patients with nephrotic syndrome were excluded from the analysis.

Pathologic findings

The histopathologic features from renal biopsies between patients with and without hypoC3 are presented in Table 2. Patients with hypoC3 had higher grade mesangial deposition of C3 (2+ to 3+) than those without hypoC3 (28.8 vs. 18.8%, P=0.011). There were no differences in mesangial hypercellularity, glomerulosclerosis, endocapillary hypercellularity, tubulointer-

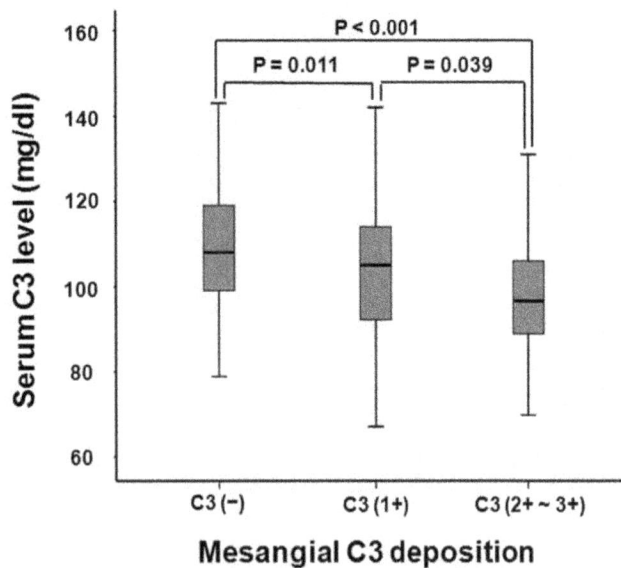

Figure 5. Comparison of serum C3 levels according to mesangial C3 deposition. Serum C3 levels decreased significantly from 0 to 2+~3+ mesangial C3 deposition (0, 111.7±18.0; 1+, 104.3±17.1; 2+~3+, 98.6±14.2 mg/dl; P<0.001).

stitial lesions, arteriosclerosis, and mesangial deposition of IgG or IgA between the two groups (Table 2). The histopathologic features were further compared according to mesangial C3 deposition. Mesangial hypercellularity (C3 deposition 0, 9.4%; 1+, 29.7%; 2+~3+, 49.3%; P<0.001) and high-grade tubular atrophy/interstitial fibrosis (C3 deposition 0, 7.5%; 1+, 10.5%; 2+~3+, 14.1%; P<0.001) were more prominent as the mesangial area of C3 deposition increased (Figure 4). However, there was no significant difference in segmental glomerulosclerosis or endocapillary hypercellularity. On the other hand, serum C3 levels decreased significantly from 0 to 2+~3+ mesangial C3 deposition (0, 111.7±18.0; 1+, 104.3±17.1; 2+~3+, 98.6±14.2 mg/dl; P<0.001) (Figure 5).

Renal Outcomes

During a mean follow-up of 53.7±30.1 months, 14 (4.1%) developed ESRD and 29 patients (8.5%) reached the end point of doubling of the baseline serum creatinine levels. There was no patient who progressed to ESRD before reaching doubling of the baseline serum creatinine. ESRD occurred in 5 patients (7.6%) with hypoC3 compared with 9 patients (3.2%) with normal C3 levels (P=0.11, Table 3). However, 12 patients (18.2%) with hypoC3 reached D-SCr compared with 17 patients (6.1%) with normal C3 levels (HR, 3.59; 95% CI, 1.56–8.28; P=0.003) (Table 3 and Table 4, Model 1) and a 10-year renal survival rate was significantly lower in the former (Figure 6A, P=0.006). In addition, the expanded mesangial deposition of C3 was associated with worse renal survival (Figure 7B). ESRD occurred in 1 (1.9%), 9 (4.1%), and 4 (5.6%) patients with mesangial C3 deposition of 0, 1+, and 2+ to 3+, respectively (P=0.30, Table 3). However, the risk of reaching D-SCr was significantly higher in patients with mesangial C3 deposition 2+ to 3+ than in patients without deposition (HR 14.24; 95% CI, 2.03–99.87; P=0.008) (Table 4, Model 2). In a multivariable model in which serum C3 levels were treated as a continuous variable, hypoC3 significantly predicted renal outcome of D-SCr (per 1 mg/dl increase of C3; HR, 0.96; 95% CI, 0.93–0.98; P=0.002) (Table 4, Model 1). When both

serum C3 levels and mesangial C3 deposition were included in a multivariate model, these two parameters remained independent predictors of adverse renal outcomes (Table 4, Model 3 and 4). In ROC curve analysis, serum C3 levels had a significant predictive value for the renal outcome (AUC=0.642, P=0.011), although the predictive value of serum C3 was lower than UPCR (AUC=0.819, P<0.001) or eGFR (AUC=0.781, P<0.001) (Figure 6). On the other hand, patients with mesangial hypercellularity, segmental glomerulosclerosis, endocapillary proliferation, and tubular atrophy/interstitial fibrosis had significantly lower renal survival than those without such findings (P<0.05) (Figure 8).

In the multivariate linear regression analysis adjusted for clinical, laboratory, and histologic factor, the decline rate of eGFR was greater in patients with hypoC3 than in patients with normal C3 levels only up to 4 years after the diagnosis. However, overall decline rate of eGFR did not differ between the two groups (Figure 9).

Discussion

This study showed that both decreased circulating C3 levels and mesangial C3 deposition were associated with deterioration of kidney function in patients with IgAN independent of heavy proteinuria and other unfavorable histopathologic features such as glomerular sclerosis or interstitial fibrosis. Our findings suggest that decreased serum C3 levels and C3 deposition within the mesangium may provide prognostic value in these patients.

In patients with IgAN, O-linked carbohydrates in the hinge region of IgA1 molecule are under-galactosylated and defective IgA1 forms circulating or *in situ* immune complexes [20]. Subsequent deposition of immune complexes within the mesangium plays a key role in the pathogenesis of IgAN. Interestingly, mesangial C3 deposits are often observed along with IgA, suggesting that complement activation may also be involved in pathogenesis. In fact, many studies have previously suggested that local complement system in the glomeruli is activated via the alternative or the mannose-binding lectin (MBL) pathway in IgAN [7–12]. Although there is a general agreement that C3 deposits are caused predominantly by complement activation via the alternative pathway in IgAN, several studies have recently suggested that the lectin pathway of complement may also be involved in the progression of disease [10–12]. In particular, Roos et al. reported that activation of the lectin pathway was associated with more severe renal damage in IgAN [11]. In their study, complement activation occurred via the alternative pathway in 75% of patients whereas glomerular deposition of MBL, L-ficolin, and C4d, which was indicative of activation of complement via the lectin pathway, was observed in 25% of patients [11]. However, it is uncertain whether such complement activation may affect the long-term outcomes in patients with IgAN. Komatsu et al. showed that C3 deposition within the mesangium significantly correlated with severe histologic lesions using kidney specimens from patients with IgAN [21]. In line with their findings, in the present study, we clearly showed that patients with higher grade mesangial deposition of C3 had worse histologic findings such as mesangial hypercellularity and tubular atrophy/interstitial fibrosis than those with lower grade deposition. Because such histologic features are apparently associated with worse prognosis [22,23], it can be presumed that patients with mesangial C3 deposition have worse renal outcomes compared with those without deposition as seen in our study. Taken together, it can be suggested that complement activation may mediate further renal injury and that mesangial C3 deposition may have prognostic value in IgAN.

Table 2. Comparison of histopathologic features from renal biopsies between patients with and without decreased C3 levels.

	All (n = 343)	C3 <90 mg/dl (n = 66)	C3 ≥90 mg/dl (n = 277)	P-value
Mesangial hypercellularity				0.81
≤50% of the glomeruli (M0)	238 (69.4%)	45 (68.2%)	193 (69.7%)	
>50% of the glomeruli (M1)	105 (30.6%)	21 (31.8%)	84 (30.3%)	
Segmental glomerulosclerosis				0.30
Absent (S0)	261 (76.1%)	47 (71.2%)	214 (77.3%)	
Present (S1)	82 (23.9%)	19 (28.8%)	63 (22.7%)	
Endocapillary hypercellularity				0.16
Absent (E0)	324 (94.5%)	60 (90.9%)	264 (95.3%)	
Present (E1)	19 (5.5%)	6 (9.1%)	13 (4.7%)	
Tubular atrophy/interstitial fibrosis				0.07
0–25% of cortical area (T0)	148 (43.1%)	23 (34.8%)	125 (45.1%)	
25–50% of cortical area (T1)	158 (46.1%)	31 (47.0%)	127 (45.8%)	
>50% of cortical area (T2)	37 (10.8%)	12 (18.2%)	25 (9.0%)	
Arteriosclerosis	70 (20.4%)	12 (18.2%)	58 (20.9%)	0.62
Mesangial IgG deposition (n, %)				0.45
Negative	204 (59.5%)	36 (54.5%)	168 (60.6%)	
1+	126 (36.7%)	26 (39.4%)	100 (36.1%)	
2+	11 (3.2%)	4 (6.1%)	7 (2.5%)	
3+	2 (0.6%)	0 (0.0%)	2 (0.7%)	
2+ and 3+	13 (3.8%)	4 (6.1%)	9 (3.2%)	
Mesangial IgA deposition (n, %)				0.77
1+	104 (30.3%)	21 (31.8%)	83 (30.0%)	
2+	168 (49.0%)	29 (43.9%)	139 (50.1%)	
3+	71 (20.7%)	16 (24.3%)	55 (19.9%)	
2+ and 3+	239 (69.7%)	45 (68.2%)	194 (70.0%)	
Mesangial C3 deposition (n, %)				0.011
Negative	53 (15.5%)	3 (4.5%)	50 (18.1%)	
1+	219 (63.8%)	44 (66.7%)	175 (63.2%)	
2+	63 (18.4%)	16 (24.3%)	47 (17.0%)	
3+	8 (2.3%)	3 (4.5%)	5 (1.8%)	
2+ and 3+	71 (20.7%)	19 (28.8%)	52 (18.8%)	

Data are presented as n (%).
Ig, immunoglobulin; C, complement.

Although previous studies demonstrated that complement activation occurred locally in IgAN, several studies reported that systemic complement activation may also be present [13,14]. In particular, Zwirner et al. showed that activated C3 levels in the plasma were elevated in patients with IgAN and correlated with deterioration in renal function [14], suggesting that systemic complement activation may also be involved in the progression of IgAN. However, measurement of activated C3 is not widely available because slow *ex vivo* generation of activated C3 can be observed even during storage at −70°C [24]. Consumption of complement factors is reflected by either decreased levels of individual proteins such as C3 and C4 or depressed total complement hemolytic activity (CH50), as well as the production of complement activation split products [25]. In this regard, decreased serum C3 levels in our 66 patients are possibly due to C3 consumption due to systemic complement activation although other components of complement cascade and C3 splits were not measured. To date, clinical implication of decreased serum C3

levels in patients with IgAN has not yet been explored. Several Japanese studies have examined the clinical utility of C3. Tomino et al. showed that serum IgA/C3 ratio might be of help in diagnosing IgAN [26]. In addition, renal survival was significantly decreased in patients with a higher serum IgA/C3 ratio than those with a lower ratio [21]. Interestingly, in a study by Komatsu et al., serum C3 levels were decreased in patients with IgAN with severe histologic lesions compared with those seen in non-IgAN. Unfortunately, they did not assess the prognostic value of decreased serum C3 levels. In the present study, we showed for the first time that patients with decreased serum C3 levels had worse renal survival than those with higher C3 levels. Moreover, decreased serum C3 levels were independently predictive of renal outcome in the multivariate analysis even after adjustment for factors known to be associated with worse prognosis such as proteinuria and decreased renal function at presentation although predictive value of low C3 levels were not so potent as these conventional factors. It should be noted that many physicians are

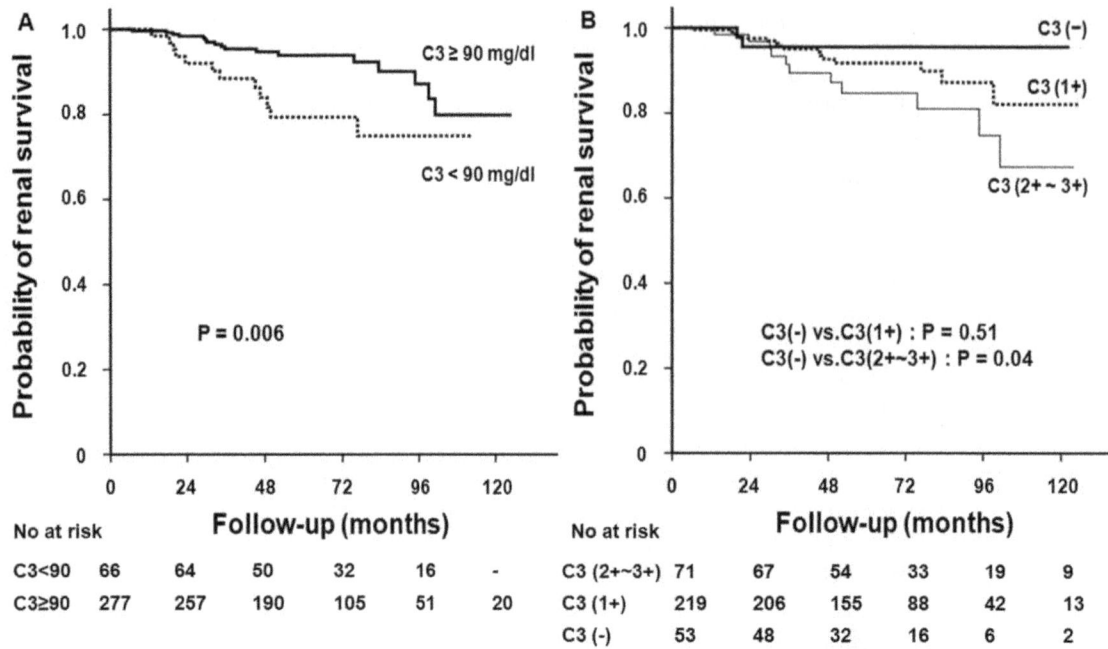

Figure 6. Kaplan-Meier analyses of cumulative renal survival of patients with IgA nephropathy based on (A) serum C3 level and (B) mesangial C3 deposition. (A) A 10-year renal survival rate was significantly lower in patients with C3 levels <90 mg/dl than those with C3 levels ≥90 mg/dl (P = 0.006). (B) A 10-year survival in patients with 2+ and 3+ mesangial deposition of C3 was lower than in those without C3 deposition (P = 0.04).

not aware of the significance of decreased serum C3 levels in patients with IgAN although hypoC3 is not common. In this regard, our findings deserve particular attention because decreased serum C3 levels may be another useful biomarker to predict progression of IgAN.

In contrast to findings by Tomino et al, in this study, IgA/C3 ratio had a trend toward poor renal outcome, but it did not reach statistical significance (data not shown). This can be explained by the fact that simply elevated IgA levels cannot reflect disease activity. In fact, although circulating IgA levels are elevated in

patients with IgAN, correlation of the elevated IgA levels with clinical features of the disease is inconsistent [27,28]. Interestingly, 40 to 50% of first degree relatives of IgAN patients have elevated IgA levels, but most of these persons do not exhibit clinical sings of renal injury [29,30]. These findings suggest that additional pathogenic factors such as generation of antibodies against IgA or immune-complex formation are required to activate the disease.

It is uncertain whether systemic and local activation of complement system coordinate together or if they exert independent effects although both types of activation have been previously

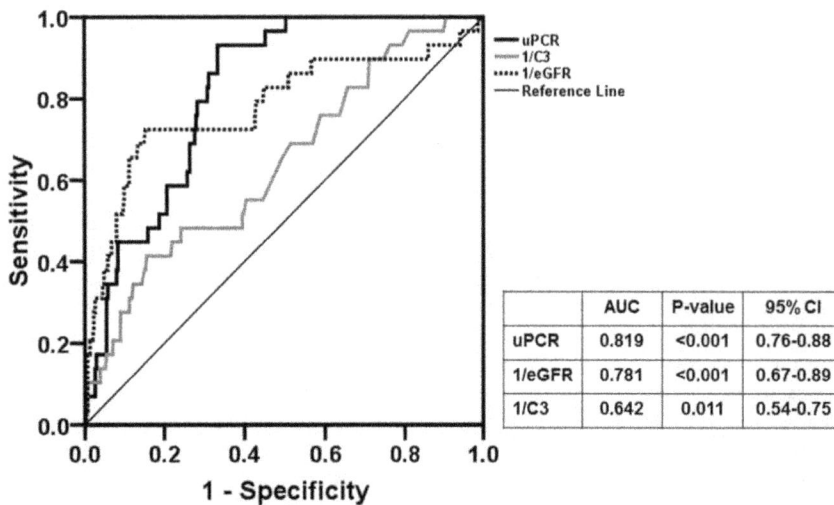

	AUC	P-value	95% CI
uPCR	0.819	<0.001	0.76-0.88
1/eGFR	0.781	<0.001	0.67-0.89
1/C3	0.642	0.011	0.54-0.75

Figure 7. ROC curve analysis for renal outcome of the doubling of the baseline serum creatinine. Serum C3 levels had a significant predictive value for renal outcome (AUC = 0.642, P = 0.011), although the predictive value of serum C3 was lower than UPCR (AUC = 0.819, P<0.001) or eGFR (AUC = 0.781, P<0.001).

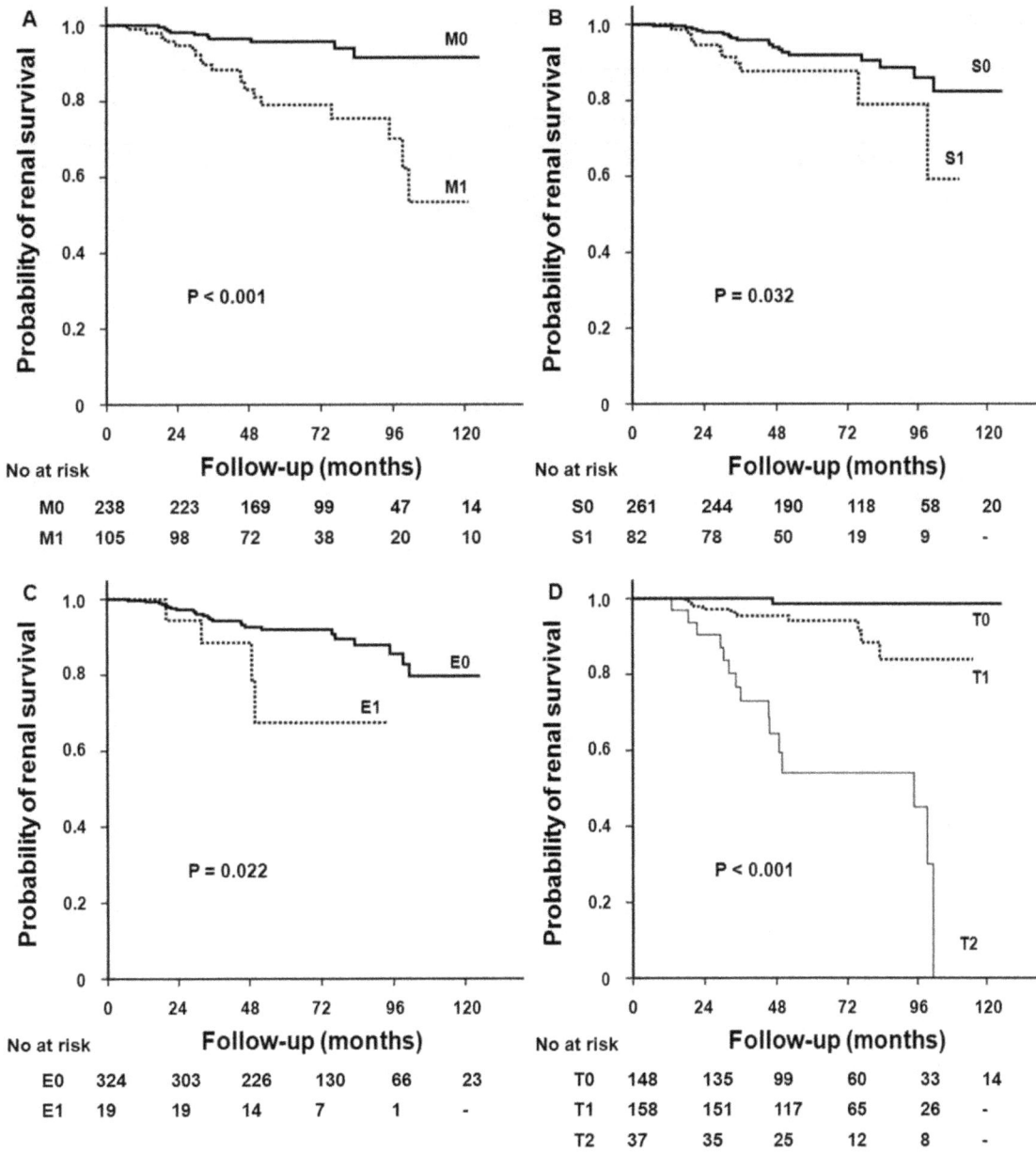

Figure 8. Kaplan-Meier analyses of cumulative renal survival of patients with IgA nephropathy according to histopathologic features including (A) mesangial hypercellularity, (B) segmental glomerulosclerosis, (C) endocapillary hypercellularity, and (D) tubular atrophy/interstitial fibrosis. Patients with mesangial hypercellularity, segmental glomerulosclerosis, endocapillary hypercellularity, and tubular atrophy/interstitial fibrosis had significantly lower renal survival than those without such findings (P<0.05).

reported in IgAN [7–14]. Activation of the complement system was common in patients with systemic lupus erythematosus (SLE), leading to hypocomplementemia and deposition of complement component at sites of tissue injury, particularly in the glomeruli and the skin [31]. This finding suggests that complement activation likely has a role in tissue damage in SLE. In addition, some studies reported that the lectin pathway of the complement system is activated in rheumatoid arthritis. Although levels of lectin pathway proteins were higher in plasma than synovial fluid, paired plasma and synovial fluid levels correlated significantly in all cases [32]. Consistent with these findings, our study showed that serum C3 levels correlated with mesangial C3 deposition, suggesting a possible link between the two complement systems. Despite such a correlation, it is possible that both factors may be

independently associated with poor renal survival because there was no significant interaction on multivariable Cox regression analysis (data not shown). However, due to the observational nature of the study, it is difficult to clarify how systemic complement activation is involved in local activation.

Interestingly, in this study, patients with C3 ≥90 mg/dl had higher BMI, blood pressure, and cholesterol levels. Recent previous studies showed that increased complement levels were related to extreme adiposity and insulin resistance [33,34]. On the contrary, a few studies suggested complement activation in patients with very low BMI such as anorexia nervosa [35–37]. All these patients exhibited decreased C3 levels, which might reflect severe comorbid conditions such as malnutrition. However, in this study, it is uncertain whether C3 levels were affected by

Table 3. Incidence of patients with doubling of serum creatinine and ESRD according to decreased C3 levels and mesangial C3 deposition.

	Serum C3						Mesangial C3 deposition						
	C3 <90 mg/d		C3 ≥90 mg/dl		P-value		C3(−)		C3(+)		C3(2+~3+)		P-value
	N (%)	/1000 patient -years	N (%)	/1000 patient -years			N (%)	/1000 patient -years	N (%)	/1000 patient -years	N (%)	/1000 patient -years	
ESRD	5 (7.6%)	15.67	9 (3.2%)	7.57	0.11		1 (1.9%)	5.05	9 (4.1%)	9.30	4 (5.6%)	11.73	0.30
Doubling of Scr	12 (18.2%)	34.48	17 (6.1%)	12.62	0.002		2 (3.8%)	5.05	16 (7.3%)	15.50	11 (15.5%)	29.33	0.016

ESRD, end-stage renal disease; C, complement; N, number; Scr, serum creatinine.

obesity or nutritional status. Mean BMI of the study subjects were 22.7 kg/m^2 and there were only 12 patients with BMI>30 kg/m^2. Even patients with C3 ≥90 mg/dl had a mean BMI of 23.2 kg/m^2, suggesting that they were not obese. In addition, serum albumin level, which is a good indicator of nutritional status, did not differ between patients with hypoC3 and patients with C3 ≥90 mg/dl. Nevertheless, to examine possible effects of these factors on outcome, we conducted a Cox regression model further adjusted for BMI, cholesterol, and serum albumin and found that decreased C3 levels and mesangial C3 deposits remained significant predictors of renal outcome (Table 4, Model 4).

Not surprisingly, we confirmed that unfavorable histologic features such as mesangial hypercellularity, glomerulosclerosis, and tubular atrophy/interstitial fibrosis, which were previously reported to be poor prognostic factors, were significantly associated with adverse renal outcomes. However, it is unclear how glomerulopathy associated with mesangial IgA deposition leads to tubulointerstitial injury although tubulointerstitial lesions are common in IgAN [38]. It is possible that glomerulotubular cross-talk with mediators such as cytokines, complement, and angiotensin II may contribute to the pathogenesis of tubulointerstitial damage in IgAN as suggested by Chan et al. [39]. Interestingly, in the present study, the severity of tubulointerstitial lesions was associated with the expansion of mesangial C3 deposition. This finding suggests that complement activation may aggravate glomerular injury, eventually resulting in the development of tubulointerstitial damage, and that the complement system may act as a mediator in glomerulotubular cross-talk.

Recent studies showed that other pathologic features such as wide areas of electron dense deposits [40] and thrombotic microangiopathy [41] were associated with adverse outcome in IgAN. Detailed analysis on relationship between mesangial C3 deposition and these pathologic features is beyond the scope of this study. However, we found that there was no correlation between intensity of C3 deposits and areas of electron dense deposits although electron dense deposits were observed in other areas besides paramesangial area. It is possible that complement activation in response to immune complex may differ depending on mesangial or paramesangial areas. In addition, thrombotic microangiopathy was found in only 25 (7.3%) patients, which is quite low compared with 53% in a study by Karoui et al. This is probably because our study subjects were relatively young and blood pressure was well controlled. In fact, in a study by Karoui et al, 71% had uncontrolled hypertension, which was associated with thrombotic microangiopathy. In contrast, only 38 (11.1%) patients in our study had systolic blood pressure >140 mmHg and intensity C3 deposits were not related with thrombotic microan-

giopathy. Furthermore, Karoui et al. found no genetic mutation of complement factor H and I in patients with severe thrombotic microangiopathy, suggesting the alternative pathway is less likely involved in this lesion. Whether complement activation can contribute to more depositions of immune-complex besides paramesangial area or thrombotic microangiopathy requires further in-depth investigations.

Limitations

Our study had several limitations. First, this was a retrospective study, thus the observational nature of the present study limits our findings suggesting that complement activation actually contributes to the progression of IgAN. Second, other complement components including activated C3, C4-C3 complexes, or soluble C5b-9 were not available. We also did not perform the additional staining for MBL, C4d, and C3c in glomeruli, which were previously suggested to be possible predictors of disease activity as alternatives to C3 [9,12]. Third, serum C3 levels were only measured at the time of renal biopsy. Thus, whether hypoC3 persisted throughout the disease course is unknown. Interestingly, there were five patients who had follow-up data for serum C3 levels with a median duration of 22 months. They had persistently decreased serum C3 levels and four of them reached the doubling of the baseline serum creatinine. Therefore, it would be helpful to monitor the level serially to further clarify the clinical implications of hypoC3 in IgAN. Fourth, serum C3 levels and mesangial C3 deposition were not associated with the development of ESRD. This finding is partly due to the fact that ESRD occurred in only 14 patients (4.2%) during the follow-up period, thus resulting in a lack of statistical power. In addition, overall decline rate of eGFR did not differ between patients with hypoC3 and patients with normal C3 levels. It should be noted that most patients with hypoC3 reached the endpoints within 4 years after the baseline evaluation. This can explain the faster decline in eGFR in these patients until 4 years. However, it is possible that small number of events did not have adequate statistical power to see the difference in eGFR decline. Fifth, the presence of other diseases exhibiting both hypoC3 and mesangial IgA deposition could not entirely be excluded. However, we conducted a thorough pathologic examination and excluded patients with conditions such as systemic lupus erythematosus and IgA-dominant acute post-infectious glomerulonephritis. Moreover, we confirmed that autoantibodies such as antinuclear antibody or anti-DNA antibody were negative in all patients with hypoC3. Sixth, intensity of immunofluorescence may not be correct because of different condition of immunofluorescent staining, storage time, or altered antigenicity of immune complex by environmental proteases. However, in our

Table 4. Cox regression models for renal outcome of the doubling of the baseline serum creatinine.

	HR	95% CI	P-value	HR	95% CI	P-value
Model 1						
eGFR (per 1 ml/min/1.73 m^2 increase)	0.96	0.93–0.98	<0.001	0.95	0.93–0.98	<0.001
Urinary PCR (per 1 mg/mg increase)	1.70	1.36–2.12	<0.001	1.52	1.26–1.82	<0.001
Serum C3 (per 1 mg/dl increase)	0.96	0.93–0.98	0.002	-	-	-
Patients with hypoC3 (vs. no)	-	-	-	3.59	1.56–8.28	0.003
Model 2						
eGFR (per 1 ml/min/1.73 m^2 increase)	0.97	0.95–0.99	0.037	-	-	-
Urinary PCR (per 1 mg/mg increase)	1.63	1.27–2.08.	<0.001	-	-	-
Tubular atrophy/interstitial fibrosis				-	-	-
0–25% of cortical area (T0)	Reference					
25–50% of cortical area (T1)	7.632	0.91–63.6	0.061	-	-	-
>50% of cortical area (T2)	35.81	4.03–217.9	0.001	-	-	-
Mesangial C3 deposition						
0	Reference					
1+	6.03	0.93–39.00	0.059	-	-	-
2+~3+	14.24	2.03–99.87	0.008	-	-	-
Model 3						
eGFR (per 1 ml/min/1.73 m^2 increase)	0.98	0.95–0.99	0.038	0.97	0.95–0.99	0.031
Urinary PCR (per 1 mg/mg increase)	1.86	1.42–2.44	<0.001	1.71	1.32–2.21	<0.001
Tubular atrophy/interstitial fibrosis						
0–25% of cortical area (T0)	Reference			Reference		
25–50% of cortical area (T1)	8.20	0.97–69.4	0.053	8.50	1.01–71.43	0.049
>50% of cortical area (T2)	35.26	4.04–207.5	0.001	34.90	3.93–209.9	0.001
Mesangial C3 deposition						
0	Reference			Reference		
1+	3.75	0.63–22.3	0.147	5.64	0.80–39.55	0.082
2+~3+	8.76	1.39–55.2	0.021	14.03	1.86–105.77	0.010
Serum C3 (per 1 mg/dl increase)	0.95	0.93–0.98	0.004	-	-	-
Patients with hypoC3 (vs. no)	-	-	-	3.35	1.41–7.99	0.006
Model 4						
eGFR (per 1 ml/min/1.73 m^2 increase)	0.97	0.95–0.99	0.030	0.97	0.95–0.99	0.021
Urinary PCR (per 1 mg/mg increase)	1.78	1.29–2.46	<0.001	1.65	1.21–2.26	0.002
Tubular atrophy/interstitial fibrosis						
0–25% of cortical area (T0)		Reference			Reference	
25–50% of cortical area (T1)	8.14	0.94–70.59	0.057	8.09	0.94–69.6	0.057
>50% of cortical area (T2)	32.41	3.61–191.44	0.002	30.42	3.31–179.2	0.003
Mesangial C3 deposition						
0		Reference			Reference	
1+	4.58	0.62–33.70	0.135	7.25	0.69–58.89	0.064
2+~3+	10.17	1.33–77.9	0.026	16.18	1.89–138.36	0.011
Serum C3 (per 1 mg/dl increase)	0.96	0.93–0.99	0.019	-	-	-
Patients with hypoC3 (vs. no)	-	-	-	2.73	1.09–6.86	0.032

Data are reported as hazard ratio (HR) and 95% confidence interval (CI).
Model 1: age, sex, presence of gross hematuria, mean arterial blood pressure, eGFR, proteinuria, treatment, and serum C3 levels.
Model 2: age, sex, presence of gross hematuria, mean arterial blood pressure, eGFR, proteinuria, treatment, and pathologic findings.
Model 3: Model 2+serum C3 levels.
Model 4: Model 3+BMI, total cholesterol, and serum albumin.
eGFR, estimated glomerular filtration rate; PCR, protein-to-creatinine ratio.

institute, immunofluorescence pictures were generally taken immediately after biopsy samples were processed. Furthermore, to quantify the immunofluorescence intensity, these pictures were converted to digital images and analyzed using ImageJ software.

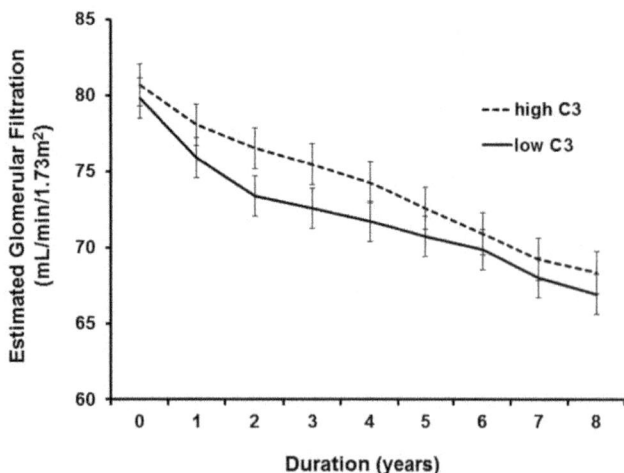

Figure 9. The decline rate of eGFR. Error bars indicate standard error.

Seventh, serum C3 levels were mildly decreased in 66 patients with hypoC3, suggesting that the disease may not truly be a 'flare-up', which can be seen in severe lupus nephritis [42]. It is unknown whether such a mild decrease in C3 levels may affect the clinical outcomes. Considering the fact that IgAN exhibits a slowly progressive course, it is possible that indolent inflammatory

process is still underway even in such a mild hypoC3status. Based on our finding that renal survival rate was lower in patients with hypoC3 compared to those with normal C3 levels although no significant difference in baseline histopathologic features was observed, we surmise that complement activation may contribute to the development of slowly progressive renal injury for an extended period of time. Finally, clinical significance of C3 levels was reported mostly from studies involving Asian population [21,26]. In addition, a prior study suggested a geographical variability in long-term outcomes of IgA nephropathy [43]. Therefore, our results may not be extrapolated to other ethnic populations.

Conclusion

This study showed that both decreased circulating C3 levels and mesangial C3 deposition were independently associated with poor renal outcome in patients with IgAN. These findings suggest that systemic and local activation of complement may play a role in the progression of IgAN and decreased serum C3 levels and mesangial C3 deposition may have prognostic value in the management of these patients.

Author Contributions

Performed the experiments: BJL HJJ. Analyzed the data: HJO DEY DHS MJL FMD. Contributed reagents/materials/analysis tools: JTP THY SWK KHC. Wrote the paper: SJK HMK SHH.

References

1. D'Amico G (1987) The commonest glomerulonephritis in the world: IgA nephropathy. Q J Med 64: 709–727.
2. D'Amico G, Colasanti G, Barbiano di Belgioioso G, Fellin G, Ragni A, et al. (1987) Long-term follow-up of IgA mesangial nephropathy: clinico-histological study in 374 patients. Semin Nephrol 7: 355–358.
3. Li PK, Ho KK, Szeto CC, Yu L, Lai FM (2002) Prognostic indicators of IgA nephropathy in the Chinese–clinical and pathological perspectives. Nephrol Dial Transplant 17: 64–69.
4. D'Amico G (2004) Natural history of idiopathic IgA nephropathy and factors predictive of disease outcome. Semin Nephrol 24: 179–196.
5. Walsh M, Sar A, Lee D, Yilmaz S, Benediktsson H, et al. (2010) Histopathologic features aid in predicting risk for progression of IgA nephropathy. Clin J Am Soc Nephrol 5: 425–430.
6. Oortwijn BD, Eijgenraam JW, Rastaldi MP, Roos A, Daha MR, et al. (2008) The role of secretory IgA and complement in IgA nephropathy. Semin Nephrol 28: 58–65.
7. Hiemstra PS, Gorter A, Stuurman ME, Van Es LA, Daha MR (1987) Activation of the alternative pathway of complement by human serum IgA. Eur J Immunol 17: 321–326.
8. Stad RK, Bruijn JA, van Gijlswijk-Janssen DJ, van Es LA, Daha MR (1993) An acute model for IgA-mediated glomerular inflammation in rats induced by monoclonal polymeric rat IgA antibodies. Clin Exp Immunol 92: 514–521.
9. Nakagawa H, Suzuki S, Haneda M, Gejyo F, Kikkawa R (2000) Significance of glomerular deposition of C3c and C3d in IgA nephropathy. Am J Nephrol 20: 122–128.
10. Endo M, Ohi H, Ohsawa I, Fujita T, Matsushita M (1998) Glomerular deposition of mannose-binding lectin (MBL) indicates a novel mechanism of complement activation in IgA nephropathy. Nephrol Dial Transplant 13: 1984–1990.
11. Roos A, Rastaldi MP, Calvaresi N, Oortwijn BD, Schlagwein N, et al. (2006) Glomerular activation of the lectin pathway of complement in IgA nephropathy is associated with more severe renal disease. J Am Soc Nephrol 17: 1724–1734.
12. Espinosa M, Ortega R, Gomez-Carrasco JM, Lopez-Rubio F, Lopez-Andreu M, et al. (2009) Mesangial C4d deposition: a new prognostic factor in IgA nephropathy. Nephrol Dial Transplant 24: 886–891.
13. Wyatt RJ, Kanayama Y, Julian BA, Negoro N, Sugimoto S, et al. (1987) Complement activation in IgA nephropathy. Kidney Int 31: 1019–1023.
14. Zwirner J, Burg M, Schulze M, Brunkhorst R, Gotze O, et al. (1997) Activated complement C3: a potentially novel predictor of progressive IgA nephropathy. Kidney Int 51: 1257–1264.
15. Nasr SH, D'Agati VD (2011) IgA-dominant postinfectious glomerulonephritis: a new twist on an old disease. Nephron Clin Pract 119: c18–25; discussion c26.
16. Giannakakis K, Faraggiana T (2011) Histopathology of lupus nephritis. Clin Rev Allergy Immunol 40: 170–180.

17. Levey AS, Bosch JP, Lewis JB, Greene T, Rogers N, et al. (1999) A more accurate method to estimate glomerular filtration rate from serum creatinine: a new prediction equation. Modification of Diet in Renal Disease Study Group. Ann Intern Med 130: 461–470.
18. Cattran DC, Coppo R, Cook HT, Feehally J, Roberts IS, et al. (2009) The Oxford classification of IgA nephropathy: rationale, clinicopathological correlations, and classification. Kidney Int 76: 534–545.
19. Kim JK, Kim JH, Lee SC, Kang EW, Chang TI, et al. (2012) Clinical features and outcomes of IgA nephropathy with nephrotic syndrome. Clin J Am Soc Nephrol 7: 427–436.
20. Floege J, Feehally J (2000) IgA nephropathy: recent developments. J Am Soc Nephrol 11: 2395–2403.
21. Komatsu H, Fujimoto S, Hara S, Sato Y, Yamada K, et al. (2004) Relationship between serum IgA/C3 ratio and progression of IgA nephropathy. Intern Med 43: 1023–1028.
22. Radford MG Jr., Donadio JV Jr., Bergstralh EJ, Grande JP (1997) Predicting renal outcome in IgA nephropathy. J Am Soc Nephrol 8: 199–207.
23. Myllymaki JM, Honkanen TT, Syrjanen JT, Helin HJ, Rantala IS, et al. (2007) Severity of tubulointerstitial inflammation and prognosis in immunoglobulin A nephropathy. Kidney Int 71: 343–348.
24. Janssen U, Bahlmann F, Kohl J, Zwirner J, Haubitz M, et al. (2000) Activation of the acute phase response and complement C3 in patients with IgA nephropathy. Am J Kidney Dis 35: 21–28.
25. Tsokos GC (2004) Exploring complement activation to develop biomarkers for systemic lupus erythematosus. Arthritis Rheum 50: 3404–3407.
26. Tomino Y, Suzuki S, Imai H, Saito T, Kawamura T, et al. (2000) Measurement of serum IgA and C3 may predict the diagnosis of patients with IgA nephropathy prior to renal biopsy. J Clin Lab Anal 14: 220–223.
27. van der Boog PJ, van Kooten C, van Seggelen A, Mallat M, Klar-Mohamad N, et al. (2004) An increased polymeric IgA level is not a prognostic marker for progressive IgA nephropathy. Nephrol Dial Transplant 19: 2487–2493.
28. Feehally J, Beattie TJ, Brenchley PE, Coupes BM, Mallick NP, et al. (1986) Sequential study of the IgA system in relapsing IgA nephropathy. Kidney Int 30: 924–931.
29. Gharavi AG, Moldoveanu Z, Wyatt RJ, Barker CV, Woodford SY, et al. (2008) Aberrant IgA1 glycosylation is inherited in familial and sporadic IgA nephropathy. J Am Soc Nephrol 19: 1008–1014.
30. Suzuki H, Kiryluk K, Novak J, Moldoveanu Z, Herr AB, et al. (2011) The pathophysiology of IgA nephropathy. J Am Soc Nephrol 22: 1795–1803.
31. Cook HT, Botto M (2006) Mechanisms of Disease: the complement system and the pathogenesis of systemic lupus erythematosus. Nat Clin Pract Rheumatol 2: 330–337.

32. Ammitzboll CG, Thiel S, Ellingsen T, Deleuran B, Jorgensen A, et al. (2011) Levels of lectin pathway proteins in plasma and synovial fluid of rheumatoid arthritis and osteoarthritis. Rheumatol Int.

33. Ohsawa I, Inoshita H, Ishii M, Kusaba G, Sato N, et al. (2010) Metabolic impact on serum levels of complement component 3 in Japanese patients. J Clin Lab Anal 24: 113–118.

34. Hernandez-Mijares A, Jarabo-Bueno MM, Lopez-Ruiz A, Sola-Izquierdo E, Morillas-Arino C, et al. (2007) Levels of C3 in patients with severe, morbid and extreme obesity: its relationship to insulin resistance and different cardiovascular risk factors. Int J Obes (Lond) 31: 927–932.

35. Palmblad J, Fohlin L, Norberg R (1979) Plasma levels of complement factors 3 and 4, orosomucoid and opsonic functions in anorexia nervosa. Acta Paediatr Scand 68: 617–618.

36. Sigal LH, Snyder BK (1989) Low serum complement levels in anorexia nervosa. Am J Dis Child 143: 1391–1392.

37. Flierl MA, Gaudiani JL, Sabel AL, Long CS, Stahel PF, et al. (2011) Complement C3 serum levels in anorexia nervosa: a potential biomarker for the severity of disease? Ann Gen Psychiatry 10: 16.

38. Roufosse CA, Cook HT (2009) Pathological predictors of prognosis in immunoglobulin A nephropathy: a review. Curr Opin Nephrol Hypertens 18: 212–219.

39. Chan LY, Leung JC, Lai KN (2004) Novel mechanisms of tubulointerstitial injury in IgA nephropathy: a new therapeutic paradigm in the prevention of progressive renal failure. Clin Exp Nephrol 8: 297–303.

40. Kusaba G, Ohsawa I, Ishii M, Inoshita H, Takagi M, et al. (2012) Significance of broad distribution of electron-dense deposits in patients with IgA nephropathy. Med Mol Morphol 45: 29–34.

41. El Karoui K, Hill GS, Karras A, Jacquot C, Moulonguet L, et al. (2012) A clinicopathologic study of thrombotic microangiopathy in IgA nephropathy. J Am Soc Nephrol 23: 137–148.

42. Birmingham DJ, Irshaid F, Nagaraja HN, Zou X, Tsao BP, et al. (2010) The complex nature of serum C3 and C4 as biomarkers of lupus renal flare. Lupus 19: 1272–1280.

43. Geddes CC, Rauta V, Gronhagen-Riska C, Bartosik LP, Jardine AG, et al. (2003) A tricontinental view of IgA nephropathy. Nephrol Dial Transplant 18: 1541–1548.

14

Male Microchimerism at High Levels in Peripheral Blood Mononuclear Cells from Women with End Stage Renal Disease before Kidney Transplantation

Laetitia Albano[1], Justyna M. Rak[2], Doua F. Azzouz[2], Elisabeth Cassuto-Viguier[1], Jean Gugenheim[3,4,5], Nathalie C. Lambert[2]*

1 UMC Transplantation Rénale, Hôpital Pasteur, Centre Hospitalo-Universitaire de Nice, Nice, France, 2 INSERM UMR1097, Parc Scientifique de Luminy, Marseille, France, 3 Service de Chirurgie et Transplantation Hépatique, Hôpital l'Archet 2, Nice, France, 4 Université de Nice Sophia Antipolis, Nice, France, 5 INSERM U526, IFR 50, Faculté de Médecine, Université de Nice Sophia Antipolis, Nice, France

Abstract

Patients with end stage renal diseases (ESRD) are generally tested for donor chimerism after kidney transplantation for tolerance mechanism purposes. But, to our knowledge, no data are available on natural and/or iatrogenic microchimerism (Mc), deriving from pregnancy and/or blood transfusion, acquired prior to transplantation. In this context, we tested the prevalence of male Mc using a real time PCR assay for DYS14, a Y-chromosome specific sequence, in peripheral blood mononuclear cells (PBMC) from 55 women with ESRD, prior to their first kidney transplantation, and compared them with results from 82 healthy women. Male Mc was also quantified in 5 native kidney biopsies obtained two to four years prior to blood testing and in PBMC from 8 women collected after female kidney transplantation, several years after the initial blood testing. Women with ESRD showed statistically higher frequencies (62%) and quantities (98 genome equivalent cells per million of host cells, gEq/M) of male Mc in their PBMC than healthy women (16% and 0.3 gEq/M, p<0.00001 and p = 0.0005 respectively). Male Mc was increased in women with ESRD whether they had or not a history of male pregnancy and/or of blood transfusion. Three out of five renal biopsies obtained a few years prior to the blood test also contained Mc, but no correlation could be established between earlier Mc in a kidney and later presence in PBMC. Finally, several years after female kidney transplantation, male Mc was totally cleared from PBMC in all women tested but one. This intriguing and striking initial result of natural and iatrogenic male Mc persistence in peripheral blood from women with ESRD raises several hypotheses for the possible role of these cells in renal diseases. Further studies are needed to elucidate mechanisms of recruitment and persistence of Mc in women with ESRD.

Editor: Cees Oudejans, VU University Medical Center, Netherlands

Funding: The authors have no support or funding to report.

Competing Interests: The authors have declared that no competing interests exist.

* E-mail: nathalie.lambert@inserm.fr

Introduction

Microchimerism (Mc) is the presence of a small amount of foreign cells or DNA within a person's circulation or tissues [1]. Mc can be acquired through iatrogenic interventions such as organ transplantation, first described in liver transplantation in 1969 [2], or blood transfusion [3]. Mc can also be naturally acquired during pregnancy due to feto-maternal traffic of cells through the placenta membrane [4]. Interestingly, these cells are not short term transitory cells as they can persist for decades in small quantities in their respective hosts [5]. Exchange of cells between fetuses can also contribute to natural Mc within an individual. They were first described between bovine dizygotic twins [6] and later in humans [7]. Recently, our group even reported the presence of cells from an unrecognized (vanished) twin in a 40-year-old man diagnosed with a scleroderma-like disease [8].

The natural phenomenon of Mc has already been investigated in whole peripheral blood [9], peripheral blood mononuclear cells (PBMC) [10] and different tissues [11] from healthy women and women with autoimmune diseases as scleroderma, dermatomyositis, thyroiditis [12,13,14,15]… Higher quantities and frequencies of male Mc observed in women with scleroderma compared to matched controls suggested a possible role for these cells in autoimmunity [12]. However it is still unclear whether the presence of Mc is the cause or the consequence of autoimmunity, whether natural Mc is present to heal or to kill (for reviews [16,17]). For example, in breast cancer, Mc was seen as a protective factor in a study by Gadi et al., where the risk of cancer was lower in women positive for male Mc at the peripheral level [18], whereas in another study, on human breast carcinoma developing during pregnancy, presence of fetal Mc in tumor sections suggested these cells played a detrimental role [19].

Evaluation of the role of fetal Mc in the context of renal diseases was mostly studied indirectly. Indeed fetal cells have been found twice as often in kidneys from women with systemic lupus erythematosus (SLE) than in normal kidneys [20], suggesting that they could play a role in renal disease and/or renal function. A prior study in patients with SLE noted a higher mean number of male equivalent cells in peripheral blood from patients with renal disease than from patients with no renal involvement (4.2 male equivalent cells vs 0.89 male equivalent cells respectively; p<0.05) [21].

When chimerism is studied in patients with renal diseases it is generally to analyze the influence of donor Mc after kidney transplantation for tolerance mechanism purposes [22], and not to analyze the potential role and fate of natural and/or iatrogenic Mc acquired prior to transplantation.

In this context, we studied the unexplored phenomenon of Mc in women with end stage renal diseases (ESRD) prior to their first kidney transplantation, by using a quantitative PCR method for male Mc detection in their PBMC. Male Mc quantification was estimated according to the source of chimerism, pregnancy or transfusion, and compared to results obtained from healthy women.

Methods

Participant' characteristics

Fifty-five women awaiting their first kidney transplantation and 82 healthy women were studied. Controls and patients came from the same geographical area between Marseille and Nice, in the south east of France.

All 55 women with chronic kidney disease were hemodialyzed except for 4 with a Cockroft and Gault creatinine clearance <15 ml/min at the time of DNA extraction. The initial nephropathies were interstitial (n = 21), glomerulonephritis (n = 11), polycystic kidney disease (n = 9), nephroangiosclerosis (n = 4), lupus nephritis (n = 3), diabetes type I (n = 2), diabetes type 2 (n = 2), hemolytic-uremic syndrome (n = 2), indeterminate (n = 1). This proportion is similar to those described in transplanted patients by the French ESRD Registry REIN 2009.

Women with ESRD and healthy women were very similar for pregnancy history and differed for transfusion history (leuko-reduced) as detailed in **Table 1**.

Ethics Statements

All controls were healthy women with no history of autoimmune disease or kidney disease. These healthy women have been used as controls in a previous published study [23]. This study received the approval from the French Ethical Committee Marseille 2 and is registered at the INSERM under the Biomedical Research Protocol number RBM-04-10. Written consent forms obtained according to the Declaration of Helsinki [24] were signed. Questionnaires with detailed information about previous transfusions, pregnancies, and existence of an older brother (as a possible source of male Mc) were filled in for each participant of the study. For one healthy control, we were not able to obtain all the information. Samples from women with ESRD were collected for HLA-typing before registration on the waiting list and then for microchimerism detection which was performed as a "res nullus" analysis. Patients were informed and acquiescent.

DNA extraction from PBMC and native kidney parenchyma

DNA extractions from PBMC for women with ESRD were performed prior to the extractions from controls obtained for a different study. Genomic DNA from patients was extracted using a "salting-out" method [25], from PBMC after EDTA blood processing by Ficoll Histopaque 1077 gradient centrifugation (Sigma-Aldrich, St Louis, MO, USA). Genomic DNA was quantified and purity was assessed by spectrophotometric absorbance at 260 and 280 nm.

Genomic DNA from controls was extracted from PBMC after EDTA blood processing by Ficoll Histopaque 1077 gradient centrifugation (Sigma-Aldrich, St Louis, MO, USA). DNA isolation was done with an EZ1 DNA Tissue Kit (Qiagen, Hilden, Germany) on a BIOROBOT® *EZ1* according to the manufacturer's instructions.

Aware that different DNA extraction methods between the two groups could lead to different results for Mc, 9 patients with ESRD with blood taken more recently had their DNA extracted with a similar method to healthy women (Qiagen kit) and were tested as a separate group to verify whether different methods lead to different results (see results).

For 5 patients, renal tissues from native kidneys were obtained by transcutaneous biopsy and cryopreserved. DNA was extracted with an EZ1 DNA Tissue kit (Qiagen, Hilden, Germany) as described above.

DYS14 real time quantitative PCR

Quantification of male Mc was obtained by real-time PCR for a Y-chromosome specific sequence DYS14 on a Light Cycler® with Light Cycler® Fast Start DNA MasterPLUS Reaction kits (Roche, Indianapolis, IN, USA) as previously described [23]. Total amount of tested DNA was measured by ß-globin, a house keeping gene, as previously described [13]. Duplicates of ß-globin were averaged

Table 1. Characteristics from healthy women and women with ESRD.

Characteristics	Women with ESRD (N = 55)	Healthy women (N = 82)	P values
Median age, range	50[14–67]	52 [37–69]	ns
Mean number of children	2	2 (N = 81)[a]	ns
Mean number of sons	1	1(N = 81)	ns
% of women with at least one son	69	62 (N = 81)	ns
Mean age of the youngest son	19	21 (N = 81)	ns
% of nulligravid women	10	6 (N = 81)	ns
% of women with early pregnancy loss	43	53 (N = 81)	ns
% of women with blood transfusion	65	12	<0.0001
Mean number of transfusions	1	0	<0.0001
Years since last transfusion: mean, [range]	5.6 [0.5–30]	24.5 [17–36]	<0.0001

[a]pregnancy and transfusion information was incomplete for one healthy woman. ns: not significant.

for each woman, giving the total number of cell equivalents multiplied by the number of wells tested.

Sensitivity of the DYS14 assay was accurate to the equivalent DNA of 1 male cell in a background equivalent DNA of 20,000 female cells. DNA from each participant was tested in ten samples with a DNA equivalent of 20,000 cells by real-time PCR for ß-globin (equivalent of 200,000 cells tested/woman). For ease of result legibility, the amount of male DNA was expressed as the number of genome equivalent male cells per million female cells (gEq/M). Because the male Mc in each well is assumed to have a Poisson distribution, the male genome equivalent cells for each subject were averaged as previously described [23]. The estimate for individuals for whom all replicates are assayed using the same number of cells per replicate is the usual Poisson estimate: $-ln$ $(1-p)/M$ where p is the fraction of samples with at least 1 male cell (the limit of p being 1 well positive out of 10 tested) and M is the number of cells in the sample (20,000 in our case). The confidence limit for calculation is when 1 well is positive out of 10, this is why as a conservative estimate of the quantity of male DNA, we required that a sample had at least two wells out of ten positive. Extreme caution was employed to avoid PCR contamination: women performed all the technical work. Pre-amplification steps were carried out in a separate room. A negative control sample was included in each experiment.

Statistical analysis

Significant differences between the two groups were detected using the Chi square test for qualitative variables (Fisher exact test) and an unpaired t-test for continuous variables with a normal distribution or if not, a non-parametric test i.e a Wilcoxon signed-rank test and a Mann-Whitney test for paired series using Statview 5 software (SAS Institute Inc;Cary, NC; USA). Logistic regression was used to assess a relationship between renal status and the presence of male DNA. For all tests, statistical significance was defined as p<0.05.

Results

Increased frequency and higher quantities of male Mc in PBMC from women with ESRD compared to controls

When both groups were analyzed as a whole, without stratifying by age, parity, or history of transfusion, as illustrated in **Figure 1**, we detected male Mc in 62% (34/55) of women with ESRD versus only 16% (13/82) of healthy women (p<0.00001). Differences in quantities of Mc between the two groups were also very significant (**Figure 1**, **Figure 2** for typical amplifications and **Table S1** for number of wells positive). Levels of Mc ranged from 0 to 1382 gEq/M in women with ESRD and from 0 to 5 gEq/M in controls with a mean number of 98 gEq/M and 0.3 gEq/M respectively (p = 0.0005). We did not find any correlation between Mc levels and the length of time since the last abortion, the number of induced or spontaneous abortions, the length of time since the last transfusion, the length of time since the birth of the last child or last son, or the number of sons or children (data not shown).There was also no relationship between the types of nephropathy (vascular, glomerular, interstitial and polycystic) and the presence or the level of Mc (data not shown).

As differences in DNA extraction methods between women with ESRD and healthy women could introduce artifacts for Mc results, we analyzed a separate subgroup of 9 patients with ESRD with blood taken more recently, for whom DNA extraction methods were identical to healthy controls. Frequency of women positive for Mc was statistically significant in this subgroup of patients with ESRD (Fisher's exact test, p = 0.013), with 5 out of 9 women with

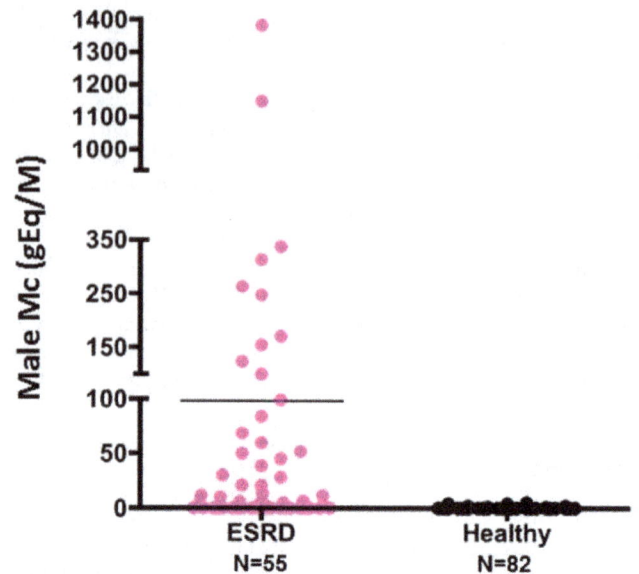

Figure 1. Male Mc quantities in PBMC from women with ESRD and healthy women.

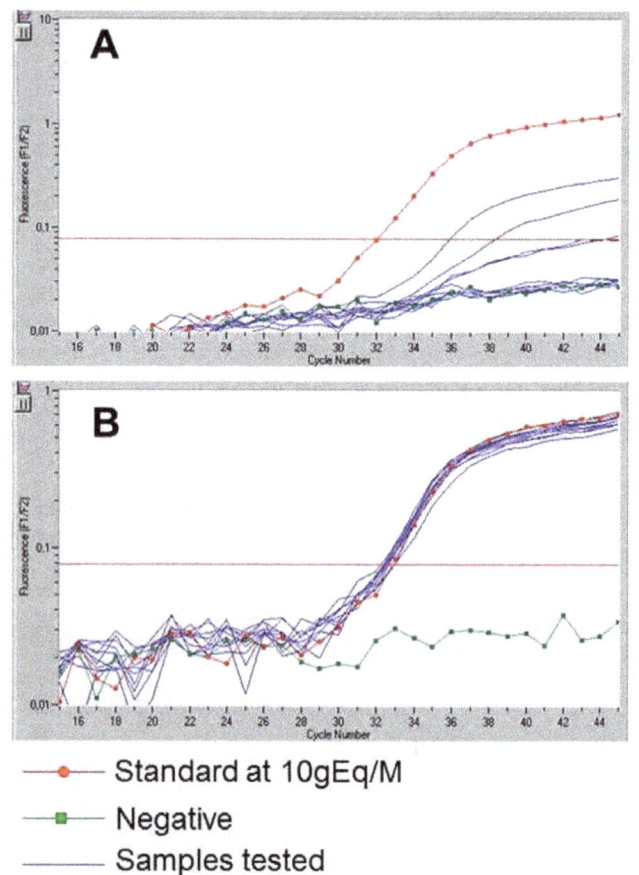

Figure 2. Typical amplifications of male Mc in female host's DNA. PBMC from a healthy woman (A) and a woman with ESRD (B) tested for male Mc in 10 samples.

ESRD positive compared to 13 out of 82 healthy women. Levels of Mc were also significantly increased (Mann Whitney, p = 0.0006) with respectively a mean of 57.0 gEq/M [95% CI: −12.46–126.6] and 0.3 gEq/M [95%.CI: 0.11–0.54]. Results of this sub-analysis exclude a possible bias due to different DNA extraction methods.

Frequencies and quantities of Mc are increased in women with ESRD whether they had or not a history of male pregnancy and/or of transfusion

Male Mc could come from natural or iatrogenic source; we therefore classified women with ESRD and healthy women according to whether they had or not a transfusion history and they had or not given birth to at least one son (**Table 2**). Non-transfused (TSF−) women with ESRD had male Mc more often than healthy matched controls, regardless of whether they had given birth to a son or not (S+ or S−), with respectively 50% and 71% compared with 18% and 14% (p = 0.02 and p = 0.001 respectively). Moreover quantities of male Mc were higher in non-transfused women with ESRD compared to matched healthy women and again differences were not due to pregnancy history as results were similarly significant whether they had or not given birth to at least one son (p = 0.0019 and <0.0001 respectively).

Similarly, transfused (TSF+) women with ESRD also had male Mc more often and in higher quantities than healthy matched controls whether they had given birth to a son, with only the former case (S+) that could be statistically evaluated (p = 0.008) due to small numbers in the latter case (S−).

Male Mc in kidney biopsies two to four years prior to blood testing

Five women were investigated for male DNA in their kidney parenchyma (**Table 3**). Renal tissues were obtained from kidney biopsies with a median time of 36 months (range from 24 to 48) prior to blood testing. Among the five patients, 1 had anti-neutrophil cytoplasmic antibodies (ANCA), 2 had systemic lupus erythematosus (SLE), 1 hemolytic-uremic syndrome (HUS), and 1 focal glomerulosclerosis (FSGS). Two of the five patients were negative for male Mc in renal parenchyma and a few years later had either 10 gEq/M in their PBMC or no male Mc. Three women carried male DNA at concentrations of 30, 10 and 3 gEq/M in renal tissue and a few years later had respectively 21, 2 and 474 gEq/M in their PBMC. No correlation was found between earlier levels in kidney biopsies and later levels of Mc in PBMC.

Clearance of male Mc after kidney transplantation in PBMC from 8 women with ESRD (Table 4)

Finally, we quantified male Mc in PBMC from 8 women with ESRD who had received a female kidney transplant (so as not to complicate Mc sources). At the time of DNA extraction from PBMC, all 8 kidney grafts were functional with a glomerular filtration rate (GFR) ranged from 25 to 70 ml/min. The immunosuppressive protocol consisted in an induction by anti-lymphocyte serum in all patients and triple drugs regimen (steroids, calcineurin inhibitors and mycophenolic acid) therapy. PBMC analysis was carried out in a median time of 4.6 years after transplantation. Among the 8 women tested, 3, negative in their PBMC prior to transplantation remained negative after transplantation, 5 positive before transplantation with, from the lowest to the highest results: 5, 14, 21, 45 and 1,149 gEq/M were all negative after transplantation except the third patient who had 6 gEq/M in her PBMC. Using a Wilcoxon signed-rank test, which is a non-parametric test, we found a marginal decrease (p = 0.04) of Mc levels in the pre to post transplantation period.

Discussion

We present the first study analyzing male Mc in PBMC from women with end stage renal disease (ESRD), prior to their first kidney transplantation. Male Mc was found significantly more often and at higher concentrations than in healthy women. Samples were collected from two independent studies and DNA extractions obtained by different methods, which could introduce artefacts in the results. Noteworthy, divergences between methods have been demonstrated with *circulating DNA* from plasma or urine samples, where small DNA fragments were lost [26] depending on DNA extraction methods but not from cell DNA samples. However to eliminate any suspicion, we tested independently a subgroup of 9 patients for whom DNA was extracted with a similar method to healthy women and found similar results to those obtained in the main group of women with ESRD.

Women with ESRD often have a history of leuko-reduced blood transfusion which could leave iatrogenic Mc as a post transfusion consequence and trigger higher levels of male Mc, when the donor was male [3]. However, we demonstrated that the difference for Mc frequency and/or quantity observed in women with ESRD was not dependent on transfusion history, as results remained significant in women who had never had a blood transfusion. Intriguingly, the difference observed did not correlate either with

Table 2. Male Mc in women with ESRD and healthy women according to pregnancy and transfusion history.

Analyzed group		Women positive for Mc # (%)	Frequency p-values	Mean quantity of male Mc (gEq/M) [range]; Median	Quantity p-values
TSF−S+	Controls (N = 44)	8 (18%)		0.3 [0–5]; 0	
	ESRD (N = 12)	6 (50%)	0.05	36.5 [0–247]; 2	0.0019
TSF−S−	Controls (N = 28)	4 (14%)		0.4 [0–4]; 0	
	ESRD (N = 7)	5 (71%)	0.006	37.4 [0–101]; 28	<0.0001
TSF+S+	Controls (N = 7)	0 (0%)		0	
	ESRD (N = 26)	17 (65%)	0.003	130 [0–1149]; 16.5	0.008
TSF+S−	Controls (N = 3)	1 (33%)		0.6 [0–2]; 0	
	ESRD (N = 10)	6 (60%)	No stats *	192.2 [0–1382]; 4.5	No stats*

TSF+: women who had received at least one blood transfusion; TSF −: women who had never received a blood transfusion; S+: women who had given birth to at least one son; S−: women who had never given birth to a son (S−);
*no stats: statistical analyses were not done due to small numbers.

Table 3. Quantification of Mc in kidney biopsies prior to transplantation from five women with ESRD.

Patients	Kidney disease	Results of male Mc in kidneys (gEq/M)	Year of kidney biopsy	Results of male Mc in PBMC (gEq/M)	Year of blood test	Months between kidney biopsy and blood test
1	ANCA*	30	1999	21	2002	36
2	SLE	0	2003	10	2005	24
3	SLE	0	1999	0	2002	36
4	HUS	10	2000	2	2004	48
5	FSGS	3	2000	474	2002	36

*ANCA: antineutrophil cytoplasmic antibodies, SLE: systemic lupus erythematosus; HUS: hemolytic-uremic syndrome, FSGS: Focal segmental glomerulosclerosis.

pregnancy history, since having given birth to a son or not had no influence on the results. Furthermore, women with ESRD who had never had a blood transfusion and never given birth to a son had male Mc more often in their PBMC and at higher quantities than healthy matched controls. These surprising results suggest they have male DNA from an incomplete pregnancy and/or an unrecognized twin as previously discussed in other studies relative to Mc [27,28]. Indeed, a non-negligible number of pregnancies end before they are clinically noticed [29] and unrecognized twinning is relatively common in healthy pregnancy [30]. In a recent study, Kremer Hovinga et al., also suspected such non-classical sources as principal causes for Mc in renal biopsies from women with lupus nephritis as they showed no significant difference between the occurrence of chimerism in the biopsies of women who had been pregnant compared with women who had not been pregnant [31].

Several hypotheses, not necessarily exclusive, could explain the higher prevalence of male Mc in women with ESRD before kidney transplant compared to healthy women.

First, high levels of male Mc observed in peripheral blood mononuclear cells could indicate a decreased capacity to eliminate male DNA, a consequence of ESRD by decrease of glomerular filtration rate. Very little is known about the life cycle, persistence and elimination process of foreign or semi-foreign cells within an individual. It has been shown that fetal DNA disappears from peripheral blood right after delivery in a very rapid, probably immunological and/or renal, process [32]. Moreover, male DNA has been found in female urine in several cases: after male kidney transplantation and during pregnancy with male fetuses [33].

However, it is still unknown how DNA crosses the normal kidney barrier and appears in the filtrate. Our initial results, on peripheral blood from 8 women who had received a female kidney transplant more than 4 years before, seem to argue in favour of a recovered capacity to eliminate male Mc after transplantation. Indeed women with ESRD who were previously positive for male Mc became negative after kidney transplant. However it is still speculative to consider that clearance of male DNA observed post-transplant in PBMC is due to restored kidney function, as patients undergoing kidney transplant are under strong immunosuppressive drugs that could also affect microchimerism levels. Illustrating this, we recently found, in women with Rheumatoid Arthritis, fluctuating levels of Mc coinciding with disease flare up and treatment [34].

A second hypothesis for high levels of Mc in blood could be a consequence of inflammation in dialysis as well as ESRD patients. It has been recognized that 30% to 50% of pre-dialysis, hemodialysis and peritoneal dialysis patients have serological evidence of an activated inflammatory response [35]. Many mechanisms can induce an inflammatory condition such as reduced renal clearance of cytokines, accumulation of advanced glycation end-products (AGEs), chronic heart failure, atherosclerosis *per se*, unrecognized persistent infections with additional causes in dialysis such as fistula infection and bioincompatibility of dialysis membrane, exposure to endotoxins [35]. High levels of cytokines and chemoattractants may possibly recruit fetal cells from their niche, for example from bone marrow or lymph nodes [36,37]. Here again the quasi-absence of Mc in PBMC after kidney transplantation could come from decreased inflammation due to strong immuno-suppression targeting T lymphocytes.

Table 4. Quantification of male Mc in PBMC from 8 women with ESRD after female kidney transplantation.

Patients	Male Mc in PBMC (gEq/M)		Years after transplantation	GFR* (ml/min) at the time of post-transplant blood test
	before transplantation	after transplantation		
1	1149	0	6	67
2	0	0	5	53
3	14	0	6	60
4	21	6	5	49
5	0	0	3	25
6	45	0	7	59
7	0	0	4	44
8	5	0	5	32

*GFR: glomerular filtration rate.
All patients from this table are different from patients presented table 3, except Patient 4 who is Patient 1 in Table 3.

Thirdly, microchimeric cells could be mobilized to repair damaged tissue and high blood levels would only be reflecting higher kidney levels. In a rat model, it has been described that fetal cells could remodel the maternal kidney after injury [38]. Therefore, the presence of male Mc in kidneys, although at low levels, could be a regenerative process. In our study, we were able to obtain 5 native kidneys biopsies taken 24 to 48 months prior to the blood test, at the time of diagnosis, and demonstrate that 3 out of 5 tested were slightly positive for Mc, but we could not demonstrate whether these cells belonged to the kidney or came from blood vessels supplying the organ. This would have to be determined in further analyses and was beyond the scope of the current study.

Finally as a fourth hypothesis, fetal cells recruited under inflammatory processes might not be bystanders in peripheral blood, or helpers, but effector cells as suggested in a recent study on kidney biopsies from patients with lupus nephritis. In these biopsies microchimeric cells were indeed shown within the hematopoietic stem cell phenotype (CD34+) as well as within T lymphocytes [20].

As anticipated, there is no single explanation for our results showing high levels of male Mc in women with ESRD. Even if we speculate that Mc cells are recruited to help the damaged organ, it is obvious that this help is not fully efficient, since the kidney is not functional in the end. However, it is to be noted that a few studies describe slower disease progression in women with chronic renal disease compared to men, which could argue for a protective role of Mc. Indeed, a meta-analysis involving 11,345 patients determined a gender effect on kidney disease progression from non-diabetic patients [39]. Men with autosomal dominant polycystic kidney disease, membranous nephropathy, or chronic kidney disease of unspecified etiology progressed to renal failure more rapidly than women. Female protection from renal disease progression is also observed in animal models of progressive renal disease [40]. Little is known about the mechanisms underlying sex differences in renal disease susceptibility [41] and it would be interesting to investigate whether chimerism could contribute to a certain "protection" and lead to a gender difference.

This article brings forward new original insights into the unexplored phenomenon of Mc in renal diseases and should initiate future research to determine mechanisms of recruitment and persistence of Mc in patients with ESRD prior to kidney transplantation.

Acknowledgments

Greatest thanks to Marion Causeret for patient recruitment.

Author Contributions

Conceived and designed the experiments: NCL. Performed the experiments: LA JMR DFA. Analyzed the data: LA EC-V JG NCL. Contributed reagents/materials/analysis tools: EC-V. Wrote the paper: LA NCL.

References

1. Rinkevich B (2011) Quo vadis chimerism? Chimerism 2: 1–5.
2. Kashiwagi N, Porter KA, Penn I, Brettschneider L, Starzl TE (1969) Studies of homograft sex and of gamma globulin phenotypes after orthotopic homotransplantation of the human liver. Surg Forum 20: 374–376.
3. Lee TH, Paglieroni T, Ohto H, Holland PV, Busch MP (1999) Survival of donor leukocyte subpopulations in immunocompetent transfusion recipients: frequent long-term microchimerism in severe trauma patients. Blood 93: 3127–3139.
4. Lo YM, Lo ES, Watson N, Noakes L, Sargent IL, et al. (1996) Two-way cell traffic between mother and fetus: biologic and clinical implications. Blood 88: 4390–4395.
5. Bianchi DW, Zickwolf GK, Weil GJ, Sylvester S, DeMaria MA (1996) Male fetal progenitor cells persist in maternal blood for as long as 27 years postpartum. Proc Natl Acad Sci U S A 93: 705–708.
6. Owen RD (1945) Immunogenetic Consequences of Vascular Anastomoses between Bovine Twins. Science 102: 400–401.
7. Dunsford I, Bowley CC, Hutchison AM, Thompson JS, Sanger R, et al. (1953) A human blood-group chimera. Br Med J 2: 80–81.
8. de Bellefon LM, Heiman P, Kanaan SB, Azzouz DF, Rak JM, et al. (2010) Cells from a vanished twin as a source of microchimerism 40 years later. Chimerism 1: 56–60.
9. Nelson JL (1998) Microchimerism and the causation of scleroderma. Scand J Rheumatol Suppl 107: 10–13.
10. Evans PC, Lambert N, Maloney S, Furst DE, Moore JM, et al. (1999) Long-term fetal microchimerism in peripheral blood mononuclear cell subsets in healthy women and women with scleroderma. Blood 93: 2033–2037.
11. Koopmans M, Kremer Hovinga IC, Baelde HJ, Fernandes RJ, de Heer E, et al. (2005) Chimerism in kidneys, livers and hearts of normal women: implications for transplantation studies. Am J Transplant 5: 1495–1502.
12. Nelson JL, Furst DE, Maloney S, Gooley T, Evans PC, et al. (1998) Microchimerism and HLA-compatible relationships of pregnancy in scleroderma. Lancet 351: 559–562.
13. Lambert NC, Lo YM, Erickson TD, Tylee TS, Guthrie KA, et al. (2002) Male microchimerism in healthy women and women with scleroderma: cells or circulating DNA? A quantitative answer. Blood 100: 2845–2851.
14. Reed AM, Picornell YJ, Harwood A, Kredich DW (2000) Chimerism in children with juvenile dermatomyositis. Lancet 356: 2156–2157.
15. Klintschar M, Schwaiger P, Mannweiler S, Regauer S, Kleiber M (2001) Evidence of fetal microchimerism in Hashimoto's thyroiditis. J Clin Endocrinol Metab 86: 2494–2498.
16. Lambert NC (2010) [Microchimerism in scleroderma: ten years later]. Rev Med Interne 31: 523–529.
17. Lee ES, Bou-Gharios G, Seppanen E, Khosrotehrani K, Fisk NM (2010) Fetal stem cell microchimerism: natural-born healers or killers? Mol Hum Reprod 16: 869–878.
18. Gadi VK, Nelson JL (2007) Fetal microchimerism in women with breast cancer. Cancer Res 67: 9035–9038.
19. Dubernard G, Aractingi S, Oster M, Rouzier R, Mathieu MC, et al. (2008) Breast cancer stroma frequently recruits fetal derived cells during pregnancy. Breast Cancer Res 10: R14.
20. Kremer Hovinga IC, Koopmans M, Baelde HJ, van der Wal AM, Sijpkens YW, et al. (2006) Chimerism occurs twice as often in lupus nephritis as in normal kidneys. Arthritis Rheum 54: 2944–2950.
21. Mosca M, Curcio M, Lapi S, Valentini G, D'Angelo S, et al. (2003) Correlations of Y chromosome microchimerism with disease activity in patients with SLE: analysis of preliminary data. Ann Rheum Dis 62: 651–654.
22. Starzl TE (2004) Chimerism and tolerance in transplantation. Proc Natl Acad Sci U S A 101 Suppl 2: 14607–14614.
23. Rak JM, Pagni PP, Tiev K, Allanore Y, Farge D, et al. (2009) Male microchimerism and HLA compatibility in French women with scleroderma: a different profile in limited and diffuse subset. Rheumatology (Oxford) 48: 363–366.
24. Vollmann J, Winau R (1996) Informed consent in human experimentation before the Nuremberg code. BMJ 313: 1445–1449.
25. Miller SA, Dykes DD, Polesky HF (1988) A simple salting out procedure for extracting DNA from human nucleated cells. Nucleic Acids Res 16: 1215.
26. Wang M, Block TM, Steel L, Brenner DE, Su YH (2004) Preferential isolation of fragmented DNA enhances the detection of circulating mutated k-ras DNA. Clin Chem 50: 211–213.
27. Yan Z, Lambert NC, Guthrie KA, Porter AJ, Loubiere LS, et al. (2005) Male microchimerism in women without sons: Quantitative assessment and correlation with pregnancy history. American Journal of Medicine 118: 899–906.
28. Lambert NC, Pang JM, Yan Z, Erickson TD, Stevens AM, et al. (2005) Male microchimerism in women with systemic sclerosis and healthy women who have never given birth to a son. Ann Rheum Dis 64: 845–848.
29. Macklon NS, Geraedts JP, Fauser BC (2002) Conception to ongoing pregnancy: the 'black box' of early pregnancy loss. Hum Reprod Update 8: 333–343.
30. Robinson HP, Caines JS (1977) Sonar evidence of early pregnancy failure in patients with twin conceptions. Br J Obstet Gynaecol 84: 22–25.

31. Kremer Hovinga IC, Koopmans M, Grootscholten C, van der Wal AM, Bijl M, et al. (2008) Pregnancy, chimerism and lupus nephritis: a multi-centre study. Lupus 17: 541–547.

32. Lo YM, Zhang J, Leung TN, Lau TK, Chang AM, et al. (1999) Rapid clearance of fetal DNA from maternal plasma. Am J Hum Genet 64: 218–224.

33. Umansky SR, Tomei LD (2006) Transrenal DNA testing: progress and perspectives. Expert Rev Mol Diagn 6: 153–163.

34. Rak JM, Maestroni L, Balandraud N, Guis S, Boudinet H, et al. (2008) Transfer of shared epitope through microchimerism in women with Rheumatoid Arthritis. Arthritis and Rheumatism in press.

35. Stenvinkel P (2002) Inflammation in end-stage renal failure: could it be treated? Nephrol Dial Transplant 17 Suppl 8: 33–38; discussion 40.

36. O'Donoghue K, Chan J, de la Fuente J, Kennea N, Sandison A, et al. (2004) Microchimerism in female bone marrow and bone decades after fetal mesenchymal stem-cell trafficking in pregnancy. Lancet 364: 179–182.

37. Koopmans M, Kremer Hovinga IC, Baelde HJ, Harvey MS, de Heer E, et al. (2008) Chimerism occurs in thyroid, lung, skin and lymph nodes of women with sons. J Reprod Immunol 78: 68–75.

38. Wang Y, Iwatani H, Ito T, Horimoto N, Yamato M, et al. (2004) Fetal cells in mother rats contribute to the remodeling of liver and kidney after injury. Biochem Biophys Res Commun 325: 961–967.

39. Neugarten J, Acharya A, Silbiger SR (2000) Effect of gender on the progression of nondiabetic renal disease: a meta-analysis. J Am Soc Nephrol 11: 319–329.

40. Ji H, Pesce C, Zheng W, Kim J, Zhang Y, et al. (2005) Sex differences in renal injury and nitric oxide production in renal wrap hypertension. Am J Physiol Heart Circ Physiol 288: H43–47.

41. Dubey RK, Jackson EK (2001) Estrogen-induced cardiorenal protection: potential cellular, biochemical, and molecular mechanisms. Am J Physiol Renal Physiol 280: F365–388.

15

Mortality of IgA Nephropathy Patients: A Single Center Experience over 30 Years

Hajeong Lee[1,2], Dong Ki Kim[1], Kook-Hwan Oh[1], Kwon Wook Joo[1,3], Yon Su Kim[1,3], Dong-Wan Chae[3,4], Suhnggwon Kim[1,2,3], Ho Jun Chin[2,3,4]*

1 Department of Internal Medicine, Seoul National University Hospital, Seoul, Korea, 2 Department of Immunology, Seoul National University College of Medicine, Seoul, Korea, 3 Kidney Research Institute, Seoul National University Hospital, Seoul, Korea, 4 Department of Internal Medicine, Seoul National University Bundang Hospital, Seongnam, Korea

Abstract

Research on the prognosis of IgA nephropathy (IgAN) has focused on renal survival, with little information being available on patient survival. Hence, this investigation aimed to explore long-term patient outcome in IgAN patients. Clinical and pathological characteristics at the time of renal biopsy were reviewed in 1,364 IgAN patients from 1979 to 2008. The outcomes were patient death and end stage renal disease (ESRD) progression. Overall, 71 deaths (5.3%) and 277 cases of ESRD (20.6%) occurred during 13,916 person-years. Ten-, 20-, and 30-year patient survival rates were 96.3%, 91.8%, and 82.7%, respectively. More than 50% patient deaths occurred without ESRD progression. Overall mortality was elevated by 43% from an age/sex-matched general population (GP) (standardized mortality ratio [SMR], 1.43; 95% confidence interval [CI], 1.04–1.92). Men had comparable mortality to GP (SMR, 1.22; 95% CI, 0.82–1.75), but, in women, the mortality rate was double (SMR, 2.17; 95% CI, 1.21–3.57). Patients with renal risk factors such as initial renal dysfunction (estimated glomerular filgration rate <60 ml/min per $1.73m^2$; SMR, 1.70; 95% CI, 1.13–2.46), systolic blood pressure ≥140 mmHg (SMR, 1.88; 95% CI, 1.19–2.82) or proteinuria ≥1 g/day (SMR, 1.66; 95% CI, 1.16–2.29) had an elevated mortality rate. Patients with preserved renal function, normotension, and proteinuria <1 g/day, however, had a similar mortality rate to GP. When risk stratification was performed by counting the number of major risk factors present at diagnosis, low-risk IgAN patients had a mortality rate equal to that of GP, whereas high-risk patients had a mortality rate higher than that of GP. This investigation demonstrated that overall mortality in IgAN patients was higher than that of GP. Women and patients with renal risk factors had a higher mortality than that of GP, Therefore, strategies optimized to alleviate major renal risk factors are warranted to reduce patient mortality.

Editor: Hamid Reza Baradaran, Tehran University of Medical Sciences, Iran (Republic of Islamic)

Funding: The authors have no support or funding to report.

Competing Interests: The authors have declared that no competing interests exist.

* E-mail: mednep@snubh.org

Introduction

IgA nephropathy (IgAN) is the most common form of glomerular disease worldwide, with an incidence that ranges from 20% to 40% in patients with primary glomerulonephritis [1]. The relative incidence of IgAN has increased recently, especially in Korea [2]. Despite the well-known heterogeneity of the disease and a generally slow course of disease progression, IgAN is a significant contributor to end stage renal disease (ESRD) progression [1,3,4]. Indeed, numerous studies have addressed the clinical [3–9] and pathological [3,10–14] risk factors linked to the risk of progression. These include initial renal impairment [3,5,9], heavier or prolonged proteinuria [4–6,8], hypertension [6,8,9], and several histological changes [3,6,8,14]. However, the mortality data are not reported in most IgAN survival studies. Patient death has been considered as one part of a composite outcome [8,12,15] or analyzed only descriptively [16]. The mortality rate or its predictors have not been addressed in previous studies. Therefore, according to the Kidney Disease: Improving Global Outcomes (KDIGO) Clinical Practice Guidelines for glomerulonephritis (to be published), there is an assumption that IgAN patients had higher mortality than the general population

(GP), and that cardiovascular morbidity and mortality increase in these patients, as in others with chronic kidney disease.

IgAN patients are usually diagnosed at a relatively young age, and most have a benign clinical course in our clinical practice. Moreover, these patients are thought to be more likely to receive transplantation because of their relatively younger age even after ESRD progression compared to their diabetic ESRD counterparts. Such clinical experiences suggest a favorable patient outcome in IgAN patients. Therefore, the rate of IgAN progression to patient death needs to be clarified, as do the clinical or pathological risk factors involved. The main purpose of this retrospective observational study was to describe the definitive patient outcome and analysis of their predictive factors, compared with renal outcome and its indicators.

Materials and Methods

Ethics statement

This investigation was approved by the institutional review board in Seoul National University Hospital and was in accordance with the principle of the Helsinki Declaration II (H-

Table 1. Baseline demographic and clinical characteristics.

Parameters	Total	Death			ESRD		
		No	Yes	P	No	Yes	P
At the time of biopsy (n)	1,364	1,276	71		1,067	277	
Age (years)	33(25–45)	32(22–44)	47(36–61)	<0.001	33(24–44)	36(28–46)	0.001
Sex (male)	682(50.0)	632(49.5)	43(60.6)	0.087	513(48.1)	161(58.1)	0.003
SBP (mmHg)	120(110–138)	120(110–130)	140(124–150)	<0.001	120(110–130)	130(120–150)	<0.001
Co-morbidity							
Diabetes	25(2.0)	22(1.9)	3(5.0)	0.120	18(1.9)	7(2.7)	0.037
Cancer	10(0.8)	4(0.3)	6(10.0)	<0.001	7(0.7)	3(1.2)	0.448
Hypertension	484(38.7)	442(37.2)	42(67.7)	<0.001	319(32.4)	165(62.3)	<0.001
Clinical manifestations							
Edema	314(24.1)	288(23.2)	26(40.0)	0.004	210(20.3)	104(38.4)	<0.001
Gross hematuria	438(33.2)	417(33.3)	21(31.3)	0.791	370(35.4)	70(25.5)	0.002
AUA	457(35.0)	442(35.6)	15(22.7)	0.034	386(37.3)	71(26.0)	<0.001
Laboratory tests							
Hemoglobin (g/dL)	13.3(11.8–14.6)	13.3(11.9–14.6)	11.7(9.4–13.9)	<0.001	13.5(12.1–14.7)	12.1(10.5–13.9)	<0.001
Albumin (g/dL)	3.9(3.5–4.2)	3.9(3.5–4.2)	3.3(2.7–3.9)	<0.001	3.9(3.6–4.2)	3.6(3.1–4.0)	<0.001
Cholesterol (mg/dL)	186(158–220)	186(158–219)	209(154–239)	0.125	184(157–216)	203(166–233)	<0.001
Creatinine (mg/dL)	1.10(1.10–1.50)	1.10(0.90–1.40)	1.50(1.20–2.15)	<0.001	1.10(0.90–1.30)	1.70(1.20–2.40)	<0.001
eGFR (mL/min/1.73m^2)	67.6(27.6)	68.7(27.4)	48.3(25.4)	<0.001	73.5(25.2)	45.7(24.9)	<0.001
24hour proteinuria (g/day)	1.30(0.56–2.50)	1.22(0.54–2.36)	2.62(1.60–5.44)	<0.001	1.11(0.50–2.12)	2.11(1.03–3.46)	<0.001
During follow-up (n)	1223	1163	60		965	258	
Development of cancer	47(3.8)	35(3.0)	12(20.0)	<0.001	30(3.1)	17(6.6)	0.016
Development of diabetes	73(6.0)	66(5.7)	7(9.6)	0.084	50(5.2)	23(8.9)	0.037
Medical treatment (n)	1050	1009	41		842	208	
Antiplatelet agents	695(64.8)	322(31.3)	6(14.0)	0.017	265(30.9)	63(29.6)	0.740
Statin	146(13.6)	142(13.8)	4(9.3)	0.501	117(13.6)	29(13.6)	1.000
RAS blockade	328(30.6)	675(65.6)	20(46.5)	0.014	557(64.9)	137(64.3)	0.873
Immunosuppressant	137(12.7)	124(12.0)	13(30.2)	0.002	103(12.0)	34(15.9)	0.137

All continuous variables are shown as mean (SD) for normal distributions, or median (interquartile range) for non-parametric variables. Categorical variables were frequency per observation (N (%)). Baseline characteristics for patients who progressed to the primary outcome were compared with those who did not using χ^2 test for dichotomous variables, and student t-test for parametric continuous variables.
Abbreviations: ESRD, end stage renal disease; BMI, body mass index; AUA, asymptomatic urinary abnormalities; SBP, systolic blood pressure; DBP, diastolic blood pressure; eGFR, estimated glomerular filtration rate; TA, tubular atrophy; RAS, renin-angiotensin system.

1010-055-336). As the study was retrospective in design and did not include any interventions, informed consent was waived.

Study subjects

From 1979 to 2008, a kidney biopsy registry was constructed using 4,998 kidney needle biopsy cases among patients aged ≥15 years at the Seoul National University Hospital. Allograft biopsy cases were excluded from this cohort. Among the retrospective cohort, a primary diagnosis of IgAN was made in 1,379 patients. Fifteen of these patients who had less than 5 glomeruli in their biopsy specimen had insufficient information for diagnosis and were excluded from this study [11,17]. The diagnosis was based on immunofluorescence microscopy showing mesangial IgA deposition as the predominant or co-dominant immunoglobulin, and on the lack of clinical or laboratory evidence of systemic lupus erythematosus, Henoch-Schonlein nephrtis, or liver cirrhosis. In case of lupus nephritis, only the patients with clinical suspicion for lupus nephritis were further tested for lupus autoantibodies.

Clinical data

Baseline demographic and clinical characteristics were obtained from a review of the medical records at the time of biopsy. Demographic and clinical parameters including age, sex, blood pressure, blood chemistry analysis and 24-h urine protein were obtained. Information about co-morbidities was also collected. Hypertension was defined as a reported history of hypertension, a systolic blood pressure (SBP) ≥140 mmHg, or a diastolic blood pressure ≥90 mmHg. Diabetes mellitus was defined as a reported history of diabetes or as the active use of an oral hypoglycemic agent or insulin. Anemia was defined as a hemoglobin level <13 g/dL for men and <12 g/dL for women. The estimated glomerular filtration rate (eGFR) was calculated by the modified modification of diet in renal disease equation after measuring serum creatinine. Data on medication were collected if any of the following was started within 6 months of renal biopsy and was prescribed for more than 3 months: renin-angiotensin system blockades, including any kind of angiotensin-converting enzyme inhibitor and angiotensin receptor

Table 2. Pathologic changes of study population.

Parameters	Total (n = 1,270)	Death			ESRD		
		No(n = 1190)	Yes(n = 67)	P	No(n = 858)	Yes(n = 219)	P
Number of glomerulus	64(21–55)	35(22–56)	26(18–43)	0.007	38(23–58)	26(17–40)	<0.001
Global sclerosis (%)	14.8(3.7–34.9)	14.3(3.4–34.2)	25(5.6–46.2)	0.020	11.3(2.4–27.2)	37.5(19.2–59.3)	<0.001
Segmental sclerosis (%)	6.8(0–14.3)	6.9(0–14.3)	3.3(0–16.7)	0.193	6.1(0–13.0)	11.2(3.4–19.1)	<0.001
Crescent (yes)	268(21.3)	246(20.7)	22(32.8)	0.022	210(21.2)	58(21.8)	0.866
TA/Interstitial fibrosis				0.004			<0.001
None	119(9.6)	114(9.7)	5(7.9)		106(10.8)	13(5.0)	
Mild	517(41.8)	498(42.4)	19(30.2)		472(48.3)	45(17.2)	
Moderate	375(30.3)	358(30.5)	17(27.0)		291(23.5)	84(32.1)	
Severe	228(18.3)	205(17.4)	22(34.9)		108(11.1)	120(45.8)	
Interstitial inflammation				0.014			<0.001
None	163(13.2)	155(13.2)	7(11.1)		133(13.6)	30(11.5)	
Mild	485(39.1)	467(39.7)	18(26.6)		447(45.8)	38(14.5)	
Moderate	380(30.7)	362(30.8)	18(26.6)		293(30.0)	87(22.9)	
Severe	211(17.0)	191(16.3)	20(31.7)		104(10.6)	107(40.8)	
Vascular change				0.042			<0.001
None	769(62.0)	736(62.7)	32(50.0)		657(67.2)	112(43.1)	
Hyalinosis	215(17.4)	199(17.0)	16(25.0)		148(15.1)	66(25.4)	
Atherosclerotic change	255(20.6)	239(20.3)	16(25.0)		173(17.7)	82(31.6)	
WHO pathologic grade (n)	1077	1027	50		858	219	
I	31(2.9)	31(3.0)	0(0.0)		29(3.4)	2(0.9)	
II	272(25.3)	267(26.0)	5(10.0)		265(30.9)	7(3.2)	
III	464(43.1)	446(43.5)	18(36.0)		398(46.4)	66(30.1)	
IV	191(17.8)	178(17.3)	13(26.0)		124(14.5)	67(30.6)	
V	118(11.0)	104(10.1)	14(11.9)		42(4.9)	77(35.2)	

All continuous variables are shown as mean (SD) for normal distributions, or median (interquartile range) for non-parametric variables. Categorical variables were frequency per observation (N (%)). Pathological characteristics for patients who progressed to the primary outcome were compared with those who did not using χ^2 test for dichotomous variables, and student t-test for parametric continuous variables. Abbreviations: ESRD, end stage renal disease; TA, tubular atrophy;

blocker; any kind of glucocorticoid; statins; and antiplatelet agents such as aspirin or clopidogrel.

To evaluate histopathological change, 2 pathologists reviewed the renal biopsy slides. In the glomerular area, the numbers of glomeruli, proportions of global sclerosis, segmental sclerosis, and crescent lesion were calculated. The percentages of glomeruli with these lesions were deduced and categorized. In the tubulointerstitial area, tubular atrophy and interstitial fibrosis, interstitial inflammatory cell infiltration, and vascular change were graded. The histopathological grades were also analyzed using the WHO grading system for IgAN.

Outcome measurement

The outcomes were the death from any cause and ESRD progression (permanent hemodialysis, peritoneal dialysis or renal transplantation) after renal biopsy. Data on mortality and cause of death were obtained from the Korean National Statistical Office (KNSO), and ESRD data were collected from the Korea ESRD registry [18]. We combined all these data according to the unique identification number held by all Koreans. In addition, the medical records were searched retrospectively to obtain additional information related to the primary outcome and the recent renal function of the patients. It was assumed that patients who had no follow-up with our institution and no follow-up creatinine values,

and who did not undergo any renal replacement therapy or a reported death did not meet the primary endpoint at the time the database closed.

Statistical analysis

The data are presented as frequencies and percentages for categorical variables. Continuous variables with normal distribution are indicated as mean ± SD, while those without normal distribution are shown as median and interquartile range (IQR). Comparisons between the outcome group and other groups were performed using the χ^2 test for dichotomous variables, Student t-test for parametric continuous variables, and Mann-Whitney test for non-parametric continuous variables.

Survival rates for ESRD, death, and composite outcome were analyzed using the Kaplan-Meier method. Survival differences were tested by the log-rank procedure. Cox proportional hazards models were used for prognostic factor assessment. Proportional hazards assumption for Cox models were tested by using log-minus-log plots. Variables that failed to satisfy the proportional hazards assumptions were analyzed by using time-dependent Cox regression analysis. Variables that showed a significant association ($P<0.10$) in the univariate analysis or that were of considerable theoretical relevance were retained as potential predictors in the multivariate model. In the forward conditional multivariate

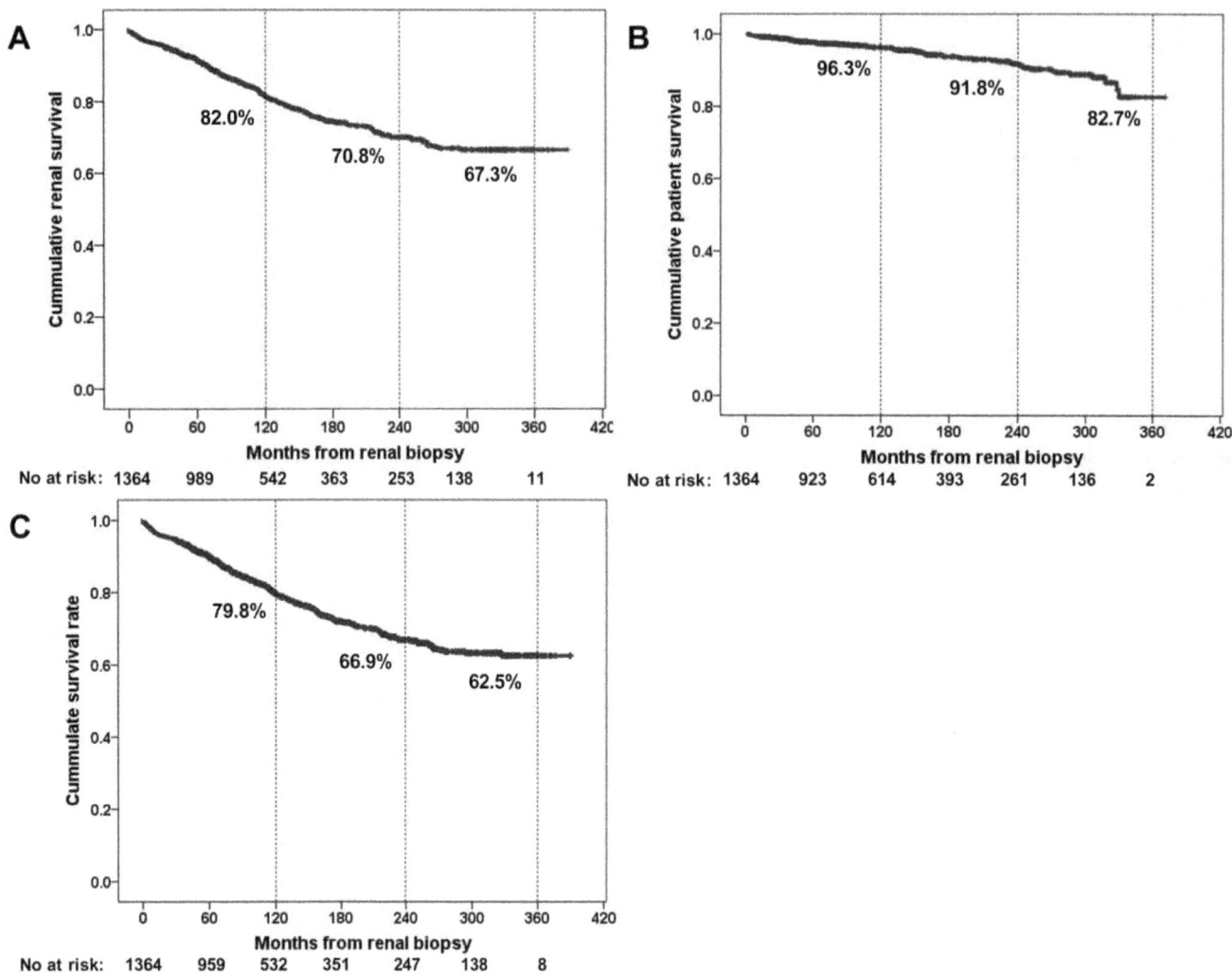

Figure 1. Cumulative renal and patient survival after renal biopsy. The primary endpoint was renal (A) and patient survival (B) and composite outcome (C). The numbers of patients remaining at 60, 120, 180, 240, 300, and 360 months of follow-up are shown at the bottom. ESRD, end stage renal disease.

models, the orders of variable selection and the values of Wald statistics helped to determine the rankings of the risk factors.

From the results of Cox-regression analyses, we identified 3 major risk factors: SBP ≥140 mmHg, proteinuria ≥1 g/day, and baseline renal insufficiency with eGFR <60 ml/min per 1.73m². These major risk factors were simplified as a sum of present risk factors as follows: low-risk group for none or one of the risk factors; intermediate-risk group for any 2 of the risk factors, and high-risk group for all their simultaneous presence. Patient survival and renal survival analyses were also performed according to the risk stratification.

To clarify the mortality rate associated with IgAN, the standardized mortality ratio (SMR) was calculated as the ratio between the observed and the expected number of deaths. The expected number of deaths was calculated by person-year methods as follows: (1) The sum of annual observed person-years was calculated during the observation period (1992–2008). (2) The expected number of deaths was calculated by multiplying the sum of annual observed person-years by sex-adjusted national mortality data in 5-year calendar periods and 5-year age groups. (3) The sum of annual expected number of deaths was calculated. Information about the annual mortality rates of the general

Korean population was collected from the KNSO. Because national mortality statistics were available from 1992, SMR was calculated in the patients who had a renal biopsy after 1992. An SMR >1.0 was considered to be an excess mortality. To calculate the 95% confidence intervals (CIs) for the SMR of each group, the Poisson-distributed number of observed cases was assumed [19]. Two-sided P values are reported, with the level of statistical significance set at 0.05. The SPSS Statistics (version 19.0, Chicago, IL, USA) package was used for statistical analysis.

Results

Baseline characteristics according to outcome development

Overall, 1,364 patients were included in the final analysis. Initial demographic and clinical data are listed in Table 1. The median age at the time of biopsy was 33 years (IQR, 25–45). The proportion of men and women was equal, although age distribution according to sex was quite different. Median age was lower in men (31 years; IQR, 22–45) than in women (35 years; IQR, 27–45). Gross hematuria was present in 33.2% of patients.

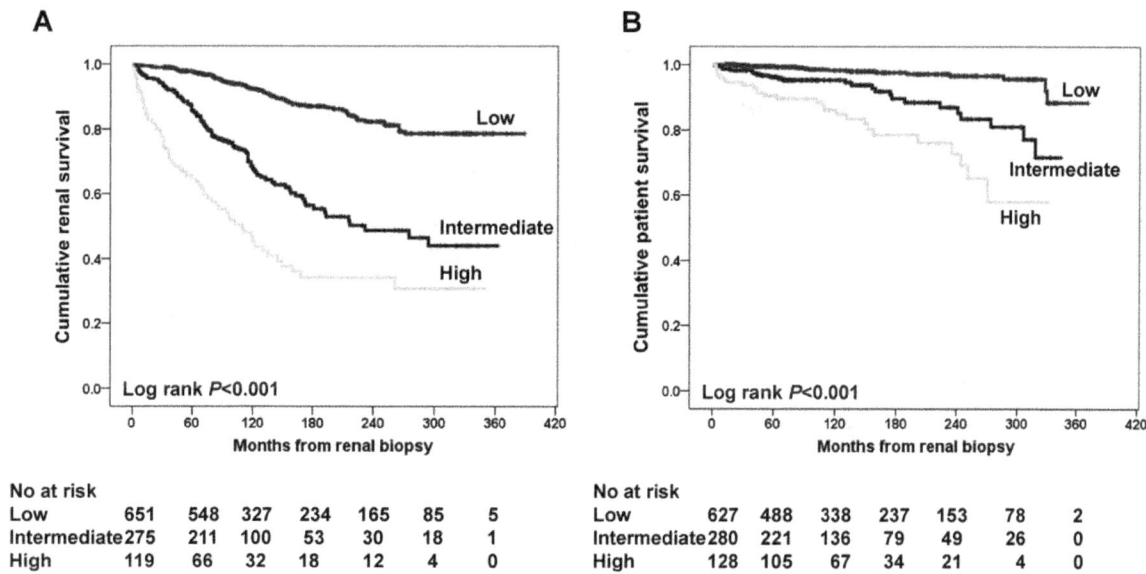

Figure 2. Cumulative renal (A) and patient survival (B) according to the risk stratification. The primary outcome is patient survival. The numbers of patients remaining at 60, 120, 180, 240, 300, and 360 months of follow-up are shown at the bottom.

The mean eGFR was 67.6 ml/min per 1.73m² and proteinuria was 1.3 g/day. In all, 137 patients were treated with immunosuppressive agents, of which 25 were treated with intravenous steroids; 130 with oral steroids; 36 with oral cyclophosphamide; 9 with cyclosporine; and 9 with mycophenolate mofetil.

The patients who died were significantly older, and had higher blood pressure, more nephrotic features and more depressed renal function at the time of biopsy than did the survivors. A higher proportion of the patients who died was managed with immunosuppressive agents before death. Patients with ESRD progression were slightly older and included a higher proportion of men than did the non-ESRD group. Nephrotic features, higher blood pressure, lower hemoglobin level and initial renal dysfunction were significantly higher in patients with renal progression. Table 2 summarizes the pathological data of the study population. The pathological changes were more severe in both glomerular and tubulointerstitial areas in ESRD patients and in those who died.

Figure 1 compares the overall renal and patient survival rates. In cases of renal survival, 277 (20.6%) patients advanced to renal death. Ten, 20- and 30-year renal survival rates were 82.0%, 70.8% and 67.3%, respectively during a median observation period of 96 (IQR, 56–187) months with 14,495 person-years. The median time to ESRD was 71 (IQR, 32–123) months. Seventy-one (5.3%) patients died during the median observation period of 100 (IQR, 51–210) months, with 13,916 person-years. The median time to death was 101 (IQR, 38–189) months. Ten, 20-, and 30-year patient survival rates were 96.3%, 91.8%, and 82.7%, respectively. For composite outcome, the median observation period was 96 months (IQR, 57–188), with 14,588 person-years. The median time to event was 69 (IQR, 31–165) months. Three-hundred and sixteen (23.2%) patients reached the composite outcome during the long-term follow-up. Ten, 20-, and 30-year patient survival rates were 79.8%, 66.9%, and 62.5%, respectively.

Comparisons of predictors according to renal and patient outcome

Risk factor assessment was performed according to ESRD, death, and composite outcome, respectively, In the univariate analysis,

renal survival was predominantly affected gradually by eGFR stage in the univariate analysis, even from an eGFR <90 ml/min per 1.73m². SBP ≥140 mmHg, proteinuria ≥1 g/day, hypoalbuminemia and edema were the next important determinants of ESRD progression. For death, age was a predominant risk factor even from the age of 40 years. Combined malignancy; SBP ≥140 mmHg; eGFR <60 ml/min per 1.73m²; nephrotic features such as edema, proteinuria, and hypoalbuminemia; and anemia were the next significant predictors of patient death. None of the medical treatment had any demonstrable effect on mortality. In addition, patient survival was influenced by glomerular changes such as global sclerosis, segmental sclerosis, and the presence of any crescent formation. Severe degrees of tubulointerstitial changes were also associated with poor patient survival. For composite outcome, the significant predictors were similar to those of ESRD.

The results of the multivariate analysis for the indicators of ESRD and patient death are summarized in Table 3. In the case of renal survival, initial renal function was the most important determinant, followed, as expected, by hypertension. Segmental sclerosis and hypoalbuminemia remained as significant predictors of renal progression. Gross hematuria was associated with a favorable renal outcome. For patient outcome, advanced age, SBP ≥140 mmHg, hypoalbuminemia and combined malignancy were identified as independent determinants. Interestingly, predictors of patient and renal death appeared to be similar, with hypoalbuminemia and hypertension (or SBP ≥140 mmHg) being common risk factors for both outcomes. Moreover, determinants of the composite outcome seemed to be the combination of the predictors of mortality and ESRD progression. When the simplified risk stratification was applied, it predicted both renal and patient outcome in IgAN patients well (Figure 2).

Subgroup analysis for patient death

Among the 71 deaths, 39(55.7%) patients died before ESRD progression. These 39 patients were significantly older (median age 49 [IQR, 38–64] vs.61 [IQR, 53–68] years, P=0.049) and showed relatively conserved renal function (median eGFR 55.8 [IQR, 39.1–71.5] vs. 37.0 [IQR, 18.3–53.7] ml/min per 1.73m²,

Table 3. Univariate and multivariate time dependent cox regression analyses for patient death and renal death.

		Univariate analysis				Multivariate analysis			
		Wald	HR	95% CI	P	Wald	HR	95% CI	P
ESRD	eGFR ≥90(mL/min/1.73m²)	Ref.	Ref.	Ref.		Ref.	Ref.	Ref.	
	60–90	14.403	4.151	1.990–8.658	<0.001	5.024	2.395	1.116–5.141	0.025
	30–60	48.996	12.988	6.335–26.627	<0.001	27.808	7.330	3.496–15.368	<0.001
	15–30	91.860	40.496	18.998–86.322	<0.001	35.737	12.828	5.557–29.612	<0.001
	<15	122.268	84.995	38.673–186.804	<0.001	69.844	41.724	17.393–100.092	<0.001
	Hypertension	57.262	2.693	2.084–3.481	<0.001	9.667	1.698	1.216–2.370	0.002
	Segmental sclerosis ≥20%	38.746	2.480	1.863–3.301	<0.001	8.063	1.674	1.173–2.389	0.005
	Gross hematuria	31.694	0.435	0.326–0.582	<0.001	5.753	0.613	0.411–0.914	0.016
	Albumin <3.5 g/dL	63.312	2.741	2.138–3.514	<0.001	4.416	1.429	1.024–1.993	0.036
Death	Age <40 years	Ref.	Ref.	Ref.		Ref.	Ref.	Ref.	
	40–59	20.440	3.718	2.104–6.571	<0.001	4.626	2.229	1.074–4.626	0.031
	≥60	101.088	24.493	13.130–45.691	<0.001	49.267	15.627	7.253–33.670	<0.001
	SBP ≥140 mmHg	28.157	3.730	2.294–6.065	<0.001	9.121	2.484	1.376–4.482	0.003
	Albumin <3.5 g/dL	39.264	4.778	2.930–7.794	<0.001	8.481	2.470	1.344–4.539	0.003
	Cancer	28.999	5.745	3.040–10.855	<0.001	3.943	2.224	1.010–4.894	0.047
Composite	Age <40 years	Ref.	Ref.	Ref.		Ref.	Ref.	Ref.	
	40–59	16.913	1.695	1.318–2.180	<0.001	1.520	0.672	0.358–1.264	0.218
	≥60	60.809	4.582	3.125–6.718	<0.001	14.317	5.351	2.244–12.757	<0.001
	Cancer	23.350	2.760	1.828–4.166	<0.001	13.545	2.882	1.640–5.064	<0.001
	eGFR ≥90 (mL/min/1.73m²)	Ref.	Ref.	Ref.		Ref.	Ref.	Ref.	
	60–90	15.181	3.523	1.870–6.639	<0.001	1.306	1.518	0.742–3.107	0.253
	30–60	58.847	11.161	6.026–20.672	<0.001	13.687	3.940	1.906–8.147	<0.001
	15–30	111.663	34.982	18.092–67.639	<0.001	18.046	6.246	2.682–14.542	<0.001
	<15	118.059	46.326	23.192–92.536	<0.001	23.710	9.675	3.881–24.120	<0.001
	WHO grade I–III	Ref.	Ref.	Ref.		Ref.	Ref.	Ref.	
	IV	83.574	4.433	3.222–6.101	<0.001	7.818	1.847	1.201–2.840	0.005
	V	231.786	11.790	8.581–16.197	<0.001	38.291	4.625	2.847–7.511	<0.001
	SBP ≥140 mmHg	62.387	2.543	2.017–3.206	<0.001	7.136	1.578	1.129–2.206	0.008

Multivariate time-dependent cox regression analysis for patient-death was included age, sex, clinical manifestations of edema/gross hematuria, co-morbidities of hypertension/cancer, BMI, GFR, anemia, albumin <3.5g/dL, SBP ≥140 mmHg, DBP ≥90 mmHg, proteinuria ≥1 g/day, and pathologic change of global sclerosis, presence of crescent, interstitial inflammation and tubular atrophy/interstitial fibrosis. Sex and global sclerosis did not meet proportional hazards assumption for Cox model. Global sclerosis interacted with GFR and interstitial inflammatory cell infiltration. BMI interacted with age. Therefore such interactions were considered in this model.
Multivariate time-dependent cox regression analysis for renal-death was included age, sex, clinical manifestations of edema/gross hematuria, co-morbidities of diabetes/hypertension/cancer, GFR, anemia, albumin <3.5g/dL, SBP ≥140 mmHg, DBP ≥90 mmHg, proteinuria ≥1 g/day, pathologic change of segmental sclerosis, and treatment history with statin and renin-angiotensin system blockades. Sex and age were considered changes of proportional hazard according to time progression. Global sclerosis and other tubulointerstitial changes were excluded in the final model because of severe interaction with GFR.
Abbreviations: SBP, systolic blood pressure; ESRD, end-stage renal disease; eGFR, estimated glomerular filtration rate; HR, Hazard ratio; CI, confidence interval.

$P = 0.004$) compared to the rest. However, other clinical factors were not different between the 2 groups). Table 4 summarizes the causes of death. The causes of death in the patients who died before advancing to ESRD progression were malignancies (12 patients, 30.8%), cardiovascular diseases (5 patients, 12.8%), and infection (6 patients, 15.8%). Death from ESRD and dialysis-related complications occurred in only 2 patients. In contrast, the deaths after ESRD progression were caused by renal disease (11 patients, 35.5%), and cardiovascular disease (5 patients, 16.1%), with only one case of cancer mortality.

As expected, ESRD progression was a significant predictor of mortality (hazard ratio, 2.593; 95% CI, 1.609–4.177; P <0.001). After ESRD progression, 25.3% patients received renal transplantation. Among the patients who received transplantation, only

3 patients died, 1 from infection and the other 2 after allograft failure and resumption of dialysis. All of them were dead by 12 years after ESRD progression. As a result, although the 10-year survival rate after ESRD was higher in all ESRD patients including transplantation recipients, than in those excluding transplantation recipients, the 20-year survival rate of ESRD was similar in both groups at about 65% (Figure 3).

Thirteen patients who were managed by immunosuppressive agents had died. Among them, 5 patients died from infection and two patients died from malignancy. Three patients whose cause of death was infection had underlying cancer (Table 5). There was no relationship between the cumulative dose of immunosuppressive agents and any death or infection-associated death (data was not shown).

Table 4. Causes of death.

Causes of death (N)	Death before ESRD (n = 39)	Death after ESRD (n = 31)	Total
Renal disease	2	11	13
Cardiovascular disease	5	5	10
Cancer	12	1	13
Infection	6	4	10
Traffic accident or injury	3	1	4
Miscellaneous	2	3	5
Unknown	9	6	15

Abbreviations: ESRD, end-stage renal diseas.

Standardized mortality ratio in IgAN

Table 6 summarizes the overall and sex-specific SMR results. The overall relative mortality rate of IgAN patients was significantly higher by 43% than that of age/sex-matched GP (SMR, 1.43; 95% CI, 1.04–1.92). Interestingly, the mortality rate was different according to subgroups. An excess mortality rate was found in women (SMR, 2.17; 95% CI, 1.21–3.57), but not in men (SMR, 1.22; 95% CI, 0.82–1.75) with IgAN. Moreover, patients with lower eGFR (<60 ml/min per1.73m^2; SMR, 1.70; 95% CI, 1.13–2.46), higher proteinuria (≥1 g/day; SMR, 1.66; 95% CI, 1.16–2.29), or higher SBP (≥140 mmHg; SMR, 1.88; 95% CI, 1.19–2.82) had an elevated mortality rate compared with their age/sex-matched GP, whereas patients without such risk factors had a similar mortality rate.

When the SMR was further classified by the simplified risk stratification, IgAN patients in the low-risk group had a similar mortality rate to the GP. In the intermediate-risk group, IgAN patients' mortality appeared higher than that in the GP, although insignificant. However, in the high-risk group, IgAN patients' mortality was significantly higher than that in the GP. Interest-

ingly, this relationship was different according to sex. Thus, risk stratification did not have any influence on the SMR in men, but SMR in women was affected significantly (Figure 4).

Discussion

Until recently, investigations on IgAN have focused on renal prognosis because it is the most common primary glomerulonephritis and a significant contributor to the development of ESRD, despite the slow rate of progression [1,20]. However, there has been no information about death, which is more definitive outcome than ESRD. In this investigation, we demonstrated that the 30-year mortality of IgAN patients was 82.7%. Moreover, we showed that mortality of IgAN patients was higher than that of the age/sex-matched GP by 43%. To the best of our knowledge, this is the first study to investigate patient survival and its predictive factors as distinguished from renal survival in IgAN patients.

The most notable finding in our survival analyses is that although the overall relative mortality of IgAN, expressed by SMR, was shown to be higher than that of the GP, the absolute mortality rate was not very high when considering the significant renal progression to ESRD. More than half of the deaths occurred even before ESRD progression and the most common cause of death was malignancy. In particular, the patients who survived and progressed to ESRD had a better survival rate than the general dialysis patients did. According to the Korean ESRD registry, the 10-year survival rate of the overall dialysis patients was about 45%, and the 10-year survival rate of the non-diabetic dialysis patients within this group was 58.5% [21]. In the 2011 US Renal Data System data, survival over the first 5 years of therapy was only 45% in the patients with glomerulonephritis [22]. Compared with the above data, the ESRD patients with IgAN in this investigation have a favorable survival rate. The relatively young age of the ESRD population in this study may have explained the favorable survival. In this study, the mean age of the 277 patients who progressed to ESRD was 45 years, which was lower than the mean age (52.1 years) of the 5,550 glomerulonephritis-induced ESRD patients in the Korean ESRD registry [21].

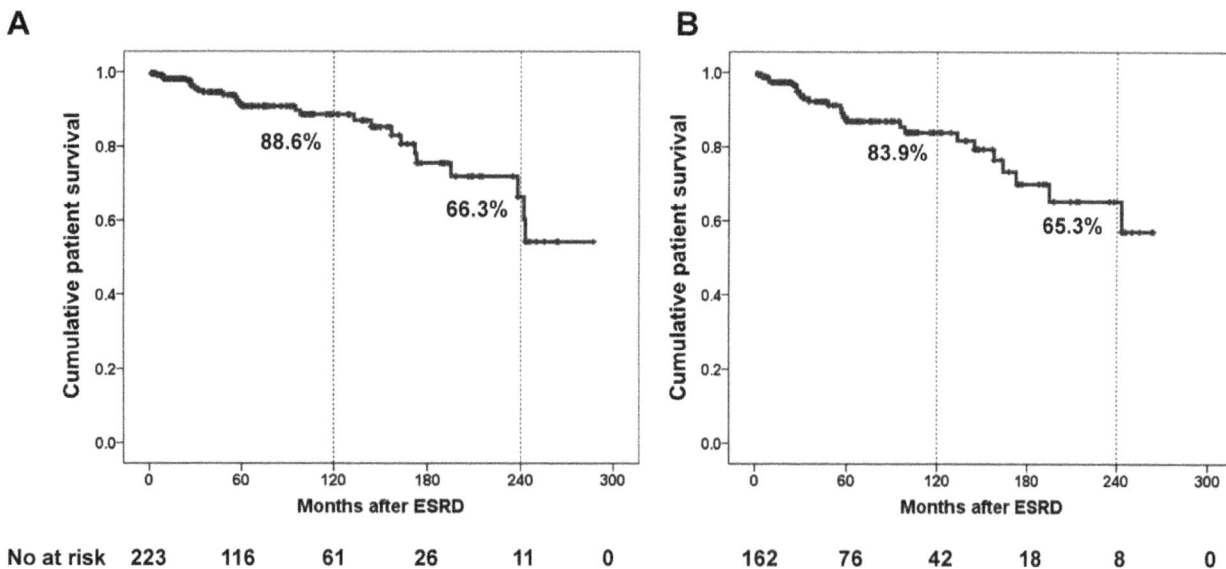

Figure 3. Cumulative patient survival after ESRD progression according to the all ESRD patients (A) and excluding transplantation recipients (B). The primary outcome is patient survival. The numbers of patients remaining at 60, 120, 180, 240, 300, and 360 months of follow-up are shown at the bottom. ESRD, end stage renal disease.

Table 5. Causes of death according to use of immunosuppressive agents.

	Steroid IV	Steroid PO	Cyclophosphamide	Calcineurin inhibitor	Mycophenolate
No of prescription	25	130	36	9	9
Cumulative dose	1187(450–2437)	3115(1519–4308)	6487(4087–10050)	1833	107000
Duration	3(1.8–6.0)	122(75–168)	80(48–123)	107	111
No of death	3	12	6	2	1
Cause of death					
Renal disease	0	0	1	0	0
Cardiovascular disease	0	1	1	0	0
Cancer	0	2	0	0	0
Infection	2	5	2	2	1
Unknown	1	4	2	0	0

Abbreviations: IV, intravenous; PO per oral;

With regard to transplantation, this may have contributed to the improved survival in the ESRD patients with IgAN for 10-year survival rate, but not the 20-year survival rate. To clarify the precise mechanisms of the fair survival rate for IgAN patients with ESRD, further well-designed investigations are needed.

Interestingly, the survival patterns differed according to the sex, renal function, proteinuria and blood pressure. Patients who were male, with preserved renal function, normotension, and proteinuria <1 g/day had a similar mortality rate compared with the GP, whereas female patients, or patients with renal dysfunction, higher blood pressure and proteinuria ≥1 g/day had significantly higher

mortality, compared with the GP. The results for the 3 subgroups (renal dysfunction, higher blood pressure, and proteinuria ≥1 g/day) were similar, although the difference according to sex was unexpected result. In the regression analysis, a sex difference was not detected even in the univariate analysis. However, men showed a comparable survival rate, whereas women tended to have a higher mortality rate compared with the age-matched Korean GP, although the actual number of patients who died was higher in men. On average, men had a 20% higher death rate than did women. The difference was increased up to 3-fold in their 40s and 50s compared with Korean GP (http://kostat.go.kr). This difference

Table 6. Standardized mortality ratios (SMRs) in overall and subpopulation of IgAN patients.

		N	Initial age	Final age	Person-year	Observed	Expected	SMR(95% CI)
Overall		1009	36.8±13.7	45.0±14.0	8134.2	44	30.7	1.43(1.04–1.92)
eGFR	≥60	606	32.9±12.2	41.3±13.2	5077.4	15	13.8	1.08(0.61–1.79)
	<60	374	43.4±13.6	50.9±13.2	2825.6	28	16.5	1.70(1.13–2.46)
Proteinuria	<1 g/day	341	33.8±13.1	41.0±13.3	2445.5	6	6.2	0.97(0.36–2.12)
	≥1 g/day	572	39.1±13.7	47.7±13.7	4941.5	36	21.7	1.66(1.16–2.29)
SBP	<140	768	35.2±13.1	42.8±13.4	5911.3	18	18.3	0.98(0.58–1.56)
	≥140	230	42.2±14.1	51.4±13.9	2125.2	23	12.3	1.88(1.19–2.82)
Men		495	36.1±14.7	45.0±15.0	4403.6	29	23.8	1.22(0.82–1.75)
eGFR	≥60	309	31.6±12.9	40.7±13.6	2827.9	10	10.2	0.98(0.47–1.81)
	<60	173	44.6±14.0	53.1±13.5	1482.8	18	13.4	1.34(0.80–2.13)
Proteinuria	<1 g/day	143	31.5±13.7	40.1±14.0	1225.5	3	1.9	1.57(0.32–4.58)
	≥1 g/day	307	38.7±14.4	47.8±14.3	2791.7	12	4.6	2.60(1.35–4.55)
SBP	<140	356	34.4±14.3	43.0±14.5	3092.0	12	14.1	0.85(0.44–1.49)
	≥140	135	40.6±14.9	50.2±14.6	1299.1	15	9.7	1.55(0.87–2.56)
Women		514	37.5±12.6	45.0±13.0	3730.6	15	6.9	2.17(1.21–3.57)
eGFR	≥60	297	34.4±11.3	41.9±12.7	2249.5	5	3.7	1.36(0.44–3.18)
	<60	201	42.4±13.2	49.0±12.8	1342.8	10	3.1	3.24(1.55–5.95)
Proteinuria	<1 g/day	198	35.5±12.4	41.6±2.9	1220.0	3	4.2	0.71(0.15–2.07)
	≥1 g/day	265	39.4±12.7	47.5±13.0	2149.8	24	17.1	1.40(0.90–2.08)
SBP	<140	412	35.9±12.0	42.7±12.4	2819.3	6	4.2	1.43(0.53–3.12)
	≥140	95	44.5±12.5	53.1±12.7	826.1	8	2.6	3.09(1.34–6.10)

Abbreviations: SMR, standardized mortality ratio; CI, confidence interval; eGFR, estimated glomerular filtration rate; SBP, systolic blood pressure.

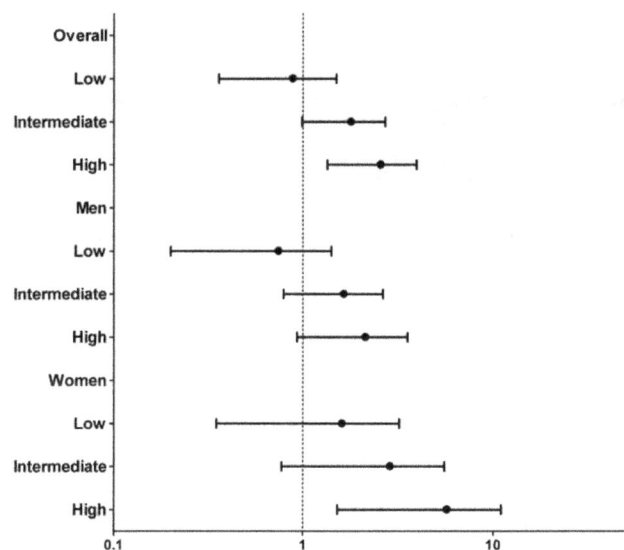

Figure 4. Standardized mortality ratio (SMR) according to risk stratification. The x-axis represents SMR with 95% confidence interval in log scale. The y-axis represents overall and gender subgroup of IgAN patients.

may cause the discordance between the relative and absolute mortality in IgAN patients. The precise mechanisms of the sex difference in relative mortality remain to be defined.

The survival pattern of IgAN patients described in this analysis suggests the need for some changes in clinical practice. Despite the high prevalence of IgAN, adequate and specific treatment intervention in the early stage of IgAN remains controversial. Therefore, both clinicians and patients tend to hesitate before following an active therapeutic approach to individual IgAN patients, even at high risk for progression. However, the decreased age at diagnosis, reduced cardiovascular risk factors and increased average life expectancies have allowed more IgAN patients to live with ESRD state for a relatively longer duration, compared with other causes of ESRD including diabetes. ESRD treatment clearly presents a considerable burden to both society and the patients [22]. The cost per person-year of ESRD was the highest and that of transplantation was the fourth highest among the 500 common

disease categories in Korea. Moreover, expenditure per person-year for ESRD has increased continuously up to US$12,639 per patient per year in 2010 (http://www.nhic.or.kr). Thus, the fair survival rate of IgAN patients also implies a substantial social cost for ESRD. Therefore, optimal treatment guidelines, including both active and supportive care need to be developed for IgAN patients according to their renal risk stratification in order to reduce renal progression.

While the present study suggested some novel findings, there are several limitations. First, this investigation was a retrospective observational study in a single center. During the long follow-up period, the general medical status and/or treatment strategy of the patients changed over time. However, we could not reflect such changes, and only took initial medical treatments into account. For this reason, the incompleteness of the data and the possibility of residual confounding cannot be excluded. For example, information about patients who received tonsillectomy was not available in our analyses. A validation study in an external cohort or a prospective multicenter study may be necessary to overcome our study limitations. The inability to elucidate reproducibility in pathological diagnosis is another weak point of our investigation.

In conclusion, we have demonstrated that the absolute 30-year survival of IgAN was 82.7%. Moreover, the relative mortality was higher than that of the age/sex-matched GP by 43%. Especially, relative mortality was higher in a subgroup with well-known renal risk factors and in women. However, patients without renal risk factors survived similarly to the GP. Considering the socioeconomic burdens of ESRD, more meticulous and active management to mitigate renal progression is warranted in IgAN patients.

Acknowledgments

We thank Ji-Soo Yang for her strenuous assistance for these extensive data collection and analyses. The authors are grateful to the cooperation of the Medical Research Collaborating Center in Seoul National University Hospital, without which this study could not have been completed.

Author Contributions

Conceived and designed the experiments: HL HJC. Analyzed the data: YSK DWC. Wrote the paper: HL HJC. Supervised this project: HJC. Gave conceptual advice and commented on the manuscript: YSK SK. Assembled input data: DKK KHO. Performed statistical analyses: KWJ.

References

1. Donadio JV, Grande JP (2002) IgA nephropathy. N Engl J Med 347: 738–748.
2. Chang JH, Kim DK, Kim HW, Park SY, Yoo TH, et al. (2009) Changing prevalence of glomerular diseases in Korean adults: a review of 20 years of experience. Nephrol Dial Transplant 24: 2406–2410.
3. Radford MG, Donadio JV, Bergstralh EJ, Grande JP (1997) Predicting renal outcome in IgA nephropathy. J Am Soc Nephrol 8: 199–207.
4. Bartosik LP, Lajoie G, Sugar L, Cattran DC (2001) Predicting progression in IgA nephropathy. Am J Kidney Dis 38: 728–735.
5. Beukhof JR, Kardaun O, Schaafsma W, Poortema K, Donker AJ, et al. (1986) Toward individual prognosis of IgA nephropathy. Kidney Int 29: 549–556.
6. Alamartine E, Sabatier JC, Guerin C, Berliet JM, Berthoux F (1991) Prognostic factors in mesangial IgA glomerulonephritis: an extensive study with univariate and multivariate analyses. Am J Kidney Dis 18: 12–19.
7. Le W, Liang S, Hu Y, Deng K, Bao H, et al. (2011) Long-term renal survival and related risk factors in patients with IgA nephropathy: results from a cohort of 1155 cases in a Chinese adult population. Nephrol Dial Transplant 27: 1479–1485.
8. Berthoux F, Mohey H, Laurent B, Mariat C, Afiani A, et al. (2011) Predicting the risk for dialysis or death in IgA nephropathy. J Am Soc Nephrol 22: 752–761.
9. Xie J, Kiryluk K, Wang W, Wang Z, Guo S, et al. (2012) Predicting Progression of IgA Nephropathy: New Clinical Progression Risk Score. PLoS ONE 7: e38904.
10. Shi SF, Wang SX, Jiang L, Lv JC, Liu LJ, et al. (2011) Pathologic predictors of renal outcome and therapeutic efficacy in IgA nephropathy: validation of the oxford classification. Clin J Am Soc Nephrol 6: 2175–2184.
11. Kang SH, Choi SR, Park HS, Lee JY, Sun IO, et al. (2011) The Oxford classification as a predictor of prognosis in patients with IgA nephropathy. Nephrol Dial Transplant 27: 252–258.
12. Walsh M, Sar A, Lee D, Yilmaz S, Benediktsson H, et al. (2010) Histopathologic features aid in predicting risk for progression of IgA nephropathy. Clin J Am Soc Nephrol 5: 425–430.
13. Tsuboi N, Kawamura T, Koike K, Okonogi H, Hirano K, et al. (2010) Glomerular density in renal biopsy specimens predicts the long-term prognosis of IgA nephropathy. Clin J Am Soc Nephrol 5: 39–44.
14. Frimat L, Briancon S, Hestin D, Aymard B, Renoult E, et al. (1997) IgA nephropathy: prognostic classification of end-stage renal failure. L'Association des Nephrologues de l'Est. Nephrol Dial Transplant 12: 2569–2575.
15. Kim JK, Kim JH, Lee SC, Kang EW, Chang TI, et al. (2012) Clinical Features and Outcomes of IgA Nephropathy with Nephrotic Syndrome. Clin J Am Soc Nephrol 7: 427–436.
16. Bjorneklett R, Vikse BE, Bostad L, Leivestad T, Iversen BM (2011) Long-term risk of ESRD in IgAN; validation of Japanese prognostic model in a Norwegian cohort. Nephrol Dial Transplant 27: 1485–1491.
17. Myllymki JM, Honkanen TT, Syrjnen JT, Helin HJ, Rantala IS, et al. (2007) Severity of tubulointerstitial inflammation and prognosis in immunoglobulin A nephropathy. Kidney Int 71: 343–348.

16

Mechanisms of Endothelial Dysfunction in Resistance Arteries from Patients with End-Stage Renal Disease

Leanid Luksha[1], Peter Stenvinkel[2], Folke Hammarqvist[3], Juan Jesús Carrero[2], Sandra T. Davidge[4], Karolina Kublickiene[1]*

1 Division of Obstetrics & Gynecology, Karolinska Institutet, Karolinska University Hospital, Department of Clinical Science, Intervention & Technology, Stockholm, Sweden, 2 Division of Renal Medicine, Karolinska Institutet, Karolinska University Hospital, Department of Clinical Science, Intervention & Technology, Stockholm, Sweden, 3 Division of Surgery, Karolinska Institutet, Karolinska University Hospital, Department of Clinical Science, Intervention & Technology, Stockholm, Sweden, 4 Department of Obstetrics and Gynecology, University of Alberta, Edmonton, Alberta, Canada

Abstract

The study focuses on the mechanisms of endothelial dysfunction in the uremic milieu. Subcutaneous resistance arteries from 35 end-stage renal disease (ESRD) patients and 28 matched controls were studied *ex-vivo*. Basal and receptor-dependent effects of endothelium-derived factors, expression of endothelial NO synthase (eNOS), prerequisites for myoendothelial gap junctions (MEGJ), and associations between endothelium-dependent responses and plasma levels of endothelial dysfunction markers were assessed. The contribution of endothelium-derived hyperpolarizing factor (EDHF) to endothelium-dependent relaxation was impaired in uremic arteries after stimulation with bradykinin, but not acetylcholine, reflecting the agonist-specific differences. Diminished vasodilator influences of the endothelium on basal tone and enhanced plasma levels of asymmetrical dimethyl L-arginine (ADMA) suggest impairment in NO-mediated regulation of uremic arteries. eNOS expression and contribution of MEGJs to EDHF type responses were unaltered. Plasma levels of ADMA were negatively associated with endothelium-dependent responses in uremic arteries. Preserved responses of smooth muscle to pinacidil and NO-donor indicate alterations within the endothelium and tolerance of vasodilator mechanisms to the uremic retention products at the level of smooth muscle. We conclude that both EDHF and NO pathways that control resistance artery tone are impaired in the uremic milieu. For the first time, we validate the alterations in EDHF type responses linked to kinin receptors in ESRD patients. The association between plasma ADMA concentrations and endothelial function in uremic resistance vasculature may have diagnostic and future therapeutic implications.

Editor: Marcelo G. Bonini, University of Illinois at Chicago, United States of America

Funding: Financial support was provided by grants from the Swedish Society of Medicine, Swedish Heart and Lung Foundation, Center for Gender Medicine at Karolinska Institutet, Loo and Hans Ostermans Foundation, the Swedish Kidney Association and the Karolinska Institute Research Funds. L. Luksha is supported by PostDoc research grants from AFA insurance and Department of Clinical Science, Intervention & Technology (CLINTEC) at Karolinska Institutet, Sweden. S. Davidge is supported by Canadian Institute for Health Research. The funders had no role in study design, data collection and analysis, decision to publish, or preparation of the manuscript.

Competing Interests: The authors have read the journal's policy and have the following conflicts: The study was partly funded by AFA Insurance. This does not alter the authors' adherence to all the PLoS ONE policies on sharing data and materials, as detailed online in the guide for authors.

* E-mail: karolina.kublickiene@ki.se

Introduction

Adverse cardiovascular events are common complications of end-stage renal disease (ESRD) and these patients are more likely to die from cardiovascular disease (CVD) than from kidney failure [1]. Although the underlying mechanisms that predispose ESRD patients to higher risk of CVD are incompletely understood, morphological and functional abnormalities of the endothelium may play an important role [2]. Endothelial dysfunction is considered an early marker of CVD [3], which facilitates the progress of atherosclerosis [4] and contributes to the development of hypertension through the enhancement of vascular resistance [5]. Thus, studies aimed to at investigating the mechanisms of endothelial dysfunction in ESRD are of importance and may provide a means to ameliorate cardiovascular complications and introduce novel treatment strategies.

Our current knowledge of endothelial dysfunction in ESRD is mainly based on findings from animal models [6], circulating plasma markers [7] and *in-vivo* assessments in the human forearm [8]. Although few attempts have been made to estimate endothelial function in resistance arteries of ESRD patients [9–11], the mechanisms of endothelial dysfunction need further clarification. NO deficiency has been considered as a principal event leading to endothelial dysfunction in the uremic milieu [12]. However, the contribution of NO to endothelium-dependent control of vascular tone is inversely associated with caliber of arteries. Another vasodilator, known as endothelium-derived hyperpolarizing factor (EDHF), seems to act as a predominant mediator of endothelium-dependent dilatation in resistance-size arteries. EDHF type responses are characterized by endothelium-dependent hyperpolarization that occurs due to direct electrical coupling via myoendothelial gap junctions (MEGJs) and/or the release of different mediators [13]. The role of EDHF in endothelial maintenance has been introduced as a back-up mechanism during NO deficiency. However when deprivation of EDHF occurs, this may further aggravate endothelial dysfunction leading to enhanced blood pressure and impaired blood flow to target organs [13].

Studies concerning the detailed mechanisms of endothelial dysfunction in resistance arteries with a focus on the relative contribution of NO and EDHF in ESRD are scarce. Current data on the contribution of EDHF to endothelium-dependent relaxation of resistance arteries in kidney failure are mainly based on animal studies and characterized by explicit heterogeneity [6,14–18]. To the best of our knowledge, the only study that has investigated the relative contribution of EDHF *vs.* NO to acetylcholine (ACh)-induced-relaxation in ESRD patients has reported an impairment in NO-mediated responses but an unchanged, or even increased, role of EDHF as assessed by forearm blood flow [19].

In this study, we hypothesized that endothelial dysfunction in resistance arteries of incident dialysis patients is not only restricted to impairment in production and/or bioavailability of NO, but EDHF type responses may also be affected by uremic milieu. To test this hypothesis we isolated arteries from subcutaneous fat to segregate pharmacologically the relative impairments in NO and EDHF type responses that confer endothelial dysfunction in ESRD. Targeted pathways of endothelial dysfunction were assessed using basal and receptor-dependent stimulation of endothelium-derived vasodilators, expression of endothelial NO synthase (eNOS), prerequisites for MEGJ, and associations between endothelium-dependent responses and plasma levels of endothelial dysfunction surrogate markers.

Results

Participants

Age, gender, and smoking status were similar between the groups. The body mass index was lower in ESRD patients *vs.* controls. Plasma levels of asymmetrical dimethyl L-arginine (ADMA), soluble vascular cell adhesion molecule-1 (sVCAM-1), interleukin-6, pentraxin-3, high sensitivity C-reactive protein (hsCRP) and lipoprotein(a) and triglycerides were elevated in ESRD. No differences in blood pressure or total cholesterol were observed between the groups (Table 1).

Vascular function

In total, 84 subcutaneous arteries with internal diameter of 209±6 μm were dissected from 35 ESRD patients and 71 arteries with internal diameter of 224±7 μm were dissected from 28 controls (P>0.05). There was no difference in the magnitude of pre-constriction 3 μmol/L norepinephrine between the groups (2.5±0.2 mN/mm² ESRD *vs.* 2.7±0.2 mN/mm² controls).

Endothelium-dependent relaxation

In controls, ACh and bradykinin (BK) caused relaxation of arteries with similar magnitude (Figure 1). However, arteries were more sensitive to BK *vs.* ACh (pEC$_{50}$, here and in the following text: BK 7.9±0.1 *vs.* ACh 7.7±0.1, P=0.01). NOS/cyclooxygenase (COX) inhibition reduced endothelium-dependent relaxation (Figure 1) and the sensitivity to agonists became similar (ACh: 7.2±0.1 *vs.* BK: 7.3±0.1, P=0.5).

Relaxation and sensitivity to both agonists was attenuated in ESRD *vs.* controls (Figure 1). In contrast to the controls, the sensitivities of ESRD arteries in PSS were similar between the agonists (ACh: 7.3±0.1 vs. BK: 7.4±0.1, P=0.2).

After NOS/COX inhibition relaxation and sensitivity to ACh and BK were attenuated in ESRD (Figure 1). The concentration-response curves after NOS/COX inhibition were shifted to the

right in ESRD *vs.* controls (Figure 1). However, the maximal EDHF type relaxation was reduced in ESRD *vs.* controls in response to BK but not to ACh (BK: P=0.003; ACh: P=0.09). Moreover, the relative contribution of EDHF was reduced in ESRD *vs.* controls in response to BK but not to ACh (Figure 2).

An inhibitor of gap junctions (18-α-glycyrrhetinic acid, 18-αGA) markedly reduced EDHF type relaxation in response to both agonists (Figure 1). There was no difference in residual relaxation after incubation with 18-αGA along with NOS inhibitor, N^ω-nitro-L-arginine-methyl ester (L-NAME) and COX inhibitor, indomethacin (Indo) between ESRD *vs.* controls (Figure 1). The relative contribution of MEGJs to EDHF type responses was similar between ESRD and controls independently of the agonist used (ACh, 1 μmol/l: 86±4 ESRD (n=16) *vs.* 80±6 controls (n=12), P=0.7; BK, 1 μmol/l: 85±5 ESRD (n=13) *vs.* 87±3 controls (n=8), P=0.9).

In order to eliminate the possible interference of co-morbidities, the responses to agonists before and after NOS/COX inhibition in ESRD patients without diabetes mellitus (DM) and CVD were compared with those of controls. In response to BK we observed similar results as above (Figure 1B). In contrast to the whole ESRD group, in arteries from ESRD without DM and CVD, ACh-induced relaxation was reduced in PSS as compared to controls but similar after NOS/COX inhibition (ACh after NOS/COX inhibition: 7±0.1 ESRD without DM and CVD (n=18) *vs.* 7.2±0.1 controls (n=23), P=0.1).

Table 1. Baseline characteristics of ESRD patients and controls.

Parameters	ESRD (n=35)	Controls (n=28)
Age (years)	57±13	54±14
Males n (%)	24 (69)	21 (75)
Body mass index (kg/m²)	24.1±3.3*	27.6±3.7
Systolic blood pressure (mmHg)	144±21	138±17
Diastolic blood pressure (mmHg)	86±11	84±11
Total cholesterol (mmol/L)	4.6±1.2*	5.1±1.0
Triglycerides (mmol/L)	1.6* (0.8–5.7)	1.3 (0.7–19)
Lipoprotein(a) (mg/L)	409 (50–2572)*	156 (50–802)
S-albumin (g/L)	34.9±3.4*	38.4±3.4
S-Creatinine (μmol/L)	620 (249–1069)*	78 (55–100)
Interleukin-6 (pg/ml)	5.0 (1.9–16.8)*	1.5 (0.4–17.1)
hsC-reactive protein (mg/L)	1.9 (0.2–24.9)*	1.4 (0.4–13.9)
Pentraxin-3 (ng/ml)	1.2 (0.5–8.3)*	0.6 (0.1–2.3)
Fibrinogen (g/L)	4.8±1.3*	3.2±1.3
Glomerular filtration rate (ml/min)	12±3*	89±3
Asymmetric Dimethylarginine (μmol/L)	0.6±0.1*	0.5±0.1
Soluble VCAM-1 (ng/ml)	1295 (637–1980)*	588 (368–830)
Soluble ICAM-1 (ng/ml)	223 (138–404)	231 (161–363)
Diabetes mellitus n, (%)	10 (29)	0
CVD, n, (%)	13 (37)	0
Antihypertensive treatment, n, (%)	33 (94)	0
Statin treatment, n, (%)	15 (43)	0

*, P<0.05.

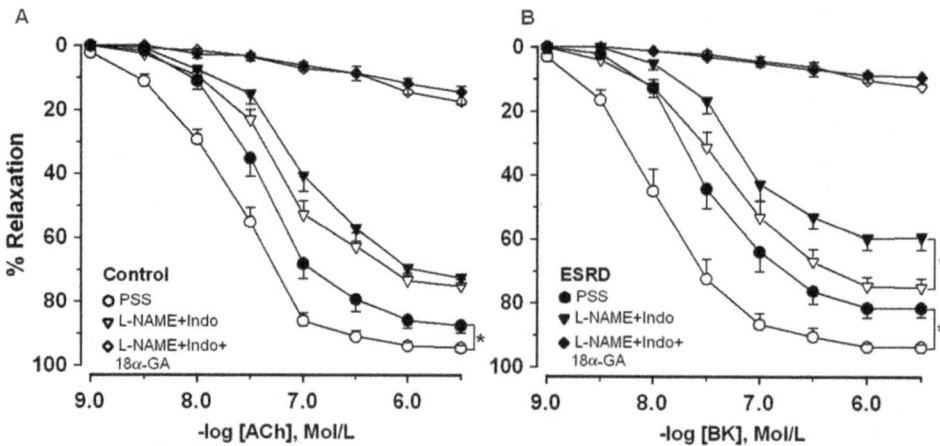

Figure 1. Concentration response curves to acetylcholine (ACh, A) and bradykinin (BK, B). Responses in physiological salt solution (PSS) and after incubation with N^{ω}-nitro-L-arginine methyl ester plus indomethacin alone (L-NAME+Indo) or together with 18α-glycyrrhetinic acid (L-NAME+Indo+18α-GA) in arteries from ESRD patients (n = 32 for ACh and n = 22 for BK) and controls (n = 23 for ACh and n = 17 for BK). * ESRD vs. controls, $P<0.05$.

Transmission electron microscopy (TEM)

Analysis of TEM images focused on morphological prerequisites for the gap junctions between EC and smooth muscle cells (SMC) in arteries from ESRD patients and controls (n = 3). The main criteria for identification of MEGJs was the presence of the characteristic pentalaminar membrane structure at points of cell to cell contact, where the central region had a higher electron opacity than the inner parts and distance between the EC and SMC plasma membranes was around 3.5 nm [20]. TEM images showed the presence of long protrusions (up to 4.5 μm) from both ECs (Figure 3A) and SMCs (Figure 3B) penetrating the internal elastic lamina and forming close contacts with each other (Figure 3C and 3D). Although the observed EC-SMC contacts did not fulfill all criteria for the characteristic pentalaminar structures, they could be considered as prerequisites for MEGJs.

Endothelium-independent relaxation

Endothelium-independent relaxation to NO donor sodium nitroprusside (SNP) was similar between the groups (pEC$_{50}$:

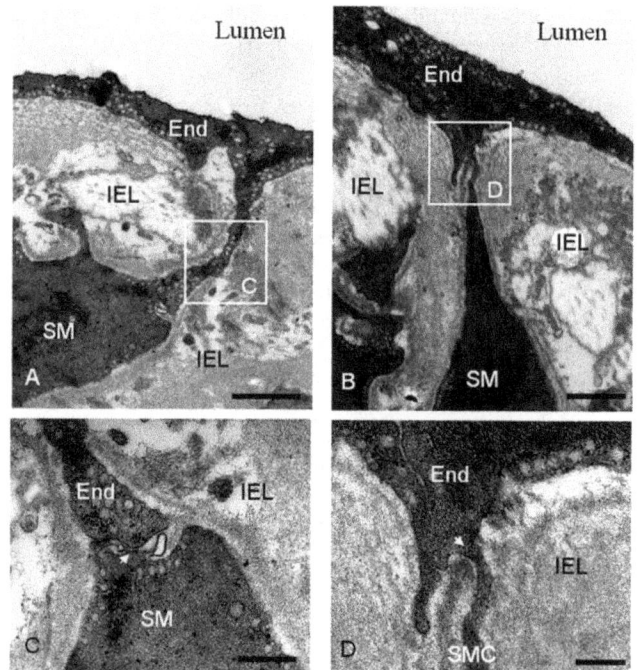

Figure 3. Transmission electron images of arteries from ESRD patients. The lower magnification pictures (A,B) show an overview of the vascular wall with endothelium (End) and smooth muscle (SM) being separated by the internal elastic lamina (IEL). The areas denoted by the boxes are magnified and show the sites of intercellular contacts that could be considered as prerequisites of myoendothelial gap junctions (C, D). The width of the gap is ~20 nm (C, arrow), ~11 nm (D, arrow). Bar: (A) 2 μm; (B) 3 μm; (C) 0.1 μm; (D) 0,2 μm.

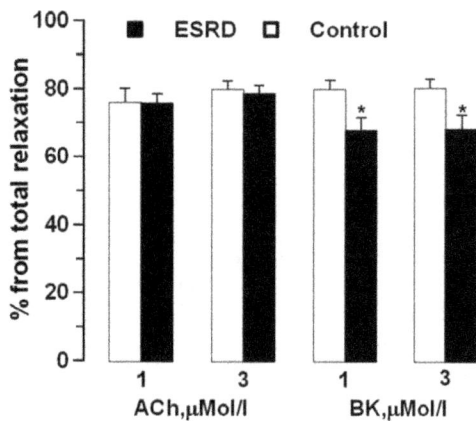

Figure 2. The relative contribution of endothelium-derived hyperpolarizing factor (EDHF). Contribution of EDHF in arteries from ESRD patients and controls in response to acetylcholine (ACh) and bradykinin (BK). * ESRD vs. controls, $P<0.05$.

6.0±0.1 ESRD (n = 17) vs. 6.2±0.2 controls (n = 13), $P = 0.6$). In ESRD patients pinacidil-induced responses were blunted as compared to controls (6.1±0.1 ESRD vs 5.7±0.1 controls, $P = 0.01$, Figure 4). NOS/COX inhibition attenuated the response in controls but not in ESRD (6.1±0.1 PSS vs 5.8±0.1 L-

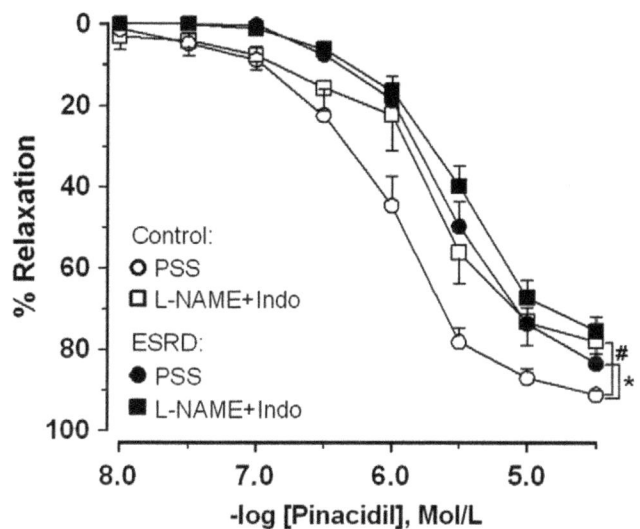

Figure 4. Concentration response curves to pinacidil. Responses in arteries from ESRD patients (n = 10) and controls (n = 7) in physiological salt solution (PSS) and after incubation with N^{ω}-nitro-L-arginine methyl ester plus indomethacin (L-NAME+Indo). * ESRD vs. controls, $P<0.05$; # before vs. after incubation with L-NAME+Indo, $P<0.05$.

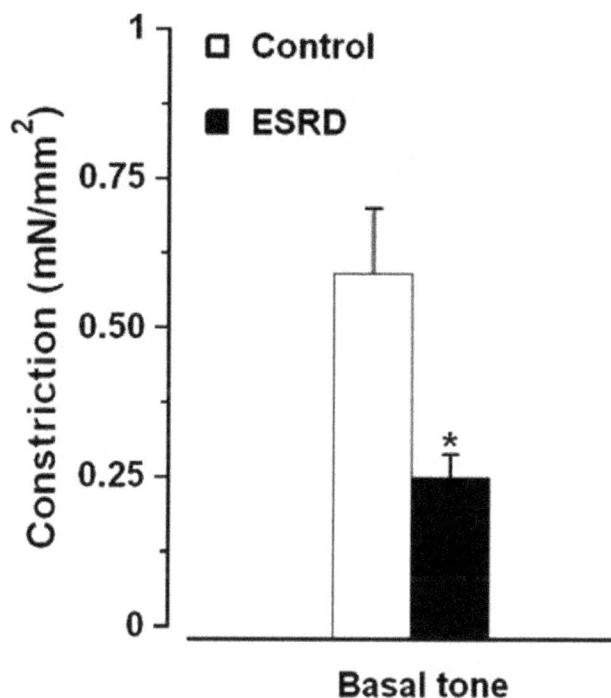

Figure 5. Contractile response to NOS/COX inhibitors of arteries from controls (n = 26) vs. ESRD patients with (n = 32). *, $P<0.05$ ESRD vs. controls.

Name+Indo, $P=0.03$ controls; 5.7 ± 0.1 vs 5.6 ± 0.1, $P=0.3$ ESRD, respectively, Figure 4). There was no difference between ESRD and controls in their responses to pinacidil after NOS/COX inhibition (Figure 4).

Influence of the endothelium-derived factors on basal tone and expression of eNOS

NOS/COX inhibitors induced constriction of arteries from both ESRD and control groups. This constriction was reduced in ESRD vs. controls (Figure 5). Exclusion of the patients with DM and CVD from ESRD group did not change the outcome (Figure 5; 0.28 ± 0.1 mN/mm^2 ESRD without DM and CVD (n = 17) vs. 0.59 ± 0.1 mN/mm^2 controls (n = 26), $P=0.02$). There was no difference in eNOS expression in ESRD vs. controls (Figure 6).

Associations between endothelium-dependent responses and plasma markers of endothelial dysfunction

The sensitivity of arteries to ACh and BK was negatively associated with plasma levels of ADMA in ESRD (Figure 7A) but not in controls (Figure 7B). There was no association between ADMA and vascular sensitivity to the endothelium-dependent agonists after NOS/COX inhibition in both groups. Similarly, sensitivity to SNP was not associated with ADMA levels (data not shown).

In contrast to the agonists-induced relaxation, constriction in response to NOS/COX inhibition was negatively associated with plasma levels of ADMA in both ESRD and controls (Figure 7C and 7D).

No relation was found between resistance artery function and other surrogate markers of endothelial dysfunction (soluble intercellular adhesion molecule-1 (sICAM-1) and sVCAM-1) in ESRD and controls (data not shown).

Discussion

In this ex-vivo study of human uremic resistance arteries we describe, for the first time, the relative role of endothelium-derived factors, agonist-specific differences and associations between endothelial function and surrogate plasma markers of endothelial dysfunction. We show that reduced EDHF type responses contribute markedly to endothelial dysfunction in ESRD. Impaired EDHF type responses in ESRD were detected with endothelium-dependent agonist BK but not ACh. Thus, we suggest that changes in signal transduction from endothelial receptors towards generation and/or transformation of hyperpolarization to the smooth muscle are differently affected by uremic toxins with a predominant impact on those mediated by kinin receptors. Diminished vasodilator influence of the endothelium on basal tone of SMCs along with enhanced plasma levels of ADMA indicates an impairment in NO-mediated control of arterial tone in ESRD. While the eNOS expression and the contribution of

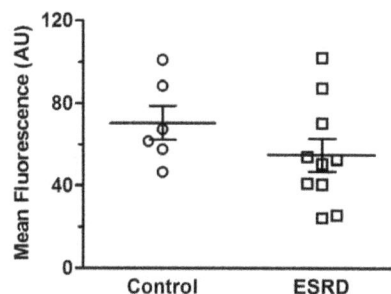

Figure 6. Endothelial nitric oxide synthase (eNOS) expression in arteries from controls (n = 6) and ESRD patients (n = 10).

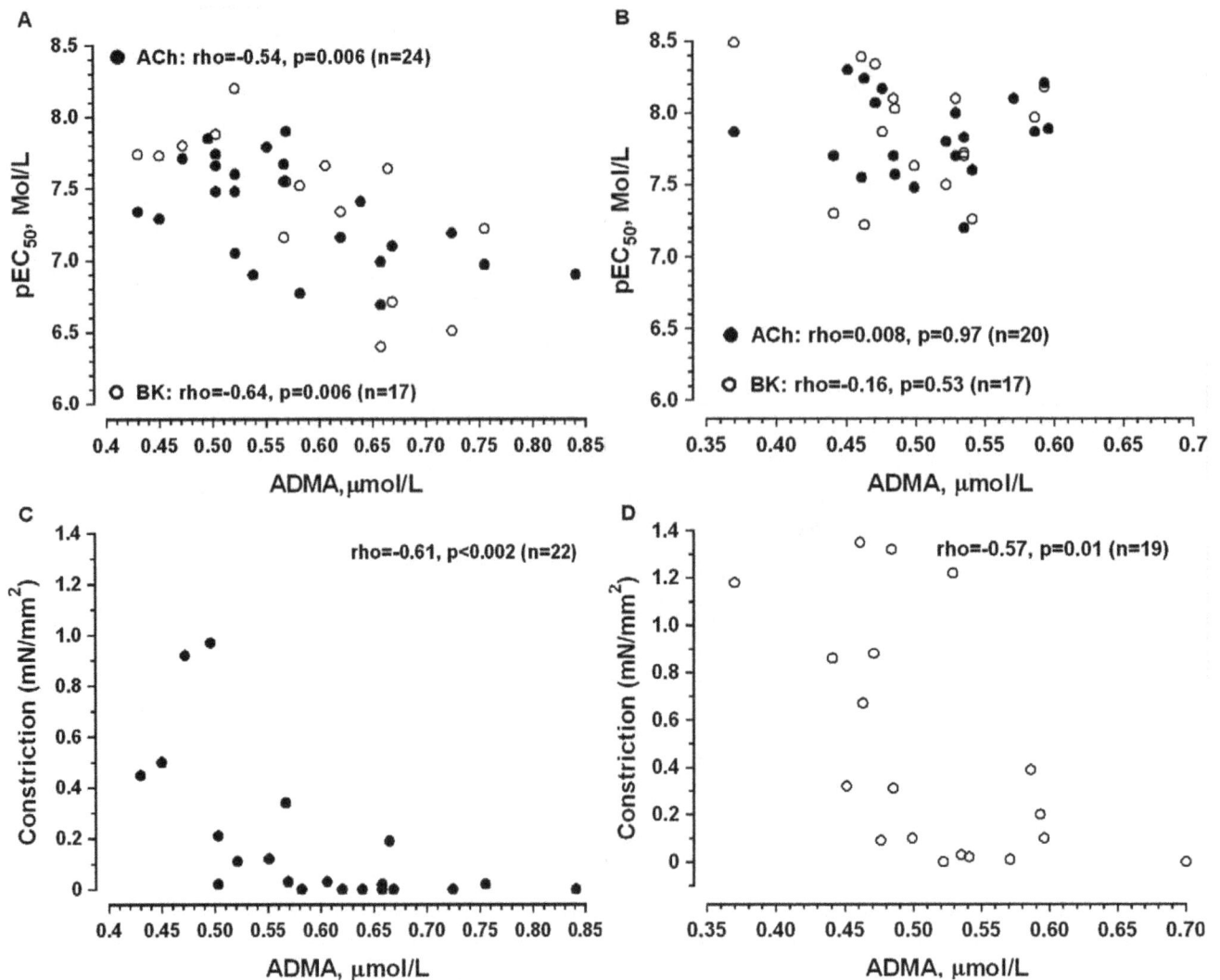

Figure 7. Spearman rank correlation between plasma levels of asymmetrical dimethyl L-arginine (ADMA, μmol/L) and artery sensitivity to endothelium-dependent vasodilators (pEC$_{50}$, A, B) or vasoconstriction in response to NOS/COX inhibition (L-NAME+Indo, C, D) in ESRD patients (A, C) and controls (B, D).

MEGJs to EDHF type responses appeared to be unaltered in uremic arteries, the upstream machinery of both endothelial pathways (i.e. NO and EDHF) were impaired. Since relaxation in response to NO donor or hyperpolarizing agent pinacidil (after NOS/COX inhibition) were similar between the groups, we confirm that the endothelium is the main target of uremic environment, whereas functional capacity of the vascular smooth muscle appeared to be rather tolerant. In accordance with our previous study [11] we corroborate a central role of the uremic milieu in the genesis of endothelial dysfunction. The present study also shows that among measured plasma markers of endothelial dysfunction only ADMA was strongly associated with the magnitude of endothelial dysfunction in uremic resistance arteries. Thus, our findings provide novel insights into the mechanisms of endothelial dysfunction in resistance circulation of ESRD patients.

The pattern of impairment of EDHF type responses after BK but not ACh stimulation in uremic arteries emphasizes the agonist-specific mechanisms of endothelial dysfunction in this toxic milieu. We speculate that conventional and/or disease-specific risk factors may differently affect kinin and muscarinic receptors and/or their

regulatory pathways. For example, endothelial dysfunction in atherosclerosis appears to be receptor-specific, involving the muscarinic receptors with relative sparing of the kinin receptor pathways. Abnormal reactivity of epicardial coronary arteries during physiologic stress is better represented by BK and not by ACh responses [21]. Moreover, differences exist between BK- and ACh- induced relaxation of the mesenteric arteries from spontaneously hypertensive rats at different ages, suggesting a more detrimental effect of increased blood pressure on BK-induced vasorelaxation [22], while selective impairment of endothelium-dependent relaxation to ACh but not BK is observed in isolated small omental arteries from women with preeclampsia [23]. Thus, prior conclusions based only on the vascular effects of one agonist (i.e. ACh) should be considered with caution. In contrast to previous studies, in which only ACh was tested [9–10], our more comprehensive analysis of pathways involved in endothelial dysfunction of resistance arteries in ESRD patients revealed an impairment of EDHF contribution coupled with stimulation of kinin receptors.

In contrast to our findings on heterogeneity of mechanisms of EDHF type responses in preeclampsia [24–25], the present data revealed MEGJs as a common pathway of EDHF in both groups. Hence, the compensatory response for preservation of endothelial function via the flexibility of mechanisms behind EDHF type responses seems to be lacking in ESRD. Since the contribution of EDHF and MEGJ to ACh-induced relaxation was similar between the two experimental groups, it is unlikely that impairment at the level of MEGJs could be linked with kinin receptors. Therefore, it can be speculated that alterations in BK-induced EDHF type responses in uremic resistance arteries may reside in the signaling sequence extending from B_2-kinin receptors to the activation of Ca^{2+}-dependent K^+-channels (K_{ca}-channels) generating hyperpolarization of the endothelium with following transformation to the smooth muscle via MEGJ. Further studies are warranted to clarify the involvement of particular endothelial K_{ca}-channels in alterations of BK-induced EDHF type responses in this patient group.

Despite the fact that EDHF normally does not act through the K_{ATP}-channels [13], pinacidil-induced responses allowed us to assess the general mechanism of relaxation induced by hyperpolarization due to outward K^+ currents at the level of the smooth muscle [26]. Moreover, an animal study of renal failure suggested that alterations in smooth muscle K^+-channels could be involved in reduced endothelium-dependent hyperpolarization [16]. In our study, relaxation to pinacidil was reduced in ESRD vs. controls but this difference disappeared after NOS/COX inhibition, which opposes the findings in the animal study [16]. Most likely basal NO had a potentiating effect on pinacidil-induced relaxation in controls but not in ESRD patients. While in general relaxation induced by K_{ATP}-channels openers has yet been considered endothelium-independent [27], the potentiating effects of endothelium-derived factors has been reported before [25,28].

Impaired endothelial influence on pinacidil-induced responses may further support our data about reduced basal release of endothelium-derived factors in ESRD. Indeed, NOS/COX inhibitors induced smaller constriction in uremic vs. control arteries. As basal vascular tone is to a large extend NO-dependent [29], our data implies a reduction in basal production of NO in ESRD. In contrast, a previous study reported increased basal NO production in the forearm of hemodialysis patients [30]. The inconsistent results may be caused by different methodology, and selection of patients. Recently, we demonstrated the lack of NO contribution to shear stress responses in subcutaneous uremic arteries [11]. In the current study, differences in sensitivity between BK and ACh, depending from NOS/COX inhibition in controls but not in ESRD, indicated on distinct NO contribution to agonist-induced relaxation between the two groups. Moreover, the negative correlation between serum ADMA levels and relaxation to ACh and BK in ESRD but not in controls further supports the impaired contribution of NO to agonists-induced responses in uremia.

Multiple mechanisms may lead to NO deficiency in renal failure [12,31]. A decreased bioavailability of NO due to increased pro-oxidative environment has been suggested [11]. Reduced expression of eNOS has been linked to a decreased NO production in an animal model of kidney failure [32]. Studies on EC cultures have shown that erythrocytes [33] or sera fractions enriched with advanced glycation end products [34] from uremic patients may directly affect expression and activity of eNOS. However, we failed to find any difference in eNOS protein expression between uremic and control arteries. Moreover, an elevated vascular expression but unchanged activity of eNOS was demonstrated in radial arteries of ESRD patients [35]. Neverthe-

less, such observations might indicate that unchanged or even increased expression of eNOS in the vascular wall could not guarantee a sufficient NO bioavailability in ESRD patients. We therefore speculate that endothelial dysfunction along with unchanged expression of eNOS, may represent a potential outcome of a reduced ability of the enzyme to generate NO via eNOS uncoupling with following decrease in NO bioavailability in uremic resistance arteries.

ADMA may serve as a feasible candidate to link the uremic environment with endothelial dysfunction in the resistance vasculature. Indeed, ADMA, as an endogenous inhibitor of eNOS that accumulates when renal function declines [36], it has been shown to induce eNOS uncoupling either via substrate reduction or via direct effect on eNOS catalysis and, as a consequence, eNOS will generate superoxide radicals instead of NO [37]. On the other hand, we cannot exclude the possibility that the effect of ADMA on endothelial superoxide generation may be due to the activation of other enzymatic sources of superoxide radicals such as NADPH oxidases. ADMA may also stimulate renin angiotensin system, and ADMA induced impairement of NO-mediated function due to increased superoxide production has been shown to occur via activation of of Ang II-NADPH oxidase pathway in isolated small vessels from rats [38]. In animal models of experimental diabetic nephropathy, AngII induced activation of NADPH oxidase and eNOS uncoupling serves as the major source of superoxide, and the blockade of AngII signaling ameliorates eNOS uncoupling by increased tetrahydrobiopterin levels with following restoration of NO bioavailability and improved glomerular hemodynamics [39–40].

Although, an association between elevated ADMA levels and endothelium-dependent dilatation in the forearm was previously reported [41], we are the first to show an association between ADMA and endothelium-dependent relaxation in uremic resistance vasculature. The inverse correlation between ADMA and changes in basal tone after NOS/COX inhibition in both experimental groups support in-vivo results demonstrating that ADMA increases vascular resistance in ESRD patients [42] and in healthy humans [43]. Taken together our data endorse the proposal that elevated ADMA may act as a potential mechanism behind the impaired NO-dependent control of uremic resistance artery tone.

On the other hand, adhesion molecules sICAM-1 and sVCAM-1, two purported biomarkers of endothelial dysfunction, did not correlate with changes in basal tone nor with responses to endothelium-dependent agonists. As ADMA is a potentially modifiable risk factor, future interventional studies primarily focusing on acute and long term L-arginine supplementation [44] or regulation of dimethylarginine dimethylaminohydrolase activity that confers the intracellular ADMA concentrations [45] are of interest.

In summary, by studying the mechanisms of endothelial dysfunction in uremic resistance arteries we were able to dissect the impairment in basal and agonist-specific effects of two endothelium-derived vasodilators - EDHF and NO. For the first time, we provided evidence of impaired EDHF type responses particularly linked to kinin receptors in ESRD. The current results support our previous findings that NO plays a critical role in uremic endothelial dysfunction in resistance circulation. The observation that preserved responses of smooth muscle to pinacidil and NO-donor indicated a decisive role of malfunctions within the endothelium and tolerance of vasodilator mechanisms to the uremic retention products at the level of smooth muscle. As this study showed an association between circulating plasma ADMA concentrations and endothelial dysfunction in uremic resistance vasculature, our findings may have diagnostic and future therapeutic implications.

Materials and Methods

Participants

The study was approved by the Ethical Committee at Karolinska University Hospital and conducted according to the principles expressed in the Declaration of Helsinki. All participants involved in the research gave written informed consent prior to enrollment.

Subcutaneous fat biopsies were obtained from 35 ESRD patients at the time of peritoneal dialysis catheter insertion. Only patients starting dialysis treatment were included. Exclusion criteria were acute infection, vasculitis or liver disease at the time of evaluation. Control tissue was obtained from 28 age-matched volunteers without renal, mental or diabetic disease who underwent hernia repair (n = 17) or laparoscopic cholecystectomy (n = 11).

Baseline Laboratory and Clinical Assessments

Clinical history of CVD or DM was obtained from medical records. CVD was defined as the presence of ischemic cardiac disease, peripheral vascular disease and/or cerebrovascular disease. Ongoing medication was collected from medical charts. Glomerular filtration rate was estimated by the mean of creatinine- and urea clearances in ESRD patients, whereas cystatin-C estimated glomerular filtration rate in the controls. Fasting venous blood samples were taken. Plasma and serum were stored at $-70°C$ pending further analyses. Serum interleukin-6 was measured on an Immulite® analyzer (Siemens Medical Solution Diagnostic, Los Angeles, CA, USA). Serum concentrations of albumin, creatinine, lipids and hsCRP were measured routinely. ADMA was assessed in serum by ELISA assays (DLD Diagnostika GMBH, Germany). Concentrations of pentraxin-3, sICAM-1 and sVCAM-1 were measured in serum (ELISA assays from R&D systems, USA).

Vascular function

Arteries were isolated and mounted on two stainless steel wires (25 μm in diameter) in the organ baths of a four-channel wire myograph (model 610, Danish Myo Technology; Aarhus, Denmark) as described previously [25]. Arteries collected from patients with ESRD we refer as "uremic arteries".

Once a sustained, steady contraction to norepinephrine (3 μmol/L) was attained, the concentration-response curves to the endothelium-dependent vasodilators ACh and BK (1 nmol/L to 3 μmol/L) or SNP (10 nmol/L to 100 μmol/L), NO-donor and an opener of ATP-sensitive K^+-channels (K_{ATP}-channels), pinacidil (10 nmol/L to 100 μmol/L), were obtained. Arteries were then incubated for 20 min with NOS inhibitor (300 μmol/L) and COX inhibitor, Indo (10 μmol/L). Subsequently, arteries were pre-constricted again and second concentration-response curve for endothelium-dependent agonists was obtained. The term "EDHF" used in this study refers to the L-NAME+Indo-insensitive component of endothelium-dependent vasodilatation. The level of increased resting tone of the arteries after incubation with L-NAME+Indo was considered as an index of vasoactive properties of the endothelium, reflecting a basal release of endothelium-derived vasoactive factors. To evaluate the contribution of gap junctions in EDHF type responses, the concentration-response curves to ACh and BK were constructed after 15 min co-incubation with 18-αGA (100 μmol/L) in the presence of L-NAME+Indo.

Fluorescence immunohistochemistry

Freshly isolated arteries where cryopreserved in optimal cutting temperature compound on dry ice. Transverse 8 μm cryosections were prepared and mounted onto slides, air-dried, and stored at $-80°C$. For immunostaining, cryosections were incubated for 1.5 hr at room temperature with the mouse polyclonal anti-eNOS antibody (1:250, BD Biosciences 610296). Incubation with the secondary goat anti-mouse antibody (Invitrogen, Alexa fluor 488 A11001) was done for 1 hr in the dark. Glass coverslips were mounted with Vectashield H-1200 Mounting Kit (Vector Laboratories). Stained sections were examined immediately under fluorescence microscope. All images presented are in (×100) magnification.

Transmission electron microscopy

Artery segments were fixed as described previously [24–25]. Serial transverse, ultra-thin sections (approximately 50–80 nm) were cut. The series consisted of 3–5 sections. For each artery such series were repeated three times after an interval of 10 μm. Sections were examined in a Tecnai 10 transmission electron microscope at 80 kV and digital images were captured.

Chemicals

The composition of PSS was (in mmol/L): NaCl 119, KCl 4.7, $CaCl_2$ 2.5, $MgSO_4$ 1.17, $NaHCO_3$ 25, KH_2PO_4 1.18, EDTA 0.026, and glucose 5.5. The chemicals were obtained from Sigma, St. Louis. To prepare stock solution, the substances were dissolved in distilled water. Indo and pinacidil were dissolved in ethanol and 18α-GA was dissolved in DMSO. Pilot studies showed that the solvents used had no effect upon vascular responses at their final concentrations.

Data analysis

In figures, results are expressed as mean ± SEM. In tables, normally distributed variables are expressed as mean ± SD, and non-normally distributed variables as medians and interquartile ranges. Baseline characteristics of the patients and arteries used and staining were analysed by conventional parametric and non-parametric methods. The isometric force developed by artery segment during application of vasoactive compounds was calculated using Myodata (Danish Myo Technology, Denmark) and expressed as mN/mm^2. Relaxation was expressed as a percentage of the pre-constriction. In order to visualize the relative contribution of EDHF or MEGJs, a percentage of the relaxation was calculated after pre-incubation with L-NAME+Indo or L-NAME+Indo+18α-GA and related to the full response in PSS or after pre-incubation with L-NAME+Indo. Negative log concentration (in mol/l) required to achieve 50% of the maximum response (pEC_{50}) was calculated by nonlinear regression analysis (BioDataFit 1.02). ANOVA was used to compare concentration-response curves before and after incubation with different inhibitors. Spearman's rank correlation was used to determine the associations between artery sensitivity (pEC_{50}) to endothelium-dependent vasodilators and plasma markers of endothelial dysfunction. Significance was taken at the 5% level for all comparisons. All statistical analyses were performed with STATISTICA (v.10.0, StatSoft, Uppsala, Sweden).

Acknowledgments

We would like to thank the patients and personnel at Karolinska University Hospital-Huddinge involved in the sample collection. Special consideration to our biochemical analysis coordinator Björn Anderstam, and Monica Eriksson and Ann-Christin Bragfors-Helin for biochemical analysis; to

John Sandberg and Olof Heimbürger for patients recruitment; to KBC (Annika Nilsson, Anki Emmot and Ulrika Jensen) for sampling protocol and coordination.

Author Contributions

Conceived and designed the experiments: LL PS KK. Performed the experiments: LL PS STD KK. Analyzed the data: LL STD KK. Contributed reagents/materials/analysis tools: LL PS JJC FH STD KK. Wrote the paper: LL PS KK. Collected biopsy material: FH.

References

1. Stenvinkel P, Pecoits-Filho R, Lindholm B (2003) Coronary Artery Disease in End-Stage Renal Disease: No Longer a Simple Plumbing Problem. J Am Soc Nephrol 14: 1927–1939.
2. Schiffrin EL, Lipman ML, Mann JF (2007) Chronic Kidney Disease: Effects on the Cardiovascular System. Circulation 116: 85–97.
3. Brocq ML, Leslie SJ, Milliken P, Megson I (2008) Endothelial Dysfunction: From Molecular Mechanisms to Measurement, Clinical Implications, and Therapeutic Opportunities. Antioxid Redox Signal 10: 1631–1674.
4. Chhabra N (2009) Endothelial dysfunction – A predictor of atherosclerosis. Internet J Med Update 4: 33–41.
5. Félétou M, Köhler R, Vanhoutte P (2010) Endothelium-derived Vasoactive Factors and Hypertension: Possible Roles in Pathogenesis and as Treatment Targets. Curr Hypertens Rep 12: 267–275.
6. Vettoretti S, Ochodnicky P, Buikema H, Henning RH, Kluppel CA, et al. (2006) Altered myogenic constriction and endothelium-derived hyperpolarizing factor-mediated relaxation in small mesenteric arteries of hypertensive subtotally nephrectomized rats. J Hypertens 24: 2215–2223.
7. Malyszko JS, Malyszko J, Hryszko T, Kozminski P, Pawlak K, et al. (2006) Markers of endothelial damage in patients on hemodialysis and hemodiafiltration. J Nephrol 19: 150–154.
8. Yilmaz MI, Saglam M, Carrero JJ, Qureshi AR, Caglar K, et al. (2008) Serum visfatin concentration and endothelial dysfunction in chronic kidney disease. Nephrol Dial Transplant 23: 959–965.
9. Morris S, McMurray J, Spiers A, Jardine AG (2001) Impaired endothelial function in isolated human uremic resistance arteries. Kidney Int 60: 1077–1082.
10. Passauer J, Pistrosch F, Lässig G, Herbrig K, Büssemaker E, et al. (2005) Nitric oxide- and EDHF-mediated arteriolar tone in uremia is unaffected by selective inhibition of vascular cytochrome P450 2C9. Kidney Int 67: 1907–1912.
11. Luksha N, Luksha L, Carrero JJ, Hammarqvist F, Stenvinkel P, et al. (2011) Impaired resistance artery function in patients with end-stage renal disease. Clin Sci (Lond) 120: 525–536.
12. Baylis C (2008) Nitric oxide deficiency in chronic kidney disease. Am J Physiol Renal Physiol 294: F1–9.
13. Luksha L, Agewall S, Kublickiene K (2009) Endothelium-derived hyperpolarizing factor in vascular physiology and cardiovascular disease. Atherosclerosis 202: 330–344.
14. Benchetrit S, Green J, Katz D, Bernheim J, Rathaus M (2003) Early endothelial dysfunction following renal mass reduction in rats. Eur J Clin Invest 33: 26–33.
15. Kohler R, Eichler I, Schonfelder H, Grgic I, Heinau P, et al. (2005) Impaired EDHF-mediated vasodilation and function of endothelial Ca2+-activated K+-channels in uremic rats. Kidney Int 67: 2280–2287.
16. Kalliovalkama J, Jolma P, Tolvanen J-P, Kähönen M, Hutri-Kähönen N, et al. (1999) Potassium channel-mediated vasorelaxation is impaired in experimental renal failure. Am J Physiol Heart Circ Physiol 277: H1622–H1629.
17. Kimura K, Nishio I (1999) Impaired endothelium-dependent relaxation in mesenteric arteries of reduced renal mass hypertensive rats. Scand J Clin Lab Invest 59: 199–204.
18. Gschwend S, Haug MB, Nierhaus M, Schulz A, Vetter R, et al. (2009) Short-term treatment with a beta-blocker with vasodilative capacities improves intrarenal endothelial function in experimental renal failure. Life Sci 85: 431–437.
19. Passauer J, Pistrosch F, Büssemaker E, Lässig G, Herbrig K, et al. (2005) Reduced Agonist-Induced Endothelium-Dependent Vasodilation in Uremia Is Attributable to an Impairment of Vascular Nitric Oxide. J Am Soc Nephrol 16: 959–965.
20. Sokoya EM, Burns AR, Marrelli SP, Chen J (2007) Myoendothelial gap junction frequency does not account for sex differences in EDHF responses in rat MCA. Microvascular Research 74: 39–44.
21. Prasad A, Husain S, Schenke W, Mincemoyer R, Epstein N, et al. (2000) Contribution of bradykinin receptor dysfunction to abnormal coronary vasomotion in humans. J Am Coll Cardiol 36: 1467–1473.
22. Wirth KJ, Linz W, Wiemer G, Schölkens BA (1996) Differences in acetylcholine- and bradykinin-induced vasorelaxation of the mesenteric vascular bed in spontaneously hypertensive rats of different ages. Naunyn Schmiedebergs Arch Pharmacol 354: 38–43.
23. Pascoal IF, Lindheimer MD, Nalbantian-Brandt C, Umans JG (1998) Preeclampsia selectively impairs endothelium-dependent relaxation and leads to oscillatory activity in small omental arteries. J Clin Invest 101: 464–470.
24. Luksha L, Luksha N, Kublickas M, Nisell H, Kublickiene K (2010) Diverse Mechanisms of Endothelium-Derived Hyperpolarizing Factor-Mediated Dilatation in Small Myometrial Arteries in Normal Human Pregnancy and Preeclampsia. Biol Reprod 83: 728–735.
25. Luksha L, Nisell H, Luksha N, Kublickas M, Hultenby K, et al. (2008) Endothelium-derived hyperpolarizing factor in preeclampsia: heterogeneous contribution, mechanisms, and morphological prerequisites. Am J Physiol Regul Integr Comp Physiol 294: R510–R519.
26. Kühberger E, Kukovetz WR, Groschner K (1993) Cromakalim Inhibits Multiple Mechanisms of Smooth Muscle Activation with Similar Stereoselectivity. J Cardiovasc Pharmacol 21: 947–954.
27. Stojnic N, Gojkovic-Bukarica L, Peric M, Grbovic L, Lesic A, et al. (2007) Potassium channel opener pinacidil induces relaxation of the isolated human radial artery. J Pharmacol Sci 104: 122–129.
28. Deka DK, Raviprakash V, Mishra SK (1998) Basal nitric oxide release differentially modulates vasodilations by pinacidil and levcromakalim in goat coronary artery. Eur J Pharmacol 348: 11–23.
29. Rees DD, Palmer RM, Moncada S (1989) Role of endothelium-derived nitric oxide in the regulation of blood pressure. Proc Natl Acad Sci USA 86: 3375–3378.
30. Passauer J, Bussemaker E, Range U, Plug M, Gross P (2000) Evidence In Vivo Showing Increase of Baseline Nitric Oxide Generation and Impairment of Endothelium-Dependent Vasodilation in Normotensive Patients on Chronic Hemodialysis. J Am Soc Nephrol 11: 1726–1734.
31. Kao M, Ang D, Pall A, Struthers AD (2009) Oxidative stress in renal dysfunction: mechanisms, clinical sequelae and therapeutic options. J Hum Hypertens 24: 1–8.
32. Kim SW, Lee JU, Paek YW, Kang DG, Choi KC (2000) Decreased nitric oxide synthesis in rats with chronic renal failure. J Korean Med Sci 15: 425–430.
33. Bonomini M, Pandolfi A, Pietro ND, Sirolli V, Giardinelli A, et al. (2005) Adherence of uremic erythrocytes to vascular endothelium decreases endothelial nitric oxide synthase expression. Kidney Int 67: 1899–1906.
34. Linden E, Cai W, He JC, Xue C, Li Z, et al. (2008) Endothelial Dysfunction in Patients with Chronic Kidney Disease Results from Advanced Glycation End Products-Mediated Inhibition of Endothelial Nitric Oxide Synthase through RAGE Activation. Clin J Am Soc Nephrol 3: 691–698.
35. Gómez-Fernández P, Pérez-Requena J, Sánchez-Margalet V, Esteban J, Murillo-Carretero M, et al. (2005) Vascular damage in chronic renal failure. The increase of vascular nitrotyrosine and cytochines accumulation is accompanied by an increase of endothelial nitric oxide synthase expression. Nefrologia 25: 155–162.
36. Billecke SS, D'Alecy LG, Platel R, Whitesall SE, Jamerson KA, et al. (2009) Blood content of asymmetric dimethylarginine: new insights into its dysregulation in renal disease. Nephrol Dial Transplant 24: 489–496.
37. Antoniades C, Shirodaria C, Leeson P, Antonopoulos A, Warrick N, et al. (2009) Association of plasma asymmetrical dimethylarginine (ADMA) with elevated vascular superoxide production and endothelial nitric oxide synthase uncoupling: implications for endothelial function in human atherosclerosis. European Heart Journal 30: 1142–1150.
38. Veresh Z, Racz A, Lotz G, Koller A (2008) ADMA Impairs Nitric Oxide-Mediated Arteriolar Function Due to Increased Superoxide Production by Angiotensin II-NAD(P)H Oxidase Pathway. Hypertension 52: 960–966.
39. Satoh M, Fujimoto S, Arakawa S, Yada T, Namikoshi T, et al. (2008) Angiotensin II type 1 receptor blocker ameliorates uncoupled endothelial nitric oxide synthase in rats with experimental diabetic nephropathy. Nephrology Dialysis Transplantation 23: 3806–3813.
40. Satoh M, Fujimoto S, Haruna Y, Arakawa S, Horike H, et al. (2005) NAD(P)H oxidase and uncoupled nitric oxide synthase are major sources of glomerular superoxide in rats with experimental diabetic nephropathy. American Journal of Physiology - Renal Physiology 288: F1144–F1152.
41. Yilmaz MI, Saglam M, Caglar K, Cakir E, Ozgurtas T, et al. (2005) Endothelial Functions Improve with Decrease in Asymmetric Dimethylarginine Levels after Renal Transplantation. Transplantation 80: 1660–1666.
42. Mittermayer F, Schaller G, Pleiner J, Vychytil A, Sunder-Plassmann G, et al. (2005) Asymmetrical Dimethylarginine Plasma Concentrations Are Related to Basal Nitric Oxide Release but Not Endothelium-Dependent Vasodilation of Resistance Arteries in Peritoneal Dialysis Patients. J Am Soc Nephrol 16: 1832–1838.
43. Achan V, Broadhead M, Malaki M, Whitley G, Leiper J, et al. (2003) Asymmetric Dimethylarginine Causes Hypertension and Cardiac Dysfunction in Humans and Is Actively Metabolized by Dimethylarginine Dimethylaminohydrolase. Arterioscler Thromb Vasc Biol 23: 1455–1459.
44. Albrecht E, van Goor H, Smit-van Oosten A, Stegeman C (2003) Long-term dietary -arginine supplementation attenuates proteinuria and focal glomerulosclerosis in experimental chronic renal transplant failure. Nitric Oxide 8: 53–58.
45. Wadham C, Mangoni AA (2009) Dimethylarginine dimethylaminohydrolase regulation: a novel therapeutic target in cardiovascular disease. Expert Opin Drug Metab Toxicol 5: 303–319.

17

Effectiveness of Influenza Vaccination in Patients with End-Stage Renal Disease Receiving Hemodialysis

I-Kuan Wang[1,2,3], Cheng-Li Lin[4,5], Po-Chang Lin[6], Chih-Chia Liang[2], Yao-Lung Liu[2], Chiz-Tzung Chang[2], Tzung-Hai Yen[7], Donald E. Morisky[8], Chiu-Ching Huang[2]*, Fung-Chang Sung[4,5]*

1 Graduate Institute of Clinical Medical Science, China Medical University College of Medicine, Taichung, Taiwan, 2 Division of Nephrology, China Medical University Hospital, Taichung, Taiwan, 3 Department of Internal Medicine, China Medical University College of Medicine, Taichung, Taiwan, 4 Management Office for Health Data, China Medical University Hospital, Taichung, Taiwan, 5 Department of Public Health, China Medical University, Taichung, Taiwan, 6 Division of Infection, China Medical University Hospital, Taichung, Taiwan, 7 Division of Nephrology, Chang Gung Memorial Hospital, Taipei and Chang Gung Univeristy College of Medicine, Taoyuan, Taiwan, 8 UCLA Fielding School of Public Health, Los Angeles, California, United States of America

Abstract

Background: Little is known on the effectiveness of influenza vaccine in ESRD patients. This study compared the incidence of hospitalization, morbidity, and mortality in end-stage renal disease (ESRD) patients undergoing hemodialysis (HD) between cohorts with and without influenza vaccination.

Methods: We used the insurance claims data from 1998 to 2009 in Taiwan to determine the incidence of these events within one year after influenza vaccination in the vaccine (N = 831) and the non-vaccine (N = 3187) cohorts. The vaccine cohort to the non-vaccine cohort incidence rate ratio and hazard ratio (HR) of morbidities and mortality were measured.

Results: The age-specific analysis showed that the elderly in the vaccine cohort had lower hospitalization rate (100.8 vs. 133.9 per 100 person-years), contributing to an overall HR of 0.81 (95% confidence interval (CI) 0.72–0.90). The vaccine cohort also had an adjusted HR of 0.85 [95% CI 0.75–0.96] for heart disease. The corresponding incidence of pneumonia and influenza was 22.4 versus 17.2 per 100 person-years, but with an adjusted HR of 0.80 (95% CI 0.64–1.02). The vaccine cohort had lowered risks than the non-vaccine cohort for intensive care unit (ICU) admission (adjusted HR 0.20, 95% CI 0.12–0.33) and mortality (adjusted HR 0.50, 95% CI 0.41–0.60). The time-dependent Cox model revealed an overall adjusted HR for mortality of 0.30 (95% CI 0.26–0.35) after counting vaccination for multi-years.

Conclusions: ESRD patients with HD receiving the influenza vaccination could have reduced risks of pneumonia/influenza and other morbidities, ICU stay, hospitalization and death, particularly for the elderly.

Editor: Li-Min Huang, National Taiwan University Hospital, Taiwan

Funding: Executive Yuan National Science Council (grant number NSC 100-2621-M-039 -001), the Department of Health (grant numbers DOH101-TD-B- 111-004 and DOH101-TD-C-111-005) and the China Medical University Hospital (grant number 1MS1). The funders had no role in study design, data collection and analysis, decision to publish, or preparation of the manuscript.

Competing Interests: The authors have declared that no competing interests exist.

* E-mail: fcsung1008@yahoo.com (F-CS); cch@mail.cmuh.org.tw (C-CH)

Introduction

The influenza virus is a common transmissible human respiratory virus that causes significant morbidity and mortality. In the Unites States, influenza can cause hospitalizations of more than 225,000 patients and 36,000 deaths annually [1,2]. The morbidity and mortality of influenza are increased in people of old ages, immunocompromised patients, and those with chronic diseases [3]. Patients with end-stage renal disease (ESRD) are also at increased risk of influenza complications [4]. Infection is the second leading cause of mortality and a major cause of morbidity in ESRD patients [5]. In addition, mortality rate related to pulmonary infection is likely 10-fold higher in ESRD patients than in the general population [6]. Immune dysfunction, older age, and comorbid conditions, such as diabetes mellitus, malnu-

trition, invasive dialysis procedures, disruption of skin and mucosa barriers, and nosocomial transmission, contribute to the high infection risk for ESRD patients [4,7]. The causes of immune dysfunction in ESRD patients include diminished functions in complement activation, neutrophil, monocyte/macrophage, T-cell, and B-cell [8].

Observation studies have reported that influenza vaccination can reduce the risk of deaths and hospitalizations among elderly and high-risk populations [9,10]. Thus, annual influenza vaccination for ESRD patients is recommended [11]. However, little is known on the effectiveness of influenza vaccine in ESRD patients. Observation studies showed conflicting results.[12,13,14,15,16] The present study aims to investigate the effectiveness of influenza vaccination in reducing morbidity and mortality for ESRD patients receiving hemodialysis (HD) using population-based universal insurance data, derived from the Taiwan National Health Insurance (NHI) program.

Materials and Methods

Data Sources

The Taiwan NHI was integrated from 13 insurance programs in 1995 in Taiwan. This insurance program has covered approximately 99% of the entire 23.74 million people in Taiwan since 1999 [17]. The Taiwan Bureau of National Health Insurance had authorized the National Health Research Institutes (NHRI) to manage reimbursement claims from hospitals and clinics. A committee at the Bureau of National Health Insurance was responsible to randomly select claims and to check the accuracy of claims. NHRI also had been authorized to established data sets for administrative and research uses. We obtained a sub-dataset with one million of population from NHRI for this study. This subset data is similar to the whole population in the distributions in gender and age. The claims data included information on demographic status, date and source of diagnosis, ambulatory care, outpatient and inpatient treatment, dental services, and physicians providing services. Claims data were randomly audited by the insurance system. Data files are linked with scrambled patient identification number to protect the privacy of the patients. The International Classification of Disease, 9th Revision, Clinical Modification (ICD-9-CM) was used to identify individual health status. This study was approved by the Institutional Review Board of China Medical University.

Study Subjects

We identified patients with ESRD newly diagnosed in 1998–2009 yearly from the sub-dataset with one million insured people. The patients who had completed the seasonal influenza vaccination (ICD-9-CM V04.7 and V04.8) were designated in the vaccine cohort, with the date of vaccination defined as the index date for measuring the follow-up period. The patients who received pneumococcal vaccine were excluded (N = 75). Newly diagnosed HD patients without both influenza and pneumococcal vaccinations were also identified annually as the non-vaccine cohort. The corresponding non-vaccine cohort was selected randomly from the same month of the index year.

Outcome Measures

Both cohorts were followed up since the index date for one year or until selected events, death, or withdrawal from the insurance. We were interested in outcome events of total hospitalization, pneumonia or influenza (ICD-9-CM codes 480-487), hospitalization for septicemia, bacteremia, or viremia (ICD-9-CM codes 038.x, 790.7, and 790.8), hospitalization for heart disease (ICD-9-CM codes 401–429), respiratory failure (ICD-9-M codes 518.81, 518.82, 518.83, 518.84, 799.1), or intensive care unit (ICU) admission or death. The history of coronary artery disease (ICD-9-CM codes 410–413, 414.01–414.05, 414.8, and 414.9), congestive heart failure (ICD-9-CM codes 428, 398.91, 402.x1), cancer (ICD-9-CM codes 140–149, 150–159, 160–165, 170–175, 179–189, 190–199, 200, 202, 203, 210–213, 215– 229, 235–239, 654.1, 654.10, 654.11, 654.12, 654.13, 654.14), hyperlipidemia (ICD-9-CM codes 272), hypertension (ICD-9-CM codes 401–405), diabetes (ICD-9-CM codes 250), atrial fibrillation (ICD-9-CM codes 427.31), stroke (ICD-9-CM codes 430–438), chronic hepatitis (ICD-9-CM codes 571, 572.2, 572.3, 572.8, 573.1, 573.2, 573.3, 573.8, 573.9), and chronic obstructive pulmonary disease (ICD-9-CM codes490, 491– 495, 496) were identified as comorbidities before the index date.

Statistical Analysis

Proportion of annual influenza vaccination in HD patients was measured chronologically from 1998–2009. Demographic characteristics of HD patients and prevalence of comorbidities were compared between the vaccine and non-vaccine cohorts, and tested using Chi-square test for categorical variables and t-test for continuous variables. Incidence rates for hospitalization events, infections (pneumonia/influenza, septicemia, bacteremia and viremia), heart disease, respiratory failure, intensive care unit (ICU) admission, and mortality were estimated for each cohort. The vaccine to non-vaccine cohort incidence rate ratio (IRR) and 95% confidence interval (CI) were estimated using Poisson regression. Cox proportional hazards regression model was also used to estimate the hazard ratio (HR) for each of these events and the corresponding 95% CI, within one year after the vaccination. The Cox proportional hazards regression model were also used to estimate pneumonia/influenza-free rates, controlling for age, sex, hyperlipidemia, hypertension, congestive heart failure, chronic hepatitis, chronic obstructive pulmonary disease and calendar year. Similarly, the probability free of respiratory failure, ICU admission, and mortality were plotted using the Cox proportional hazards regression model. The influenza vaccination changed annually, we used the time-dependent Cox model to further evaluate the mortality risk related to the vaccination for multiple years. SAS version 9.1 (SAS Institute, Cary, NC, USA) was used for data analyses; p <0.05 was considered to indicate statistical significance.

Results

From 1998 to 2009, new patients receiving HD increased annually from 264 cases in 1998 to a peak of 368 cases in 2007, and then declined to 347 cases in 2009 (Table 1). The proportion of patients receiving influenza vaccine increased from 1.14% to a peak of 38.0% in 2009. A total of 29 patients received both seasonal influenza and influenza A (H1N1) vaccines in 2009. A total of 103 patients received seasonal influenza vaccination only (data not shown). Overall, 831 patients were in the influenza vaccine cohort, which comprised less portion of women than 3187 patients in the non-vaccine comparison cohort (Table 2). The

Table 1. Proportion of annual influenza vaccination in hemodialysis patients.

| Year | Influenza vaccine | | | |
	N	Yes	No	Proportion (%)
1998	264	3	261	1.14
1999	270	16	254	5.93
2000	313	50	263	15.97
2001	315	48	267	15.24
2002	335	80	255	23.88
2003	361	90	271	24.93
2004	363	78	285	21.49
2005	397	89	308	22.42
2006	355	90	265	25.35
2007	368	70	298	19.02
2008	330	85	245	25.76
2009	347	132	215	38.04

Table 2. Demographic status and comorbidity at baseline in hemodialysis patients with and without influenza vaccination.

	Influenza vaccine		p-value
	Yes (n = 831)	No (n = 3187)	
Age, mean ± SD	70.2±9.96	59.4±14.5	<0.0001[#]
Stratify age			
18–39	8(0.96)	284(8.91)	<0.0001
40–64	127(15.3)	1714(53.8)	
65+	696(83.8)	1189(37.3)	
Gender			
Women	413(49.7)	1635(51.3)	0.41
Men	418(50.3)	1552(48.7)	
Comorbidity			
CAD	401(48.3)	997(31.3)	<0.0001
CHF	253(30.5)	672(21.1)	<0.0001
Cancer	82(9.87)	236(7.41)	0.02
Hyperlipidemia	466(56.1)	1342(42.1)	<0.0001
Hypertension	776(93.4)	2795(87.7)	<0.0001
Diabetes	552(66.4)	1694(53.2)	<0.0001
Atrial fibrillation	26(3.13)	67(2.10)	0.08
Chronic hepatitis	323(38.9)	874(27.4)	<0.0001
COPD	356(42.8)	917(28.8)	<0.0001

Abbreviations: CAD, coronary artery disease; CHF, congestive heart failure; COPD; chronic obstructive pulmonary disease
Chi-square test; [#]: Two-sample t-test

vaccine cohort mainly included the elderly, with the mean age much higher than that of the non-vaccine cohort (70.2± 9.96 vs. 59.4±14.5 years). The vaccine cohort also tended to be more prevalent with comorbidities. There was no patient who received transplantation or was shifted to peritoneal dialysis during the follow-up period.

The analysis for age-specific hospitalization shows that most of patients hospitalized were the elderly (≥ 65 years) (Table 3). The overall crude hospitalization rate was 11.0% higher in the vaccine cohort than in the non-vaccine cohort (99.4 vs. 89.4 per 100 person-years). However, the vaccine cohort had an adjusted HR of 0.81(95% CI = 0.72–0.90) after controlling for sex, age, coronary artery disease; congestive heart failure; chronic obstructive

pulmonary disease, cancer, stroke, and calendar year. The elderly with vaccination had significant lower rate than those without (100.8 vs. 133.9 per 100 person-years), with an adjusted IRR of 0.73 (95% CI 0.64–0.82).

Table 4 shows that the incidence of heart disease, the major cause of hospitalization, was higher in the vaccine cohort than in the non-vaccine cohort (65.3 vs. 51.7 per 100 person-years). However, the adjusted HR of the vaccine cohort was 0.85 (95% CI 0.75–0.96). The incidence rates of pneumonia/influenza, hospitalization for septicemia/bacteremia/viremia, and respiratory failure were also higher in the vaccine cohort than in the non-vaccine cohort. However, adjusted HRs also demonstrated protective association from the vaccination. Compared with the patients in the non-vaccine cohort, those in the vaccine cohort were less likely to be admitted in the ICU [2.6 vs. 6.8 per 100 person-years; adjusted HR 0.2 (95% CI 0.12–0.33)] and to be deceased [18.5 vs. 21.0 per 100 person-years; adjusted HR 0.50 (95% CI 0.41–0.60)].

The evaluation for only the elderly also showed that those with vaccination were at lower risks of pneumonia/influenza, hospitalization for septicemia/bacteremia/viremia, and heart disease, ICU admission, respiratory failure, and death (data not shown). The time-dependent Cox model revealed that the overall adjusted HR for mortality associated with the vaccination reduced to 0.30 (95% CI 0.26–0.35), compared with non-vaccinated persons (Table 5).

Figures 1A trough 1D show that, compared with the non-vaccine cohort, the vaccine cohort had significantly lower rates of pneumonia/influenza (P-value = 0.02) (Figure 1A), respiratory failure (P-value <0.0001) (Figure 1B), ICU stay (Figure 1C) (P-value <0.0001), and mortality (Figure 1D) (P-value <0.0001).

Discussion

Our study demonstrated that influenza vaccination for ESRD patients receiving HD was associated with lower morbidities, including total hospitalization, ICU admission, pneumonia/influenza, septicemia/bacteremia/viremia, respiratory failure, and heart disease. In addition, influenza vaccination was also associated with lower all-cause mortality risk for 50%. The mortality risk decreased further to have an overall adjusted HR of 0.30 as subjects with vaccinations for multiple years were counted. Consistent with the present study, a previous research in the US reported that the risks of hospitalization and death for HD patients vaccinated against influenza are lower than those of unvaccinated patients, with odds ratios of 0.93 (95% 0.90–0.95) and 0.77 (0.73–

Table 3. Comparison in hospitalization rates between hemodialysis patients with and without influenza vaccination.

Outcome	Vaccine			Non-vaccine			IRR[*](95% CI)	Adjusted IRR(95% CI)	Adjusted HR (95% CI)
	Event	PY	Rate[#]	Event	PY	Rate[#]			
Total Hospitalization	459	462	99.4	1688	1888	89.4	1.11(0.96, 1.28)	0.80(0.69, 0.94)	0.82(0.73, 0.91)
Age, years									
18–39	1	5	20	113	205	55.1	0.40(0.03, 5.54)	0.36(0.03, 4.76)	0.36(0.05, 2.62)
40–64	59	62	95.2	820	1118	73.3	1.31(0.92, 1.86)	1.22(0.86, 1.74)	1.16(0.89, 1.52)
65+	399	396	100.8	755	564	133.9	0.75(0.64, 0.89)	0.70(0.59, 0.82)	0.73(0.64, 0.82)

Rate[#], incidence rate, per 100 person-years; IRR[*], incidence rate ratio;
HR, hazard ratio adjusted for sex, age, coronary artery disease; congestive heart failure; chronic obstructive pulmonary disease, cancer, stroke, and calendar year

Table 4. Hospitalization, intensive care unit utilization, and mortality comparison between hemodialysis patients with and without influenza vaccination.

Outcome	Vaccine			Non-vaccine			IRR*(95% CI)	Adjusted IRR (95% CI)	Adjusted HR (95% CI)
	Event	PY	Rate#	Event	PY	Rate#			
Pneumonia/influenza[†]	139	620	22.4	445	2584	17.2	1.30(1.08, 1.56)	0.77(0.64, 0.93)	0.78(0.64, 0.96)
Septicemia, bacteremia, and viremia[†]	103	637	16.2	347	2661	13.0	1.24(1.02, 1.50)	0.66(0.47, 0.92)	0.72(0.56, 0.88)
Heart disease[†]	341	522	65.3	1138	2203	51.7	1.26(1.08, 1.47)	0.83(0.71, 0.97)	0.85(0.75, 0.96)
Respiratory Failure[†]	66	653	10.1	262	2697	9.7	1.04(0.84, 1.29)	0.52(0.42, 0.64)	0.53(0.41, 0.70)
Intensive care unit admission[†]	17	660	2.6	184	2696	6.8	0.38(0.27, 0.53)	0.19(0.14, 0.27)	0.20(0.12, 0.33)
Mortality[†]	123	665	18.5	581	2765	21.0	0.88(0.73, 1.07)	0.49(0.41, 0.59)	0.50(0.41, 0.60)

Rate#, incidence rate, per 100 person-years; IRR*, incidence rate ratio
Hospitalization[†]: adjusted for age, CAD, CHF, cancer, COPD, stroke, and calendar year
Hospitalization for pneumonia/influenza[†]: adjusted for age, sex, CAD, CHF, cancer, diabetes, atrial fibrillation, COPD, and calendar year
Hospitalization for septicemia, bacteremia, and viremia[†]: adjusted for age, cancer, diabetes, atrial fibrillation, and calendar year
Hospitalization for heart disease[†]: adjusted for age, CAD, CHF, hypertension, diabetes, atrial fibrillation, chronic hepatitis, and calendar year
Respiratory Failure[†]: adjusted for age, sex, CAD, cancer, CHF, diabetes, hypertension, chronic hepatitis, and calendar year
Intensive care unit[†]: adjusted for age, cancer, hyperlipidemia, hypertension, diabetes, atrial fibrillation, chronic hepatitis, and calendar year
Mortality[†]: adjusted for age, sex, CAD, cancer, CHF, diabetes, hyperlipidemia, hypertension, chronic hepatitis, atrial fibrillation, COPD, and calendar year

0.81), respectively [14]. Moreover, they found that vaccination was significantly associated with lower risks of cause-specific mortality, including cardiac and infectious deaths. Recent reports demonstrated that influenza vaccination was associated with a lower mortality risk [12,13]. The mortality hazard was reduced further for patients receiving both pneumococcal and influenza vaccinations. On the contrary, McGrath et al. recently reported little clinical benefits of influenza vaccination on preventing hospitalization and death [16]. However, their study did not consider the confounding effect of pneumococcal vaccination. Therefore, our study observed closely the effectiveness of influenza vaccination, by excluding the effect of pneumococcal vaccine. In addition, these studies analyzed prevalent ESRD patients. Length of time with ESRD may have confounding effect on the outcomes.

Compared with healthy control subjects, ESRD patients possess suboptimal immune response rates but develop satisfying protection rates to influenza vaccination [18,19,20,21,22]. The antibody response rates to influenza vaccination (defined as a four-fold increase in hemagglutination inhibition titers) vary from 7% to 89% [18,19,20,21,22]. The seroprotection rates (defined as hemagglutination inhibition titers≥40) range from 46% to 93%, depending on the specific strain measured [18,19,20,21,22]. Booster vaccination fails to improve the immune response [20,21,23]. Influenza vaccination is safe without causing major adverse effects in HD patients [20,23], and the number of minor adverse reactions is low [20].

Since 1998, the Taiwan NHI program has started to offer influenza vaccinations to high-risk subjects, including ESRD patients and the elderly subjects. Majority of the vaccinated subjects receive this service annually between October 1 and December 31. However, the influenza vaccination rate in this study was low for incident HD patients, especially in the beginning years (1998 and 1999). The higher vaccination rate in 2009 was likely due to the pandemic novel influenza A (H1N1) in April 2009 [24]. The low vaccination rate may be attributed to the lack of awareness on its benefit, fear of adverse reactions, and lack of physician recommendation [25]. The goal of the World Health Organization is to increase the annual influenza vaccination rate to 90% by 2010 for ESRD patients.

Influenza may lead to viral pneumonia and bacterial superinfection. HD patients are susceptible to pulmonary infection. Transient hypoxemia occurs during dialysis because of leukocyte migration in the pulmonary vasculature and loss of carbon dioxide [6]. In addition, HD patients are exposed to other patients and medical staff. Our study demonstrated that influenza vaccination was associated with a lower risk of pneumonia/influenza during the first 3 months after vaccination (data not shown). Seroprotection was maintained at least for 3 months and up to 6 months after influenza vaccination in patients with renal diseases [26].

Consistent with the findings of the present study, Gilbertson reported that influenza vaccination is associated with a lower risk of heart disease in ESRD patients [14]. For patients with chronic kidney disease, an association between influenza vaccination and atherosclerotic heart disease event rates also exists [27]. Systemic inflammation caused by influenza infection may lead to endothelial injury, impaired vasodilatation, and enhanced thrombosis formation [28]. Inflammation is highly associated with increasing cardiovascular mortality [29,30].

The current study has several limitations. First, the NHI database provided limited information on socio-demographic characteristics, with unavailable information on marital status, educational level, smoking habit, body-mass index, and laboratory

Table 5. Time-dependent Cox model estimated hazard ratios and 95% confidence intervals of mortality risk associated with the vaccination.

	Hazard ratio(95% CI)	
	Crude	Adjusted[†]
Vaccination	0.47(0.41, 0.55)	0.30(0.26, 0.35)

Adjusted HRs[†]: adjusted for age, sex, CHF, diabetes, hyperlipidemia, hypertension, chronic hepatitis, and atrial fibrillation

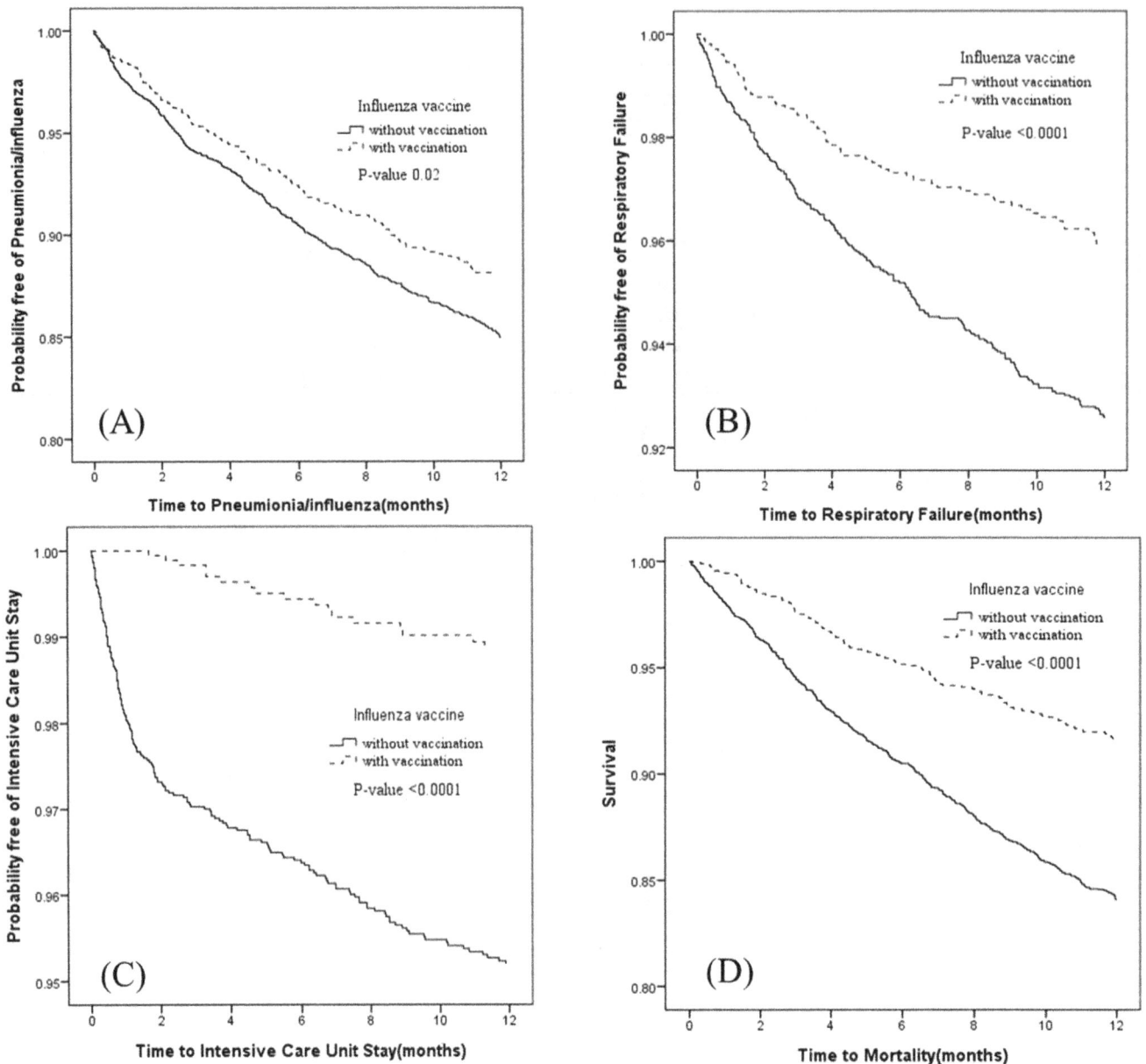

Figure 1. The probability free of pneumonia/influenza, respiratory failure, intensive care unit stay, and mortality for hemodialysis patients with (dashed line) or without (solid line) influenza vaccination.

data, such as hemoglobin, albumin, and residual renal function. These variables cannot be adjusted in the analysis. Furthermore, certain information on chronic conditions, such as hyperlipidemia and hypertension, were not available for some individuals. However, HD patients were visited by health care professionals frequently, the claim data were reliable. Moreover, the decision to receive vaccination may have been affected by socioeconomic status, as well as availability of health care and medical providers. Although multivariate analysis was used, selection bias may occur. Fourth, this study focused only on all-cause mortality because the cause of death cannot be obtained from the database. Finally, the strain and virulence of the predominant virus and the match between the circulating virus strain and the virus strain selected in

the vaccine varied from year to year. Therefore, we adjusted the calendar year for temporal effect.

Conclusions

Our study provides evidence that influenza vaccination is associated with the reduction of mortality and morbidity in HD patients. Thus, HD patients should be vaccinated annually. More large-scale prospective studies are necessary to analyze the issue.

Author Contributions

Conceived and designed the experiments: IKW CLL PCL CCL YLL CTC THY. Analyzed the data: CLL. Wrote the paper: IKW CCH FCS DEM.

References

1. Thompson WW, Shay DK, Weintraub E, Brammer L, Cox N, et al. (2003) Mortality associated with influenza and respiratory syncytial virus in the United States. JAMA 289: 179–186.
2. Thompson WW, Shay DK, Weintraub E, Brammer L, Bridges CB, et al. (2004) Influenza-associated hospitalizations in the United States. JAMA 292: 1333–1340.
3. Fiore AE, Uyeki TM, Broder K, Finelli L, Euler GL, et al. (2010) Prevention and control of influenza with vaccines: recommendations of the Advisory Committee on Immunization Practices (ACIP), 2010. MMWR Recomm Rep 59: 1–62.
4. Naqvi SB, Collins AJ (2006) Infectious complications in chronic kidney disease. Adv Chronic Kidney Dis 13: 199–204.
5. Collins AJ, Foley RN, Herzog C, Chavers BM, Gilbertson D, et al. (2010) Excerpts from the US Renal Data System 2009 Annual Data Report. Am J Kidney Dis 55: S1–420, A426–427.
6. Sarnak MJ, Jaber BL (2001) Pulmonary infectious mortality among patients with end-stage renal disease. Chest 120: 1883–1887.
7. Vanholder R, Van Biesen W (2002) Incidence of infectious morbidity and mortality in dialysis patients. Blood Purif 20: 477–480.
8. Descamps-Latscha B (1993) The immune system in end-stage renal disease. Curr Opin Nephrol Hypertens 2: 883–891.
9. Hak E, Nordin J, Wei F, Mullooly J, Poblete S, et al. (2002) Influence of high-risk medical conditions on the effectiveness of influenza vaccination among elderly members of 3 large managed-care organizations. Clin Infect Dis 35: 370–377.
10. Hak E, Buskens E, van Essen GA, de Bakker DH, Grobbee DE, et al. (2005) Clinical effectiveness of influenza vaccination in persons younger than 65 years with high-risk medical conditions: the PRISMA study. Arch Intern Med 165: 274–280.
11. Johnson DW, Fleming SJ (1992) The use of vaccines in renal failure. Clin Pharmacokinet 22: 434–446.
12. Bond TC, Spaulding AC, Krisher J, McClellan W (2012) Mortality of dialysis patients according to influenza and pneumococcal vaccination status. Am J Kidney Dis 60: 959–965.
13. Gilbertson DT, Guo H, Arneson TJ, Collins AJ (2011) The association of pneumococcal vaccination with hospitalization and mortality in hemodialysis patients. Nephrol Dial Transplant 26: 2934–2939.
14. Gilbertson DT, Unruh M, McBean AM, Kausz AT, Snyder JJ, et al. (2003) Influenza vaccine delivery and effectiveness in end-stage renal disease. Kidney Int 63: 738–743.
15. McGrath LJ, Kshirsagar AV (2012) Influenza and pneumococcal vaccination in dialysis patients: merely a shot in the arm? Am J Kidney Dis 60: 890–892.
16. McGrath LJ, Kshirsagar AV, Cole SR, Wang L, Weber DJ, et al. (2012) Influenza vaccine effectiveness in patients on hemodialysis: an analysis of a natural experiment. Arch Intern Med 172: 548–554.
17. Lu JF, Hsiao WC (2003) Does universal health insurance make health care unaffordable? Lessons from Taiwan. Health Aff (Millwood) 22: 77–88.
18. Antonen JA, Hannula PM, Pyhala R, Saha HH, Ala-Houhala IO, et al. (2000) Adequate seroresponse to influenza vaccination in dialysis patients. Nephron 86: 56–61.
19. Cavdar C, Sayan M, Sifil A, Artuk C, Yilmaz N, et al. (2003) The comparison of antibody response to influenza vaccination in continuous ambulatory peritoneal dialysis, hemodialysis and renal transplantation patients. Scand J Urol Nephrol 37: 71–76.
20. Scharpe J, Peetermans WE, Vanwalleghem J, Maes B, Bammens B, et al. (2009) Immunogenicity of a standard trivalent influenza vaccine in patients on long-term hemodialysis: an open-label trial. Am J Kidney Dis 54: 77–85.
21. Song JY, Cheong HJ, Ha SH, Kee SY, Jeong HW, et al. (2006) Active influenza immunization in hemodialysis patients: comparison between single-dose and booster vaccination. Am J Nephrol 26: 206–211.
22. Vogtlander NP, Brown A, Valentijn RM, Rimmelzwaan GF, Osterhaus AD (2004) Impaired response rates, but satisfying protection rates to influenza vaccination in dialysis patients. Vaccine 22: 2199–2201.
23. Tanzi E, Amendola A, Pariani E, Zappa A, Colzani D, et al. (2007) Lack of effect of a booster dose of influenza vaccine in hemodialysis patients. J Med Virol 79: 1176–1179.
24. (2009) 2009 pandemic influenza A (H1N1) virus infections - Chicago, Illinois, April-July 2009. MMWR Morb Mortal Wkly Rep 58: 913–918.
25. Kausz A, Pahari D (2004) The value of vaccination in chronic kidney disease. Semin Dial 17: 9–11.
26. Brydak LB, Roszkowska-Blaim M, Machala M, Leszczynska B, Sieniawska M (2000) Antibody response to influenza immunization in two consecutive epidemic seasons in patients with renal diseases. Vaccine 18: 3280–3286.
27. Snyder JJ, Collins AJ (2009) Association of preventive health care with atherosclerotic heart disease and mortality in CKD. J Am Soc Nephrol 20: 1614–1622.
28. Nichol KL, Nordin J, Mullooly J, Lask R, Fillbrandt K, et al. (2003) Influenza vaccination and reduction in hospitalizations for cardiac disease and stroke among the elderly. N Engl J Med 348: 1322–1332.
29. Engstrom G, Stavenow L, Hedblad B, Lind P, Eriksson KF, et al. (2003) Inflammation-sensitive plasma proteins, diabetes, and mortality and incidence of myocardial infarction and stroke: a population-based study. Diabetes 52: 442–447.
30. Libby P (2002) Inflammation in atherosclerosis. Nature 420: 868–874.

18

Evaluation of Candidate Nephropathy Susceptibility Genes in a Genome-Wide Association Study of African American Diabetic Kidney Disease

Nicholette D. Palmer[1,2,3]*, Maggie C. Y. Ng[2,3], Pamela J. Hicks[1], Poorva Mudgal[3], Carl D. Langefeld[4], Barry I. Freedman[2,3,5], Donald W. Bowden[1,2,3,5]

1 Department of Biochemistry, Wake Forest School of Medicine, Winston-Salem, North Carolina, United States of America, 2 Center for Genomics and Personalized Medicine Research, Wake Forest School of Medicine, Winston-Salem, North Carolina, United States of America, 3 Diabetes Research Center, Wake Forest School of Medicine, Winston-Salem, North Carolina, United States of America, 4 Center for Public Health Genomics and Department of Biostatistical Sciences, Wake Forest School of Medicine, Winston-Salem, North Carolina, United States of America, 5 Department of Internal Medicine, Wake Forest School of Medicine, Winston-Salem, North Carolina, United States of America

Abstract

Type 2 diabetes (T2D)-associated end-stage kidney disease (ESKD) is a complex disorder resulting from the combined influence of genetic and environmental factors. This study contains a comprehensive genetic analysis of putative nephropathy loci in 965 African American (AA) cases with T2D-ESKD and 1029 AA population-based controls extending prior findings. Analysis was based on 4,341 directly genotyped and imputed single nucleotide polymorphisms (SNPs) in 22 nephropathy candidate genes. After admixture adjustment and correction for multiple comparisons, 37 SNPs across eight loci were significantly associated ($1.6E-05 < P_{emp} < 0.049$). Among these, variants in *MYH9* were the most significant ($1.6E-05 < P_{emp} < 0.049$), followed by additional chromosome 22 loci (*APOL1*, *SFI1*, and *LIMK2*). Nominal signals were observed in *AGTR1*, *RPS12*, *CHN2* and *CNDP1*. Additional adjustment for *APOL1* G1/G2 risk variants attenuated association at *MYH9* ($P_{emp} = 0.00026-0.043$) while marginally improving significance of other *APOL1* SNPs (rs136161, rs713753, and rs767855; $P_{emp} = 0.0060-0.037$); association at other loci was markedly reduced except for *CHN2* (chimerin; rs17157914, $P_{emp} = 0.029$). In addition, SNPs in other candidate loci (*FRMD3* and *TRPC6*) trended toward association with T2D-ESKD ($P_{emp} < 0.05$). These results suggest that risk contributed by putative nephropathy genes is shared across populations of African and European ancestry.

Editor: Giuseppe Remuzzi, Mario Negri Institute for Pharmacological Research and Azienda Ospedaliera Ospedali Riuniti di Bergamo, Italy

Funding: Genotyping services were provided by the Center for Inherited Disease Research (CIDR), which is fully funded through a federal contract from the National Institutes of Health (NIH) to The Johns Hopkins University, contract number HHSC268200782096C. This work was supported by NIH grants K99 DK081350 (NDP), R01 DK066358 (DWB), R01 DK053591 (DWB), R01 HL56266 (BIF), R01 DK 070941 (BIF), R01 DK 084149 (BIF) and in part by a grant from the General Clinical Research Center of the Wake Forest School of Medicine, M01 RR07122. The funders had no role in study design, data collection and analysis, decision to publish, or preparation of the manuscript.

Competing Interests: Nicholette D. Palmer is currently an Academic Editor at PLoS One. This does not alter the authors' adherence to all the PLoS ONE policies on sharing data and materials.

* E-mail: nallred@wakehealth.edu

Introduction

Diabetes-associated kidney disease (DKD) is the most common cause of nephropathy in western societies, present in approximately 40% of patients with type 2 diabetes (T2D) [1]. Patients with DKD account for half of the incident cases of end-stage kidney disease (ESKD) in the United States. T2D-ESKD is a devastating complication with five year survivals in the range of 30% [2]. Current trends suggest that the prevalence of DKD will continue to increase [1] constituting a significant socioeconomic burden on the healthcare system and resulting in increased morbidity and mortality.

T2D-ESKD is a complex disorder resulting from genetic and environmental factors [reviewed in [3]]. Among population groups, African Americans have the highest incidence and prevalence and the rate of new ESKD cases has grown by 7.0% since 2000 [2]. In contrast to risk for non-diabetic ESKD in African Americans, which is powerfully associated with genetic variants in the apolipoprotein L1 gene (*APOL1*; [4]), evidence to date suggests that T2D-ESKD has multi-factorial genetic risk.

The purpose of this study was to extend analysis of data from a previous genome-wide association study (GWAS) of T2D-ESKD in the African American population [5] with detailed assessment of genes previously implicated in ESKD susceptibility while accounting for the effects observed at the *APOL1* locus. The value of this dataset has been enhanced through imputation of genotypes for over 2.2 million additional single nucleotide polymorphisms (SNPs) in the GWAS subjects which facilitates a comprehensive evaluation of putative susceptibility genes for association with T2D-ESKD in African Americans.

Results

Clinical Characteristics of Study Samples

The clinical characteristics of study participants included in the GWAS are shown in **Table 1**. T2D-ESKD cases tended to have a higher proportion of females (P = 0.076), possibly reflecting the increased prevalence of T2D among African American women [6], participation bias, and survival. In addition, the age at enrollment for T2D-ESKD subjects is older than that for the control groups (P<0.0001); however, the age at enrollment for the control groups is older than the age of T2D diagnosis in T2D-ESKD subjects (P<0.0001). Notably, the use of population-based controls has not precluded the identification of trait associations in other investigations (e.g. [7]). Both cases and controls were overweight or obese at the time of enrollment (P = 0.30).

GWAS

A total of 832,357 directly genotyped autosomal SNPs passed quality control and were tested for association in 965 T2D-ESKD cases and 1029 controls lacking T2D and ESKD. Only a modest increase in the inflation factor was noted with inclusion of related individuals (1.04 versus 1.06) therefore, cryptic first degree relatives (n = 54) were retained in the analysis. In addition, >2.28 million SNPs were imputed from HapMap II release 22. Results from twenty-two T2D-DKD candidate loci with 10 kb flanking sequence upstream and downstream (n = 4333 SNPs; **Table S1**) were selected for subsequent analysis.

T2D-ESKD Candidate Loci

We defined T2D-ESKD candidate loci as genes which have been implicated in ESKD (diabetes associated or non-diabetes associated) either through direct (e.g. *CNDP1*, *APOL1*) genetic analysis or through compelling functional relationships (e.g. *REN*). In addition, candidates highlighted from a previous genome-wide association study (GWAS) of T2D-ESKD in this African American population [5] were included (i.e. *RPS12*, *LIMK2*, and *SFI1*). Analysis of the twenty two loci (n = 4333 SNPs) using PC1 as a covariate revealed nominal association (P<0.05) at 20 loci (n = 382 SNPs; **Table S1 and Figure S1**). Correction for multiple comparisons using the number of independent tests at each locus identified eight loci (38 SNPs) with empiric p-values less than 0.05 (P_{emp}<0.05; **Table 2**). The most significant signal (rs5750250, P_{emp} = 1.6E-05, OR (95% CI) = 0.72 (0.63–0.81)) was observed in intron 13 of the non-muscle myosin heavy chain 9 (*MYH9*) gene. Of the 157 SNPs evaluated in *MYH9* resulting in 56 independent SNPs, 12 SNPs had P_{emp}<0.05 and were modestly correlated

(0.02<r^2<0.89; **Figure S2**). Association was also observed with three additional loci on chromosome 22: apolipoprotein L1 (*APOL1*; P_{emp} = 0.0068–0.045; 0.03<r^2<0.82, **Figure S2**), LIM domain kinase 2 (*LIMK2*; P_{emp} = 0.020–0.024; r^2>0.99, **FigureS 2**), and Sfi1 homolog (*SFI1*; P_{emp} = 0.044). Among other significant loci, two SNPs (rs9493454 and rs7769051; r^2 = 0.67) in the ribosomal protein S12 (*RPS12*) gene were associated with T2D-ESKD (P_{emp} = 0.0071 and 0.0083, respectively). Imputation revealed two SNPs (rsq>0.90) in moderate LD (r^2 = 0.49) located in the cytosol nonspecific dipeptidase 1 (*CNDP1*) gene which remained significant after correction for 45 effective SNPs tested (rs4892249, P_{emp} = 0.043 and rs6566815, P_{emp} = 0.0076). Additionally, nominal signals were observed at the angiotensin II receptor type 1 (*AGTR1*; P_{emp} = 0.018) and chimerin 2 (*CHN2*; P_{emp}<0.044; 0.00<r^2<0.05) genes.

T2D-ESKD Candidate Loci with Adjustment for APOL1 G1 and G2 Variants

Adjustment for the *APOL1* G1 and G2 nephropathy risk variants [4] marginalized but did not abolish the significant evidence of associations observed at three loci (P_{emp}<0.048; n = 5 SNPs; **Table 3**). The strongest signal observed was located downstream of the *CNDP1* gene (rs6566815, P_{emp} = 0.011). Three signals of association were observed at the *CHN2* locus (rs17157914, P_{emp} = 0.026; rs3793313, P_{emp} = 0.043; rs17157908, P_{emp} = 0.048). Two of these signals, which were highly correlated (rs17157908 and rs17157914, r^2 = 0.94), emerged only after adjustment for *APOL1* G1/G2 (rs17157914, P_{emp} = 0.091 and rs17157908, P_{emp} = 0.14 prior to *APOL1* G1/G2 adjustment) while the initial signal at rs3793313 maintained the same level of significance (P_{emp} = 0.043). The previous single signal of association observed in the *AGTR1* gene remained significant (rs12695897, P_{emp} = 0.032) after accounting for the effects at the *APOL1* locus. In contrast, the previously observed significant association in the *MYH9* gene was abolished (rs5750250, P_{emp} = 0.20) as were other signals observed on chromosome 22 (P_{emp}>0.099).

Discussion

The goal of this study was to perform a detailed genetic analysis of reported ESKD susceptibility genes in a large African American cohort. Previous studies have been few in number and limited in scope focusing on divergent populations and evaluating relatively few variants by modern day standards. Advantages of this study include a comprehensive evaluation of genetic variation at each susceptibility locus using directly genotyped and imputed SNPs in analysis. In addition, this study uses a single population in which to compare and contrast findings from all reported loci.

After correction for the effective number of variants tested at each locus (**Table 2**), we identified eight susceptibility loci as nominally associated with T2D-ESKD. Examination of the risk allele burden of these variants (n = 37) in the eight loci revealed an increased risk allele burden (P<0.0001) with cases, on average, carrying 50.2 risk alleles while controls carried 47.0 (data not shown). The most significant signal was observed at the *MYH9* locus (rs5750250, P_{emp} = 1.6E-05) although this signal was abolished (P_{emp} = 0.20) after adjustment for the *APOL1* G1/G2 risk alleles. While this finding could be attributed to the potential inclusion of non-diabetic ESKD cases samples, the vast majority (>74%) of the case population had a duration of T2D greater than 5 years before initiating renal replacement therapy. Notably, this variant was the most significant SNP from our T2D-ESKD GWAS [5] despite inclusion of additional imputed variants to

Table 1. Clinical Characteristics of Study Participants.

	T2D-ESKD	Control	p-value
N	965	1029	
Female (%)	61.2%	57.3%	0.076
Age at Enrollment (years)	61.6±10.5	49.0±11.9	<0.0001
Age at T2D Diagnosis (years)	41.6±12.4	-	<0.0001*
Age at ESKD Diagnosis (years)	58.0±10.9	-	<0.0001*
T2D to ESKD Duration (years)	16.2±10.9	-	
Retinopathy (n)	507	0	
BMI (kg/m²)	29.7±7.0	30.0±7.0	0.30

*compared to control subjects.

Table 2. Association of Candidate Diabetic Kidney Disease Loci with T2D-ESKD.

SNP	Position[1]	Gene	Eff[2]	RA[3]	OR[4]	95% CI[5]	P$_{Add}$[6]	P$_{emp}$[7]
rs12695897	3:149927874	AGTR1	40	T	0.58	0.43–0.79	0.00046	0.018
rs9493454	6:133186322	RPS12	13	C	1.25	1.10–1.42	0.00055	0.0071
rs7769051	6:133188489	RPS12	13	A	1.26	1.10–1.44	0.00063	0.0083
rs3793313	7:29272298	CHN2	194	T	1.40	1.17–1.68	0.00023	0.044
rs2057737	7:29385620	CHN2	194	A	1.79	1.32–2.44	0.00020	0.038
rs3729621*	7:29487958	CHN2	194	G	1.57	1.24–1.99	0.00019	0.037
rs4892249*	18:70404575	CNDP1	45	G	1.25	1.09–1.42	0.00095	0.043
rs6566815*	18:70406087	CNDP1	45	T	1.31	1.14–1.51	0.00017	0.0076
rs2413035	22:29930460	LIMK2	20	T	0.60	0.44–0.82	0.0012	0.024
rs737888*	22:29941549	LIMK2	20	A	0.60	0.44–0.81	0.00099	0.020
rs5753521*	22:29968027	LIMK2	20	T	0.60	0.44–0.81	0.00099	0.020
rs2283879*	22:29968448	LIMK2	20	G	0.60	0.44–0.81	0.00099	0.020
rs2106294	22:29975759	LIMK2	20	C	0.60	0.44–0.81	0.00099	0.020
rs4820043	22:29977094	LIMK2	20	A	0.60	0.44–0.81	0.00099	0.020
rs2078803*	22:29982852	LIMK2	20	G	0.60	0.44–0.81	0.00099	0.020
rs2073857*	22:29988281	LIMK2	20	A	0.60	0.44–0.81	0.00099	0.020
rs737684*	22:29989827	LIMK2	20	C	0.60	0.44–0.81	0.00099	0.020
rs4141404*	22:30005185	LIMK2	20	A	0.60	0.44–0.81	0.00099	0.020
rs1858821*	22:30006454	LIMK2	20	T	0.60	0.44–0.81	0.00099	0.020
rs2040533*	22:30009110	LIMK2	20	G	0.60	0.44–0.81	0.00099	0.020
rs5753543*	22:30015458	LIMK2	20	G	0.60	0.44–0.81	0.0012	0.023
rs5749286	22:30230359	SFI1	27	A	0.62	0.46–0.84	0.0016	0.044
rs136161	22:34987378	APOL1	9	C	0.77	0.67–0.90	0.00076	0.0068
rs713753	22:34988480	APOL1	9	T	0.79	0.67–0.92	0.0032	0.029
rs767855*	22:35002241	APOL1	9	T	0.68	0.52–0.89	0.0050	0.045
rs735853	22:35009161	MYH9	56	G	0.68	0.55–0.84	0.00034	0.019
rs6000229	22:35016105	MYH9	56	T	0.75	0.66–0.86	2.3E-05	0.0013
rs2071730*	22:35019972	MYH9	56	C	0.79	0.69–0.91	0.00087	0.049
rs16996648	22:35022698	MYH9	56	C	1.29	1.12–1.48	0.00028	0.016
rs4821480*	22:35025193	MYH9	56	T	0.73	0.64–0.84	5.1E-06	0.00029
rs4821481*	22:35025888	MYH9	56	T	0.73	0.64–0.84	4.8E-06	0.00027
rs5750248*	22:35032838	MYH9	56	C	0.74	0.65–0.85	7.7E-06	0.00043
rs1557529*	22:35035475	MYH9	56	A	1.35	1.17–1.56	4.1E-05	0.0023
rs2157256	22:35037607	MYH9	56	G	0.80	0.70–0.91	0.00085	0.048
rs5750250	22:35038429	MYH9	56	A	0.72	0.63–0.81	2.9E-07	1.6E-05
rs5756152*	22:35042418	MYH9	56	A	1.39	1.17–1.64	0.00015	0.0086
rs2239784*	22:35044581	MYH9	56	C	0.73	0.61–0.87	0.00049	0.027

[1]hg18;
[2]Eff, effective number of SNPs per locus;
[3]RA, reference allele;
[4]OR, odds ratio;
[5]95% CI, 95% confidence interval;
[6]P$_{Add}$, additive p-value;
[7]P$_{emp}$, empiric p-value;
*imputed SNPs.

increase coverage in the current study, i.e. GWAS coverage of *MYH9* with an $r^2>0.73$ with 46 of 166 SNPs versus GWAS and imputed data coverage of *MYH9* with an $r^2>0.99$ with 156 of 166 SNPs. SNP rs5750250 lies within the genomic interval spanned by the four SNPs (rs4821480, rs2032487, rs4821481, and rs3752462) composing the E1 risk haplotype [8] however, individually none of

these variants were associated with T2D-ESKD (P$_{emp}>0.53$). Interestingly, evidence of association at the *APOL1* locus was reduced in comparison to *MYH9* (P$_{emp}<0.045$) despite impressive associations previously observed with kidney disease in African Americans [4]. These results suggest that kidney disease, in general, is a heterogeneous class of diseases, consistent with the

Table 3. Association of Candidate Diabetic Kidney Disease Loci with T2D-ESKD after Adjustment for *APOL1* G1/G2.

SNP	Position[1]	Gene	Eff[2]	RA[3]	Covariates: PC1				Covariates: PC1 and *APOL1* G1/G2			
					OR[4]	95% CI[5]	P_{Add}[6]	P_{emp}[7]	OR[4]	95% CI[5]	P_{Add}[6]	P_{emp}[7]
rs12695897	3:149927874	*AGTR1*	40	T	0.58	(0.43–0.79)	4.6E-04	0.018	0.58	(0.43–0.80)	7.9E-04	0.032
rs3793313	7:29272298	*CHN2*	194	T	1.40	(1.17–1.68)	4.6E-04	0.044	1.43	(1.18–1.72)	2.2E-04	0.043
rs17157908	7:29413882	*CHN2*	194	C	0.70	(0.57–0.86)	7.3E-04	0.14	0.66	(0.53–0.83)	2.5E-04	0.048
rs17157914	7:29414945	*CHN2*	194	A	0.69	(0.56–0.85)	4.7E-04	0.091	0.65	(0.52–0.81)	1.3E-04	0.026
rs6566815*	18:70406087	*CNDP1*	45	T	1.31	(1.14–1.51)	1.6E-04	0.076	1.32	(1.14–1.53)	2.5E-04	0.011

[1]hg18;
[2]Eff, effective number of SNPs per locus;
[3]RA, reference allele;
[4]OR, odds ratio;
[5]95% CI, 95% confidence interval;
[6]P_{Add}, additive p-value;
[7]P_{emp}, empiric p-value;
*imputed SNP.

observation of differential odds ratios (ORs) reported for *APOL1* in HIV-associated nephropathy (OR = 29), focal segmental glomerulosclerosis (FSGS; OR = 17) and hypertension-attributed end-stage kidney disease (H-ESKD; OR = 7.3) [4,9].

The most significant signal of association observed after adjustment for the *APOL1* G1/G2 variants was rs6566815 (P_{emp} = 0.011; **Table 3**) which lies 2.8 kb downstream of the *CNDP1* locus on chromosome 18. This region has been linked to DKD in multiple populations [10,11,12], and *CNDP1* was later implicated as the basis of the linkage peak [13]. In addition, a single variant on chromosomes 3 in the *AGTR1* gene was observed to be associated with T2D-ESKD (rs12695897, P_{emp} = 0.032). The angiotensin II receptor type 1 gene product is an interesting biological candidate involved in the renin-angiotensin system (reviewed in [14]). Among 98 genotyped and imputed SNPs tested (40 effective tests), only the imputed SNP rs12695897 remained nominally associated. rs12695897 was a low frequency variant (MAF = 0.05) with good imputation quality (rsq = 0.95) which would have been missed without imputation since it was omitted from current GWAS arrays. The remaining three signals that survived multiple comparisons correction and adjustment for *APOL1* were located in the *CHN2* gene. The initial variant (rs3793313) observed in the PC-adjusted analysis remained significant and two additional correlated variants (rs17157908 and rs17157914) increased in significance. This locus has been reported to be modestly associated with DKD in European-derived studies of type 1 diabetes [15] however, their seminal SNP rs39059 was not associated in our analysis (P_{emp} = 0.61).

Despite improvements in coverage afforded through imputation, this GWAS is not without limitations. A primary limitation related to study design is the inclusion of 965 T2D-ESKD cases and 1029 population-based controls. While it is possible that T2D variants would be identified, in practice this has not been the case [5,16]. This study had >80% power to detect common variants (MAF>0.10) with a detectable OR of 1.33, consistent with common disease, when considering a significance threshold of 0.05 (**Table S2**). An advantage of our study design is the focus on loci with a priori evidence of association thus limiting the need for more stringent genome-wide significance thresholds. Although this study included evaluation of putative T2D-ESKD susceptibility loci that were identified within the same dataset, the current analyses extend those findings by increasing coverage and as was observed with *CHN2*, increased the number of variants observed with association. Related to the analytical approach, the current analysis is derived from imputation using the HapMap Phase II reference panel. Recent technological advancements have lead the way for development of more superior reference panels that allow for a more comprehensive imputation of variants across the allele spectrum. As such, these additional low frequency variants may contribute to the underlying genetic architecture of disease and deserve further evaluation in larger sample sets that are more adequately powered to examine their contribution.

In conclusion, we performed a detailed genetic analysis of T2D-ESKD susceptibility genes identified from literature searches in a large African American cohort. This study demonstrates the need for more comprehensive genotyping arrays, especially in the African American population, and confirms the utility of imputation to increase coverage in existing datasets. These findings support the hypothesis that genetic variation contributes to risk of T2D-ESKD through the combined impact of multiple genetic variants contributing modest individual risk.

Methods

Ethics Statement

Recruitment and sample collection procedures were approved by the Institutional Review Board at Wake Forest School of Medicine. Written informed consent was obtained from all study participants.

Clinical Characteristics of Study Samples

This cross-sectional case-control study was designed to examine the genetics of T2D and ESKD in African Americans [5]. Patients with T2D-ESKD were recruited from dialysis facilities. T2D was diagnosed in African Americans who reported developing T2D after the age of 25 years and did not receive only insulin therapy since diagnosis. In addition, cases had at least one of the following three criteria for inclusion: a) T2D diagnosed at least 5 years before initiating renal replacement therapy, b) background or greater diabetic retinopathy by self-report and/or c) ≥100 mg/dl proteinuria on urinalysis in the absence of other causes of nephropathy. Unrelated African American controls without a current diagnosis of diabetes or renal disease were recruited from the community and internal medicine clinics. All T2D-ESKD cases and controls lacking T2D and ESKD were born in North Carolina, South Carolina, Georgia, Tennessee or Virginia. DNA extraction was performed using the PureGene system (Gentra Systems; Minneapolis, MN).

Genotyping, Imputation, and Variant Selection

As reported previously [5], genotyping was performed on the Affymetrix Genome-wide Human SNP array 6.0 (Affy6.0). Genotypes were called using Birdseed version 2; APT 1.10.0 by grouping samples by DNA plate to determine the genotype cluster boundaries. All autosomal SNPs (n = 868,157) were included in analysis. Imputation was performed for autosomes using MACH (version 1.0.16, http://www.sph.umich.edu/csg/abecasis/MaCH/). SNPs with minor allele frequency (MAF) ≥1%, call rate ≥95% and Hardy–Weinberg p-value≥10^{-4} were used for imputation. A 1:1 mixture of the HapMap II release 22 (NCBI build 36) CEU:YRI consensus haplotypes (http://mathgen.stats.ox.ac.uk/impute/) was used as a reference panel. Imputation was performed in two steps. For the first step, 484 unrelated African American samples were randomly selected to calculate recombination and error rate estimates. In the second step, these rates were used to impute all samples across the SNPs in the entire reference panel. Imputation results were filtered at an rsq threshold of ≥0.3 and a MAF ≥0.05. Adjustment for the APOL1 G1/G2 risk variants was performed by direct genotyping of two SNPs in the APOL1 G1 nephropathy risk variant (rs73885319; rs60910145) and an indel for the G2 risk variant (rs71785313) [4] on the Sequenom platform (San Diego, CA).

SNPs in twenty two genes with prior evidence of association with nephropathy were examined. These included genes located within linkage peaks from family-based linkage analysis (NPHS1/2, TRPC6 and CNDP1/2), candidate gene studies (AGTR1, NOS3, ACACB and ACTN4), gene expression studies (PLCE1), admixture mapping (APOL1 and MYH9), and GWAS (CPVL, CHN2, ELMO1, FRMD3, CARS, PVT1, and ACE) including candidates highlighted from a previous genome-wide association study (GWAS) of T2D-ESKD in this African American population [5] (i.e. RPS12, LIMK2, and SFI1). (**Table S1**).

Statistical Analysis

Principal Component Analysis (PCA). To address the effect of admixture in this African American dataset we performed a Principal Components Analysis (PCA) using all GWAS SNPs that passed quality control, excluding regions of high linkage disequilibrium (LD) and inversions. This approach was an iterative process whereby all high quality autosomal SNPs were used to calculate the top 50 principal components. Once calculated, the principal components were examined to determine if they were narrowly associated to specific regions of the genome. If so, those SNPs were excluded and the analysis repeated. The first principal component (PC1) explained the largest proportion of variation at 22% and was used as a covariate in all analyses. A direct comparison of the PCA with FRAPPE [17] analysis of 70 ancestry informative markers (AIMs; [18]) resulted in a high correlation between PC1 and the AIMs ancestry estimates, $r^2 = 0.87$. The mean (SD) African ancestry proportion in 965 T2D-ESKD cases and 1,029 controls was 0.80±0.11 and 0.78±0.11, respectively, as estimated by FRAPPE analysis. The remaining principal components explained markedly less variation and were associated with specific regions of the genome not in proximity to the candidate genes of interest; thus, not relecting either global or local ancestry [19]. Therefore, PC1 was used as a covariate in the association analyses to adjust for population substructure.

Locus-specific Analysis. Twenty-two previously reported T2D-DKD susceptibility loci were evaluated (**Table S1**). For regional analysis, each gene was defined as +/−10 kb from the longest annotated transcript. To test for an association with T2D-ESKD a logistic regression model was computed adjusting for PC1 and assuming an additive genetic model for each SNP individually using SNPGWA (www.phs.wfubmc.edu; [20]) with adjustment for PC1. In addition, variants were tested for association after adjusting for the influence of the APOL1 G1/G2 risk variants. Based on the known linkage disequilibrium pattern where G1 and G2 risk variants are very rarely observed on a single chromosome, we constructed a binary variable representing the compound G1/G2 risk across these three markers, modeling APOL1 risk for all individuals with recessive haplotypes at either G1 or G2 or heterozygosity at both G1 and G2. APOL1 has been shown to be powerfully associated with non-diabetic ESKD [4] and has been demonstrated to confound evidence of association in T2D-ESKD [21]. A Bonferroni P value (P_{emp}) <0.05 corrected for the effective number of SNPs at each locus, i.e. independent SNPs in each locus was counted using the Li and Ji method [22] implemented in Sequential Oligogenic Linkage Analysis Routines (SOLAR), was considered statistically significant. Each locus was evaluated for the effective number of SNPs under the assumption of distinct pathways ultimately contributing to the overarching disease examined herein, diabetic nephropathy.

Power. The power of the tests of association were calculated using the genetic power calculator [23]. Estimates were based on a a sample of 965 T2D-ESKD cases and 1029 controls lacking T2D and ESKD under and additive genetic model assuming and $r^2 = 1$ of the genotyped variant with the causal variant for a disease prevalence of T2D-ESKD estimated at 1% in the African American population [24].

Supporting Information

Figure S1   Regional association plots for proposed T2D-ESRD susceptibility loci.

Figure S2   LD Structure among associated T2D-ESRD susceptibility loci.

Table S1   Proposed T2D-ESRD susceptibility loci identified for follow-up study in the African American T2D-ESRD cohort.

Table S2   Power calculations for a sample of 965 T2D-ESKD cases and 1029 controls lacking T2D and ESKD under and additive genetic model assuming and $r^2 = 1$ of the genotyped variant with the causal variant for a disease prevalence of T2D-ESKD estimated at 1%.

Acknowledgments

We wish to thank the patients, their relatives and staff of the Southeastern Kidney Council, Inc./ESRD Network 6 for their participation.

Author Contributions

Conceived and designed the experiments: NDP DWB BIF. Performed the experiments: NDP PJH. Analyzed the data: MCYN PM CDL. Contributed reagents/materials/analysis tools: NDP MCYN PM CDL BIF DWB. Wrote the paper: NDP MCYN BIF DWB.

References

1. de Boer IH, Rue TC, Hall YN, Heagerty PJ, Weiss NS, et al. (2011) Temporal trends in the prevalence of diabetic kidney disease in the United States. JAMA 305: 2532–2539.

2. System URD (2010) USRDS 2010 Annual Data Report: Atlas of Chronic Kidney Disease and End-Stage Renal Disease in the United States. Bethesda, MD: US Renal Data System.

3. Palmer ND, Freedman BI (2012) Insights into the genetic architecture of diabetic nephropathy. Curr Diab Rep 12: 423–431.

4. Genovese G, Friedman DJ, Ross MD, Lecordier L, Uzureau P, et al. (2010) Association of trypanolytic ApoL1 variants with kidney disease in African Americans. Science 329: 841–845.

5. McDonough CW, Palmer ND, Hicks PJ, Roh BH, An SS, et al. (2011) A genome-wide association study for diabetic nephropathy genes in African Americans. Kidney Int 79: 563–572.

6. Wild S, Roglic G, Green A, Sicree R, King H (2004) Global prevalence of diabetes: estimates for the year 2000 and projections for 2030. Diabetes Care 27: 1047–1053.

7. (2007) Genome-wide association study of 14,000 cases of seven common diseases and 3,000 shared controls. Nature 447: 661–678.

8. Kopp JB, Smith MW, Nelson GW, Johnson RC, Freedman BI, et al. (2008) MYH9 is a major-effect risk gene for focal segmental glomerulosclerosis. Nat Genet 40: 1175–1184.

9. Kopp JB, Nelson GW, Sampath K, Johnson RC, Genovese G, et al. (2011) APOL1 genetic variants in focal segmental glomerulosclerosis and HIV-associated nephropathy. J Am Soc Nephrol 22: 2129–2137.

10. Vardarli I, Baier LJ, Hanson RL, Akkoyun I, Fischer C, et al. (2002) Gene for susceptibility to diabetic nephropathy in type 2 diabetes maps to 18q22.3-23. Kidney Int 62: 2176–2183.

11. Iyengar SK, Abboud HE, Goddard KA, Saad MF, Adler SG, et al. (2007) Genome-wide scans for diabetic nephropathy and albuminuria in multiethnic populations: the family investigation of nephropathy and diabetes (FIND). Diabetes 56: 1577–1585.

12. Bowden DW, Colicigno CJ, Langefeld CD, Sale MM, Williams A, et al. (2004) A genome scan for diabetic nephropathy in African Americans. Kidney Int 66: 1517–1526.

13. Janssen B, Hohenadel D, Brinkkoetter P, Peters V, Rind N, et al. (2005) Carnosine as a protective factor in diabetic nephropathy: association with a leucine repeat of the carnosinase gene CNDP1. Diabetes 54: 2320–2327.

14. Crowley SD, Coffman TM (2012) Recent advances involving the renin-angiotensin system. Exp Cell Res 318: 1049–1056.

15. Pezzolesi MG, Poznik GD, Mychaleckyj JC, Paterson AD, Barati MT, et al. (2009) Genome-wide association scan for diabetic nephropathy susceptibility genes in type 1 diabetes. Diabetes 58: 1403–1410.

16. Palmer ND, McDonough CW, Hicks PJ, Roh BH, Wing MR, et al. (2012) A genome-wide association search for type 2 diabetes genes in African Americans. PLoS One 7: e29202.

17. Tang H, Peng J, Wang P, Risch NJ (2005) Estimation of individual admixture: analytical and study design considerations. Genet Epidemiol 28: 289–301.

18. Keene KL, Mychaleckyj JC, Leak TS, Smith SG, Perlegas PS, et al. (2008) Exploration of the utility of ancestry informative markers for genetic association studies of African Americans with type 2 diabetes and end stage renal disease. Hum Genet 124: 147–154.

19. Patterson N, Hattangadi N, Lane B, Lohmueller KE, Hafler DA, et al. (2004) Methods for high-density admixture mapping of disease genes. Am J Hum Genet 74: 979–1000.

20. Harley JB, Alarcon-Riquelme ME, Criswell LA, Jacob CO, Kimberly RP, et al. (2008) Genome-wide association scan in women with systemic lupus erythematosus identifies susceptibility variants in ITGAM, PXK, KIAA1542 and other loci. Nat Genet 40: 204–210.

21. Freedman BI, Langefeld CD, Lu L, Divers J, Comeau ME, et al. (2011) Differential effects of MYH9 and APOL1 risk variants on FRMD3 Association with Diabetic ESRD in African Americans. PLoS Genet 7: e1002150.

22. Li J, Ji L (2005) Adjusting multiple testing in multilocus analyses using the eigenvalues of a correlation matrix. Heredity (Edinb) 95: 221–227.

23. Skol AD, Scott LJ, Abecasis GR, Boehnke M (2006) Joint analysis is more efficient than replication-based analysis for two-stage genome-wide association studies. Nat Genet 38: 209–213.

24. System USRD (2013) USRDS 2013 Annual Data Report: Atlas of Chronic Kidney Disease and End-Stage Renal Disease in the United States. Bethesda, MD: National Institutes of Health, National Institute of Diabetes and Digestive and Kidney Diseases.

19

Effects of Hemodiafiltration and High Flux Hemodialysis on Nerve Excitability in End-Stage Kidney Disease

Ria Arnold[1], Bruce A. Pussell[2,3], Timothy J. Pianta[2,3], Virginija Grinius[2], Cindy S-Y. Lin[1], Matthew C. Kiernan[3,4], James Howells[5], Meg J. Jardine[6], Arun V. Krishnan[1]*

1 Translational Neuroscience Facility, University of New South Wales, Sydney, New South Wales, Australia, 2 Department of Nephrology Prince of Wales Hospital, Sydney, New South Wales, Australia, 3 Prince of Wales Clinical School, University of New South Wales, Sydney, New South Wales, Australia, 4 Neuroscience Research Australia, Sydney, New South Wales, Australia, 5 The University of Sydney and Institute of Clinical Neurosciences, Royal Prince Alfred Hospital, Sydney, New South Wales, Australia, 6 Department of Nephrology Concord Repatriation General Hospital and The George Institute for Global Health, Sydney, New South Wales, Australia

Abstract

Objectives: Peripheral neuropathy is the most common neurological complication in end-stage kidney disease. While high flux hemodialysis (HFHD) and hemodiafiltration (HDF) have become the preferred options for extracorporeal dialysis therapy, the effects of these treatments on nerve excitability have not yet been examined.

Methods: An observational proof-of-concept study of nerve excitability and neuropathy was undertaken in an incident dialysis population (n = 17) receiving either HFHD or HDF. Nerve excitability techniques were utilised to assess nerve ion channel function and membrane potential, in conjunction with clinical assessment and standard nerve conduction studies. A mathematical model of axonal excitability was used to investigate the underlying basis of the observed changes. Nerve excitability was recorded from the median nerve, before, during and after a single dialysis session and correlated with corresponding biochemical markers. Differences in nerve excitability were compared to normal controls with longitudinal follow-up over an 18 month period.

Results: Nerve excitability was performed in patient cohorts treated with either HFHD (n = 9) or online HDF (n = 8), with similar neuropathy status. Nerve excitability measures in HDF-treated patients were significantly closer to normal values compared to HFHD patients obtained over the course of a dialysis session ($p < 0.05$). Longitudinal studies revealed stability of nerve excitability findings, and thus maintenance of improved nerve function in the HDF group.

Conclusions: This study has provided evidence that nerve excitability in HDF-treated patients is significantly closer to normal values prior to dialysis, across a single dialysis session and at longitudinal follow-up. These findings offer promise for the management of neuropathy in ESKD and should be confirmed in randomised trials.

Editor: Robert Chen, University of Toronto, Canada

Funding: RA and TP were each supported by an Australian Postgraduate Award from the University of New South Wales. AK was supported by a Career Development Award from the National Health and Medical Research Council of Australia (grant 568680). MJ was supported by a Jacquot Research Establishment Award. Grant support was provided by the National Health and Medical Research Council of Australia (grant 630425). The funders had no role in study design, data collection and analysis, decision to publish, or preparation of the manuscript.

Competing Interests: The authors have declared that no competing interests exist.

* E-mail: arun.krishnan@unsw.edu.au

Introduction

Neurological complications are a major cause of physical disability in patients with end-stage kidney disease (ESKD). Of the many neurological complications that can occur in ESKD [1], peripheral neuropathy remains the most common long-term disorder [2–4]. Clinical features of neuropathy include sensory loss, paraesthesia, impaired vibration sense, reduced deep tendon reflexes, muscle wasting and weakness [4,5]. Despite the considerable advances that have occurred in the use of renal replacement therapies (RRT), neuropathy rates remain high affecting 70 to 100% of dialysis patients [2–4,6]. Moreover, neuropathy remains essentially untreatable in the majority of ESKD patients. As such, further investigation into the most beneficial treatment for ESKD patients with neuropathy is a matter of high priority.

The two preferred options for extracorporeal dialysis therapy among renal physicians are high flux hemodialysis (HFHD) and hemodiafiltration (HDF) [7]. While recent ongoing randomized trials have thus far failed to show survival benefit with HDF treatment, there remains widespread interest in the potential clinical advantages of HDF [8,9]. HDF has been reported to achieve better clearance of "clinically relevant" middle molecules [10] and studies have suggested that on-line HDF may have a positive effect on inflammatory status [11,12], oxidative stress [13] and small solute clearance [14–16]. Previous studies have not however addressed neurological function in patients treated with online HDF and HFHD forms of RRT.

While traditional nerve conduction studies demonstrate minimal change over a dialysis session [3], nerve excitability studies have demonstrated prominent abnormalities prior to dialysis that are rapidly reversed by dialysis [17–19]. These techniques are sophisticated neurophysiological measures that provide insights into ion channel function and membrane potential in human peripheral nerves. As such, nerve excitability techniques have been widely used in clinical neurophysiological research and have proven highly sensitive to the alterations in nerve function that occur with therapeutic interventions, such as hemodialysis [17], chemotherapy administration [20] and immunological therapy [21]. The present study was undertaken to investigate whether there were differences in peripheral nerve excitability studies in patients treated with HDF and HFHD.

Methods

Ethics Statement

The studies were approved by the South East Sydney Area Health Service Human Research Ethics Committee (Northern Section) and the Human Research Ethics Committee of the University of New South Wales. Participants gave written informed consent to the procedures in accordance with the Declaration of Helsinki.

An observational, proof-of-concept, clinical study of nerve excitability and neuropathy was undertaken in an incident dialysis population at a tertiary referral centre from 2010–2012. Eligibility criteria included ESKD patients aged 18–75 years, able to give

Table 1. Patient Characteristics.

	HDF	HFHD	p
Demographics			
Age	61 (14)	62 (14)	0.87
Sex	6M : 2F	7M : 2F	
Diabetes	4Y : 4N	4Y : 5N	
Neuropathy Status			
Total Neuropathy Score	9.9 (3.5)	7.3 (2.7)	0.46
Total Neuropathy Grade	1.7 (0.5)	1.1 (0.4)	0.46
Sural Nerve Amplitude (μV)	6.7 (2.0)	7.5 (2.3)	0.61
Tibial Motor Nerve Amplitude (mV)	4.3 (3.5)	5.8 (5.1)	0.66
RRT measures			
Years on RRT	3.9 (2.4)	4.2 (2.8)	0.79
Hours on RRT (per session)	4.9 (0.5)	4.7 (0.4)	0.54
Equilibrated KT/V	1.81 (0.44)	2.28 (0.76)	0.15
Urea Reduction Ratio	0.79 (0.06)	0.81 (0.13)	0.28
Pre-RRT serum biochemistry			
Sodium (mmol/L)	138(3)	139 (2)	0.70
Potassium (mmol/L)	4.5 (0.7)	5.3 (0.8)	0.03*
Chloride (mmol/L)	100 (3.7)	103 (3.8)	0.14
Bicarbonate (mmol/L)	25.6 (2.4)	23.6 (2.1)	0.08
Serum Urea Nitrogen (mg/dL)	61.1 (30.1)	65.8 (14.0)	0.68
Creatinine (μmol/L))	807 (344)	882 (236)	0.60
Calcium (mmol/L)	2.23 (0.17)	2.27 (0.15)	0.65
Magnesium (mmol/L)	1.01 (0.13)	1.09 (0.14)	0.28
Serum Phosphorus (mmol/L)	1.36 (0.61)	1.53 (0.50)	0.52
Parathyroid hormone (ng/L)	351 (380)	261 (305)	0.56

All values given as mean (±SD). *$p<0.05$ Biochemical values all taken pre-RRT after a 56 hour inter-dialytic period.

informed consent and who were maintained on HFHD or HDF dialysis modality for a continuous period of at least 6 months. Sensory and motor nerve conduction studies, including sensory comparison studies, were undertaken in all patients to exclude the presence of carpal tunnel syndrome. Patients who had alterations in median sensory or motor conduction, suggestive of carpal tunnel syndrome, were excluded from the study. Study sample size was based on calculations of changes in threshold electrotonus parameters (α error level of 5% and a statistical power of 80%) from previous studies of nerve excitability undertaken in dialysis populations [17–19].

Clinical assessment and neurophysiological studies were undertaken in 17 ESKD patients receiving 4–6 hour, thrice-weekly RRT. Nine patients were treated with HFHD and eight with online post dilution HDF with at least 20 litres of fluid replacement. In order to minimise baseline differences, groups were matched for age, gender, disease duration, presence of diabetes and current neuropathy status. Neurophysiological tests were also undertaken in 20 age and gender matched normal subjects. The two study groups were similar in age, gender, neuropathy status, and diabetic status (Table 1). The causes of ESKD included diabetes, glomerulonephritis, lithium toxicity, amyloid, obstructive nephropathy, interstitial nephritis, reflux nephropathy and in four the cause was unknown. Longitudinal assessment of these tests was undertaken 18 months later in 13 of the 17 patients.

Enrolled patients had been maintained on their respective form of RRT consistently for the previous six months. The dialyzers used were Polyflux® 201H (surface area 2.1 m^2) with either a Gambro® 200S dialysis machine for HFHD or a Gambro® AK 200Ultra for online HDF (Gambro, Hechingen, Germany). HDF machines dialysed against ultrapure water, while HFHD used pure water and both modalities used Gambro® Select Bag AX250G dialysis concentrate containing sodium (Na$^+$) 140 mmol/L, bicarbonate 34 mmol/L, potassium (K$^+$) 2.0 mmol/L, calcium 1.5 mmol/L, magnesium 0.50 mmol/L and glucose 1.0 g/L. All patients were adequately dialysed as verified by eKT/V (>1.05) and URR (>65%) [9,22].

To ensure groups were matched for severity of pre-existing neuropathy, clinical neurological assessment was undertaken in all patients. Neuropathy was graded using a modified version of the Total Neuropathy Score [23]. This scale is a validated measure of neuropathy severity that assigns a neuropathy grade from 0 (no neuropathy) to 4 (disabling neuropathy), based on clinical features and the results of nerve conduction studies [23]. Nerve conduction studies were conducted using a Medelec Synergy system (Oxford Instruments, Abingdon, United Kingdom).

Motor nerve excitability studies were obtained from the non-fistula arm of ESKD patients before, during and after a single RRT session. All excitability recordings were conducted following a 56-hour interdialytic period. Compound muscle action potentials were recorded from the abductor pollicis brevis muscle following median nerve stimulation using previously published protocols [17,19,24]. Multiple excitability parameters were recorded, including threshold electrotonus and current threshold recordings which provide information on nodal and internodal conductances. The protocol also assessed recovery cycle parameters (refractoriness, superexcitability and late subexcitability), which provide information regarding changes in Na$^+$ and K$^+$ channel function and membrane potential [25]. Skin temperature was monitored close to the site of stimulation for the duration of the study. Serum electrolytes, urea, creatinine, calcium, magnesium, phosphate and parathyroid hormone were collected at time intervals corresponding to nerve excitability studies.

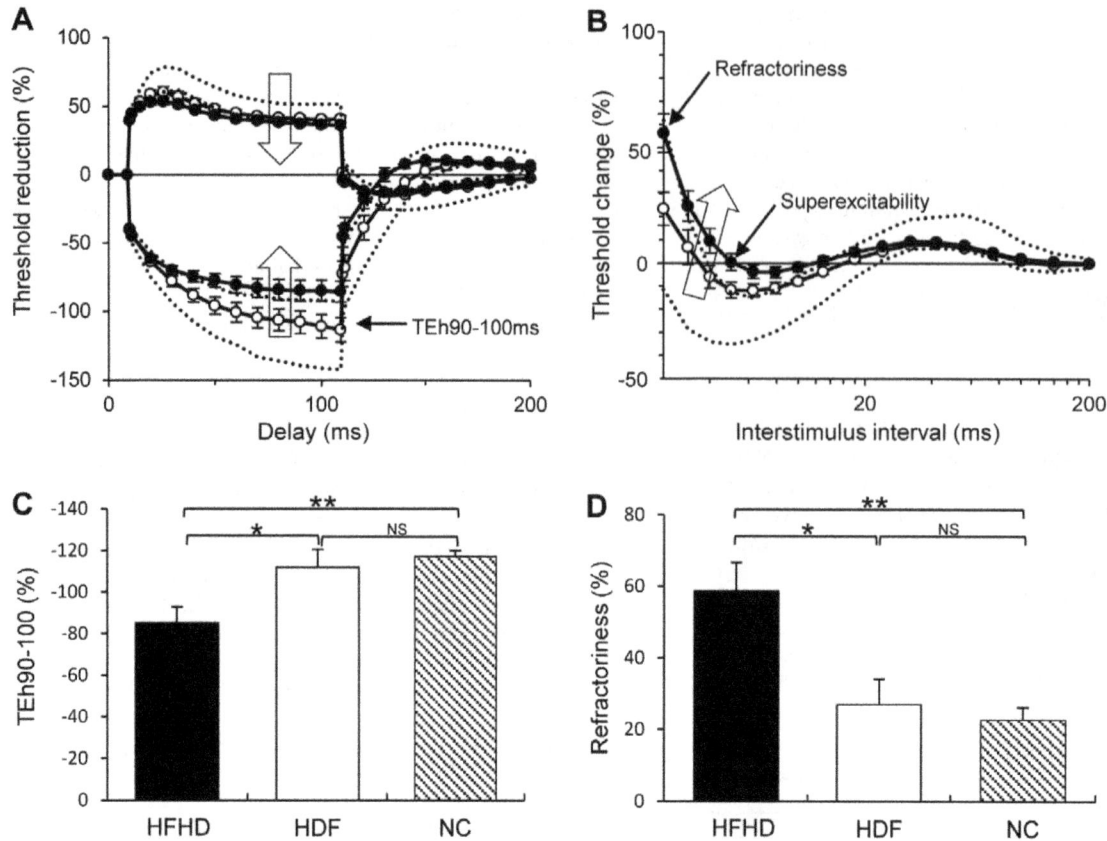

Figure 1. Pre-RRT nerve excitability recordings. Patients receiving hemodiafiltration (HDF) (empty circles) and standard high-flux HD (black filled circles) compared to 95% limits for healthy controls (dashed lines). (A) Depolarising and hyperpolarising threshold electrotonus curves. (B) Recovery cycle curve of excitability, large empty arrows indicate the direction of change with axonal depolarization. In both figures (A) and (B) the HDF group demonstrate results significantly closer to normal values than the HFHD group, specifically at hyperpolarising threshold electrotonus 90–100 ms (TEh90–100 ms), refractoriness and superexcitability. Figures (C) and (D) demonstrate the group differences in TEh90–100 ms and refractoriness in histogram format. *$p<0.05$, **$p<0.001$.

Mathematical Modelling

An established model of axonal excitability [26–30] was used to assess whether changes in extracellular K^+ concentration alone could account for the observed differences in excitability between the two groups of patients. This model consists of nodal and internodal compartments linked by a paranodal pathway through and under the myelin sheath [31]. Voltage-gated Na^+ channels (both transient and persistent), K^+ channels (slow and fast) were modelled on the nodal axolemma, while the internode incorporated both slow and fast K^+ channels and the hyperpolarization-activated cation current I_h. Separate leak conductances, Na^+/K^+-ATPase pump currents and axolemmal capacitances were modelled at both the node and internode.

Statistical Analysis

All statistical analyses were performed using IBM SPSS Statistics Package version 20 (SPSS Inc, Chicago, Illinois) with statistical significance defined as $p \le 0.05$. Clinical variables were expressed as mean±standard deviation (SD) and neurophysiological measures, figures and graphs are expressed as mean±standard error of the mean (SEM). Prior to analysis all nerve excitability data was checked for normality using Shapiro Wilks' test. Direct comparison of pre-RRT recordings with normal controls and analysis of between-group variables was undertaken using ANOVA or Kruskal-Wallis Test. To determine between group

differences post-hoc analysis was undertaken. Two-factor mixed model ANOVA analysis was used to investigate differences throughout the dialysis session recordings. Correlation analyses were used to explore relationships between potential uremic toxins and nerve excitability parameters. Longitudinal analyses were undertaken using Wilcoxon Signed Rank test and Mann-Whitney U test was used for intention to treat analyses.

Results

Clinical Findings

Table 1 demonstrates the clinical and biochemical characteristics for HDF and HFHD patient groups. There were no significant differences between the two groups for age, gender, neuropathy status, and diabetic status. Additionally, there were no significant differences between groups for years on dialysis (HDF 3.9±2.4 years; HFHD 4.2±2.8 years), dialysis duration (HDF 4.9±0.5 hours; HFHD 4.7±0.4 hours) or dialysis adequacy as measured by URR (HDF 0.79±0.06; HFHD 0.81±0.13) or eKT/V (HDF 1.81±0.44; HFHD 2.28±0.76). In keeping with previous studies, the prevalence of neuropathy in this ESKD cohort (defined as a total neuropathy score >1) [23] was ~70% [3,4,19]. The groups demonstrated similar severity of pre-existing neuropathy, with no significant baseline differences for total neuropathy score (HDF 9.9±3.5; HFHD 7.3±2.7) or total neuropathy grade (HDF 1.7±0.5; HFHD 1.1±0.4).

Table 2. Pre-RRT nerve excitability results for HDF and HFHD groups compared to controls.

	Normal controls	HDF	HFHD	ANOVA F, p
Recovery Cycle				
Refractoriness (%)	19.3 ($\pm$2.9)	27.0 ($\pm$7.2)	60.4 ($\pm$8.4)[a,b]	15.4, <0.001
Superexcitability (%)	−21.7 ($\pm$1.5)	−12.2 ($\pm$2.3)[a]	−2.0 ($\pm$2.5)[a,b]	29.0, <0.001
Threshold Electrotonus				
TEh (90–100 ms) (%)	−117 ($\pm$3)	−112 ($\pm$9)	−85 ($\pm$8)[a,b]	9.7, <0.001
TEd (10–20 ms) (%)	68.4 ($\pm$1.0)	59.6 ($\pm$3.6)[a]	53.1 ($\pm$2.4)[a]	17.7, <0.001
TEd (90–100 ms) (%)	45.4 ($\pm$0.7)	40.6 ($\pm$2.2)[a]	36.4 ($\pm$1.6)[a]	12.2, <0.001
Current Threshold				
Resting I/V slope	0.60 ($\pm$0.01)	0.67 ($\pm$0.07)	0.84 ($\pm$0.07)[a,b]	8.3, 0.001

All values given as mean ($\pm$SEM). By convention threshold electrotonus, refractoriness and superexcitability are expressed as percentage change in threshold. TEd, depolarising threshold electrotonus; TEh, hyperpolarising threshold electrotonus; I/V, current threshold. [a]Significantly different to controls, [b]significantly different to HDF.

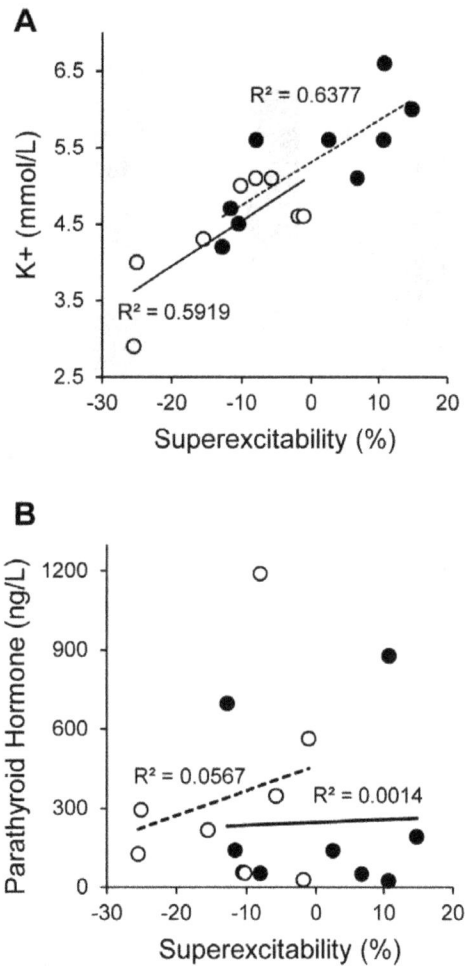

Figure 2. Relationship of pre-RRT bloods and superexcitability; a sensitive measure of membrane potential. (A) Pre-RRT serum K^+ concentrations for both HDF (empty circles) and HFHD (black filled circles) demonstrated multiple significant correlations with nerve excitability parameters including superexcitability. (B) In contrast pre-RRT serum parathyroid hormone concentrations showed no correlation.

Baseline Nerve Excitability Findings

To assess acute changes in nerve excitability across a dialysis session, recordings were conducted before, during and after a single RRT session. When compared to normal controls (NC), pre-RRT recordings in both groups demonstrated multiple abnormalities with the overall pattern of change consistent with nerve membrane depolarization (Fig. 1) [17,32], a finding that has been previously reported in studies of excitability in ESKD patients dialyzed with conventional semi-permeable membranes [17,19]. Specifically, comparison across the three groups (NC, HDF and HFHD) demonstrated significant differences for multiple nerve parameters; refractoriness, a marker of Na^+ channel inactivation [33], superexcitability, a marker of the function of fast K^+ channels [33], depolarising threshold electrotonus at the 10–20 ms interval (TEd10–20), hyperpolarising threshold electrotonus at the 90–100 ms interval (TEh90–100 ms) and resting current threshold slope (all ANOVA $p=0.001$), markers of internodal ion channel function and membrane potential [32] (Table 2). Taken together, reductions in these parameters are reflective of nerve membrane depolarization [32].

Critically, further analysis revealed that pre-RRT values in the HDF group were not significantly different to controls for several neurophysiological measures sensitive to alterations in nerve membrane potential (Fig. 1), namely refractoriness, TEh90–100 ms and resting I/V slope (Table 2). In contrast, the HFHD group demonstrated significantly impaired nerve excitability when compared to both normal controls and the HDF group. This was noted for refractoriness (NC; HFHD, $p<0.001$: HFHD; HDF, $p<0.05$), TEh90–100 ms (NC; HFHD, $p<0.001$: HFHD; HDF, $p<0.05$) and resting IV slope (NC;HFHD, $p<0.001$: HFHD; HDF, $p<0.05$) (Fig. 1, Table 2). Superexcitability demonstrated significant differences across all three groups, with a progressive worsening from normal controls to HDF to HFHD (NC

−21.7$\pm$1.5%; HDF −12.2$\pm$2.3%: HD −3.0$\pm$2.5%; $p<0.05$). While depolarising threshold electrotonus 10–20 and 90–100 ms values also demonstrated a progressive worsening from controls to HDF to HFHD, there was no significant difference between RRT modes (Table 2). Thus, in total, HDF-treated patients demonstrated improved nerve excitability following a 56 hour interdialytic period when compared to patients receiving HFHD.

In addition to the pre-RRT findings, the HDF group demonstrated significantly greater normalisation of nerve excitability when assessed across the duration of a dialysis session. While both groups demonstrated significant improvement of nerve excitability abnormalities during and post-RRT, these changes were greater in the HDF group (refractoriness, F = 4.87, $p<0.05$; superexcitability, F = 11.52, $p<0.05$; resting I/V slope, F = 5.39, $p<0.05$), compared to HFHD. This enhanced normalisation in the HDF group was further supported by significantly greater superexcitability in the HDF group when compared to the HFHD group in studies undertaken at the conclusion of RRT (HDF −23.1$\pm$2.0: HFHD −18.1$\pm$1.4; $p<0.05$).

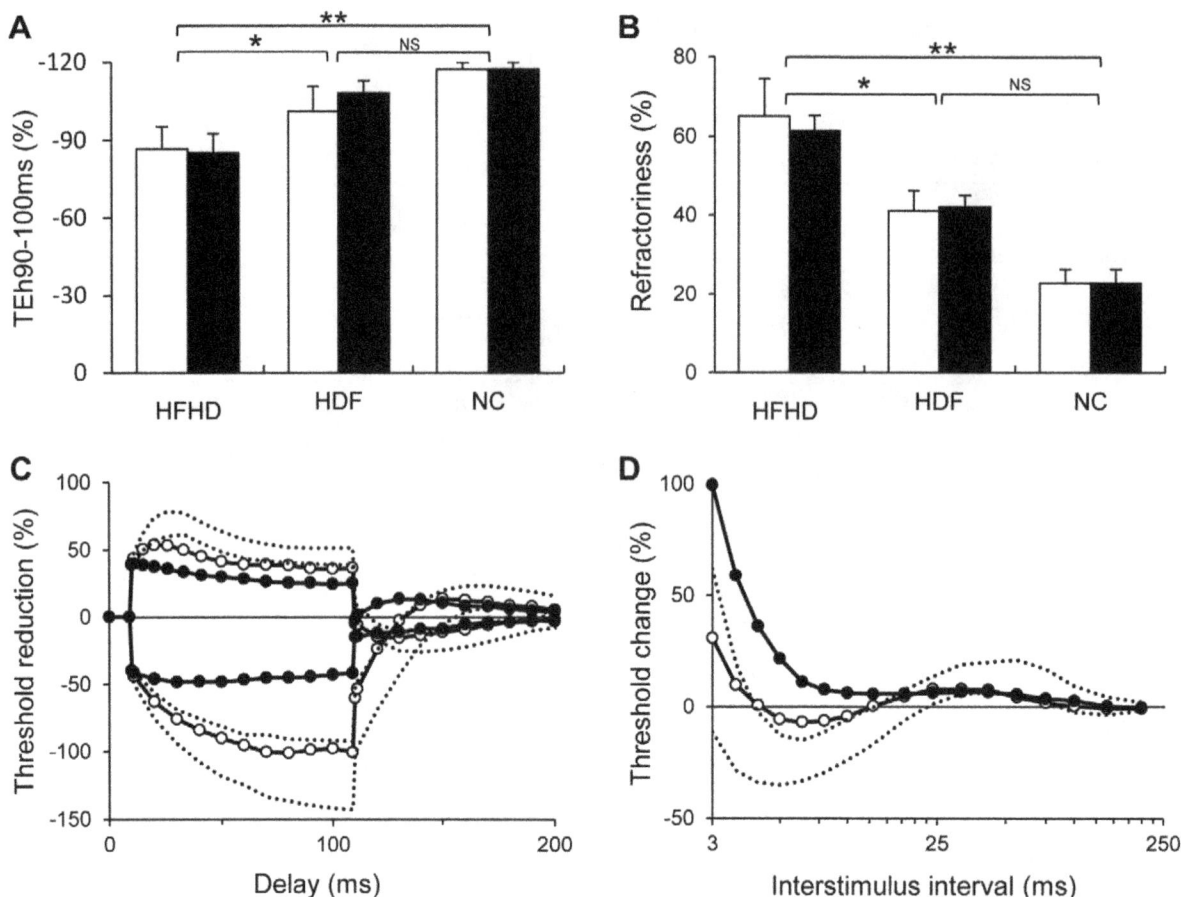

Figure 3. Longitudinal follow-up 18 months of patients who remained on their respective treatment (HDF n = 4 and HFHD n = 7).
Panels (A) and (B) demonstrate a relative stability of nerve excitability results in patients who remained on their respective treatments at baseline (white bars) and longitudinal follow-up (black bars). Additionally these graphs depict the sustained significant difference between HDF and HFHD in both hyperpolarising threshold electrotonus 90–100 ms (TEh90–100 ms) and refractoriness. *$p < 0.05$, **$p < 0.001$. Panels (C) and (D) show the results of a single patient switched from HDF to HFHD. Threshold electrotonus (C) and recovery cycle parameters (D) demonstrate the profound abnormalities at longitudinal follow-up on HFHD.

Correlation between Changes in Nerve Excitability and Levels of Uremic Toxins

Correlations were undertaken to investigate the potential relationship between changes in nerve parameters and potential neurotoxins, including small solutes and middle molecules. There were no significant correlations noted between excitability parameters and concentrations of parathyroid hormone which has previously been suggested as a possible underlying cause of nerve dysfunction in ESKD [34,35]. Pre-dialysis excitability parameters were however strongly correlated with pre-RRT serum K^+ (Fig. 2), a finding that has been demonstrated in more recent studies of nerve excitability in dialysis [17–19]. Specifically, correlations were noted between pre-RRT serum K^+ and refractoriness (HDF r = 0.76; $p < 0.05$: HFHD r = 0.69; $p < 0.05$) and superexcitability (HDF r = 0.77; $p < 0.05$: HFHD r = 0.80; $p < 0.05$). Serum K^+ also strongly correlated with several threshold electrotonus parameters including TEh90–100 (HDF r = 0.59; $p = 0.12$: HFHD r = 0.74; $p < 0.05$). Importantly, pre-RRT serum K^+ concentration was significantly different between the groups (HDF 4.5±0.7 mmol/L: HFHD 5.3±0.8 mmol/L; $p < 0.05$), a finding that was also noted on longitudinal follow-up (HDF 4.7±0.2 mmol/L: HFHD 5.6+0.6 mmol/L; $p < 0.05$). Aside from K^+, there were no significant differences between the groups for

other biochemical measures (Table 1), including urea (HDF 21.8+3.8 mmol/L; HFHD 23.5+1.7 mmol/L), creatinine (HDF 807.4±121.7 µmol/L; HFHD 882.4±78.7 µmol/L) and parathyroid hormone (HDF 351±380 ng/L; HFHD 261±305 ng/L).

Longitudinal Assessment of Nerve Excitability

Longitudinal assessments were conducted at 18 months on 13 patients. Of the four remaining patients, one received a renal transplant, two died and one declined further testing. There were no significant differences in baseline values between patients lost to follow-up those in whom longitudinal follow-up was undertaken, including serum K^+ (4.9 mmol/L: 5.1 mmol/L), TNS (5.7:9.4) and dialysis hours (4.5 hours: 4.8 hours) respectively. Of the original HDF group, four had remained on HDF while two were switched to HFHD, due to changes in equipment availability. Excitability values in both HDF and HFHD groups demonstrated no significant difference from those obtained at baseline (Fig. 3). Importantly, HDF patients maintained significant improvements in nerve excitability, when compared to the HFHD group, with pre-RRT recordings demonstrating sustained differences in superexcitability ($p < 0.05$) and TEh 90–100 ms ($p < 0.05$). When these variables were assessed using intention to treat analysis, significant differences remained between the two groups (superexcitability,

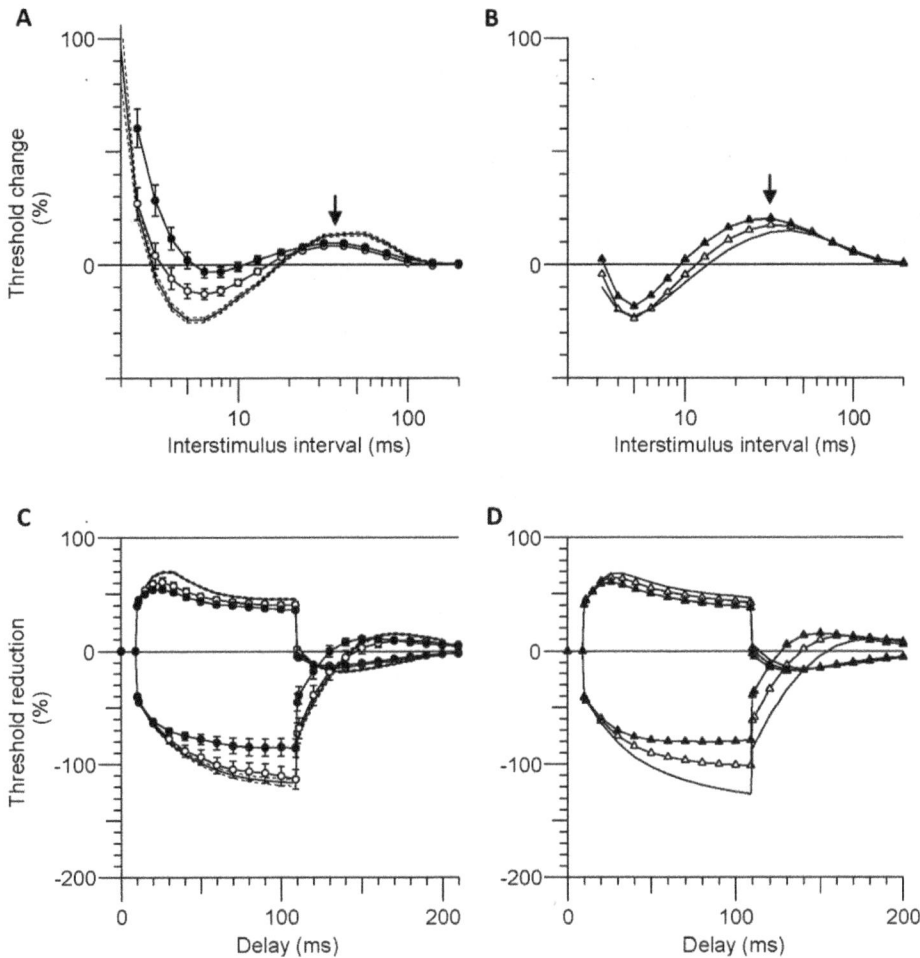

Figure 4. Mathematical model of depolarized axons. The observed excitability (mean ± SEM) is shown in panels (A) and (C) comparing HFHD patients (filled circles) and HDF (empty circles) to the healthy controls (solid and dashed lines). Panels (B) and (D) compare the modelled excitability of a healthy human motor axon (solid line) to the same model with: $[K^+]_o$ increased to 5.3 mmol/L (empty triangles); and with $[K^+]_o$ = 5.3 mmol/L and resting membrane potential further depolarized by 1 mV (filled triangles). The model provides a good fit to the changes in the threshold electrotonus data (C,D) but not the recovery cycle (A,B), particularly the extent of the changes in the refractory period, superexcitability and late subexcitability. Late subexcitability increased in the model (arrow in B) and decreased in the ESKD patients (arrow in A).

$p = 0.05$; TEh90–100, $p = 0.05$). In two patients who were changed from HDF to HFHD, deterioration in nerve excitability was noted at 18-month follow-up, with no change in lower limb motor and sensory nerve conduction amplitudes or latency (Patient #1 Sural 22.4 μV, 57 m/s vs 24.0 μV, 56 m/s and distal tibial motor amplitude 10.8 mV, 4.6 m/s vs 11.6 mV, 4.5 m/s; Patient #2 had no measurable distal tibial motor or sural response at both time points). In patient #1 (a non-diabetic), the deterioration in neurophysiological parameters was accompanied by the onset of diffuse sensory neuropathic symptoms.

Mathematical Modelling

A model of human motor axons was used to explore the underlying mechanisms for the differences between the two patient groups and the healthy controls. In the model, an increase in extracellular K^+ from 4.5 to 5.3 mmol/L alone depolarized resting membrane potential (RMP) by 2.8 mV, with the modelled changes in both threshold electrotonus and the recovery cycle consistent with depolarization (empty triangles in Fig. 4B & D). An additional 1-mV depolarization of RMP modelled threshold electrotonus better for the HFHD data (filled triangles in

Fig. 4D). Pure depolarization of RMP however increased late subexcitability, in agreement with the findings of Kiernan and Bostock [2000] [32]. However in the ESKD patients subexcitability was decreased, and there were smaller changes in the other recovery cycle measures (compare arrows in Fig. 4B & A; see discussion).

Discussion

The present study investigated the effects of HDF and HFHD on peripheral nerve excitability in incident ESKD patients. The study has demonstrated that neurophysiological measures of nerve function, specifically those sensitive to changes in nerve membrane potential, were significantly closer to normal in patients receiving HDF compared to the HFHD group. Furthermore, patients who remained on HDF maintained a more normal study profile compared to those on HFHD at long-term follow-up.

Overall, the pattern of change in excitability measures was consistent with nerve membrane depolarisation [32], an abnormality that has been demonstrated in previous studies of ESKD patients, undertaken during the era of conventional semi-permeable membranes [17–19]. Greater normality of nerve excitability results was noted in pre-RRT recordings and following a single RRT session in the HDF group, suggesting that HDF may achieve greater clearance of neurotoxic substances.

The implications of these findings are significant as maintenance of nerve membrane potential is essential for normal biochemical homeostasis and therefore axonal survival. [36,37]. Chronic changes in neural excitability over time may trigger a cascade of events leading to axonal degeneration and development of symptoms of clinical neuropathy, such as numbness and muscle weakness, major causes of disability in ESKD [38]. Moreover, previous studies have demonstrated a direct relationship between neuropathic symptoms and pre-RRT excitability values [18]. The limitations of this study, including the small samples size and the largely cross-sectional nature of the data, suggest that longitudinal studies investigating the effects of nerve excitability changes and dialysis mode on the development of neuropathy are required.

While the HDF group demonstrated greater normality of nerve excitability, the underlying basis for this remains unclear. A potential explanation for the differential effects of HDF and HFHD on nerve excitability relates to the correlation that was noted between parameters of nerve excitability and serum K^+ concentration. This correlation is consistent with the findings of recent studies that have suggested that hyperkalaemia may play an important role in the development of neuropathy in ESKD [17–19,39]. Despite these lines of evidence, a causal relationship between elevated serum K^+ concentration and neurological dysfunction has not yet been established. Moreover, mathematical modelling of data in the present study suggested that while changes in serum K^+ may have played a role in the development of the abnormalities, the changes in excitability in the HFHD group were not explicable solely by increased K^+ concentration. In particular, the significantly reduced super- and late sub- excitability in the ESKD patients may be due to a smaller time-integral of the action current, possibly a consequence of smaller Na^+ currents [27,30].

Given that both HDF and HFHD treatments in this study used the same membrane (Polyflux® 201H), dialysate flow rate (Q_D 500 mL/min) and dialysate concentrations of K^+, Na^+, bicarbonate, calcium, magnesium and glucose, another potential explanation for the differences may relate to the dilutional effects of hemofiltration. The ultrafiltration setting in HDF allows for greater hemofiltration to occur in addition to the hemodialysis component. HDF is achieved with inline fluid replacement and ultrafiltration (UF) of 60 mL/min compared to UF of 0 mL/min for HFHD. Backfiltration of up to 10 litres can be achieved with HFHD whereas the hemofiltration in HDF delivers an average of 20 litres of inline fluid re-infused, which possibly contributes to a dilutional effect on overall clearances.

While previous studies have emphasised the role of middle molecules as a cause of nerve dysfunction in ESKD [40,41], there was no significant correlation between PTH, a middle molecule assayed in this study, and pre-RRT measures of nerve excitability. However, while K^+ was closely related to pre-RRT excitability differences, it cannot explain the during and post-RRT differences between groups. Furthermore, mathematical modelling demonstrated that an additional 1 mV depolarization was required to better model the threshold electrotonus data obtained in HFHD patients, suggesting that a synergistic effect of another neurotoxin may be required to induce nerve dysfunction in ESKD, a view that has been supported by previous neurophysiological studies [19,42]. Given the known superiority of HDF in terms of middle molecule clearance and inflammatory status [12–15], future studies may need to explore a wider range of middle molecules and inflammatory mediators as potential contributors to nerve dysfunction in ESKD patients.

In conclusion, the present study provides evidence that ESKD patients treated with HDF demonstrate more normal nerve excitability both prior to RRT, across a single RRT session and at long-term follow-up compared to HFHD. These results suggest that HDF may help maintain normal nerve excitability in ESKD. The use of HDF for the clinical management of neuropathy in ESKD should be investigated further in large scale randomised trials.

Author Contributions

Contributed to revising the article and approving final version: AK BP VG CL MCK MJJ TJP JH. Conceived and designed the experiments: RA AK BP MK. Performed the experiments: RA VG. Analyzed the data: RA AK CL TJP MCK MJJ JH. Wrote the paper: RA AK BP JH.

References

1. Krishnan AV, Kiernan MC (2009) Neurological complications of chronic kidney disease. Nat Rev Neurol 5: 542–551.
2. Van den Neucker K, Vanderstraeten G, Vanholder R (1998) Peripheral motor and sensory nerve conduction studies in haemodialysis patients. A study of 54 patients. Electromyogr Clin Neurophysiol 38: 467–474.
3. Laaksonen S, Metsarinne K, Voipio-Pulkki LM, Falck B (2002) Neurophysiologic parameters and symptoms in chronic renal failure. Muscle Nerve 25: 884–890.
4. Hojs-Fabjan T, Hojs R (2006) Polyneuropathy in hemodialysis patients: the most sensitive electrophysiological parameters and dialysis adequacy. Wien Klin Wochenschr 118 Suppl 2: 29–34.
5. Krishnan AV, Kiernan MC (2007) Uremic neuropathy: clinical features and new pathophysiological insights. Muscle Nerve 35: 273–290.
6. Tilki HE, Akpolat T, Coskun M, Stalberg E (2009) Clinical and electrophysiologic findings in dialysis patients. J Electromyogr Kinesiol 19: 500–508.
7. Ledebo I, Ronco C (2008) The best dialysis therapy? Results from an international survey among nephrology professionals. NDT Plus 1: 403–408.
8. Canaud B, Bragg-Gresham JL, Marshall MR, Desmeules S, Gillespie BW, et al. (2006) Mortality risk for patients receiving hemodiafiltration versus hemodialysis: European results from the DOPPS. Kidney Int 69: 2087–2093.
9. Eknoyan G, Beck GJ, Cheung AK, Daugirdas JT, Greene T, et al. (2002) Effect of dialysis dose and membrane flux in maintenance hemodialysis. N Engl J Med 347: 2010–2019.
10. Cheung AK, Rocco MV, Yan G, Leypoldt JK, Levin NW, et al. (2006) Serum beta-2 microglobulin levels predict mortality in dialysis patients: results of the HEMO study. J Am Soc Nephrol 17: 546–555.
11. Guth HJ, Gruska S, Kraatz G (2003) On-line production of ultrapure substitution fluid reduces TNF-alpha- and IL-6 release in patients on hemodiafiltration therapy. Int J Artif Organs 26: 181–187.
12. Carracedo J, Merino A, Nogueras S, Carretero D, Berdud I, et al. (2006) On-line hemodiafiltration reduces the proinflammatory CD14+CD16+ monocyte-derived dendritic cells: A prospective, crossover study. J Am Soc Nephrol 17: 2315–2321.
13. Filiopoulos V, Hadjiyannakos D, Metaxaki P, Sideris V, Takouli L, et al. (2008) Inflammation and oxidative stress in patients on hemodiafiltration. Am J Nephrol 28: 949–957.
14. Ward RA, Schmidt B, Hullin J, Hillebrand GF, Samtleben W (2000) A comparison of on-line hemodiafiltration and high-flux hemodialysis: a prospective clinical study. J Am Soc Nephrol 11: 2344–2350.
15. Schiffl H (2007) Prospective randomized cross-over long-term comparison of online haemodiafiltration and ultrapure high-flux haemodialysis. Eur J Med Res 12: 26–33.
16. Lin CL, Yang CW, Chiang CC, Chang CT, Huang CC (2001) Long-term on-line hemodiafiltration reduces predialysis beta-2-microglobulin levels in chronic hemodialysis patients. Blood Purif 19: 301–307.
17. Kiernan MC, Walters RJL, Andersen KV, Taube D, Murray NMF, et al. (2002) Nerve excitability changes in chronic renal failure indicate membrane depolarization due to hyperkalaemia. Brain 125: 1366–1378.
18. Krishnan AV, Phoon RK, Pussell BA, Charlesworth JA, Kiernan MC (2006) Sensory nerve excitability and neuropathy in end stage kidney disease. J Neurol Neurosurg Psychiatry 77: 548–551.
19. Krishnan AV, Phoon RK, Pussell BA, Charlesworth JA, Bostock H, et al. (2005) Altered motor nerve excitability in end-stage kidney disease. Brain 128: 2164–2174.

20. Park SB, Goldstein D, Lin CS, Krishnan AV, Friedlander ML, et al. (2009) Acute abnormalities of sensory nerve function associated with oxaliplatin-induced neurotoxicity. J Clin Oncol 27: 1243–1249.

21. Lin CS, Krishnan AV, Park SB, Kiernan MC (2011) Modulatory effects on axonal function after intravenous immunoglobulin therapy in chronic inflammatory demyelinating polyneuropathy. Arch Neurol 68: 862–869.

22. Daugirdas JT, Depner TA, Gotch FA, Greene T, Keshaviah P, et al. (1997) Comparison of methods to predict equilibrated Kt/V in the HEMO Pilot Study. Kidney Int 52: 1395–1405.

23. Cornblath DR, Chaudhry V, Carter K, Lee D, Seysedadr M, et al. (1999) Total neuropathy score: validation and reliability study. Neurology 53: 1660–1664.

24. Kiernan MC, Burke D, Andersen KV, Bostock H (2000) Multiple measures of axonal excitability: a new approach in clinical testing. Muscle Nerve 23: 399–409.

25. Krishnan AV, Lin CS, Park SB, Kiernan MC (2008) Assessment of nerve excitability in toxic and metabolic neuropathies. J Peripher Nerv Syst 13: 7–26.

26. Bostock H, Baker M, Reid G (1991) Changes in excitability of human motor axons underlying post-ischaemic fasciculations: evidence for two stable states. J Physiol 441: 537–557.

27. Kiernan MC, Isbister GK, Lin CS, Burke D, Bostock H (2005) Acute tetrodotoxin-induced neurotoxicity after ingestion of puffer fish. Ann Neurol 57: 339–348.

28. Jankelowitz SK, Howells J, Burke D (2007) Plasticity of inwardly rectifying conductances following a corticospinal lesion in human subjects. J Physiol (Lond) 581: 927–940.

29. Lin CS, Krishnan AV, Lee M-J, Zagami AS, You H-L, et al. (2008) Nerve function and dysfunction in acute intermittent porphyria. Brain 131: 2510–2519.

30. Howells J, Trevillion L, Bostock H, Burke D (2012) The voltage dependence of I(h) in human myelinated axons. J Physiol (Lond) 590: 1625–1640.

31. Barrett EF, Barrett JN (1982) Intracellular recording from vertebrate myelinated axons: mechanism of the depolarizing afterpotential. J Physiol 323: 117–144.

32. Kiernan MC, Bostock H (2000) Effects of membrane polarization and ischaemia on the excitability properties of human motor axons. Brain 123 Pt 12: 2542–2551.

33. Burke D (1993) Microneurography, impulse conduction, and paresthesias. Muscle Nerve 16: 1025–1032.

34. Goldstein DA, Chui LA, Massry SG (1978) Effect of parathyroid hormone and uremia on peripheral nerve calcium and motor nerve conduction velocity. J Clin Invest 62: 88–93.

35. Slatopolsky E, Martin K, Hruska K (1980) Parathyroid hormone metabolism and its potential as a uremic toxin. Am J Physiol 239: F1–12.

36. Vogel W, Schwarz JR (1995) Voltage-clamp studies on axons: macroscopic and single-channel currents. In: Waxman SG, Kocsis JD, Stys PK, editors. The axon: Oxford University Press.

37. Lehning EJ, Doshi R, Isaksson N, Stys PK, LoPachin RM Jr (1996) Mechanisms of injury-induced calcium entry into peripheral nerve myelinated axons: role of reverse sodium-calcium exchange. J Neurochem 66: 493–500.

38. Stys PK (2005) General mechanisms of axonal damage and its prevention. J Neurol Sci 233: 3–13.

39. Bostock H, Walters RJ, Andersen KV, Murray NM, Taube D, et al. (2004) Has potassium been prematurely discarded as a contributing factor to the development of uraemic neuropathy? Nephrol Dial Transplant 19: 1054–1057.

40. Malberti F, Surian M, Farina M, Vitelli E, Mandolfo S, et al. (1991) Effect of hemodialysis and hemodiafiltration on uremic neuropathy. Blood Purif 9: 285–295.

41. Babb AL, Ahmad S, Bergstrom J, Scribner BH (1981) The middle molecule hypothesis in perspective. Am J Kidney Dis 1: 46–50.

42. Krishnan AV, Phoon RK, Pussell BA, Charlesworth JA, Bostock H, et al. (2006) Ischaemia induces paradoxical changes in axonal excitability in end-stage kidney disease. Brain 129: 1585–1592.

20

Should We Still Focus that much on Cardiovascular Mortality in End Stage Renal Disease Patients? The CONvective TRAnsport STudy

Claire H. den Hoedt[1,2], Michiel L. Bots[3]*, Muriel P. C. Grooteman[4,5], Albert H. A. Mazairac[2], E. Lars Penne[4], Neelke C. van der Weerd[4], Piet M. ter Wee[4,5], Menso J. Nubé[4,5], Renée Levesque[6], Peter J. Blankestijn[2], Marinus A. van den Dorpel[1], for the CONTRAST investigators[¶]

1 Department of Internal Medicine, Maasstad Hospital, Rotterdam, The Netherlands, 2 Department of Nephrology, UMC Utrecht, Utrecht, The Netherlands, 3 Julius Center for Health Sciences and Primary Care, UMC Utrecht, Utrecht, The Netherlands, 4 Department of Nephrology, VU Medical Center, Amsterdam, The Netherlands, 5 Institute for Cardiovascular Research VU Medical Center (ICaR-VU), VU Medical Center, Amsterdam, The Netherlands, 6 Department of Nephrology, Centre Hospitalier de l'Université de Montréal, St-Luc Hospital, Montréal, Canada

Abstract

Background: We studied the distribution of causes of death in the CONTRAST cohort and compared the proportion of cardiovascular deaths with other populations to answer the question whether cardiovascular mortality is still the principal cause of death in end stage renal disease. In addition, we compared patients who died from the three most common death causes. Finally, we aimed to study factors related to dialysis withdrawal.

Methods: We used data from CONTRAST, a randomized controlled trial in 714 chronic hemodialysis patients comparing the effects of online hemodiafiltration versus low-flux hemodialysis. Causes of death were adjudicated. The distribution of causes of death was compared to that of the Dutch dialysis registry and of the Dutch general population.

Results: In CONTRAST, 231 patients died on treatment. 32% died from cardiovascular disease, 22% due to infection and 23% because of dialysis withdrawal. These proportions were similar to those in the Dutch dialysis registry and the proportional cardiovascular mortality was similar to that of the Dutch general population. cardiovascular death was more common in patients <60 years. Patients who withdrew were older, had more co-morbidity and a lower mental quality of life at baseline. Patients who withdrew had much co-morbidity. 46% died within 5 days after the last dialysis session.

Conclusions: Although the absolute risk of death is much higher, the proportion of cardiovascular deaths in a prevalent end stage renal disease population is similar to that of the general population. In older hemodialysis patients cardiovascular and non-cardiovascular death risk are equally important. Particularly the registration of dialysis withdrawal deserves attention. These findings may be partly limited to the Dutch population.

Editor: Utpal Sen, University of Louisville, United States of America

Funding: CONTRAST is financially supported by a grant from the Dutch Kidney Foundation (Nierstichting Nederland, grant C02.2019) and unrestricted grants from Fresenius Medical Care (The Netherlands) and Gambro Lundia AB (Sweden). Additional support was received from the Dr. E.E. Twiss Fund, Roche Netherlands; the International Society of Nephrology/Baxter Extramural Grant Program; the Dutch Organization for Health Research and Development (ZonMW, grant 17088.2802). The funders had no role in study design, data collection and analysis, decision to publish, or preparation of the manuscript.

Competing Interests: CH den Hoedt, ML Bots, NC van der Weerd, EL Penne and AHA Mazairac report receiving no lecture fees, no consulting support, or grant support. MPC Grooteman reports research funded by Fresenius, Gambro and Baxter. PJ Blankestijn reports research funded by Fresenius, Gambro, Roche, Amgen and Novartis, consultant fee and honoraria for lectures from Fresenius, Gambro, Solvay, Medtronic and Novartis. R Lévesque reports research funded by Amgen Canada. PM ter Wee reports research funded by Abbott, Baxter, Gambro, Fresenius and Roche; honoraria for lectures received from Amgen, Roche, Genzyme, Fresenius. MJ Nubé reports research funded by Baxter and Fresenius; honoraria for lectures received from Fresenius and Baxter. MA van den Dorpel reports research funded by Amgen. Furthermore, this does not alter the authors' adherence to all the PLOS ONE policies on sharing data and materials.

* E-mail: m.l.bots@umcutrecht.nl

¶ Membership of the CONTRAST investigators is provided in Appendix S1.

Introduction

End-stage renal disease (ESRD) patients have a high cardiovascular (CV) mortality rate, which is substantially higher compared to the general population, especially in young subjects[1;2]. The United States (US) renal data system registry reports 43% of deaths to be cardiovascular [3]. However, mortality patterns differ considerably between ESRD patients from the US, Europe and Asia [4]. Differences in patients who start with dialysis, in selection of patients for transplantation and peritoneal dialysis (PD) and in life expectancy between the areas greatly affect mortality rates and cause specific mortality distribution [4]. In the Dutch CONvective TRAnsport STudy (CONTRAST) we found an incidence of CV mortality of 34/1000 person years in the patients treated with online hemodiafiltration (HDF) and 42/1000 person years in the patients treated with low-flux hemodialysis (HD) [5]. Whereas the US HEMO study reported 66 cardiac deaths per 1000 patients years [6] and the ERA-EDTA reported a unstandardized CV mortality rate of 74.9 CV deaths per 1000 persons years for the period 1994–2004 in European patients [7]. The latter study showed that patients starting dialysis have a generally increased risk of death that is not specifically caused by excess CV mortality [7].

The first objective of the present analysis was to compare the distribution of death causes, in particular CV deaths, in the CONTRAST cohort to the Dutch HD population and to the Dutch general population. The second objective was to study potential differences in risk factors between those who died from cardiovascular disease (CVD), from infections or from dialysis withdrawal. The third objective was to assess factors related to dialysis withdrawal.

Methods

Study design and methods of CONTRAST have been published before [5;8]. In short, CONTRAST was a randomized controlled trial comparing effects of online HDF versus low-flux HD on all-cause mortality and CV morbidity and mortality. Patients with end-stage renal disease undergoing chronic intermittent HD for at least two months and aged 18 years or above were enrolled from June 2004 until January 2010 in twenty-nine dialysis centers in The Netherlands (n = 26), Canada (n = 2), and Norway (n = 1). Patients were eligible for inclusion if they were treated two or three times per week with low-flux HD. Exclusion criteria were: treatment with hemo(dia)filtration or high-flux HD in the six months preceding randomization, a life expectancy less than three months due to non-renal disease, participation in another clinical intervention trial evaluating cardiovascular outcomes and severe non-adherence regarding frequency and/or duration of dialysis treatment.

The study was conducted in accordance with the Declaration of Helsinki and approved by the medical ethics review boards of all participating hospitals. Written informed consent was obtained from all patients prior to enrolment.

Dialysis Procedures

Online HDF was performed in the post-dilution mode, with synthetic high-flux dialyzers [5]. HD patients were treated with synthetic low-flux dialyzers. All patients were treated with ultrapure dialysis fluids, defined as less than 0.1 colony forming units per mL and less than 0.03 endotoxin units per mL. Routine patient care was performed according to national and international Quality of Care Guidelines.

Data Collection

Standardized forms were used to collect demographical, clinical and laboratory data. Type of vascular access, duration of dialysis (dialysis vintage), medical history (presence of diabetes mellitus (DM) and previous CVD), were recorded. CVD was defined as previous stroke or transient ischemic attack, peripheral vascular disease and/or coronary heart disease (CHD), including history of angina pectoris, myocardial infarction or prior coronary revascularization. Dialysis vintage was determined as the sum of time patients were treated with HD or PD before inclusion. At each three monthly visit, occurrence of clinical events was recorded. Routine blood samples were drawn prior to dialysis. Patients with a urinary production of less than 100 mL per day were considered anuric.

Health Related Quality of Life 36 (SF-36)

Health related quality of life (HRQOL) was assessed with the validated KDQOL-SF version 1.3 (http://www.rand.org/health/surveys_ tools/kdqol.html) [9;10], which contains the SF-36 version 1 [11]. The eight domains of the SF-36 were summarized into a physical functioning (Physical Component Summary – PCS) and a mental functioning (Mental Component Summary – MCS) score. These summaries are constructed so that a score of 50 represents the mean of the general United States population with a standard deviation of 10 [12]. A difference of 3 points in the summary score has been proposed to be clinically relevant [11;12].

Laboratory Measurements

Routine measurements were done in the participating hospitals using standard techniques. Serum albumin was measured in local hospitals with the bromcresol green method or bromcresol purple method and samples that were measured with the bromcresol purple method were converted to bromcresol green concentrations with the formula: bromcresol green = bromcresol purple+5.5 [13]. Inflammatory markers from 405 patients were measured centrally. hsCRP (mg/L) was measured with a particle-enhanced immuno-turbidimetric assay on a Roche-Hitachi analyzer (Roche Diagnostics GmbH, Mannheim, Germany), with a lower quantification limit of 0.1 mg/L. IL-6 (pg/mL) was measured with an ELISA (Sanquin, Amsterdam, The Netherlands), with a lower quantification limit of 0.35 pg/mL.

Outcome

Cardiovascular deaths were defined as death from CV causes, which included myocardial infarction, ischemic or haemorrhagic stroke, sudden death (unexpected death within an hour of symptom onset or unwitnessed, unexpected death without obvious non-cardiac cause in patients known to be well within the past 24 hours), heart failure or other CV causes. Non-CV causes were defined as death from infections, cancer, dialysis withdrawal, unnatural deaths and other non CV causes, such as gastrointestinal haemorrhage or respiratory insufficiency. If no documentation on the event was available, death was categorized as unknown cause. An independent Endpoint Adjudication Committee reviewed source documentation (mostly discharge letters from admissions to the hospital) for all deaths, to adjudicate the cause of death using their clinical experience. Each case was reviewed by three or, if necessary, four medical doctors and the cause of death was defined when two doctors agreed. We made no priory definition to adjudicate deaths as 'dialysis withdrawal'. For patients whose cause of death was adjudicated as dialysis withdrawal, we retrieved source documentation and explored circumstances and the interval between dialysis withdrawal and death.

The present analyses were restricted to patients who died either during treatment with HD or HDF or who died within 28 days after censoring due to transplantation, switch to PD, switch to other hospital or stopping because of other reasons. The survivor group consisted of patients who remained on HD or HDF during the study up to the end of follow-up, or up to censoring.

Comparison CONTRAST with Other Registries

Renine. Renine is the nation-wide Dutch registry for HD patients with a 100% coverage [14]. We used data from the year 2008, because patients in CONTRAST were included between 2004–2010. Cause of death was coded using the ERA-EDTA codes [15]. Code 11 denotes acute myocardial infarction, code 22 strokes and codes 12 and 15 sudden death. Codes 14, 16 and 18 denote heart failure and codes 13, 26 and 29 other CV causes. We used code 30–39 for infections, code 66 and 67 for cancer and code 51, 53 and 61 for withdrawal from HD. Code 17, 21, 23–25, 27–28, 41–44, 46, 62–64, 69–73, 90 and 102 were categorized as other non CV death. Code 52 and 80–82 were categorized as unnatural event and code 99 and 0 and 'cause of death not yet registered' were classified as unknown cause of death.

General population of the Netherlands. Causes of death of the general population were obtained at the central office of statistics of the Netherlands [16]. Eurostat ICD codes were used to classify causes of death in 2008 [17]. To determine the number of deaths from a CVD cause we used the number from 'total deaths from CV diseases' (ICD-10 I00-I99) minus the numbers of deaths caused by pulmonary embolism or other diseases of pulmonary origin (I26–28), or by infectious causes of heart disease, such as endocarditis (I33, 38–41), or by diseases from veins, arterioles, capillaries and lymph vessels I78–89 and by hypotension (I95).

Data Analysis

Comparison CONTRAST with the Dutch general population. We multiplied the 5 year age and sex specific mortality rates from the Dutch population with the age and sex specific number of person years in CONTRAST to obtain an estimate of the number of CV deaths and total deaths expected, had the Dutch mortality rate be applicable for CONTRAST. Next we summed the age and sex specific expected numbers of death to obtain an overall number of CV and total deaths. Next, the proportion of expected CV death/total expected death was estimated to come up with a proportion CV death in CONTRAST, had the general population mortality rates been applicable for the CONTRAST population.

Baseline characteristics of patients in CONTRAST by cause of death. To compare the baseline characteristics of the patients by cause of death, we ran multivariable regression models, adjusted for age and sex. To compare medication use between the different causes of death, we additionally adjusted for history of CVD. We performed Chi square test to explore differences in causes of death by the age groups younger than 60, 60–75 and older than 75 years. Two sided P-values below 0.05 were considered statistically significant. These analyses were conducted with SPSS software (version 18.0; SPSS Inc. Headquarters, Chicago, Illinois, US).

Results

Baseline characteristics are given in Table 1.

Causes of Death in CONTRAST

Two hundred thirty one patients died. Seventy-four patients (32%) died from CV causes and 142 patients (62%) died from non CV causes. Infections (22% of all deaths) and dialysis withdrawal (23% of all deaths) were the main non CV causes of death. In 7% of cases the cause of death was unknown (Table 2).

Death Causes in Renine

Renine comprised 4921 patients at the first of January 2008, with a mean age of 64.4 years and 59.7% men. 27% of deaths was of CV origin. Sudden death was the cause of death in 9% of cases. Sixteen percent of patients died from an infection and 19% withdrew from dialysis treatment. In 25% the death cause was unknown (Table 2).

Table 1. Baseline characteristics of the CONTRAST participants.

Variable	CONTRAST participants = 714
Age (years)	64.1±13.7
Male sex - no. (%)	445 (62)
Region	
- Netherlands – no. (%)	597 (84)
- Canada- no. (%)	102 (14)
- Norway – no. (%)	15 (14)
History of cardiovascular disease – no. (%)	313 (44)
Diabetes mellitus – no. (%)	170 (24)
Dialysis vintage (years)	2 (1–4)
Systolic blood pressure (mmHg)~	147±21
Diastolic blood pressure (mmHg)~	75±12
Body weight (kg)	72.4±14.4
BMI after dialysis (kg/m^2)	25.4±4.8
Residual kidney function – no. (%)*	376 (53)
eGFR (ml/min/1.73 m^2)	3.2 (1.3–5.5)
Treatment frequency	
3x/week – no. (%)	668 (94)
–2x/week – no. (%)	44 (6)
Duration of a dialysis session – min	226±23
Bloodflow (mL/min)	308±39
Dialysis access – no. (%)	
-Fistula	567 (80)
-Graft	100 (14)
-Central catheter	47 (6)
spKt/V$_{urea}$	1.40±0.22
Hemoglobin (mmol/L)	7.3±0.78
Phosphorus – mmol/L	1.64±0.49
Beta-2-microglobulin – mg/L	31.5±14
Albumin (g/L)^	40.4±3.8
Creatinine (μmol/L), pre-dialysis	861±255
C-reactive protein mg/L (n = 405)	3.9 (1.4–10.4)
Interleukin-6 pg/mL (n = 403)	2.1 (1.2–3.8)
Quality of life	
Physical Composite score	39±11
Mental Composite score	50±12
Prescribed medication – no. of patients(%)	
Beta blocker	53
Alfa blocker	10
RAAS inhibitor	49
Statin	51
Platelet aggregation inhibitor	31

Values are means ±SD, median (interquartile range) or number (percentage).
~pre-dialysis.
*residual kidney function if diuresis >100 ml/24 h.
^albumin concentrations measured with the bromcresolpurple method have been converted to the bromcresolgreen method.
eGFR = estimated glomerular filtration rate; RAAS = renine angiontensin aldosterone system.
To convert hemoglobin in mmol/L to g/dL divide by 0.62; phosphorus in mmol/L to mg/dL, divide by 0.323; albumin in g/L to g/dL, divide by 10; creatinine in μmol/L to mg/dL divide by 88.4.

Table 2. Causes of death in CONTRAST and Renine.

Cause of Death	CONTRAST deaths			Renine deaths of 2008[¥]		
Cardiovascular	n	%	95% CI of %	n	%	95% CI of %
Acute Myocardial Infarction	8	3.5	(1.1–5.8)	73	6.5	(5.0–7.9)
Cerebrovascular Accident[^]	6	2.6	(0.5–4.6)	41	3.6	(2.5–4.7)
Sudden death	37	16.0	(11.3–20.7)	105	9.3	(7.6–11.0)
Heart failure	11	4.8	(2.0–7.5)	62	5.5	(4.2–6.8)
Other cardiovascular	12	5.2	(2.3–8.1)	27	2.4	(1.5–3.3)
Total cardiovascular	**74**	**32.0**	**(26.0–38.0)**	**308**	**27.2**	**(24.6–29.8)**
Non cardiovascular						
Infection	51	22.1	(16.7–27.4)	180	15.9	(13.8–18.0)
Cancer	14	6.1	(3.0–9.1)	81	7.2	(5.7–8.7)
Unnatural death	3	1.3	(0–2.8)	8	0.7	(0.2–1.2)
Dialysis withdrawal	54	23.4	(17.9–28.8)	217	19.2	(16.9–21.5)
Other non cardiovascular	20	8.7	(5.0–12.3)	59	5.2	(3.9–6.5)
Total non cardiovascular	**142**	**61.5**	**(55.2–67.7)**	**545**	**51.0**	**(45.2–51.1)**
Unknown	15	6.5	(3.3–9.7)	247	21.8	(19.4–24.2)
Miscellaneous	n.a.	n.a.	n.a.	32	2.8	(1.9–3.8)
Total number of deaths	*231*	*100*		*1132*	*100*	

[¥]Renine population January 1st 2008: 4921 hemodialysis patients, mean age 64.4 years, 59.7% male.
[^]Cerebrovascular accident ischemic or hemorrhagic.
n.a. = not applicable.

The Percentage CV Death in CONTRAST when Dutch General Population Rates Apply

The expected number of CV- deaths in CONTRAST when the general population mortality rates were applied was 10.2; 7.7 in men and 2.5 in women. The expected number of all cause death was 35.5; 26.4 in men and 9.2 in women. The contribution of CV-death to all-cause death would therefore be 27.8% (95% CI 13.1–42.4%) based on general population mortality rates. In CONTRAST the proportion of CV-death was 32.0% (95% CI 26.0–38.0%). (Table 3).

Baseline Characteristics of Patients in CONTRAST by Cause of Death

Patients that died from CVD were younger (age at time of death: 71.1 (IQR 65.9–78.9)) than patients dying from infections (76.9 (70.3–81.4)) or after dialysis withdrawal (76.4 (69.2–80.6) (Table 4). The proportion of CV death was larger in patients younger than 60 years old than in patients aged 60–75 and older than 75 years (Figure 1, $P = 0.02$).

After adjustment for age and sex, patients dying from CVD had a significantly higher prevalence of previous CVD and CHD compared to patients dying from infections. Patients who died from infection were more likely to have a graft as vascular access than the patients who died from CVD or dialysis withdrawal. They also had higher β2-microglobulin (β2m) levels at baseline. Patients, who died after dialysis withdrawal, had the most co-morbidity at baseline, namely more often a history of CVD, more specifically previous CHD, cerebral vascular disease or peripheral arterial disease. Also their prevalence of DM was higher. Their mental quality of life at baseline, as reflected by the MCS, was significantly worse than in survivors.

Exploration of those who died after Dialysis Withdrawal

Dying of patients after dialysis withdrawal (n = 54) was often preceded by a (long) hospital stay. Three factors associated with dialysis withdrawal were identified: acute complications, chronic complications and low quality of life. In 18 patients dialysis was stopped in a period in which an acute complication occurred: in 11 patients an infection was present or suspected, 7 patients had peripheral vascular disease with a need for intervention and 7 patients had a gastrointestinal or shunt bleeding. Some patients suffered from combined complications. In 25 patients dialysis was stopped because of chronic complications: in 4 patients cancer was suspected, in others cachexia, dementia, poor general condition, pain, dyspnea, hypotension (in 3 patients due to aorta-valve stenosis) and infections were associated with dialysis withdrawal. Eleven patients withdrew from dialysis because of a low quality of life. The median number of days between withdrawal and death was 6 (IQR 2–9)(these data were available for 39 patients). 46% died within 5 days after the last dialysis session.

Discussion

In this study we found that in ESRD patients approximately one third of deaths was of CV origin. The proportion of CV death was comparable with that in Dutch registry of dialysis patients (Renine), and in the general population. The contribution of CV death was larger in younger patients. The other main causes of death were withdrawal from dialysis (23%) and infection (22%). Patients, who withdrew from dialysis, had considerable co-morbidity.

Compared to other studies in dialysis patients the proportion CVD deaths in CONTRAST was low [3;18;19]. Our study seems representative for the Dutch situation, given the comparability with death causes registered in Renine. The European ERA-EDTA registry reported a CV death proportion of 39% [7]. In the

Table 3. Comparison of cardiovascular and non cardiovascular death rates of CONTRAST patients and the Dutch general population.

Age category	Dutch general population					CONTRAST			Standardized G.P.	
	People at risk	CV deaths n	Total deaths	Rate of CV death/personyear[a]	Rate of all cause death/personyear[b]	Personyears lived[c]	CV deaths n	Total deaths	Expected CVD deaths (n)[d]	Expected total deaths (n)[e]
Men										
40–44	660 196	177	897	0.00026810	0.00135868	53.00	1	2	0.01420	0.07201
45–49	631 041	333	1379	0.00052769	0.00218527	66.03	3	3	0.03484	0.14429
50–54	573 890	530	2222	0.00092352	0.00387182	79.74	1	3	0.07364	0.30873
55–59	549 639	792	3404	0.00144094	0.00619315	89.82	2	10	0.12942	0.55626
60–64	499 340	1219	5119	0.00244122	0.01025153	117.47	8	17	0.28677	1.20424
65–69	356 075	1494	5937	0.00419574	0.01667345	109.29	9	19	0.45855	1.82224
70–74	274 517	2130	7812	0.00775908	0.02845725	185.03	10	36	1.43566	5.26544
75–79	206 572	3180	10614	0.01539414	0.05138160	149.88	8	41	2.30727	7.70107
80–84	125 720	3567	11335	0.02837257	0.09016067	69.64	6	21	1.97586	6.27878
85–89	57 780	2964	9008	0.05129802	0.15590169	17.50	2	7	0.89771	2.72827
90–94	15 560	1292	4012	0.08303341	0.25784061	1.07	0	1	0.08884	0.27588
Total	3950330	17678	61739			938.47	50	160	7.7028	26.3573
Women										
40–44	642 708	79	643	0.00012291	0.00100045	33.11	0	0	0.00406	0.03312
45–49	621 972	154	1143	0.00024760	0.00183770	45.24	0	0	0.01120	0.08313
50–54	567 963	211	1697	0.00037150	0.00298787	52.39	3	4	0.01946	0.15653
55–59	540 372	284	2412	0.00052556	0.00446359	47.31	2	5	0.02486	0.21117
60–64	495 939	503	3424	0.00101423	0.00690407	50.59	3	8	0.05131	0.34927
65–69	369 384	667	3692	0.00180570	0.00999501	94.83	5	14	0.17123	0.94782
70–74	314 518	1235	5185	0.00392664	0.01648554	97.57	1	11	0.38312	1.60849
75–79	278 271	2407	8231	0.00864984	0.02957907	86.76	7	19	0.75046	2.56628
80–84	216 243	4168	12480	0.01927461	0.05771285	43.76	3	10	0.84345	2.52551
85–89	132 311	5338	14778	0.04034434	0.11169139	6.24	0	0	0.25174	0.69695
90–94	51 771	3791	10478	0.07322632	0.20239130	0	0	0	0	0
Total	4231452	18846	64163			557.8	24	71	2.5109	9.1783

[a] calculated by the total number of people that died of cardiovascular disease (CVD) in the general population in 2008 divided by total number of people at risk.
[b] calculated by the total number of people that died in the general population in 2008 divided by total number of people at risk.
[c] number of personyears lived during CONTRAST.
[d] rate of cardiovascular (CV) death in the general population multiplied by the number of person years lived in CONTRAST.
[e] rate of all cause death in the general population multiplied by the number of person years lived in CONTRAST.
G.P. = general population.

Table 4. Baseline characteristics of patients who died during follow-up, from cardiovascular death, infection or dialysis withdrawal and of patients who survived (on treatment analysis).

Characteristics	Cardiovascular death (n = 74)		Fatal infection (n = 51)		Dialysis withdrawal (n = 54)		Survivors (n = 483)	
	Mean/ Median	SD or IQR	Mean/ Median	SD or IQR	Mean/ Median	SD or IQR	Mean/ Median	SD or IQR
Demographic								
Age at randomisation (yrs)	69.4^	10	72.9^	10	72.9^	8	60.4	14
Age at time of death	71.3	10	75.1	10	74.7	8	n.a.	
Sex (% man)	67.6		68.6		66.7		59.0	
Systolic BP (mmHg)	150	21	146	25	146	21	147	21
Diastolic BP (mmHg)	74	11	74	13	71	11	77	12
History of CVD (%)	66.2¶^		47.1#		64.8¶^		36.0	
AMI	23.3¶		10		22.2		11.4	
CHD	47.3¶^		32		48.2^		23.2	
Stroke/TIA	19.4		16		27.8^		12.5	
PAD	21.6		23.5		29.6^		11.8	
DM (%)	27.4		22#		41.5¶^		23.1	
BMI (kg/m²)	24.9	4	25.8	6	25.7	6	25.5	5
Smoking (%yes)	25.4		16		13.5		19.5	
RKF (%yes)	48.7		41.2^		46.3^		54.5	
Dialysis related								
Dialysis vintage at randomization (yrs)	1.6	(1.1–3.7)	2.8	(1.0–5.7)	2.9	(1–4.5)	1.9	(1.0–3.9)
Total dialysis vintage at death* (yrs)	3.9	(2.3–5.8)	4.1	(2.4–6.1)	4.7	(3.2–6.1)	4.6	(3.0–6.3)
Vascular access (%)								
AV-fistula	81.1		68.6		75.9		81.0	
CVC	4.1		3.9		11.1		6.4	
Graft	13.5¶		27.5#^		13.0		12.0	
Laboratory								
Hemoglobin (mmol/L)	7.3	0.7	7.4	0.8	7.3	0.8	7.3	0.8
Albumin (g/L)	39^	4	40	4	39^	4	41	4
Creatinin (µmol/L)	792	244	794	220	742^	231	902	257
Calcium (mmol/L)	2.3	0.2	2.3	0.1	2.3	0.2	2.3	0.2
Phosphorus (mmol/L)	1.6	0.4	1.6	0.5	1.6	0.5	1.7	0.5
Parathyroid hormone (pmol/L)	22.1	(3.9–33)	16.3	(9–32)	17.5	(10–31)	21.9	(11–38)
B2-microgobulin (mg/L)	30.6¶	14	35.9^	15	30.7	13	31.3	14
Hs-CRP (mg/L)	8.9^n =	(2.3–17.1)	5.7^n =	(3.2–14.2)	9.3^	(4.2–25.2)	3.0	(1.0–7.3)
IL-6 (pg/mL)	2.5^n =	(1.9–4.0)	3.7^	(2.5–4.5)	3.6^	(1.5–8.7)	1.7	(1.1–2.9)
Quality of Life								
SF-36 PCS	37^	11	37^	11	33^	8	42	10
SF-35 MCS	52#	11	51^	11	50^	16	53	11
Medication (% yes)								
Calcium antagonist	39#		36#		15		32	
Beta blocker	62#		52		41^		52	
RAAS blocker	47.3		34^		35^		53.3	
Alfa blocker	9		6		2		11	
Statin	58#		42^		39^		52	
Platelet aggregation inhibitor	42		34		37		29	

n.a. = not applicable; CVD = cardiovascular disease; AMI = acute myocardial infarction; CHD = coronary heart disease; TIA = transient ischemic accident; PAD = peripheral artery disease; DM = diabetes mellitus; BMI = body mass index; RKF = residual kidney function; AV = arterio-venous; CVC = central venous catheter; CRP = C- reactive protein;

IL-6 = interleukin-6; PCS = physical composite score; MCS = mental composite score; RAAS = renin angiotensin aldosterone system.

^significantly different as compared to survivors, after adjustment for age and sex.

#significantly different as compared to deaths due to dialysis withdrawal, after adjustment for age and sex.

¶significantly different as compared to deaths due to infection, after adjustment for age and sex.

*total vintage at time of end of study or date of drop-out for survivors.

Death causes < 60 yrs

Death causes 60-75 yrs

Death causes > 75 yrs

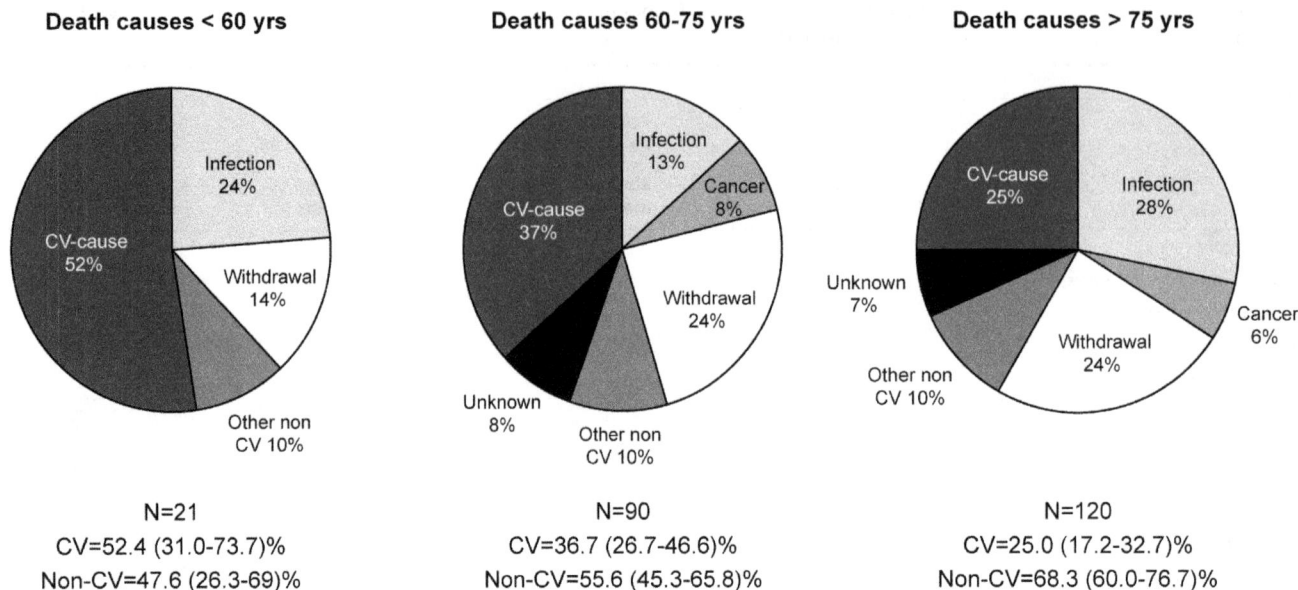

N=21
CV=52.4 (31.0-73.7)%
Non-CV=47.6 (26.3-69)%

N=90
CV=36.7 (26.7-46.6)%
Non-CV=55.6 (45.3-65.8)%

N=120
CV=25.0 (17.2-32.7)%
Non-CV=68.3 (60.0-76.7)%

Figure 1. The distribution of death causes across age groups at time of death.

4D study and in the United States Renal Data System (USRDS) CV deaths accounted for approximately 50% of all deaths [3;18]. In DOPPS III, CV death ranged from 29% in patients older than 75 years in Australia and New Zealand to 41% in patients aged 45–75 years in Europe and 56% in patients younger than 45 years in North America [19]. The discrepancies between our study and US studies are larger than between our study and other European studies. The differences between the US and the Netherlands may be a result of differences in patient selection for HD and transplantation, as well as differences in clinical practice.

Importantly, the proportion of CV deaths was not different from what would have been expected using the general population estimates. This is in agreement with the EDTA registry data, showing that CV and non CV death are similarly distributed among incident dialysis patients and the general population [7]. As in CONTRAST, they showed that in patients older than 65 years, the excess non CV death was higher than the excess CV death. Similar data were found in DOPPS III [19]. Our data might underestimate CV mortality, since only prevalent patients were included and there are data showing high rates of CV mortality in the first year of dialysis [20–22]. However, mortality in the first year of dialysis is greatly dependent on the characteristics of the patients who are selected to start dialysis and pre-dialysis care they have received [20].

Except for age, no large differences in baseline characteristics were found between the patients dying from CVD, infection or withdrawal. The higher prevalence of grafts in patients dying from infections is in agreement with studies showing a higher incidence of vascular access related infections in patients with synthetic grafts as compared to native fistulas [23;24]. Furthermore, higher β2m levels associated with infectious mortality were reported in the HEMO study [25].

Withdrawal from dialysis was much more frequent than anticipated. The death attributed to dialysis withdrawal varies highly among studies. Among elderly patients in DOPPS the proportion of death due to dialysis withdrawal varied between 1–4% in Europe, to a maximum of 8% in North America and 14% in Australia and New Zealand [19]. The proportion reported in other studies from the US varied from 6 to 22% [26;27].and the

European ERA-EDTA reported a proportion of 5.2%, which became 9.1% when the category 'Suicide/refusal of treatment' was added [7]. The 19% in Renine and the 20% in a French study were in agreement with our study [28]. The large proportion of patients dying from dialysis withdrawal was not limited to the Dutch patients in our trial, suggesting that withdrawal is not only an issue in a country where euthanasia has been legalized.

The varying percentage of patients dying after withdrawal of dialysis treatment probably reflects differences in registration practices. So far death due to dialysis withdrawal is poorly defined. Dialysis withdrawal will not always be the cause of death when dialysis is discontinued before death [29]. Notably, in case of severe co-morbidity the co-morbid conditions rather than the dialysis withdrawal itself may be the cause of death, especially when patients die within 3 days after a decision to stop dialysis is made [29].

In our study, deaths were adjudicated as 'withdrawal from dialysis', if two or three out of three members of the adjudication committee agreed on this. However, at the start of the study, no clear cut criteria were given to define this aspect. Our findings with respect to determinants of 'death due to dialysis withdrawal' were similar to that reported by a study from the US identifying old age and chronic diseases as risk factors for dialysis withdrawal [26]. Data from DOPPS III and the ERA-EDTA registry also showed that the proportion of patients who stopped, increased with older age [7;19]. Although patients who withdrew from dialysis had much baseline co-morbidity in common, the factors associated to withdrawal from dialysis were quite heterogeneous. CVD was often one of the acute or chronic reasons to decide to stop HD treatment. However, a broad scala of disease conditions was present at the time of dialysis withdrawal. Until now little attention has been paid to dialysis withdrawal in the nephrology community. In the US written policies about appropriate initiation and withdrawal from dialysis have been made [30]. Patients who refuse dialysis, who are terminally ill or permanently unconscious are patients for whom dialysis is inappropriate [30]. Before these guidelines existed, fifteen percent of nephrologists reported in a questionnaire to have written policies on dialysis withdrawal, after these guidelines, still only a minority (30) of nephrologists reported to have such a written policy [31].

Although the young dialysis patients still have a high CV risk, the strong emphasis on the risk of CV death in dialysis patients might be less justified in today's European dialysis populations [32]. Non CV causes of death and particularly withdrawal from dialysis deserve more attention, particularly in the elderly.

In view of the importance of withdrawal from dialysis in daily practice, well-defined criteria for the registration of dialysis withdrawal are warranted. We would like to propose to define death due to dialysis withdrawal as 'death occurring more than 5 days after the last dialysis treatment which has been assigned as such by patient and doctor'. A clear definition of dialysis withdrawal is a needed to investigate the incidence and risk factors for dialysis withdrawal. Mostly combinations of several co-morbidities exist, such as CVD, infections, malnutrition, and low quality of life. Regarding malnutrition, we previously showed that nutritional status relates to quality of life [33], whereas reaching clinical performance targets does not [34]. Possibly, less focus on biochemical outcome targets for patients at high risk for dialysis withdrawal, such as elderly dialysis patients might lead to a better quality of life [35]. Potentially, less dietary restrictions and les medication prescriptions might improve nutritional status. Potentially treatable symptoms in hemodialysis, such as bone pain, insomnia and emotional symptoms are undertreated, and if they are treated, then mostly by primary care providers [36]. These kinds of symptoms deserve more attention, since they are part of patients' quality of life.

Strengths of the present study are the availability of many patient characteristics, which were collected in a standardized way and second the adjudication process for causes of death by an adjudication committee. However, a limitation in the adjudication process was the lack of criteria to adjudicate deaths as 'dialysis withdrawal', which might have led to an overestimation. Using our proposed definition would probably lead to a lower percentage of dialysis withdrawal, however we do not have data to make this distinction retrospectively and therefore used the death causes as adjudicated by the committee.

Another limitation is that we did not have individual patient records from patients registered in Renine, therefore we were not able to adjust for potential differences in age and sex distribution between Renine and CONTRAST. Finally, the generalizability to other populations may be considered as a limitation, since the study population mainly consisted of Dutch patients.

In conclusion, although the absolute risk of death is much higher, the proportion of CV deaths in a prevalent ESRD population is similar to that of the general population. In older HD patients CV and non-CV death risk are equally important. Particularly the registration of dialysis withdrawal deserves attention.

Acknowledgments

The authors are grateful to patients and nursing staff participating in this project. **Canada:** Georges-L Dumont Regional Hospital, Moncton – M Dorval; CHUM St Luc Hospital, Montréal – R Lévesque; **The Netherlands:** Academic Medical Center, Amsterdam – MG Koopman; Catharina Hospital, Eindhoven – CJAM Konings; Dialysis Clinic Noord, Beilen – WP Haanstra; Dianet Dialysis Centers, Utrecht – M Kooistra and B van Jaarsveld; Fransiscus Hospital, Roosendaal – T Noordzij; Gelderse Vallei Hospital, Ede – GW Feith; Groene Hart Hospital, Gouda – HG Peltenburg; Haga Hospital, The Hague – M van Buren; Isala Clinics, Zwolle – JJG Offerman; Jeroen Bosch Hospital, 's Hertogenbosch – EK Hoogeveen; Maasland Hospital, Sittard – F de Heer; Maasstad Hospital, Rotterdam – PJ van de Ven; Martini Hospital, Groningen – TK Kremer Hovinga; Medical Center Alkmaar, Alkmaar – WA Bax; Onze Lieve Vrouwe Gasthuis, Amsterdam – JO Groeneveld; Oosterschelde Hospital, Goes – ATJ Lavrijssen; Rijnland Hospital, Leiderdorp – AM Schrander-Van der Meer; Rijnstate Hospital, Arnhem – LJM Reichert; Slingeland Hospital, Doetinchem – J Huussen; St Elisabeth Hospital, Tilburg – PL Rensma; St Fransiscus Gasthuis, Rotterdam – Y Schrama; University Medical Center St Radboud, Nijmegen –HW van Hamersvelt; University Medical Center Utrecht, Utrecht – WH Boer; VieCuri Medical Center, Venlo – WH van Kuijk; VU University Medical Center, Amsterdam – MG Vervloet; Zeeuws-Vlaanderen Hospital, Terneuzen – IMPMJ Wauters. **Norway:** Haukeland University Hospital, Bergen – I Sekse.

Author Contributions

Conceived and designed the experiments: MLB MPCG PMtW MN RL PJB MAvdD. Performed the experiments: CHdH MPCG AHAM ELP NCvdW PMtW MN RL PJb MAvdD. Analyzed the data: CHdH MLB MPCG. Contributed reagents/materials/analysis tools: CHdH MLB MPCG. Wrote the paper: CHdH MLB MPCG MAvdD. Critical review of the manuscript: CHdH MLB MPCG AHAM ELP NCvdW PMtW MN RL PJb MAvdD.

References

1. Roberts MA, Polkinghorne KR, McDonald SP, Ierino FL (2011) Secular trends in cardiovascular mortality rates of patients receiving dialysis compared with the general population. Am J Kidney Dis 58: 64–72.
2. Foley RN, Gilbertson DT, Murray T, Collins AJ (2011): Long interdialytic interval and mortality among patients receiving hemodialysis. N Engl J Med 365: 1099–1107.
3. Ritz E, Bommer J (2009) Cardiovascular problems on hemodialysis: current deficits and potential improvement. Clin J Am Soc Nephrol 4 Suppl 1: S71–S78.
4. Robinson BM, Port FK (2009) International hemodialysis patient outcomes comparisons revisited: the role of practice patterns and other factors. Clin J Am Soc Nephrol 4 Suppl 1: S12–S17.
5. Grooteman MP, van den Dorpel MA, Bots ML, Penne EL, van der Weerd NC, et al. (2012) Effect of Online Hemodiafiltration on All-Cause Mortality and Cardiovascular Outcomes. J Am Soc Nephrol 23: 1087–1096.
6. Cheung AK, Sarnak MJ, Yan G Berkoben M, Heyka R, et al. (2004) Cardiac diseases in maintenance hemodialysis patients: results of the HEMO Study. Kidney Int 65: 2380–2389.
7. de Jager DJ, Grootendorst DC, Jager KJ, van Dijk PC, Tomas LM, et al. (2009) Cardiovascular and non cardiovascular mortality among patients starting dialysis. JAMA 302: 1782–1789.
8. Penne EL, Blankestijn PJ, Bots ML van den Dorpel MA, Grooteman MP, et al. (2005) Effect of increased convective clearance by on-line hemodiafiltration on all cause and cardiovascular mortality in chronic hemodialysis patients - the

Dutch CONvective TRAnsport STudy (CONTRAST): rationale and design of a randomised controlled trial [ISRCTN38365125]. Curr Control Trials Cardiovasc Med 6: 8.
9. Hays RD, Kallich JD, Mapes DL Coons SJ, Carter WB (1994) Development of the kidney disease quality of life (KDQOL) instrument. Qual Life Res 3: 329–338.
10. Korevaar JC, Merkus MP, Jansen MA, Dekker FW, Boeschoten EW, et al. (2002) Validation of the KDQOL-SF: a dialysis-targeted health measure. Qual Life Res 11: 437–447.
11. Ware JE, Snow KK, Kosinski M Gandek B (1993) SF-36 Health Survey-Manual and Interpretation Guide.
12. Ware JE, Kosinski M, Keller SD (1994). SF-36 physical and mental health summary scales: a user's manual. 2nd ed.
13. Clase CM, St Pierre MW, Churchill DN (2001) Conversion between bromcresol green- and bromcresol purple-measured albumin in renal disease. Nephrol Dial Transplant 16: 1925–1929.
14. Stichting RENINE. Renine website (Registration of Renal Replacement Therapy in the Netherlands). Available: www.renine.nl. Accessed 2012 Dec 1.
15. ERA-EDTA. European Renal Association-European Dialysis and Transplant Association (ERA-EDTA) Registry (2009). ERA-EDTA Registry 2009 Annual Report. Amsterdam, the Netherlands. 129.
16. Central Office of Statistics, The Netherlands. STATLINE website. Available: http://statline.cbs.nl/StatWeb/Assessed 2012 Dec 1.

17. World Health Organization. International Statistical Classification of Diseases, 10th Revision (ICD-10). Geneva, Switzerland. 1990.

18. Wanner C, Krane V, Marz W, Olschewski M, Mann JF, et al. (2005) Atorvastatin in patients with type 2 diabetes mellitus undergoing hemodialysis. N Engl J Med 353: 238–248.

19. Canaud B, Tong L, Tentori F, Akiba T, Karaboyas A, et al. (2011) Clinical practices and outcomes in elderly hemodialysis patients: results from the Dialysis Outcomes and Practice Patterns Study (DOPPS). Clin J Am Soc Nephrol 6: 1651–1662.

20. Bradbury BD, Fissell RB, Albert JM, Anthony MS, Critchlow CW, et al. (2007) Predictors of early mortality among incident US hemodialysis patients in the Dialysis Outcomes and Practice Patterns Study (DOPPS). Clin J Am Soc Nephrol 2: 89–99.

21. Collins AJ, Foley RN, Gilbertson DT, Chen SC (2009) The state of chronic kidney disease, ESRD, and morbidity and mortality in the first year of dialysis. Clin J Am Soc Nephrol 4 Suppl 1: S5–11.

22. Lukowsky LR, Kheifets L, Arah OA, Nissenson AR, Kalantar-Zadeh K (2012) Patterns and predictors of early mortality in incident hemodialysis patients: new insights. Am J Nephrol 35: 548–558.

23. Schild AF, Perez E, Gillaspie E, Seaver C, Livingstone J, et al. (2008) Arteriovenous fistulae vs. arteriovenous grafts: a retrospective review of 1,700 consecutive vascular access cases. J Vasc Access 9: 231–235.

24. Akoh JA (2009) Prosthetic arteriovenous grafts for hemodialysis. J Vasc Access 10: 137–147.

25. Cheung AK, Greene T, Leypoldt JK, Yan G, Allon M, et al. (2008) Association between serum 2-microglobulin level and infectious mortality in hemodialysis patients. Clin J Am Soc Nephrol 3: 69–77.

26. Leggat JE Jr, Bloembergen WE, Levine G, Hulbert-Shearon TE, Port FK (1997) An analysis of risk factors for withdrawal from dialysis before death. J Am Soc Nephrol 8: 1755–1763.

27. Cohen LM, Bostwick JM, Mirot A (2007) A psychiatric perspective of dialysis discontinuation. J Palliat Med 10: 1262–1265.

28. Birmele B, Francois M, Pengloan J, Français P, Testou D (2004) Death after withdrawal from dialysis: the most common cause of death in a French dialysis population. Nephrol Dial Transplant 19: 686–691.

29. Holley JL (2002) A single-center review of the death notification form: discontinuing dialysis before death is not a surrogate for withdrawal from dialysis. Am J Kidney Dis 40: 525–530.

30. Moss AH (2001) Shared decision-making in dialysis: the new RPA/ASN guideline on appropriate initiation and withdrawal of treatment. Am J Kidney Dis 37: 1081–1091.

31. Holley JL, Davison SN, Moss AH (2007) Nephrologists' changing practices in reported end-of-life decision-making. Clin J Am Soc Nephrol 2: 107–111.

32. Krediet RT, Boeschoten EW, Dekker FW (2012) Are the high mortality rates in dialysis patients mainly due to cardiovascular causes? Nephrol Dial Transplant 27: 481–483.

33. Mazairac AH, de Wit GA, Penne EL, van der Weerd NC, Grooteman MP, et al (2011) Protein-energy nutritional status and kidney disease-specific quality of life in hemodialysis patients. J Ren Nutr 21: 376–386.

34. Mazairac AH, de Wit GA, Grooteman MP, Penne EL, van der Weerd NC, et al (2011) Clinical Performance Targets and Quality of Life in Hemodialysis Patients. Blood Purif 33: 73–79.

35. Jassal SV, Watson D (2009) Dialysis in late life: benefit or burden. Clin J Am Soc Nephrol 4: 2008–2012.

36. Claxton RN, Blackhall L, Weisbord SD, Holley JL (2010) Undertreatment of symptoms in patients on maintenance hemodialysis. J Pain Symptom Manage 39: 211–218.

21

Urinary Concentration of Monocyte Chemoattractant Protein-1 in Idiopathic Glomerulonephritis

Rafid Tofik[1], Sophie Ohlsson[1], Omran Bakoush[1,2]*

1 Department of Nephrology, Lund University, Lund, Sweden, **2** Department of Internal Medicine, UAE University, Al-Ain, United Arab Emirates

Abstract

Background: Monocyte chemoattractant protein-1 (MCP-1), which is up regulated in kidney diseases, is considered a marker of kidney inflammation. We examined the value of urine MCP-1 in predicting the outcome in idiopathic glomerulonephritis.

Methods: Between 1993 and 2004, 165 patients (68 females) diagnosed with idiopathic proteinuric glomerulopathy and with serum creatinine <150 μmol/L at diagnosis were selected for the study. Urine concentrations of MCP-1 were analyzed by ELISA in early morning spot urine samples collected on the day of the diagnostic kidney biopsy. The patients were followed until 2009. The progression rate to end-stage kidney disease was calculated using Kaplan–Meier survival analysis. End-stage kidney disease (ESKD) was defined as the start of kidney replacement therapy during the study follow-up time.

Results: Patients with proliferative glomerulonephritis had significantly higher urinary MCP-1 excretion levels than those with non-proliferative glomerulonephritis (p<0.001). The percentage of patients whose kidney function deteriorated significantly was 39.0% in the high MCP-1 excretion group and 29.9% in the low MCP-1 excretion group. However, after adjustment for confounding variables such as glomerular filtration rate (GFR) and proteinuria, there was no significant association between urine MCP-1 concentration and progression to ESKD, (HR = 1.75, 95% CI = 0.64–4.75, p = 0.27).

Conclusion: Our findings indicate that progression to end-stage kidney disease in patients with idiopathic glomerulopathies is not associated with urine MCP-1 concentrations at the time of diagnosis.

Editor: Delia Goletti, National Institute for Infectious Diseases (L. Spallanzani), Italy

Funding: This study was supported by ALF grants from Lund University Research Fund. The funders had no role in study design, data collection and analysis, decision to publish, or preparation of the manuscript.

Competing Interests: The authors have declared that no competing interests exist.

* E-mail: Omran.Bakoush@uaeu.ac.ae

Introduction

Glomerular diseases, including idiopathic glomerulonephritis, are major causes of end-stage kidney disease (ESKD). Clinically, they are manifested with haematuria, proteinuria and declining kidney function. Histopathologically, they are associated with inflammation and proliferation of the glomerular tissue and enhanced glomerular and interstitial production of inflammatory mediators, such as monocyte chemoattractant protein-1 (MCP-1) [1,2].

Inflammatory cytokines, including MCP-1, play an important role in glomerular inflammation. MCP-1 is produced by macrophages, vascular endothelial cells, monocytes and fibroblasts. It triggers migration and retention of monocytes and transformation of fibroblasts in the glomeruli [3–5].

The urinary concentration of MCP-1 increases with increased activity of glomerular diseases (GN) [6]. It is associated with flares of systemic lupus erythematosus (SLE) and small vessel vasculitis [7,8]. In diabetic nephropathy, increased urinary MCP-1 is associated with faster disease progression to kidney failure [9]. However, the prognostic utility of urinary MCP-1 in primary proteinuric glomerulonephritis has not received much attention.

Therefore, we evaluated the utility of urine MCP-1 as a potential predictor of disease outcome in a longitudinal cohort of patients with idiopathic chronic glomerulonephritis.

Methods

Patients

The patients were enrolled in the large glomerular disease investigation program that was conducted at the Nephrology Department, Lund University Hospital, Sweden. The cohort and the controls (healthy blood donors) have been described in detail [10,11].

Of the patients investigated between August 1993 and February 2004, 189 patients (76 females) had initial serum creatinine <150 μmol/L at the time of kidney biopsy. Of these, urine samples were available from 165 patients (68 females) for MCP-1 analysis. The study was approved by the regional ethical committee of Lund (LU 47-02), and all patients gave informed written consent.

Examination of the biopsies showed or confirmed the following diagnoses: mesangial proliferative glomerulonephritis (n = 64), IgA nephropathy (*n* = 28), membranous glomerulonephritis (*n* = 15),

Table 1. Baseline characteristics of 165 (68 female) patients with idiopathic chronic glomerulonephritis divided according to the urine MCP-1 concentrations (low <0.05 mg/mmol and high >0.05 mg/mmol).

Variables	Low MCP-1	High MCP-1	P-value
Gender (M/F)	79 (55/24)	86 (42/44)	
Age (years)	48.0 (33.0–55.0)	50.0 (31.8–66.0)	0.26
Follow-up (years)	9.4 (5.9–10.5)	6.4 (3.9–8.9)	0.001*
MAP (mm Hg)	100.0 (93.3–110.0)	106.7 (94.2–116.5)	0.06
S. creatinine (μmol/L)	85.5 (72.0–112.3)	93.0 (73.5–115.0)	0.24
GFR (ml/min/1.73)	72.4 (54.7–92.6)	63.0 (46.4–83.8)	0.02*
S. albumin (g/L)	34.0 (28.0–40.0)	29.0 (19.0–34.0)	<0.001*
IgG-uria (mg/mmol)	3.8 (1.1–7.3)	7.8 (2.7–24.2)	<0.001*
HC-uria (mg/mmol)	0.82 (0.5–1.6)	1.9 (0.7–4.3)	0.001*
ACR (mg/mmol)	53.7 (7.2–150.9)	161.9 (58.6–475.7)	<0.001*

Data are presented as median and inter-quartile range (in parentheses).
MAP = mean arterial blood pressure; GFR = glomerular filtration rate; ACR = urine albumin/creatinine ratio; HC-uria = urine alpha-1 microglobulin/creatinine ratio.
*The difference between the groups is statistically significant.

minimal change nephropathy (MCN, $n = 30$), focal segmental glomerulosclerosis (FSGS, $n = 5$), and nephrosclerosis ($n = 23$). We excluded patients with severe kindey failure on admission (serum creatinine >150 μmol/L), diabetic nephropathy, crescentic glomerulonephritis, and other secondary causes such as SLE, and small vessel vasculitis associated with antineutrophil cytoplasmic antibodies (ANCA).

Blood pressure was measured using a mercury sphygmomanometer with the patients in a supine position. The diastolic blood pressure was measured at Korotkoff phase V. Mean arterial blood pressure (MAP) was calculated by adding one third of the pulse pressure to the diastolic blood pressure. The kidney biopsies were evaluated for the percentage of global glomerulosclerosis (GGS) and the extent of tubulo-interstitial damage. Interstitial fibrosis was

scored semi quantitatively as 0 (absent), 1 (focal) or 2 (diffuse). All patients were followed regularly at the nephrology outpatient clinic of Lund University Hospital and were on a normal protein diet. Clinical data, including measures of serum creatinine, were collected during the scheduled clinic visits. The patients were followed until the last planned follow-up visit in 2009. The primary end point was end-stage kidney disease (ESKD) defined as the start of kidney replacement therapy.

Laboratory analysis

Blood samples and the first voided urine specimens were obtained in the morning of the day of the kidney biopsy. The patients had no signs of urinary tract infection in urinalysis examination performed at admission. The urinary albumin-to-creatinine ratio (ACR), measured in a spot morning urine sample, was used as a reliable estimate of the degree of proteinuria [12]. ACR (mg/mmol) is the ratio of urine albumin (mg/L) to urine creatinine (mmole/L), IgG-uria (mg/mmol) is defined as the ratio of urine IgG (mg/L) to urine creatinine (mmole/L), and HC-uria (mg/mmol) is defined as the ratio of urine protein HC (alpha-1 microglobulin) (mg/L) to urine creatinine (mmol/L).

Serum and urine creatinine were determined enzymatically using a Kodak Ektachem 700 XR-C system. Serum and urine albumin, IgG, and urine protein HC (alpha-1 microglobulin) were determined by immunoturbidimetry using a Cobas Mira S system (Roche Inc.) and monospecific rabbit antisera obtained from Dako (Copenhagen, Denmark) [13–15]. Urine MCP-1 was measured by an ELISA described in detail earlier [11]. Glomerular filtration rate (GFR) was estimated using the Lund-Malmö formula [16,17]: eGFR for patients with plasma creatinine (pCr) <150 μmol/L $= e^{4.62 - 0.0112*pCr - 0.0124*age + 0.339*ln(age) - 0.2226 \text{ (if female)}}$.

Statistical methods

The data are expressed as medians and interquartile ranges. Baseline characteristics of the patients' subgroups were compared with non-parametric Mann-Whitney U Test. Correlation was tested using Spearman's correlation coefficient. Multivariate Cox proportional hazards regression analysis was performed to examine the association of the urine-MCP-1 and IgG-uria with the progression to ESKD. Survival analysis was performed using

Table 2. The follow-up data of 165 (68 female) patients with idiopathic chronic glomerulonephritis divided according to the urine MCP-1 concentrations (low <0.05 mg/mmol and high >0.05 mg/mmol).

Variables	Low MCP-1	High MCP-1	P-value
	(n = 79)	(n = 86)	
Follow-up years	9.4 (5.9–10.5)	6.4 (3.9–8.9)	0.001*
Treatment:			
ACE inhibitors	65 (83.3%)	61 (73.5%)	0.18, ns
Immunosuppressives	18 (23%)	33 (38%)	0.023*
Corticosteroids	18	33	
Calcineurin inhibitors	4	6	
Cyclophosphamide	6	11	
EndGFR ml/min/1.73	63.2 (40.5–86.0)	56.3 (24.0–81.2)	0.25, ns
CV Death	6 (7.8%)	8 (9.6%)	0.14, ns
ESKD	8 (10.4%)	16 (19%)	0.18, ns

Data are presented as number and percentage (in parentheses) and median with inter-quartile range (in parentheses) when appropriate.
ACE = angiotensin converting enzyme; End GFR = glomerular filtration rate at the study end; CV = cardiovascular; ESKD = End-stage kidney disease
*The difference between the groups is statistically significant.

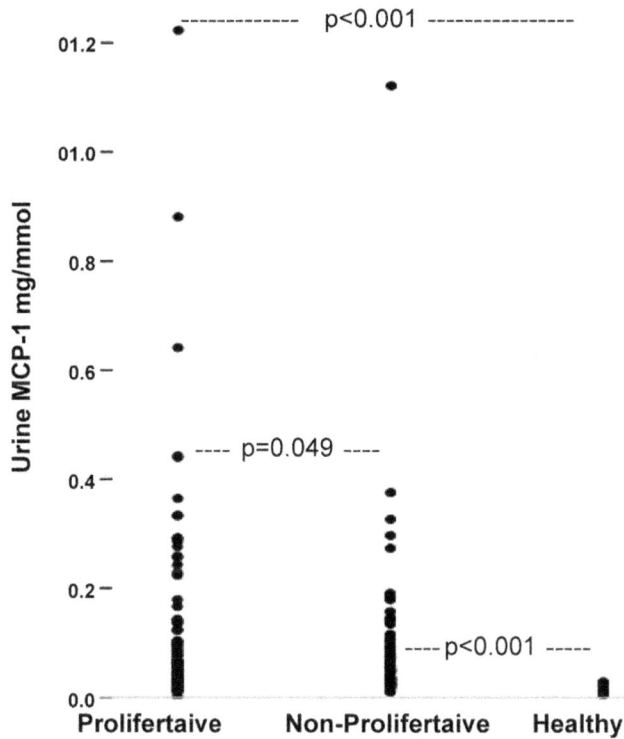

Figure 1. The urine concentrations of MCP-1 in proliferative and non-proliferative forms of glomerulonephritis compared to the urine concentrations of MCP-1 in healthy individuals, *p*<0.001 with Bonferroni-Holm corrections.

the Kaplan–Meier method. Log rank test was used to assess differences in survival. All statistics were performed using SPSS software, version 17.0 (Chicago, IL, USA). *P*<0.05 was selected as level of significance. The P-values were adjusted for multiple comparisons using Bonferroni-Holm adjustment method. Patients were divided into low and high MCP-1 groups according to the median urine concentration of MCP-1 at 0.05 mg/mmol creatinine (Tables 1 and 2).

Results

Urinary MCP-1 levels were significantly higher in patients with proliferative glomerulonephritis (IgA and mesangioproliferative)

than in those with non-proliferative forms of glomerulonephritis (membranous, FSGS, and MCN), (0.061 (IQ 0.032–0.133) mg/mmol creatinine *vs.* 0.039 (IQ 0.027–0.085) mg/mmol creatinine, $p = 0.049$ with Bonferroni-Holm correction; (Figure 1), and both had significantly higher urine MCP-1 concentrations than healthy controls: 0.01 mg/mmol creatinine (IQ 0.008–0.023, *p*<0.001 with Bonferroni-Holm correction (Figure 1). The albuminuria was significantly higher in non-proliferative glomerulonephritis than in proliferative glomerulonephritis ($p = 0.002$). However, there was no statistical difference in the kidney function ($p = 0.58$) or IgG-uria *(p = 0.33)* between proliferative and non-proliferative glomerulonephritis.

During the study, 126 patients were treated with angiotensin converting enzyme inhibitors or angiotensin II receptor antagonist; 51 patients were treated with immunosuppressive drugs (Table 3). There is no difference in the number of patients treated with angiotensin converting enzyme inhibitors in the high and low MCP-1 groups (73.5% *vs* 83.3%, $p = 0.18$; Table 2). However, more patients in the high MCP-1 group were treated with immunosuppressive drugs than those in the low MCP-1 group (46.3% *vs* 25.0%, respectively, *p = 0.008*; Table 2).

Urine MCP-1 was correlated to the degree of IgG-uria, HC-uria and ACR ($r = 0.45$, 0.38 and 0.41, respectively, $p = 0.01$), but not to the degree of interstitial fibrosis ($r = 0.06$, $p = 0.5$). Patients with severe glomerulosclerosis (global sclerosis >20% of glomeruli) had lower urine MCP-1 concentrations than those with a lesser degree of glomerulosclerosis (0.037: IQ 0.026–0.069) *vs.* 0.06: IQ 0.033–0.142, $p = 0.003$).

Kidney Survival

The kidney function of 32.8% of the patients deteriorated significantly (>3 ml/min/year) during the follow-up time. However, the percentages in the high and the low MCP-1 groups were not significantly different: they were 39% in the high MCP-1 group and 29.9% in the low MCP-1 group ($p = 0.25$, data not shown). Likewise, there was no difference in percentage of patients with deteriorated in kidney function between patients with low or high HC-uria (42.5% *vs.* 27.5%, $p = 0.1$, data not shown), or between patients with low or high ACR (39.5% *vs.* 27.8%, $p = 0.1$, data not shown). On the other hand, during the study follow-up time kidney function deteriorated significantly more frequently ($p = 0.001$) in patients with high IgG-uria (45.5%) than in patients with low IgG-uria (19.4%), data not shown.

During the study follow-up time, 24 patients (9 females) reached ESKD, 14 (4 female) died of cardiovascular events, and 4 (3 females) were lost from follow up (Table 2). Univariate regression

Table 3. The histological diagnosis and the frequency of treatment with angiotensin converting enzyme inhibitors and immunosuppressive drugs given to 165 (68 female) patients with idiopathic chronic glomerulonephritis.

Condition	N	ACEi	Steroids	Steroids+CPh	Steroids+CI	Total IS
Mesangio-proliferative GN	64	46	5	8	4	17
IgA-nephropathy	28	22	1	2	-	3
MCN	30	17	9	3	5	17
FSGS	5	5	1	1	-	2
Membranous nephropathy	15	15	8	3	1	12
Nephrosclerosis	23	21	-	-	-	-
Total	165	126	24	17	10	51

N = number; ACEI = angiotensin-converting enzyme inhibitor; CPh = cyclophosphamide; CI; calcineurin inhibitors; IS= immunosuppressive drugs; MCN = minimal change nephropathy; FSGS = focal segmental glomerulosclerosis.

Table 4. Univariate Cox regression analysis for the outcome of end-stage kidney disease in 165 (68 female) patients with idiopathic chronic glomerulnephritis.

Variables	Beta	SE	P-value	HR	95% CI
Age (2gp)	0.33	0.39	0.40	1.39	0.64–3.01
GFR (2gp)	2.59	0.74	<0.001	13.40	3.13–57.44
Albumin-uria (2gp)	0.73	0.41	0.075	2.08	0.93–4.67
HC-uria (2gp)	1.06	0.40	0.008	2.89	1.32–6.35
IgG-uria (2gp)	1.75	0.55	<0.001	5.73	1.96–16.72
MCP-uria (2gp)	0.88	0.44	0.042	2.42	1.03–5.68

2gp = the cohort was divided into two groups based on the median value of the variable; Beta = regression coefficient; SE = standard error; HR = hazard ratio; CI = confidence interval.

analysis revealed that eGFR, urine MCP-1, HC-uria, albuminuria, and IgG-uria are predictors of the outcome of ESKD (Table 4, Figure 2). However, after adjustment for the above-mentioned key confounding variables in a forward conditional stepwise multivariate Cox regression analysis, urine MCP-1 was not significantly associated with the outcome of ESKD (HR = 1.75, 95% CI = 0.64–4.75, $p = 0.27$). Only eGFR and IgG-uria remained as significant predictors for the outcome of ESKD (Table 4, Figure 2).

Discussion

Mounting evidence shows that urine MCP-1 is a potential diagnostic and prognostic marker in a variety of kidney diseases. Our results confirmed the previous reports of increased urine MCP-1 excretion in patients with glomerulonephritis and its correlation with on-going glomerular inflammation [18–20].

Contrary to our expectation, urine MCP-1 was not an independent predictor of long-term outcome in this cohort of patients with idiopathic chronic glomerulonephritis, while IgG-uria was [10]. This seems to contradict previous reports on the prognostic value of urine MCP-1 in patients with systemic diseases [11,21–24]. However, it is more likely that the levels of urine MCP-1 reflect ongoing acute glomerular and tubular inflammation, while IgG-uria reflects the severity of the glomerular damage in both the acute and chronic stages [6,25].

Proteinuria, including the IgG-uria, is associated with induction of chemokines, accumulation of fibroblasts, and progressive glomerular and interstitial injuries, which ultimately lead to ESKD [26]. Whether or not the glomerular damage is acute or chronic, the glomerular capillary wall loses its size selectivity, allowing leakage of large proteins such as IgG into urine [27]. Many studies have shown that IgG-uria is a powerful predictor of disease outcome in glomerulonephritis [25,28].

Furthermore, patients with active glomerulonephritis are more likely to receive immune-suppressive therapy. These drugs, as well as the antiproteinuric medications, such as angiotensin converting enzyme inhibitors, block the effect of the inflammatory chemokines and thereby alter the course of glomerulonephritis, diminishing the association between urine MCP-1 level and progression of kidney disease [26,29,30].

In our study we measured urine MCP-1 only once, which might have caused misclassification of patients who remitted rapidly and those with repeated flare-ups of glomerulonephritis. However, the cohort was large enough to allow the study of the predictive value of urine biomarkers at the time of diagnosis. Further studies should examine the value of repeated measurement of MCP-1 in idiopathic chronic glomerulonephritis patients, especially for monitoring the treatment response.

In summary, although urine MCP-1 concentration is increased, we found that urine MCP-1 at the time of diagnosis is not a powerful predictor of long-term kidney disease outcome in patients with idiopathic glomerulonephritis. Future studies are needed to investigate the utility of repeated measurement of urine MCP-1 in patients with idiopathic chronic glomerulonephritis.

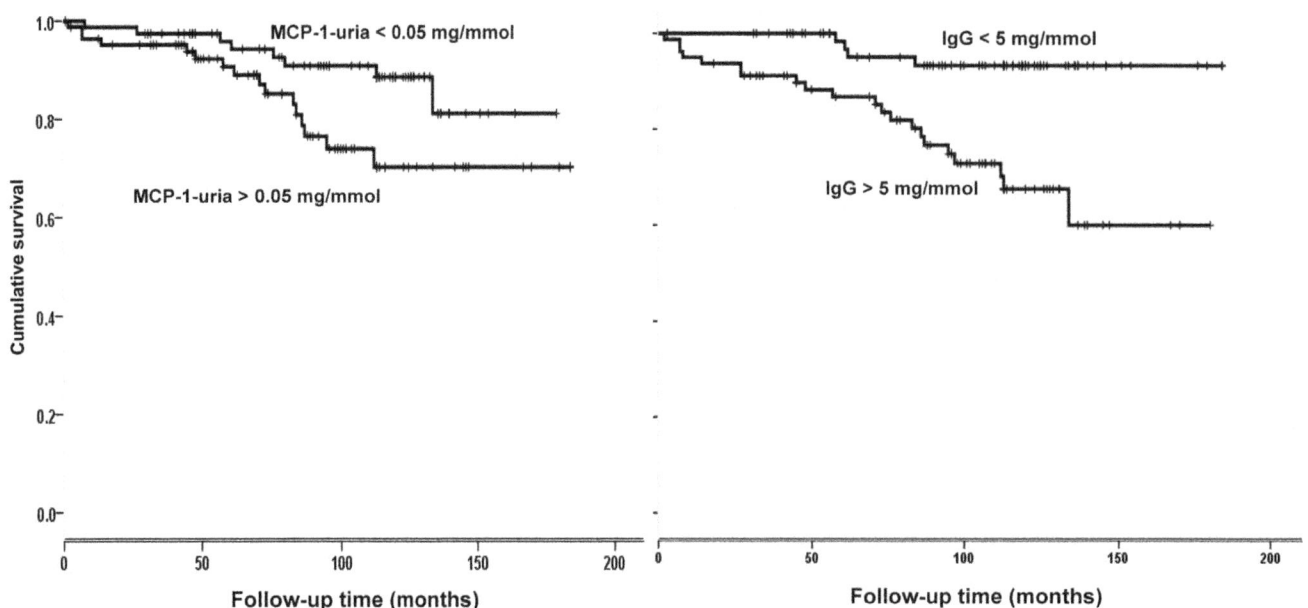

Figure 2. The cumulative risk for end-stage kidney disease according to the IgG-uria and U-MCP-1 in 165 (68 female) patients with idiopathic chronic glomerulonephritis and serum creatinine <150 μmol/L.

Acknowledgments

We wish to thank the medical staff at the outpatient Nephrology Clinic for their great assistance in collecting the patients' urine and blood samples. We wish to thank Dr. Abderrahim Oulhaj, Institute for Public Health, UAEU, for critical review of the statistical analysis, and Dr. Amin Bredan for writing assistance.

References

1. Rovin BH, Doe N, Tan LC (1996) Monocyte chemoattractant protein-1 levels in patients with glomerular disease. Am J Kidney Dis 27: 640–646.
2. Lepenies J, Eardley KS, Kienitz T, Hewison M, Ihl T, et al. (2011) Renal TLR4 mRNA expression correlates with inflammatory marker MCP-1 and profibrotic molecule TGF-beta in patients with chronic kidney disease. Nephron Clin Pract 119: c97–c104.
3. Wu CC, Chen JS, Lu KC, Chen CC, Lin SH, et al. (2010) Aberrant cytokines/ chemokines production correlate with proteinuria in patients with overt diabetic nephropathy. Clin Chim Acta 411: 700–704.
4. Furuichi K, Wada T, Iwata Y, Kitagawa K, Kobayashi K, et al. (2003) Gene therapy expressing amino-terminal truncated monocyte chemoattractant protein-1 prevents renal ischemia-reperfusion injury. J Am Soc Nephrol 14: 1066–1071.
5. Kulkarni O, Pawar RD, Purschke W, Eulberg D, Selve N, et al. (2007) Spiegelmer inhibition of CCL2/MCP-1 ameliorates lupus nephritis in MRL-(Fas)lpr mice. J Am Soc Nephrol 18: 2350–2358.
6. Kim MJ, Tam FW (2011) Urinary monocyte chemoattractant protein-1 in renal disease. Clin Chim Acta 412: 2022–2030.
7. Lieberthal JG, Cuthbertson D, Carette S, Hoffman GS, Khalidi NA, et al. (2013) Urinary Biomarkers in Relapsing Antineutrophil Cytoplasmic Antibody-associated Vasculitis. J Rheumatol 40: 674–683.
8. Rosa RF, Takei K, Araujo NC, Loduca SM, Szajubok JC, et al. (2012) Monocyte chemoattractant-1 as a urinary biomarker for the diagnosis of activity of lupus nephritis in Brazilian patients. J Rheumatol 39: 1948–1954.
9. Titan SM, Vieira JM, Jr., Dominguez WV, Moreira SR, Pereira AB, et al. (2012) Urinary MCP-1 and RBP: independent predictors of renal outcome in macroalbuminuric diabetic nephropathy. J Diabetes Complications 26: 546–553.
10. Tofik R, Aziz R, Reda A, Rippe B, Bakoush O (2011) The value of IgG-uria in predicting renal failure in idiopathic glomerular diseases. A long-term follow-up study. Scand J Clin Lab Invest 71: 123–128.
11. Ohlsson S, Bakoush O, Tencer J, Torffvit O, Segelmark M (2009) Monocyte chemoattractant protein 1 is a prognostic marker in ANCA-associated small vessel vasculitis. Mediators Inflamm 2009: 584916.
12. Miller WG, Bruns DE, Hortin GL, Sandberg S, Aakre KM, et al. (2009) Current issues in measurement and reporting of urinary albumin excretion. Clin Chem 55: 24–38.
13. Tencer J, Thysell H, Grubb A (1996) Analysis of proteinuria: reference limits for urine excretion of albumin, protein HC, immunoglobulin G, kappa- and lambda-immunoreactivity, orosomucoid and alpha 1-antitrypsin. Scand J Clin Lab Invest 56: 691–700.
14. Price CP, Spencer K, Whicher J (1983) Light-scattering immunoassay of specific proteins: a review. Ann Clin Biochem 20 Pt 1: 1–14.
15. Svendsen P, Blirup-Jensen S (1991) Determination of human plasma proteins by turbidimetry and nephelometry. Copenhagen, Dako.
16. Bjork J, Back SE, Sterner G, Carlson J, Lindstrom V, et al. (2007) Prediction of relative glomerular filtration rate in adults: new improved equations based on Swedish Caucasians and standardized plasma-creatinine assays. Scand J Clin Lab Invest 67: 678–695.
17. Nyman U, Bjork J, Sterner G, Back SE, Carlson J, et al. (2006) Standardization of p-creatinine assays and use of lean body mass allow improved prediction of calculated glomerular filtration rate in adults: a new equation. Scand J Clin Lab Invest 66: 451–468.
18. Nam BY, Paeng J, Kim SH, Lee SH, Kim do H, et al. (2012) The MCP-1/CCR2 axis in podocytes is involved in apoptosis induced by diabetic conditions. Apoptosis 17: 1–13.
19. Melgarejo E, Medina MA, Sanchez-Jimenez F, Urdiales JL (2009) Monocyte chemoattractant protein-1: a key mediator in inflammatory processes. Int J Biochem Cell Biol 41: 998–1001.
20. Kim MJ, Tam FW (2011) Urinary monocyte chemoattractant protein-1 in renal disease. Clin Chim Acta 412: 2022–2030.
21. Barbado J, Martin D, Vega L, Almansa R, Goncalves L, et al. (2012) MCP-1 in urine as biomarker of disease activity in Systemic Lupus Erythematosus. Cytokine 60: 583–586.
22. Murea M, Register TC, Divers J, Bowden DW, Carr JJ, et al. (2012) Relationships between serum MCP-1 and subclinical kidney disease: African American-Diabetes Heart Study. BMC Nephrol 13: 148.
23. Titan SM, Vieira JM Jr., Dominguez WV, Moreira SR, Pereira AB, et al. (2012) Urinary MCP-1 and RBP: independent predictors of renal outcome in macroalbuminuric diabetic nephropathy. J Diabetes Complications 26: 546–553.
24. Singh RG, Usha, Rathore SS, Behura SK, Singh NK (2012) Urinary MCP-1 as diagnostic and prognostic marker in patients with lupus nephritis flare. Lupus 21: 1214–1218.
25. Bazzi C, Rizza V, Casellato D, Stivali G, Rachele G, et al. (2012) Validation of some pathophysiological mechanisms of the CKD progression theory and outcome prediction in IgA nephropathy. J Nephrol 25: 810–818.
26. Anders HJ, Vielhauer V, Schlondorff D (2003) Chemokines and chemokine receptors are involved in the resolution or progression of renal disease. Kidney Int 63: 401–415.
27. Bakoush O, Grubb A, Rippe B, Tencer J (2001) Urine excretion of protein HC in proteinuric glomerular diseases correlates to urine IgG but not to albuminuria. Kidney Int 60: 1904–1909.
28. McQuarrie EP, Shakerdi L, Jardine AG, Fox JG, Mackinnon B (2011) Fractional excretions of albumin and IgG are the best predictors of progression in primary glomerulonephritis. Nephrol Dial Transplant 26: 1563–1569.
29. Abbate M, Zoja C, Remuzzi G (2006) How does proteinuria cause progressive renal damage? J Am Soc Nephrol 17: 2974–2984.
30. Yu C, Gong R, Rifai A, Tolbert EM, Dworkin LD (2007) Long-term, high-dosage candesartan suppresses inflammation and injury in chronic kidney disease: nonhemodynamic renal protection. J Am Soc Nephrol 18: 750–759.

Author Contributions

Conceived and designed the experiments: RT SO OB. Performed the experiments: RT SO OB. Analyzed the data: RT OB. Contributed reagents/materials/analysis tools: RT SO OB. Wrote the paper: RT SO OB.

22

Role of the Functional Toll-Like Receptor-9 Promoter Polymorphism (-1237T/C) in Increased Risk of End-Stage Renal Disease: A Case-Control Study

Hsin-Yi Yang[1], Kuo-Cheng Lu[2], Herng-Sheng Lee[3], Shih-Ming Huang[4], Yuh-Feng Lin[5,6], Chia-Chao Wu[6], Donald M. Salter[7], Sui-Lung Su[1]*

1 School of Public Health, National Defense Medical Center, Taipei, Taiwan, Republic of China, **2** Division of Nephrology, Department of Medicine, Cardinal Tien Hospital, School of Medicine, Fu Jen Catholic University, New Taipei City, Taiwan, Republic of China, **3** Department of Pathology, Tri-Service General Hospital, National Defense Medical Center, Taipei, Taiwan, Republic of China, **4** Department of Biochemistry, National Defense Medical Center, Taipei, Taiwan, Republic of China, **5** Division of Nephrology, Department of Medicine, Shuang Ho Hospital, Graduate Institute of Clinical Medicine, Taipei Medical University, New Taipei City, Taiwan, Republic of China, **6** Division of Nephrology, Department of Medicine, Tri-Service General Hospital, National Defense Medical Center, Taipei, Taiwan, Republic of China, **7** Center for Molecular Medicine, MRC IGMM, University of Edinburgh, Edinburgh, United Kingdom

Abstract

Inflammation induced by infectious and noninfectious triggers in the kidney may lead to end stage renal disease (ESRD). Toll-like receptor 9 (TLR-9) a receptor for CpG DNA is involved in activation of immune cells in renal disease and may contribute to chronic inflammatory disease progression through an interleukin-6 (IL-6) dependent pathway. Previous studies indicate that -1237T/C confers regulatory effects on TLR-9 transcription. To date the effect of TLR-9 polymorphisms on ESRD remains unknown. We performed a case-control study and genotyped 630 ESRD patients and 415 controls for -1237T/C, -1486T/C and 1635G/A by real-time PCR assays and assessed plasma concentration of IL-6 by ELISA. Haplotype association analysis was performed using the Haploview package. A luciferase reporter assay and real-time PCR were used to test the function of the -1237T/C promoter polymorphism. A significant association between -1237T/C in TLR-9 and ESRD was identified. The TCA, TTA and CCA haplotype of TLR-9 were associated with ESRD. ESRD patients carrying -1237TC had a higher mean plasma IL-6 level when compared with -1237TT. The TLR-9 transcriptional activity of the variant -1237CC allele is higher than the -1237TT allele. The results indicate that in a Han Chinese population the presence of the C allele of -1237T/C in the TLR-9 gene increases susceptibility towards development of ESRD. In vitro studies demonstrate that -1237T/C may be involved in the development of ESRD through transcriptional modulation of TLR-9.

Editor: Qing-Yi Wei, The University of Texas MD Anderson Cancer Center, United States of America

Funding: This study was supported by grants from the National Science Council, National Defense Medical Center, Tri-Service General Hospital and Cardinal Tien Hospital, Taiwan, ROC (NSC99-2314-B-016-001, NSC 99-2815-C-016-002-B, TSGH-C100-007-009-10-S03, CTH- NC10007, MAB101-29). The funders had no role in study design, data collection and analysis, decision to publish, or preparation of the manuscript.

Competing Interests: The authors have declared that no competing interests exist.

* E-mail: a131419@gmail.com

Introduction

In Taiwan chronic kidney disease (CKD) is a major public health problem due to its high prevalence, high rates of healthcare utilization, high risk of progression to end-stage renal disease (ESRD) and poor prognosis [1]. The rising tide of CKD not only adds burden to global health-care resources but also has major impact on patients and their families. CKD is classified as a multifactorial disease as a combination of genetic and environmental factors influence the onset and development of ESRD [2,3]. It is now recognized that inflammation may be established before the onset of renal disease and could be a causal factor in the development of CKD. Sensors of the innate immune system, including Toll-like receptors (TLRs), provide danger recognition platforms on immune and renal cells. These can integrate and translate the diverse triggers of renal inflammation by regulating cell activation and production of proinflammatory cytokines and chemokines [4–6].

Mammalian TLRs comprise a large family of at least 11 members. Members of the TLR family play an important role in both innate and adaptive immune responses. Their genes have been found to be polymorphic [7]. TLRs recognize a wide variety of pathogen associated molecular patterns (PAMPs) from bacteria, viruses and fungi as well as some host molecules. TLR-9, expressed within the endosomal compartment, recognizes unmethylated CpG motifs present in bacterial DNA and intracellular viral antigens [8]. Recent studies have suggested roles for TLR-9 in the development of renal diseases such as glomerulonephritis [9] and lupus nephritis [10]. Single nucleotide polymorphisms (SNPs) in TLR genes affect the susceptibility to and severity of inflammatory diseases by influencing the function of these receptors. The profile of currently known genetic polymorphisms in TLR-9 has been proposed to associate with severe clinical phenotypes [11,12] and TLR-9 polymorphisms appear to affect IgA nephropathy progression [13].

In a human embryonic kidney cell line (HEK293) model system the ability to respond to physiological and therapeutic TLR-9 ligands depends on TLR-9 SNPs [14]. -1237T/C confers regulatory effects on TLR-9 transcription [15]. Indeed the C allele of the -1237T/C polymorphism generates several regulatory sites, including an IL-6-responsive element [16] and was associated with chronic renal disease in a limited candidate gene study [17]. The affect of TLR-9 polymorphisms on ESRD however remains unknown. Therefore we investigated the predictive value of TLR-9 gene polymorphisms on ESRD in a Han Chinese population and undertook in vitro experiments to study potential mechanisms of any associations.

Methods

Study Subjects

This case-control study included 630 ESRD patients (325 females and 305 males; age 64.62 ± 14.51 years) recruited from the Cardinal Tien Hospital and five hemodialysis centers in Taipei, Taiwan. CKD was defined according to KDOQI (Kidney Disease Outcomes Quality Initiative) definitions and estimated glomerular filtration rate (eGFR) was calculated using the Modification of Diet in Renal Disease (MDRD) Study equation [18]. ESRD was defined as eGFR <15 ml/min/1.73 m^2 associated with clinical signs of uremic syndrome requiring dialysis. The enrolled patients were stable (without clinical complications), aged over 20 and had been on hemodialysis (HD) for more than 6 months. Patients with autoimmune disease, malignancy and acute or chronic infection were excluded. The causes of ESRD were diabetes mellitus in 244 patients (38.7%), chronic glomerulonephritis in 199 patients (31.6%), hypertensive nephropathy in 76 patients (12.1%), systemic nephropathy in 51 patients (8.1%) and other and unknown causes in 60 patients (9.5%). The 415 healthy control subjects (217 females and 198 males; age 74.91 ± 7.50 years) with no history of renal disease and whose eGFR was ≥ 60 ml/min/ 1.73 m^2 were recruited from the Center of Physical Examination at Cardinal Tien Hospital. The healthy control subjects showed no microalbuminuria, proteinuria or hematuria and had normal abdominal/renal ultrasonography. 24.5% healthy controls reported a history for hypertension and 13.3% for diabetes mellitus.

Ethics Statement

The study was reviewed and approved by the institutional ethical committee of Cardinal Tien Hospital (CTH-98-3-5-045). After full explanation of the study written informed consent was obtained from all participants. All clinical and biological samples were collected and DNA was genotyped following patient consent.

SNP Genotyping

Genomic DNA was extracted from the peripheral blood of patients and controls using the QIAamp DNA Blood Mini Kit (QIAGEN Inc., Hilden, Germany) according to the manufacturer's instructions. Genotyping for the TLR-9 -1237T/C (rs5743836), -1486T/C (rs187084) and -1635G/A (rs352140) was performed by real-time polymerase chain reaction (PCR). Genotypes were determined using the LightCycler 1.2 System (Roche Diagnostics, Salt Lake City, UT, USA). Primer and detection probes for each polymorphism were based on Hamann et al. and Soriano-Sarabia et al. [19,20]. Melting curve analyses for TLR genes were performed using 2.5 mM of each detection probe. After an initial denaturation at $95°C$ for 10 minutes at a ramp rate of $4.4°C/s$, temperature was dropped to $45°C$ at a ramp rate of $1°C/s$ and finally led to $80°C$ with one acquisition per degree Celsius. Genotyping was done by laboratory personnel blinded to case status and a random 10% of the samples were repeated to validate genotyping procedures.

Peripheral blood mononuclear cell Culture and Plasma Interleukin-6 Concentration

Peripheral blood mononuclear cells (PBMCs) were prepared from venous blood by Ficoll-Hypaque density-gradient centrifugation (Amersham Pharmacia Biotech, Little Chalfont, UK). PBMCs were plated at a density of 1×10^6 cells/ml in 12-well cell culture plates with RPMI 1640 supplemented with 10% heat-inactivated fetal calf serum (FCS) and 100 μg/ml streptomycin. Plasma concentration of interleukin-6 (IL-6) was determined by ELISA using human Quantikine ELISA kit (R&D Systems, Minneapolis, MN, USA).

Expression Analysis by Real-time Quantitative Reverse Transcription Polymerase Chain Reaction

1×10^6 PBMCs cultured as above were serum starved and treated with 100 pg/ml IL-6 for 24 hours. Total RNA was isolated using TriZOL reagent (Invitrogen Cor., Carlsbad, CA, USA). Two microgram of total RNA was reverse transcribed by use of the High Capacity cDNA Reverse Transcription Kit (Applied Biosystems, Foster City, CA, USA) into cDNA. Real-time PCR was performed with the Maxima® SYBR green qPCR master mix (Fermentas, Glen Burnie, MD, USA), using an ABI 7500 real-time PCR system (Applied Biosystems). Primer sequences were as follows: TLR-9 forward 5'-CCCGCTACTGGTGCTATCC-3' and reverse 5'-CCTTCCTCTTTCCACTCCC-3'; β-actin forward 5'-AGTTGCGTTACACCCTTTCTTG-3' and reverse 5'-TCACCTTCACCGTTCCAGTTT-3'. Thermocycling was performed at $95°C$ for 10 min, 40 cycles of $95°C$ for 15 s and $60°C$ for 60 s to measure the fluorescence signal. The dissociation stages, melting curves and quantitative analyses of the data were performed using 7500 system software v1.2.3 (Applied Biosystems). Expression of β-actin was used as internal control. TLR-9 gene expression normalized by β-actin was calculated by using the $2^{-\Delta\Delta Ct}$ method.

Transient Transfection and Luciferase Assay

Two TLR-9 promoter reporters (from 52260706 to 52260840, 135 bp), TLR-9-1237TT-LUC and TLR-9-1237CC-LUC, were amplified by PCR from human genomic DNA including the SNP of interest (-1237T/C) and subcloned into a pGL3 basal reporter cut at XhoI and HindIII sites. The 5' and 3' primers used for PCR were: 5'- CCgCTCgAgATGGGAGCAGAGACATAATGGA-3' and 5'-CCCAAgCTTCTGCTTGCAGTTGACTGTGT-3'. HEK293 cells were grown in Dulbecco's modified Eagle's medium (DMEM) supplemented with 10% charcoal/dextran-treated fetal bovine serum. The cells in each well (24-well plate) were transfected with jetPEI (PolyPlus-transfection, Illkirch, France) according to the manufacturer's protocol; total DNA was adjusted to 1.0 μg by addition of the pGL3 reporter. 24 hours post transfection HEK293 cells were treated with IL-6 (5 ng/ml) for an additional 18 hours. Luciferase activity was assessed using the Promega Luciferase Assay kit and expressed as mean relative light units (RLU) of two transfected sets. Results shown are representative of at least three independent experiments.

Statistical Analysis

Statistical analysis was performed with SPSS for windows version 18.0 (SPSS, Chicago, IL, USA). Demographic, clinical data and plasma IL-6 concentration between groups were compared by Student's t test or Mann-Whitney U test. The results for continuous variables are given as means ± SD. The genotype distributions were tested for Hardy-Weinberg equilibrium. The comparison of the allele and genotype frequencies between the different groups was evaluated by Chi-square test or Fisher's exact test when appropriate. The odds ratios (ORs) and corresponding 95% confidence intervals (CIs) for assessing the effect of the genotype distribution and allele frequencies on ESRD were calculated by logistic regression analysis with adjustment for relevant significant variables. Statistical significance was defined at the 95% level (P<0.05). Linkage disequilibrium (LD) and haplotype analyses were performed using Haploview software [21] (http://www.broad.mit.edu/mpg/haploview/) and WHAP (http://pngu.mgh.harvard.edu/~purcell/whap/), respectively. Associations of TLR-9 promoter polymorphism with TLR-9 mRNA expression were assessed by the Kruskal-Wallis (K-W) test.

Results

Demographic Characteristics

The characteristics of the 1,045 subjects are presented in Table 1. There was no significant difference in gender and diastolic blood pressure between the two groups. Significant differences in age, BMI, smoking history, systolic blood pressure, fasting blood sugar, eGFR, BUN, serum creatinine, total cholesterol and triglycerides were observed between ESRD patients and controls (P<0.001).

Association Analyses of TLR-9 Gene Polymorphisms with Susceptibility to ESRD

The distributions of TLR-9 -1237T/C, -1486T/C and 1635G/A genotypes and allele frequencies were compared between ESRD patients and controls (Table 2). The genotypic distributions of the gene polymorphisms in the patients and controls fit the Hardy-Weinberg equilibrium. The genotype and allelic distributions of -1237T/C in TLR-9 was significantly different between the patients and healthy controls (adjusted OR = 4.49, 95%

CI = 1.75–11.49, P = 0.002 and adjusted OR = 4.36, 95% CI = 1.72–11.08, P = 0.002, respectively). There were no significant differences of genotypic and allelic frequencies in either the TLR-9 -1486T/C or 1635G/A between ESRD patients and controls. The dominant genetic models showed that -1486T/C may be a protective factor for ESRD (adjusted OR = 0.71, 95% CI = 0.53–0.97, P = 0.03).

Although a higher eGFR was observed for patients with the TLR-9 -1237TT genotype this did not reach statistical significance and overall there was no significant association between TLR-9 -1237T/C and the degree of renal function in the ESRD group (results not shown). Stratifying patients by the underlying cause of their renal disease demonstrated marginal associations with genotype and both glomerulonephritis (p = 0.04) and hypertension (P = 0.03) but not with diabetic (P = 0.08) or systemic nephropathy (P = 0.13) (results not shown).

Haplotype Analysis of TLR-9

The haplotype analysis of TLR-9 polymorphisms in ESRD patients and control subjects is shown in Table 3. The frequency of haplotype "TCA" was 27.8% in the ESRD patients compared to 34.6% in the controls (OR = 0.73, 95% CI = 0.60–0.88, P = 0.001). In contrast haplotypes TTA and CCA were more common in ESRD patients (6.5% and 2.5%, respectively) than in controls (1.9% and 0.6%, respectively) (OR = 3.47 and 4.45, 95% CI = 2.02–5.97 and 1.70–11.67, P<0.001 and <0.001, respectively). Other haplotypes showed no significant difference (Table 3).

Association of TLR-9 -1237 T/C Polymorphism with Plasma IL-6 Level

We evaluated whether the TLR-9 -1237 T/C polymorphism might be associated with IL-6 levels in the plasma of ESRD patients. Data are shown in figure 1. Compared to healthy controls (1.56±0.24 pg/ml) the ESRD patients (4.54±0.38 pg/ml) showed a significantly higher level of plasma IL-6 (P<0.001, figure 1A). The plasma IL-6 level did not differ significantly in healthy controls between different TLR-9 -1237T/C genotypes (TT: 1.55±0.10 pg/ml; TC: 1.60±0.11 pg/ml, P = 0.87, figure 1B). The ESRD patients carrying -1237TC had a higher mean plasma IL-6 level (5.47±0.56 pg/ml) when compared with -1237TT (3.71±0.40 pg/ml; P = 0.01, figure 1C). No significant association was shown for other TLR-9 polymorphisms with plasma IL-6 concentration (results not shown).

TLR-9 mRNA Expression in PBMCs

The results of TLR-9 gene expression among 32 ESRD patients are shown in figure 2. Under basal conditions and following IL-6 treatment there was no significant difference in the expression of TLR-9 mRNA between the TT (n = 18) and TC (n = 14) genotypes (basal condition, TT = 1.09±0.09, TC = 1.21±0.25; IL-6 treatment, TT = 1.04±0.08, TC = 1.08±0.21. mean ± SEM relative mRNA expression). Similar results were seen in samples from healthy controls (TT = 8, TC = 7) (results not shown). Under basal conditions or following IL-6 treatment there was no significant difference in the expression of TLR-9 mRNA between the genotypes (mean ± SEM relative mRNA expression: basal condition, TT = 1.12±0.15, TC = 1.19±0.18; IL-6 treatment: TT = 1.08±0.19, TC = 1.16±0.21).

Comparison of Promoter Activity of TT and CC Alleles of the TLR-9 Promoter -1237T/C

To establish whether the TLR-9 SNPs were functionally important we investigated whether IL-6 influenced TLR-9

Table 1. Clinical and biochemical parameters in ESRD patients and control subjects.

	Patients n = 630	Controls n = 415	P value
Male (%)	48.4	47.6	0.80
Age (yrs)	64.62±14.51	74.91±7.50	<0.001
Body mass index (kg/m²)	21.71±5.39	24.18±3.11	<0.001
Current or former smoker (%)	22.8	14.0	<0.001
Systolic blood pressure (mmHg)	140.86±33.25	129.14±15.64	<0.001
Diastolic blood pressure (mmHg)	75.39±10.84	75.14±11.96	0.72
Fasting plasma glucose (mg/dL)	143.76±56.94	102.56±22.59	<0.001
eGFR	7.81±8.33	84.67±16.90	<0.001
BUN (mg/dL)	65.53±19.10	16.27±6.22	<0.001
Serum creatinine (mg/dL)	9.40±2.60	0.86±0.32	<0.001
Serum total cholesterol (mg/dL)	166.49±33.38	187.44±32.98	<0.001
Serum triglycerides (mg/dL)	152.33±95.92	116.50±58.55	<0.001

Quantitative data are mean ± SD.

Table 2. Genotype distributions and allele frequencies for the TLR-9 gene in ESRD patients and control subjects.

Genotypes	Patients n or (%)	Controls n or (%)	Crude OR (95% CI)	P value	*Adjusted OR (95% CI)	P value
T-1237C				<0.001		
TT	591	408	1		1	
TC	39	7	3.85 (1.70–8.68)	0.001	4.49 (1.75–11.49)	0.002
Alleles						
T-allele	97%	99%	1		1	
C-allele	3%	1%	3.76 (1.67–8.44)	0.001	4.36 (1.72–11.08)	0.002
T-1486C				0.10		
TT	276	155	1		1	
TC	290	208	0.78 (0.60–1.02)	0.07	0.72 (0.52–1.00)	0.05
CC	64	52	0.69 (0.46–1.05)	0.08	0.68 (0.41–1.13)	0.14
Alleles						
T-allele	67%	62%	1		1	
C-allele	33%	38%	0.82 (0.69–0.99)	0.04	0.80 (0.64–1.00)	0.05
#D model	276/354	155/260	0.77 (0.59–0.99)	0.04	0.71 (0.53–0.97)	0.03
&R model	566/64	363/52	0.79 (0.54–1.17)	0.23	0.81 (0.51–1.30)	0.39
G1635A				0.90		
GG	245	158	1		1	
GA	306	206	0.96 (0.73–1.25)	0.75	0.94 (0.68–1.30)	0.72
AA	79	51	1.00 (0.67–1.50)	0.99	0.97 (0.59–1.58)	0.90
Alleles						
G-allele	63%	63%	1		1	
A-allele	37%	37%	0.99 (0.82–1.19)	0.90	0.97 (0.78–1.21)	0.81
#D model	245/385	158/257	0.97 (0.75–1.25)	0.79	0.95 (0.70–1.29)	0.73
&R model	551/79	364/51	1.02 (0.70–1.49)	0.90	1.00 (0.63–1.58)	0.99

*Data are expressed as n or (%) and have been adjusted by gender, age, BMI, and smoking status.
#D model = Dominant model.
&R model = Recessive model.

promoter activity using a luciferase reporter assay in HEK293 cells. The results are shown in figure 3. The luciferase activity of the C allele was significantly higher in the absence (10.50±1.06) and presence of IL-6 (11.15±0.16) in comparison to that of the T allele (basal condition 5.61±0.29 and following IL-6 treatment 6.61±0.12) (P = 0.01). However there was no significant difference in TLR-9 promoter activity between -1237TT and -1237TC following IL-6 treatment (P = 0. 10 and 0.49, respectively).

Table 3. Haplotype frequencies in TLR-9 of ESRD patients and control subjects.

Haplotype			Frequencies			
T-1237C	T-1486C	G1635A	Patients	Controls	P value	OR (95% CI)
T	T	G	0.603	0.603	0.90	1.00 (0.83–1.19)
T	C	A	0.278	0.346	0.001	0.73 (0.60–0.88)
T	T	A	0.065	0.019	<0.001	3.47 (2.02–5.97)
T	C	G	0.023	0.023	0.90	1.02 (0.57–1.83)
C	C	A	0.025	0.006	<0.001	4.45 (1.70–11.67)

Discussion

Based on a previous study by our group [17] we have examined possible associations between three TLR-9 SNPs and ESRD in a Han Chinese population. Furthermore, in view of the known interactions between TLR-9 and IL-6 we also studied the association between TLR-9 -1237T/C and plasma IL-6 levels in ESRD and performed functional studies using this SNP. Our study has shown a statistically significant association between a polymorphism in the promoter of TLR-9 gene (-1237T/C) and ESRD. A weaker association between TLR-9 -1486T/C and ESRD was seen in dominant genetic models. The study groups were matched for sex but there were significant differences in BMI, smoking status and age between ESRD patients and healthy controls. Indeed it is recognized that patients with ESRD are often malnourished [22,23] and malnourishment is associated with poor survival in these patients [24]. We have used a non-matched case-control design and applied multiple logistic regression to adjust for confounders. Interestingly a study analyzing the quality of life of irritable bowel syndrome patients compared results when groups were matched and non-matched and found identical results. Indeed the matching procedure slightly diminished the statistical power of the results [25]. In the current study the frequency of TLR9 -1237T/C was 1%. The allele frequency of this SNP in the Han Chinese population (0.007–0.03) [17,26,27] is significantly different from Caucasians (0.10–0.15) and African Americans

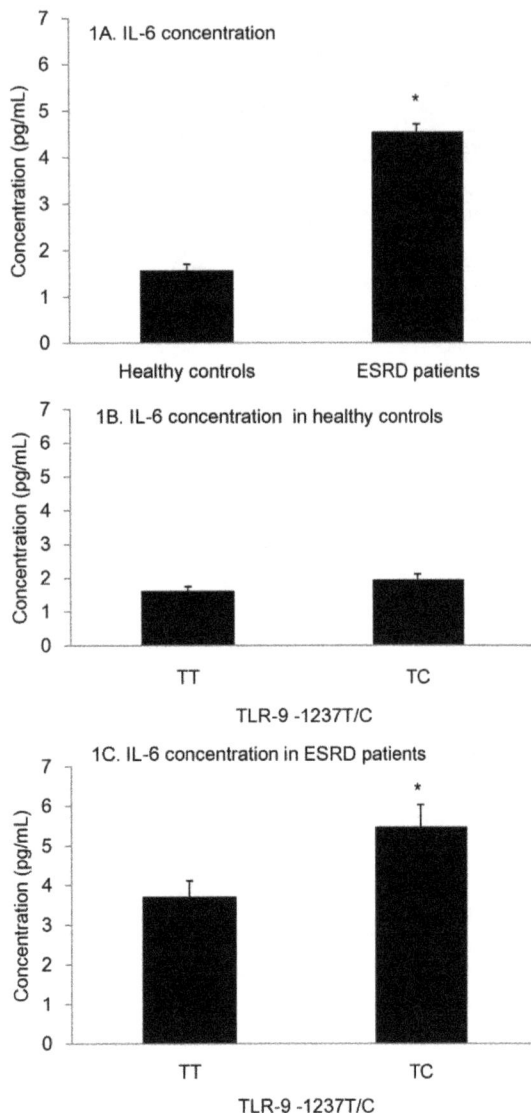

Figure 1. Effects of TLR-9 -1237T/C genotype on the level of plasma IL-6 in healthy controls and ESRD patients. IL-6 concentration was quantified by ELISA. Results are expressed as mean ± SEM. The columns represent the mean value and the lines represent standard error of mean. A: Compared to the healthy controls, the ESRD patients showed a significant increase in plasma IL-6 level (P<0.001). B: The difference of mean level of IL-6 between TT (n = 22) and TC (n = 7) carriers was not significant (P = 0.87) in healthy controls. C: The difference of mean level of IL-6 between TT (n = 18) and TC (n = 14) carriers showed significant difference (P = 0.01) in ESRD patients. *P<0.05.

(0.25–0.39) [28,29]. This indicates the existence of a geographic/ethnic-specific difference in TLR-9 genotypes that may in part reflect ethnic diversity to ESRD susceptibility or other conditions where TLR-9 pathways may be involved.

There is emerging evidence that TLR-9 may play an important role in renal disease and a number of inflammatory conditions of other organ systems. Activation of TLR-9 induces progression of renal disease in MRL-Fas (lpr) mice [30]. TLR-9 has been shown to be involved in antigen-induced immune complex glomerulonephritis and lupus nephritis through regulation of both humoral and cellular immune responses [31]. With respect to TLR-9 SNPs, the

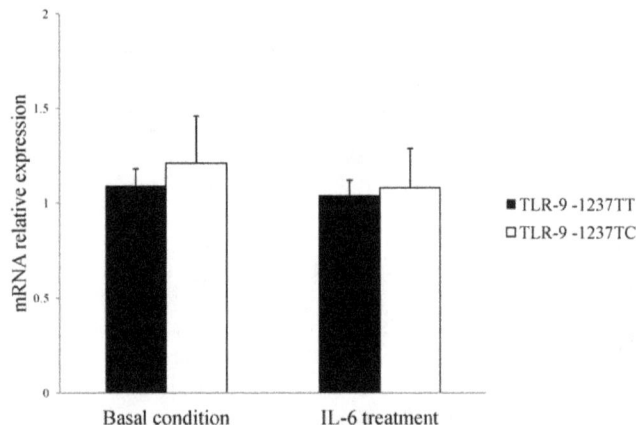

Figure 2. Comparison of PBMC TLR-9 mRNA expression between different genotypes of -1237T/C. β-actin gene expression was used as an internal control gene. TLR-9 mRNA expression in TT or TC PBMCs in the absence or presence of IL-6 (100 pg/ml) treatment was assessed. Values shown are mean ± SEM. Experiments were performed in triplicate.

-1237T/C polymorphism has been shown to be associated with asthma [29], Crohn's disease [32] and HIV infection [33]. The TLR-9 2848 AA genotype is associated with significantly higher expression of TLR-9 and the frequency of intracellular IgM positive B cells in patients with Primary Biliary Cirrhosis [34] whilst the TLR-9 1635G/A polymorphism appears to play a role in the susceptibility to Systemic lupus erythematosus (SLE) in a Chinese population [35]. Less is known regarding TLR-9 SNPs and renal disease. We have previously identified an association between CKD and the -1237T/C of TLR-9 [17] whilst another group has shown that +1174A/G is associated with increased risk for progression of IgA nephropathy in Japanese patients [36] and patients with a TT genotype at 1635G/A show more severe renal damage and poorer therapeutic outcomes [37].

The haplotype of three polymorphisms in TLR-9 was associated with ESRD in the current study. Our data indicate that ESRD

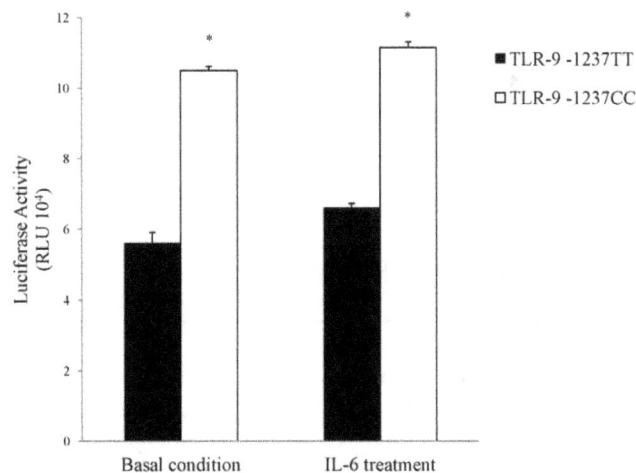

Figure 3. Effects of the -1237T/C genotype in TLR-9 promoter on luciferase activity in cultured HEK293 cells. Luciferase reporters containing a TLR-9 promoter sequence with the wild-type T allele or risk C allele at SNP -1237T/C were transfected into HEK293 cells. The mean ± SEM is given for each construct from three experiments. *P<0.05.

patients carrying the TCA haplotype had a lower risk of ESRD than those not carrying this haplotype whilst patients carrying the TTA or CCA haplotype had a higher risk of ESRD than those not carrying these haplotypes. Holla et al. (2009) demonstrated previously that the TLR-9 TTA haplotype may increase susceptibility to chronic periodontitis whereas the TLR-9 TCG haplotype has a protective effect against this condition [38]. Specific haplotypes in the TLR-9 gene might affect host defense mechanisms and influence susceptibility or resistance to infections. Common TLR-9 alleles with a frequency higher than 5% however do not appear to contribute significantly to the genetic risk involved in susceptibility to SLE or lupus nephritis [39]. Further work is required to fully understand the role of TLR-9 haplotypes on the genetic susceptibility to ESRD.

TLR-9 has been mapped to chromosome 3p21.3. It spans approximately 5 kb and has two exons, the second of which is the major coding region. To date several transcription factors such as AP-1, Sp-1, NF-κB, GATA and CRE are recognized to regulate expression of the TLR-9 gene [40]. In the current study we assessed the functionality of the TLR-9 -1237T/C polymorphism for effects on transcriptional activity. Our data suggest that transcriptional activity of the variant C allele is higher than that of the wild-type T allele. This may be a consequence of creation of an NF-κB binding site with the C allele [41]. Indeed higher transcriptional activity was seen in the presence of the CC allelic variant. These results are consistent with observations of a moderate increase in promoter activity associated with the -1237CC genotype of TLR-9 in asthma patients [15]. Higher promoter activity of the TT allelic variant at -1237T/C in atopic eczema [42] may relate to different pathogenic mechanisms and indicate the need for further investigation in this area. In silico analysis of the human TLR-9 promoter reveals that the C allele of the -1237T/C polymorphism generates several new regulatory sites including an IL-6-responsive element [16]. In the study of Carvalho et al (2011) PBMCs containing the TC allele but not those with the TT allele increased TLR-9 gene expression in response to IL-6 [16]. In contrast no association between -1237T/ C genotype and TLR-9 mRNA level or promoter activity

following IL-6 treatment was identified in the current study. The reason for this discrepancy is not clear but differences in cell sources, detection methods, and time course of experiments in addition to the complexity of gene regulation in vivo may be relevant.

IL-6 is a pleiotropic cytokine that plays a central role in modulating inflammatory responses. Several studies have indicated that IL-6 is a reliable predictor of mortality in ESRD [43,44]. B-cell activation with a TLR-9 agonist significantly increases production of IL-6 in ESRD patients when compared to normal age-matched controls [45]. Associations between genetic polymorphisms and plasma IL-6 levels have been identified [46]. SNPs in the IL-6 gene are associated with plasma IL-6 in myocardial infarction survivors [47] and IL-6 plasma levels are modulated by a polymorphism in the NF-κB1 gene [48]. Our data revealing that ESRD patients carrying -1237TC in TLR-9 gene had a higher mean plasma IL-6 level than those carrying -1237TT are consistent with previous observations [16]. SNPs in the promoter region affecting TLR-9 transcriptional activity might explain inter-individual variability in the production of IL-6 in ESRD patients. However whether a TLR-9/IL-6 signal amplification loop such as that which regulates B cell proliferation [16] is active in patients with renal disease remains to be investigated.

In conclusion, we found the -1237T/C SNP of the TLR-9 gene is significantly associated with ESRD in a Han-Chinese population and that -1237T/C may be involved in the development of ESRD through transcriptional modulation of TLR-9. These observations provide new insights into the role of TLR-9 polymorphisms in renal disease that have the potential to provide new avenues for treatment and may also allow identification of individuals at risk.

Author Contributions

Conceived and designed the experiments: HYY KCL HSL DMS SLS. Performed the experiments: HYY KCL SMH YFL CCW. Analyzed the data: HYY HSL SMH YFL CCW SLS. Contributed reagents/materials/ analysis tools: KCL HSL SMH YFL SLS. Wrote the paper: HYY HSL SMH DMS SLS.

References

1. Wen CP, Cheng TY, Tsai MK, Chang YC, Chan HT, et al. (2008) All-cause mortality attributable to chronic kidney disease: a prospective cohort study based on 462 293 adults in Taiwan. Lancet 371: 2173–2182.
2. Satko SG, Sedor JR, Iyengar SK, Freedman BI (2007) Familial clustering of chronic kidney disease. Semin Dial 20: 229–236.
3. Adler S (2006) Renal disease: environment, race, or genes? Ethn Dis 16: S2-35-39.
4. Eleftheriadis T, Lawson BR (2009) Toll-like receptors and kidney diseases. Inflamm Allergy Drug Targets 8: 191–201.
5. Smith KD (2009) Toll-like receptors in kidney disease. Curr Opin Nephrol Hypertens 18: 189–196.
6. Koc M, Toprak A, Arikan H, Odabasi Z, Elbir Y, et al. (2011) Toll-like receptor expression in monocytes in patients with chronic kidney disease and haemodialysis: relation with inflammation. Nephrol Dial Transplant 26: 955–963.
7. Schwartz DA, Cook DN (2005) Polymorphisms of the Toll-like receptors and human disease. Clin Infect Dis 41 Suppl 7: S403–407.
8. Dalpke A, Zimmermann S, Heeg K (2002) CpG DNA in the prevention and treatment of infections. Bio Drugs 16: 419–431.
9. Summers SA, Steinmetz OM, Ooi JD, Gan PY, O'Sullivan KM, et al. (2010) Toll-like receptor 9 enhances nephritogenic immunity and glomerular leukocyte recruitment, exacerbating experimental crescentic glomerulonephritis. Am J Pathol 177: 2234–2244.
10. Summers SA, Hoi A, Steinmetz OM, O'Sullivan KM, Ooi JD, et al. (2010) TLR9 and TLR4 are required for the development of autoimmunity and lupus nephritis in pristane nephropathy. J Autoimmun 35: 291–298.
11. Bochud PY, Hersberger M, Taffe P, Bochud M, Stein CM, et al. (2007) Polymorphisms in Toll-like receptor 9 influence the clinical course of HIV-1 infection. AIDS 21: 441–446.
12. Krayenbuehl PA, Hersberger M, Truninger K, Mullhaupt B, Maly FE, et al. (2010) Toll-like receptor 4 gene polymorphism modulates phenotypic expression

in patients with hereditary hemochromatosis. Eur J Gastroenterol Hepatol 22: 835–841.
13. Suzuki H, Suzuki Y, Narita I, Aizawa M, Kihara M, et al. (2008) Toll-like receptor 9 affects severity of IgA nephropathy. J Am Soc Nephrol 19: 2384–2395.
14. Kubarenko AV, Ranjan S, Rautanen A, Mills TC, Wong S, et al. (2010) A naturally occurring variant in human TLR9, P99L, is associated with loss of CpG oligonucleotide responsiveness. J Biol Chem 285: 36486–36494.
15. Lange NE, Zhou X, Lasky-Su J, Himes BE, Lazarus R, et al. (2011) Comprehensive genetic assessment of a functional TLR9 promoter polymorphism: no replicable association with asthma or asthma-related phenotypes. BMC Med Genet 12: 26.
16. Carvalho A, Osorio NS, Saraiva M, Cunha C, Almeida AJ, et al. (2011) The C allele of rs5743836 polymorphism in the human TLR9 promoter links IL-6 and TLR9 up-regulation and confers increased B-cell proliferation. PLoS One 6: e28256.
17. Lu KC, Yang HY, Lin YF, Kao SY, Lai CH, et al. (2011) The T-1237C polymorphism of the Toll-like receptor-9 gene is associated with chronic kidney disease in a Han Chinese population. Tohoku J Exp Med 225: 109–116.
18. Levey AS, Bosch JP, Lewis JB, Greene T, Rogers N, et al. (1999) A more accurate method to estimate glomerular filtration rate from serum creatinine: a new prediction equation. Modification of Diet in Renal Disease Study Group. Ann Intern Med 130: 461–470.
19. Hamann L, Hamprecht A, Gomma A, Schumann RR (2004) Rapid and inexpensive real-time PCR for genotyping functional polymorphisms within the Toll-like receptor -2, -4, and -9 genes. J Immunol Methods 285: 281–291.
20. Soriano-Sarabia N, Vallejo A, Ramirez-Lorca R, Rodriguez Mdel M, Salinas A, et al. (2008) Influence of the Toll-like receptor 9 1635A/G polymorphism on the CD4 count, HIV viral load, and clinical progression. J Acquir Immune Defic Syndr 49: 128–135.

21. Barrett JC, Fry B, Maller J, Daly MJ (2005) Haploview: analysis and visualization of LD and haplotype maps. Bioinformatics 21: 263–265.

22. Kopple JD, Greene T, Chumlea WC, Hollinger D, Maroni BJ, et al. (2000) Relationship between nutritional status and the glomerular filtration rate: results from the MDRD study. Kidney Int 57: 1688–1703.

23. Gama-Axelsson T, Heimburger O, Stenvinkel P, Barany P, Lindholm B, et al. (2012) Serum albumin as predictor of nutritional status in patients with ESRD. Clin J Am Soc Nephrol 7: 1446–1453.

24. Jansen MA, Korevaar JC, Dekker FW, Jager KJ, Boeschoten EW, et al. (2001) Renal function and nutritional status at the start of chronic dialysis treatment. J Am Soc Nephrol 12: 157–163.

25. Faresjo T, Faresjo A (2010) To match or not to match in epidemiological studies–same outcome but less power. Int J Environ Res Public Health 7: 325–332.

26. Ng MW, Lau CS, Chan TM, Wong WH, Lau YL (2005) Polymorphisms of the toll-like receptor 9 (TLR9) gene with systemic lupus erythematosus in Chinese. Rheumatology (Oxford) 44: 1456–1457.

27. Wu JF, Chen CH, Ni YH, Lin YT, Chen HL, et al. (2012) Toll-like receptor and hepatitis B virus clearance in chronic infected patients: a long-term prospective cohort study in Taiwan. J Infect Dis 206: 662–668.

28. Velez DR, Wejse C, Stryjewski ME, Abbate E, Hulme WF, et al. (2010) Variants in toll-like receptors 2 and 9 influence susceptibility to pulmonary tuberculosis in Caucasians, African-Americans, and West Africans. Hum Genet 127: 65–73.

29. Lazarus R, Klimecki WT, Raby BA, Vercelli D, Palmer LJ, et al. (2003) Single-nucleotide polymorphisms in the Toll-like receptor 9 gene (TLR9): frequencies, pairwise linkage disequilibrium, and haplotypes in three U.S. ethnic groups and exploratory case-control disease association studies. Genomics 81: 85–91.

30. Anders HJ, Vielhauer V, Eis V, Linde Y, Kretzler M, et al. (2004) Activation of toll-like receptor-9 induces progression of renal disease in MRL-Fas(lpr) mice. FASEB J 18: 534–536.

31. Anders HJ, Banas B, Schlondorff D (2004) Signaling danger: toll-like receptors and their potential roles in kidney disease. J Am Soc Nephrol 15: 854–867.

32. Török HP, Glas J, Endres I, Tonenchi L, Teshome MY, et al. (2009) Epistasis between Toll-like receptor-9 polymorphisms and variants in NOD2 and IL23R modulates susceptibility to Crohn's disease. Am J Gastroenterol 104: 1723–1733.

33. Soriano-Sarabia N, Vallejo A, Ramírez-Lorca R, Rodríguez MM, Salinas A, et al. (2008) Influence of the Toll-like receptor 9 1635A/G polymorphism on the CD4 count, HIV viral load, and clinical progression. J Acquir Immune Defic Syndr 49: 128–135.

34. Kikuchi K, Lian ZX, Kimura Y, Selmi C, Yang GX, et al. (2005) Genetic polymorphisms of toll-like receptor 9 influence the immune response to CpG and contribute to hyper-IgM in primary biliary cirrhosis. J Autoimmun 24: 347–352.

35. Xu CJ, Zhang WH, Pan HF, Li XP, Xu JH, et al. (2009) Association study of a single nucleotide polymorphism in the exon 2 region of toll-like receptor 9 (TLR9) gene with susceptibility to systemic lupus erythematosus among Chinese. Mol Biol Rep 36: 2245–2248.

36. Suzuki H, Suzuki Y, Narita I, Aizawa M, Kihara M, et al. (2008) Toll-like receptor 9 affects severity of IgA nephropathy. J Am Soc Nephrol 19: 2384–2395.

37. Sato D, Suzuki Y, Kano T, Suzuki H, Matsuoka J, et al. (2012) Tonsillar TLR9 expression and efficacy of tonsillectomy with steroid pulse therapy in IgA nephropathy patients. Nephrol Dial Transplant 27: 1090–1097.

38. Holla LI, Vokurka J, Hrdlickova B, Augustin P, Fassmann A (2009) Association of Toll-like receptor 9 haplotypes with chronic periodontitis in Czech population. J Clin Periodontol 37: 152–159.

39. De Jager PL, Richardson A, Vyse TJ, Rioux JD (2006) Genetic variation in toll-like receptor 9 and susceptibility to systemic lupus erythematosus. Arthritis Rheum 54: 1279–1282.

40. Takeshita F, Suzuki K, Sasaki S, Ishii N, Klinman DM, et al. (2004) Transcriptional regulation of the human TLR9 gene. J Immunol 173: 2552–2561.

41. Ng MT, Van't Hof R, Crockett JC, Hope ME, Berry S, et al. (2010) Increase in NF-kappaB binding affinity of the variant C allele of the toll-like receptor 9 -1237T/C polymorphism is associated with Helicobacter pylori-induced gastric disease. Infect Immun 78: 1345–1352.

42. Novak N, Yu CF, Bussmann C, Maintz L, Peng WM, et al. (2007) Putative association of a TLR9 promoter polymorphism with atopic eczema. Allergy 62: 766–772.

43. Hasuike Y, Nonoguchi H, Ito K, Naka M, Kitamura R, et al. (2009) Interleukin-6 is a predictor of mortality in stable hemodialysis patients. Am J Nephrol 30: 389–398.

44. Zoccali C, Tripepi G, Mallamaci F (2006) Dissecting inflammation in ESRD: Do cytokines and C-reactive protein have a complementary prognostic value for mortality in dialysis patients? J Am Soc Nephrol 17: S169–S173.

45. Pahl MV, Gollapudi S, Sepassi L, Gollapudi P, Elahimehr R, et al. (2010) Effect of end-stage renal disease on B-lymphocyte subpopulations, IL-7, BAFF and BAFF receptor expression. Nephrol Dial Transplant 25: 205–212.

46. Smith AJ, Humphries SE (2009) Cytokine and cytokine receptor gene polymorphisms and their functionality. Cytokine Growth Factor Rev 20: 43–59.

47. Ljungman P, Bellander T, Nyberg F, Lampa E, Jacquemin B, et al. (2009) DNA variants, plasma levels and variability of interleukin-6 in myocardial infarction survivors: results from the AIRGENE study. Thromb Res 124: 57–64.

48. Giachelia M, Voso MT, Tisi MC, Martini M, Bozzoli V, et al. (2012) Interleukin-6 plasma levels are modulated by a polymorphism in the NF-kappaB1 gene and are associated with outcome following rituximab-combined chemotherapy in diffuse large B-cell non-Hodgkin lymphoma. Leuk Lymphoma 53: 411–416.

23

HLA Polymorphism and Susceptibility to End-Stage Renal Disease in Cantonese Patients Awaiting Kidney Transplantation

Qiong Cao[1]*, Di Xie[2], Jiangmei Liu[3], Hongyan Zou[4], Yinze Zhang[4], Hong Zhang[1], Zhimei Zhang[1], Hao Xue[1], Jiyuan Zhou[3], Pingyan Chen[3]*

1 Division of Tissue Typing Center, Nanfang Hospital, Southern Medical University, Guangdong, Guangzhou, China, 2 Division of Nephrology, Nanfang Hospital, Southern Medical University, Guangdong, Guangzhou, China, 3 Department of Biostatistics, School of Public Health and Tropical Medicine, Southern Medical University, Guangdong, Guangzhou, China, 4 HLA High-Resolution Confirmatory Typing Laboratory, Shenzhen Blood Center, Shenzhen, China

Abstract

Background: End-Stage Renal Disease (ESRD) is a worldwide public health problem. Currently, many genome-wide association studies have suggested a potential association between human leukocyte antigen (HLA) and ESRD by uncovering a causal relationship between HLA and glomerulonephritis. However, previous studies, which investigated the HLA polymorphism and its association with ESRD, were performed with the modest data sets and thus might be limited. On the other hand, few researches were conducted to tackle the Chinese population with ESRD. Therefore, this study aims to detect the susceptibilities of HLA polymorphism to ESRD within the Cantonese community, a representative southern population of China.

Methods: From the same region, 4541 ESRD patients who were waiting for kidney transplantation and 3744 healthy volunteer bone marrow donors (controls) were randomly chosen for this study. Polymerase chain reaction-sequence specific primer method was used to analyze the HLA polymorphisms (including HLA-A, HLA-B and HLA-DRB1 loci) in both ESRD patients and controls. The frequencies of alleles at these loci and haplotypes were compared between ESRD patients and controls.

Results: A total of 88 distinct HLA alleles and 1361 HLA A-B-DRB1 haplotypes were detected. The frequencies of five alleles, HLA-A*24, HLA-B*55, HLA-B*54, HLA-B*40(60), HLA-DRB1*04, and one haplotype (HLA-A*11-B*27-DRB1*04) in ESRD patients are significantly higher than those in the controls, respectively.

Conclusions: Five HLA alleles and one haplotype at the HLA-A, HLA-B and HLA-DRB1 loci appear to be associated with ESRD within the Cantonese population.

Editor: Clive M. Gray, University of Cape Town, South Africa

Funding: This study was supported by the National Natural Science Foundation of China (Numbers 30972554 and 81273191) granted to Pingyan Chen and the National Natural Science Foundation of China (Numbers 81373098 and 81072386) granted to Prof. Jiyuan Zhou. The funders had no role in study design, data collection and analysis, decision to publish, or preparation of the manuscript.

Competing Interests: All the authors declared no competing interests.

* E-mail: chenpy99@126.com (PC); caoliy2000@126.com (QC)

Introduction

With a high incidence, end-stage renal disease (ESRD) becomes a worldwide public health problem [1]. ESRD is a condition where a patient is permanently dependent on renal replacement in order to avoid life-threatening uremia. The incidence of ESRD has been increasing in Europe and United States over the past decade, with doubling the number of patients [2]. In China, there is a rising incidence of ESRD, too. The number of the registered ESRD patients who were treated by hemodialysis was 41,755 in 1999, and this number was even more than 120,000 in 2008 [3]. The annual incidence of ESRD that needed hemodialysis therapy was estimated to be as high as 36.1 per million population (pmp) in China [4].

Many patients with chronic kidney disease (CKD) can progress to ESRD despite receiving intensive therapy, and the rate of progression varies from person to person. Exploring those specific genetic-variants in ESRD patients can benefit the development of novel strategies to detect and prevent ESRD at the early stage. Unlike developed countries, in which the major causes of ESRD are diabetes mellitus and hypertension, the leading cause of ESRD in China remains glomerulonephritis, which accounts for 49.9% of total kidney diseases [4–6]. Recently, many genome-wide association studies have detected a strong association between the human leukocyte antigen (HLA) and glomerulonephritis [7–10], indicating a potential association between HLA and ESRD. HLA is located at chromosome 6p21.31 [11]. People with certain HLA types are more likely to developing autoimmune diseases such as type I diabetes. Moreover, HLA has a gene-dense region, and its mutation is also linked to autoimmune diseases [11]. Therefore, HLA plays a critical role in the immune responses, which are crucial in ESRD processing. Exploring the specific genetic-variants of HLA in ESRD patients may benefit the development of novel strategies to detect and prevent ESRD at the early stage. Thus, this study expands our knowledge by analyzing the association between HLA polymorphism and ERSD, and detects the mechanisms underlying initiation and progression of renal failure.

Currently, there have been several studies to indicate the association between HLA alleles/haplotypes and ESRD [12,13]. However, these findings were based on the modest data sets and thus might be limited. On the other hand, little is known about the association between HLA polymorphism and ESRD within the Chinese population, specifically in the Cantonese patients. In order to enrich the knowledge of HLA polymorphism in the Cantonese population and detect its susceptibilities to ESRD, the frequencies of alleles at the HLA-A, -B and -DRB1 loci and haplotypes in both ESRD patients who are waiting for kidney transplantation and healthy volunteer bone marrow donors (controls) from the same region of Southern China were investigated.

Methods

Patients and control donors

4541 Cantonese patients in 1996–2010, who were diagnosed with ESRD and waiting for a cadaveric kidney, were selected from the Transplantation Center of Nanfang Hospital for this study. As the largest transplantation center of Southern China, Transplantation Center of Nanfang Hospital holds the database of tissue typing, and it also provides HLA-A, -B and -DRB1genotype data of the patients. The medical records of the patients such as age, gender, and primary cause of ESRD were extracted from Nanfang Hospital. All the data were collected by a research nurse, who is a non-investigator in this study. In order to preserve patients' privacy, all data are anonymous.

Based on the database of HLA High-Resolution Confirmatory Typing Laboratory of Shenzhen Blood Center, a total 3744 unrelated, healthy, and volunteer bone marrow donors were selected as controls from the same Southern Chinese population. The age, gender, HLA-A, -B and -DRB1 genotype data of the donors were acquired from a registry system database. The laboratory of Shenzhen Blood Center is one of seven HLA high-resolution confirmatory typing laboratories of the China Marrow Donor Program, which is a non-profit sub-organization of the Red Cross Society of China. All the data of the controls were hosted by Shenzhen Blood Center. All the identifying information of volunteers was removed in the final dataset for analysis in order to preserve patients' privacy.

The entire study protocol was approved by the Nanfang Ethics Committee, and the whole research process was supervised by Nanfang Ethics Committee.

DNA extraction

Whole blood samples were collected from the participants and stored at $-20°C$ until DNA extraction. Genomic DNA was extracted from whole blood samples containing ethylene diamine tetraacetic acid (EDTA) by QIAamp DNA blood Mini Kit (QIAGEN GmbH, Hilden, Germany), which can yield good quality high molecular weight DNA suitable for analysis [14].

Polymerase chain reaction-sequence specific primer based typing at HLA-A, -B and–DRB1 loci

The genotyping at the HLA-A, -B, and -DRB1 loci was performed by the Tissue Typing Center affiliated to the Transplantation Center of Nanfang Hospital. The Tissue Typing Center uses a standardized set of HLA typing program, provided by National Center for Clinical Laboratory of China. Polymerase chain reaction (PCR) amplification was performed using a GeneAmp PCR system 9700 (Applied Biosystems, Foster city CA, USA). According to the manufacturer's instructions, sequence specific primer (SSP) analysis was performed with a mixture of nucleotides and dNTPs by HLA-ABDR GeneType analysis kit (Biotest AG, Dreieich, Germany). All amplifications were performed in a thermocycler using the following conditions: initial denaturation 94°C for 2 minutes, denaturation 94°C for 10 seconds, annealing and extension 65°C for 1 minute, 10 cycles, followed by 94°C for 10 seconds, 61°C for 50 seconds, 72°C of 30 seconds for 20 cycles, and stored at 4°C. Primer set amplified single amplicons as demonstrated by agarose gel electrophoresis. The PCR products were pre-stained with SYBR Green I (0.5 µl/ 100 ml gel), loaded in agarose gels, and then electrophoresed for 10 minutes at 10V/cm in 0.5×TBE (Tris-Boric acid-EDTA) buffer. The agarose gels were examined under UV illumination and documented by photography. The exact HLA type was investigated by Biotest HLA-SSP Typing software 1.1.

Statistical methods

Data are described with arithmetic mean, standard deviation, median, range and absolute number of the subjects. The frequencies of the alleles at the HLA-A, -B and -DRB1 loci were estimated using SAS9.17®. The frequencies of the HLA-A-B-DRB1 haplotypes were calculated by the expectation maximization (EM) algorithm using Arlequin software 3.5 (Switzerland). The exact test was used to evaluate the assumption of Hardy-Weinberg equilibrium (HWE) as described by Guo and Thomson [15]. The linkage disequilibrium coefficient between any two alleles at these loci is measured by Lewontin D' [16]. The frequencies of the HLA-A, -B, -DRB1 alleles and HLA-A-B-DRB1 haplotypes were compared between ESRD patients and controls by Fisher's exact test or Pearson chi-square test with the Bonferroni correction for multiple testing [17]. A 5% significance level was considered sufficient to reject the null hypothesis.

Results

Characteristics of patients and control donors

A total of 4541 Cantonese ESRD patients were selected from the database of the tissue typing center affiliated with the Transplantation Center of Nanfang Hospital, including 2754 (60.65%) males. The median age of patients was 40 (mean±sd: 40±12, min-max: 7–81). Among those patients, 1975 (43.5%) patients have glomerulonephritis, which is the most common cause of ESRD. A total of 3744 healthy volunteer bone marrow donors were included in this study. All donors were unrelated, and from the same southern Chinese population, including 1994 (53.26%) males. The median age was 31.0 (mean±sd: 32±8, min-max: 18–55).

Hardy-Weinberg equilibrium tests at HLA-A,-B and -DRB1 loci

In 4541 ESRD patients, there were 21 HLA-A, 47 HLA-B and 14 HLA-DRB1 alleles to occur. In 3744 control donors, there were 17 HLA-A, 41 HLA-B and 16 HLA-DRB1 alleles to occur.

In both groups, a total of 88 distinct HLA alleles occurred including 21 HLA-A, 51 HLA-B and 16 HLA-DRB1 alleles (see Table 1). The most frequent alleles which occurred at the HLA-A, -B and–DRB1 loci of all subjects were consistent with a previous study conducted within the Cantonese population [18]. The HWE tests at the HLA-A, -B and -DRB1 loci showed the violation of HWE in both the ESRD patients and the controls (P<0.05).

Allele frequency at HLA-A, -B and -DRB1 loci in kidney transplant recipients and control donors

The frequencies of alleles at the HLA-A, -B and -DRB1 loci obtained by DNA typing are summarized in Table 2. In the most frequent alleles (top 20% of all the allele frequencies) which occurred at the HLA-A (n = 4), -B (n = 10) and -DRB1 (n = 4) loci in the ESRD patients or in the controls, the frequencies of HLA-A*24, HLA-B*55, HLA-B*54, HLA-B*40(60), HLA-DRB1*04 were significantly higher in ESRD patients than those in controls, respectively.

HLA-A-B-DRB1 haplotype frequencies and association analysis

Using the EM algorithm, a total of 1361 HLA A-B-DRB1 haplotypes were detected, where there were 974 haplotypes identified in 4541 ESRD patients, and 887 haplotypes identified in 3744 control donors, respectively. Moreover, the frequencies of the three most common haplotypes HLA-A*02-B*46-DRB1*09, HLA-A*33-B*58-DRB1*03(17), and HLA-A*11-B*15(75)-DRB1*12 were 4.42%, 3.97%, and 3.18% in ESRD patients, respectively. Additionally, the above three haplotypes were also the most common haplotypes in the controls, with the frequencies of 4.97%, 5.01%, and 3.61%, respectively. These results were consistent with a previous study conducted within the Cantonese population [18].

For the most frequent HLA-A-B-DRB1 haplotypes (top 5% of all the haplotypes), the haplotype distribution in ESRD patients (n = 50) was significantly different from that in the controls (n = 21), as shown in Table 3. HLA-A*11-B*27-DRB1*04 is one of the common haplotypes in ESRD patients, with the frequency being 0.426%. However, the frequency of the same haplotype was 0.086% in the controls, which was much smaller than that in ESRD patients (P<0.05). This result indicated that HLA-A*11-B*27-DRB1*04 haplotype appears to be associated with ESRD within the Cantonese population.

Discussion

Our study has academic significance. Due to the importance of the immune response in the processing of ESRD, genes located on HLA potentially contribute to the ESRD processing. The identification and analysis of HLA polymorphism are important not only for the study of the ESRD susceptibility, but also for the

tissue transplantation in ESRD patients. A key step for tissue transplantation is histocompatibility testing, which is crucial in the selection of tissue receptors and tissue donors. Our study provides useful information for the selection of donor kidneys in Cantonese ESRD patients, who are waiting for kidney transplantation. In these patients, grafted kidney may survive better through selecting donor kidneys without susceptible haplotypes of ESRD, although the efficacy of such an approach for improving the prognosis of kidney transplantation need be supported by further investigations.

Our present study was distinct because we found several HLA alleles/haplotypes which appear to be associated with ESRD. Specifically, significantly higher frequencies of five alleles (HLA-A*24, HLA-B*55, HLA-B*54, HLA-B*40(60) and HLA-DRB1*04) and one haplotype (HLA-A*11-B*27-DRB1*04) (see Tables 2 and 3) in Cantonese ESRD patients were observed, respectively. To further explore specific HLA alleles/haplotypes for specific renal diseases, a subgroup analysis was performed based on definite pathologic diagnosis for the case of enough sample size. Among 4541 ESRD patients, 399 patients received renal biopsy previously and were diagnosed definitely as glomerulonephritis (n = 265), hypertensive nephropathy (n = 32), diabetic nephropathy (n = 39), chronic interstitial nephritis (n = 36), hereditary or other kidney disorders (n = 27), separately. Note that the analysis results based on data sets with small sample size may not be so reliable and thus we only conducted the subgroup analysis based on 265 patients with glomerulonephritis. The frequencies of three alleles (HLA-A*11, HLA-B*58 and HLA-DRB1*04) and one haplotype (HLA-A*02-B*40(61)-DRB1*04) in the 265 patients were significantly higher than those in the controls, respectively (Table 4).

Note that the polymorphism of HLA-DRB1 is considered as a susceptible genetic marker for several autoimmune conditions and diseases, such as type I diabetes and dilated cardiomyopathy [19,20]. As such, among the above identified HLA alleles and haplotype, it is worthy to pay close attention to HLA-DRB1*04 which has the frequency of 14.21% in ESRD patients. In our study, either in the analysis for pooled ESRD patients or in subgroup analysis, the frequency of HLA-DRB1*04 in ESRD patients was significantly higher than that in the controls and HLA-DRB1*04 was also included in the HLA-A-B-DRB1 haplotypes which distributed significantly differently between ESRD patients and controls (in the pooled ESRD: HLA-A*11-B*27-DRB1*04; in the glomerulonephritis subgroup: HLA-A*02-B*40(61)-DRB1*04). Another interesting issue is HLA-B*40, with a frequency of 16.26% in ESRD patients, which is identified as a susceptible allele for IgA nephropathy in Han Chinese through a genome-wide association study [8]. HLA associated IgA nephropathy has a high prevalence in Asia, and it is the primary reason for glomerulonephritis among individuals undergoing renal biopsy [21,22]. Approximately 15–40% patients with HLA associated IgA nephropathy can progress to ESRD within 20 years [23,24].

Table 1. Numbers of HLA-A, -B and -DRB1 alleles in ESRD patients and controls.

Locus	No. of alleles		
	ESRD patients	Controls	Both groups
HLA-A	21	17	21
HLA-B	47	41	51
HLA-DRB1	14	16	16

Table 2. Allele frequencies at HLA-A, -B and -DRB1 loci in ESRD patients and controls (ordered by statistical significance for each locus).

Allele	ESRD patients [a] (n = 4541*2)	Controls [a] (n = 3744*2)	P [b]	Adjusted P [c]
HLA-A (%)				
*24	17.45	15.37	0.0003	0.0055
HLA-B (%)				
*55	3.50	2.50	0.0002	0.0071
*54	3.70	2.67	0.0002	0.0076
*40(60)	16.26	14.37	0.0008	0.0297
HLA-DRB1 (%)				
*04	14.21	10.24	<0.0001	<0.0001

[a]Listed are only the most frequent (top 20%) alleles for each HLA locus in the ESRD patients and controls, respectively.
[b]Using Fisher exact test.
[c]P values were adjusted by Bonferroni method. Multiplicative factor was used for each allele.

In brief, compared to previous studies, our study detected a similar relationship between HLA polymorphism and ESRD incidence. However, discrepancies occurred between our results and other results. For example, compared to the controls, the frequencies of HLA-B*78 and -DRB1*11 significantly increased in 105 Brazilian patients with ESRD; while the frequency of HLA-B*14 was significantly lower in them [12]. Moreover, a study of 1620 IgA nephropathy ESRD patients from Eurotranplant found that the frequencies of HLA-B35 and DR5 (by HLA antigen typing) were significantly increased in these patients, and HLA-A2-B5-DR5 was identified as a susceptible haplotype in ESRD patients [13]. Although further studies are needed, HLA alleles and haplotype which were found to be associated with ESRD in our study may contribute to be susceptible markers for ESRD patients in the Chinese people, especially in the Cantonese people.

CKD is becoming the major pathogenic hypothesis for kidney damage with abnormalities in both humoral and cellular responses, and CKD can progress to the ESRD over a period of time. Logically, the processing of ESRD should be: HLA polymorphism and susceptibility→a disease (one by one) → CKD →ESRD. Regardless of the primary underlying disease, chronically injured kidneys are histomorphologically characterized by tubulointerstitial fibrosis which is considered the common pathway of chronic progressive kidney disease. Recent studies provided the evidence that genetic polymorphism and epigenetic variations determine the individual susceptibility of patients to develop rapid progressive kidney disease [25]. In this study, we focused on the final outcomes of ESRD in order to avoid unexplained causes contributed by many known or unknown diseases. From the results, HLA polymorphism and their susceptibility to ESRD are an indicator rather than the direct causes of ESRD. Glomerulonephritis remained the leading cause of ESRD in 2008, although the contribution of diabetes and hypertension to the ESRD slightly increased according to the national survey [4]. In spite of the continuous change in the patient population with time, analysis done in our study was still stylish because the characteristics of ESRD patients are not substantially changed over years [4]. The number of patients having definite causes for ESRD confirmed by previous renal biopsy was too small to conduct disease specific analysis. In spite of

Table 3. Frequency of the susceptible three-locus HLA haplotypes in ESRD patients and controls (ordered by statistical significance for susceptible haplotypes).

HLA haplotype [a]	ESRD patients (n = 4541*2)	Controls (n = 3744*2)	P [b]	Adjusted P [c]
Susceptible HLA A-B-DRB1 haplotype (%)				
A*11-B*27-DRB1*04	0.426	0.086	<0.0001	0.0036
A*24-B*40(60)-DRB1*08	0.605	0.216	0.0001	0.0514
A*02-B*40(60)-DRB1*11	0.850	0.397	0.0003	0.1450
A*24-B*40(60)-DRB1*04	0.847	0.480	0.0043	1.0000
A*11-B*55-DRB1*04	0.557	0.279	0.0062	1.0000
A*11-B*40(60)-DRB1*04	1.615	1.127	0.0076	1.0000
A*24-B*40(60)-DRB1*15	0.645	0.366	0.0120	1.0000
A*24-B*46-DRB1*09	0.810	0.530	0.0300	1.0000
A*24-B*13-DRB1*15	0.793	0.521	0.0352	1.0000
A*02-B*40(60)-DRB1*12	0.588	0.359	0.0426	1.0000

[a]Listed are only the top 5% of all the HLA-A-B-DRB1 haplotypes with significant uncorrected P-value.
[b]Using Fisher exact test.
[c]P values were adjusted by Bonferroni method. Multiplicative factor was used for each haplotype.

Table 4. Allele and haplotype frequencies at HLA-A, -B and -DRB1 loci in ESRD patients with definite pathologic diagnosis of glomerulonephritis and controls.

Allele/Haplotype	ESRD patients [a] (n = 265*2)	Controls [a] (n = 3744*2) P [b]		Adjusted P [c]
HLA-A*11 (%)	38.68	32.39	0.0035	0.0104
HLA-B *58 (%)	5.84	9.51	0.0050	0.0241
HLA-DRB1 *04 (%)	14.15	10.24	0.0065	0.0196
HLA-A*02-B*40(61)-DRB1*04(%)	1.077	0.126	0.0002	0.0100

[a]Listed are only the most frequent (top 20%) alleles for each HLA locus in the ESRD patients and controls, respectively and a HLA-A-B-DRB1 haplotype with significant uncorrected P-value.
[b]Using Fisher exact test.
[c]P values were adjusted by Bonferroni method. Multiplicative factor was used for each allele or haplotype.

this limitation, our results still provided valuable information. Furthermore, little is known about the working mechanism of HLA genes, and further studies are required to develop the methods for predicting and preventing ESRD at early stages.

This study has a number of statistical strengths. First, this analysis was based on the Cantonese population, and reduced the effect of geographic and population diversity on the results. Second, the present study was conducted in a very large population, and only the most frequent (top 20%) HLA alleles and the most frequent (top 5%) HLA haplotypes were chosen for analysis. With those strict requirements, this study can generate sufficiently statistical power to detect a slight effect, and can avoid generating a fluctuated risk estimate [26]. In addition, only the P values of less than 0.05 (after the Bonferroni correction for multiple comparisons) were considered statistically significant; therefore, the efficacy of test is kept.

This study also had a few limitations in its design. Controls were healthy volunteer bone marrow donors, but we could not entirely rule out the possibility of the incidence of ESRD in the future. However, the prevalence of ESRD in Cantonese people is low (about 0.1%) [3]; therefore, the selection bias for future incidence of ESRD is negligible. In addition, the China Marrow Donor Program only collected the age, gender, and HLA genotype data of donors. It is hard to compare other important ESRD risk factors such as hypertension, diabetes mellitus, albuminuria, dyslipidemia, hyperuricemia, and smoking to those of ESRD patients. Also, our study was not as systematic as genome-wide association studies, and further studies should analyze the association of other HLA antigens and other non-HLA antigens in ESRD patients. More studies by HLA typing are required to confirm the current findings in other independent individuals. Another limitation is the EM algorithm in our study. EM algorithm was used to estimate the frequencies of HLA A-B-DRB1 haplotypes, and this approach is usually used for diploid genotype data under the condition of HWE in the pooled data of the patients and controls. However,

our results revealed that the frequency distribution of HLA alleles was inconsistent with the HWE in both ESRD patients and controls. The accuracy of the frequency estimates derived from the EM algorithm may be queried in our study. However, Fallin et al [27] suggested that the frequency estimates in individual haplotypes *via* the EM algorithm deviate their true values in 5% range for large samples (>100) in unphased diploid genotype data, even in the worst cases. Although there may be a problem for detecting very rare haplotypes among the sampled individuals (frequency in the sample <0.1%), the likelihood that such extremely rare haplotypes contribute appreciably to the risk of disease among the affected individuals in the samples may be very low. Schmidt [28] indicated that the violation of HWE could be ignored if the sample size is large enough. Therefore, EM algorithm can be used to analyze unphased diploid genotype data for determining the disease-predisposing haplotypes in this study.

In summary, this study detected the association between HLA polymorphism and ESRD and its susceptibilities for ESRD within the Cantonese population. Five susceptible alleles and one susceptible haplotype were detected in Cantonese ESRD patients awaiting kidney transplantation. These HLA alleles and haplotype might serve as susceptible genetic marker for ESRD within the Cantonese population. Results from our study should be confirmed in further investigations.

Acknowledgments

The authors gratefully acknowledge Dr. Ying Guan for her comments and constructive suggestions for improving the manuscript.

Author Contributions

Conceived and designed the experiments: QC PC. Analyzed the data: JL PC. Wrote the paper: QC DX. Reviewed/edited manuscript: PC JZ QC. Collected data: QC DX HZ YZ HZ ZZ HX.

References

1. Levey AS, Atkins R, Coresh J, Cohen EP, Collins AJ, et al. (2007) Chronic kidney disease as a global public health problem: approaches and initiatives – a position statement from Kidney Disease Improving Global Outcomes. Kidney Int 72: 247–259.
2. van Dijk PC, Jager KJ, de Charro F, Collart F, Cornet R, et al. (2001) Renal replacement therapy in Europe: the results of a collaborative effort by the ERA-EDTA registry and six national or regional registries. Nephrol Dial Transplant 16: 1120–1129.
3. Zuo L, Wang M (2010) Current burden of ESRD in China and it is estimated to be increasing faster in the near future. Chinese Journal of Blood Purification 9: 47–49.
4. Zuo L, Wang M (2010) Current burden and probable increasing incidence of ESRD in China. Clin Nephrol 74 Suppl 1: S20–22.
5. Chen N, Wang W, Huang Y, Shen P, Pei D, et al. (2009) Community-based study on CKD subjects and the associated risk factors. Nephrol Dial Transplant 24: 2117–2123.
6. Chen W, Wang H, Dong X, Liu Q, Mao H, et al. (2009) Prevalence and risk factors associated with chronic kidney disease in an adult population from southern China. Nephrol Dial Transplant 24: 1205–1212.
7. Stanescu HC, Arcos-Burgos M, Medlar A, Bockenhauer D, Kottgen A, et al. (2011) Risk HLA-DQA1 and PLA(2)R1 alleles in idiopathic membranous nephropathy. N Engl J Med 364: 616–626.
8. Yu XQ, Li M, Zhang H, Low HQ, Wei X, et al. (2011) A genome-wide association study in Han Chinese identifies multiple susceptibility loci for IgA nephropathy. Nat Genet 44: 178–182.

9. Gharavi AG, Kiryluk K, Choi M, Li Y, Hou P, et al. (2011) Genome-wide association study identifies susceptibility loci for IgA nephropathy. Nat Genet 43: 321–327.

10. Feehally J, Farrall M, Boland A, Gale DP, Gut I, et al. (2010) HLA has strongest association with IgA nephropathy in genome-wide analysis. J Am Soc Nephrol 21: 1791–1797.

11. Erlich HA, Opelz G, Hansen J (2001) HLA DNA typing and transplantation. Immunity 14: 347–356.

12. Crispim JC, Mendes-Junior CT, Wastowski IJ, Palomino GM, Saber LT, et al. (2008) HLA polymorphisms as incidence factor in the progression to end-stage renal disease in Brazilian patients awaiting kidney transplant. Transplant Proc 40: 1333–1336.

13. Doxiadis, II, De Lange P, De Vries E, Persijn GG, Claas FH (2001) Protective and susceptible HLA polymorphisms in IgA nephropathy patients with end-stage renal failure. Tissue Antigens 57: 344–347.

14. Miller SA, Dykes DD, Polesky HF (1988) A simple salting out procedure for extracting DNA from human nucleated cells. Nucleic Acids Res 16: 1215.

15. Guo SW, Thompson EA (1992) Performing the exact test of Hardy-Weinberg proportion for multiple alleles. Biometrics 48: 361–372.

16. Lewontin RC (1988) On measures of gametic disequilibrium. Genetics 120: 849–852.

17. Perneger TV (1998) What's wrong with Bonferroni adjustments. BMJ 316: 1236–1238.

18. Zhu WG, Bao ZQ, Lan YX, Jin SZ, Li Z, et al. (2009) Sequence analysis and haplotpye diversity of human leukocyte antigen -A, -B, -DRB1 genes in Han population from southern China. Chin J Blood Transfusion 22: 893–897.

19. Zhang XM, Wang HY, Luo YY, Ji LN (2009) HLA-DQ, DR allele polymorphism of type 1 diabetes in the Chinese population: a meta-analysis. Chin Med J (Engl) 122: 980–986.

20. Jin B, Ni H, Geshang Q, Li Y, Shen W, et al. (2011) HLA-DR4 antigen and idiopathic dilated cardiomyopathy susceptibility: a meta-analysis involving 11,761 subjects. Tissue Antigens 77: 107–111.

21. D'Amico G (1987) The commonest glomerulonephritis in the world: IgA nephropathy. Q J Med 64: 709–727.

22. Barratt J, Feehally J (2005) IgA nephropathy. J Am Soc Nephrol 16: 2088–2097.

23. Donadio JV, Grande JP (2002) IgA nephropathy. N Engl J Med 347: 738–748.

24. Hsu SI, Ramirez SB, Winn MP, Bonventre JV, Owen WF (2000) Evidence for genetic factors in the development and progression of IgA nephropathy. Kidney Int 57: 1818–1835.

25. Tampe B, Zeisberg M (2013) Contribution of genetics and epigenetics to progression of kidney fibrosis. Nephrol Dial Transplant. Epub ahead of print.

26. Wacholder S, Chanock S, Garcia-Closas M, El Ghormli L, Rothman N (2004) Assessing the probability that a positive report is false: an approach for molecular epidemiology studies. J Natl Cancer Inst 96: 434–442.

27. Fallin D, Schork NJ (2000) Accuracy of haplotype frequency estimation for biallelic loci, via the expectation-maximization algorithm for unphased diploid genotype data. Am J Hum Genet 67: 947–959.

28. Schmidt AH, Baier D, Solloch UV, Stahr A, Cereb N, et al. (2009) Estimation of high-resolution HLA-A, -B, -C, -DRB1 allele and haplotype frequencies based on 8862 German stem cell donors and implications for strategic donor registry planning. Hum Immunol 70: 895–902.

24

Regional Homogeneity Changes in Hemodialysis Patients with End Stage Renal Disease: *In Vivo* Resting-State Functional MRI Study

Cheng Li[1]❾, Huan-Huan Su[2]❾, Ying-Wei Qiu[2], Xiao-Fei Lv[3], Sheng Shen[1], Wen-Feng Zhan[2], Jun-Zhang Tian[2], Gui-Hua Jiang[2]*

1 Department of Renal Transplantation, Guangdong No.2 Provincial People's Hospital, Guangzhou, People's Republic of China, 2 Department of Medical Imaging, Guangdong No.2 Provincial People's Hospital, Guangzhou, People's Republic of China, 3 State Key Laboratory of Oncology in South China and Department of Medical Imaging and Interventional Radiology, Sun Yat-Sen University Cancer Center, Guangzhou, People's Republic of China

Abstract

Objective: To prospectively investigate and detect early cerebral regional homogeneity (ReHo) changes in neurologically asymptomatic patients with end stage renal disease (ESRD) using in vivo resting-state functional MR imaging (Rs-fMRI).

Methods: We enrolled 20 patients (15 men, 5 women; meanage, 37.1 years; range, 19–49 years) with ESRD and 20 healthy controls (15 men, 5 women; mean age, 38.3 years; range, 28–49 years). The mean duration of hemodialysis for the patient group was 10.7 ± 6.4 monthes. There was no significant sex or age difference between the ESRD and control groups. Rs-fMRI was performed using a gradient-echo echo-planar imaging sequence. ReHo was calculated using software (DPARSF). Voxel-based analysis of the ReHo maps between ESRD and control groups was performed with a two-samples t test. Statistical maps were set at P value less than 0.05 and were corrected for multiple comparisons. The Mini-Mental State Examination (MMSE) was administered to all participants at imaging.

Results: ReHo values were increased in the bilateral superior temporal gyrus and left medial frontal gyrus in the ERSD group compared with controls, but a significantly decreased ReHo value was found in the right middle temporal gyrus. There was no significant correlation between ReHo values and the duration of hemodialysis in the ESRD group. Both the patients and control subjects had normal MMSE scores (≥ 28).

Conclusions: Our finding revealed that abnormal brain activity was distributed mainly in the memory and cognition related cotices in patients with ESRD. The abnormal spontaneous neuronal activity in those areas provide information on the neural mechanisms underlying cognitive impairment in patients with ESRD, and demonstrate that Rs-fMRI with ReHo analysis is a useful non-invasive imaging tool for the detection of early cerebral ReHo changes in hemodialysis patients with ESRD.

Editor: Xi-Nian Zuo, Institute of Psychology, Chinese Academy of Sciences, China

Funding: This work was supported by the Guangdong Provincial Science and Technology (Grant number: 2012B031800170). The funders had role in data collection and analysis, decision to publish and preparation of the manuscript.

Competing Interests: The authors have declared that no competing interests exist.

* E-mail: 112662748@qq.com

❾ These authors contributed equally to this work.

Introduction

End stage renal disease (ESRD) is defined as a glomerular filtration rate (GFR) less than 15 mL/min/1.73 m^2, or chronic renal failure that has progressed to the point at which the kidneys are permanently functioning at less than 10% of their capacity. Patients with ESRD usually have central nervous system abnormalities, some related to ESRD itself and others related to problems secondary to hemodialysis [1,2,3,4]. These Patients with ESRD often present with neurological complications such as focal white matter lesions, cerebral atrophy, osmotic demyelination syndrome, dialysis encephalopathy, hypertensive encephalopathy, intracranial hemorrhage, infarction, sinus thrombosis, and infection [1,2,3,4]. Furthermore, among patients with ESRD, depres-sion and cognitive impairment are the most common causes of neuropsychiatric illness [5]. Cognitive deficits may occur in patients with ESRD long before any overt neurological symptoms are observed. Depression and cognitive impairment are considered important factors for the determination of a patient's survival and prognosis. Thus, it is important to elucidate the mechanism of depression and cognitive impairment in Patients with ESRD.

Previous studies of brain changes that accompany or follow ESRD have mainly used brain computed tomography (CT) or conventional magnetic resonance imaging (MRI) [6,7,8,9,10]. Computed tomography can be used to assess neurological complications, such as intracranial hemorrhage and cerebral infarction. MRI is a sensitive imaging tool for the neurological evaluation of patients with ESRD [11]. Because the clinical evaluation and ongoing assessment of ESRD are complicated, so it has been suggested that MRI be used before the onset of therapy, so that these initial findings can serve as a basis for later comparisons [3,4,11]. For example, conventional MRI studies have shown focal white matter lesions to be more common in patients undergoing hemodialysis (56%) than in the normal population (27%) [11]. In the past decade, functional imaging studies about ESRD have consistently demonstrated regional microscopic structure and metabolic abnormalities in the white matter. Hsieh et al, who used diffusion tensor imaging to measure fractional anisotropy (FA) values in patients with ESRD, reported that patients with ESRD have significant lower FA values than healthy control subjects [12]. Chiu et al reported that significant elevations of the choline/phosphatidylcholine (Cho)/total choles-terol (tCr) and myo-inositol (mI)/tCr ratios in the frontal grey matter, frontal white matter, and temporal white matter as well as in the basal ganglia were found in ESRD group compared with controls [13]. However, these brain imaging methods have limitation in that they are not capable of estimation and visualization of neural activity.

Functional brain imaging studies have suggested that the brain is not inactive during rest, but rather shows a default state of activation [14,15,16,17,18]. Low frequency oscillations (ranging from 0.01 to 0.1 Hz) of resting-state functional MRI (Rs-fMRI) time-series are known to show correlated patterns between anatomically separated brain regions [18,19,20]. It has been suggested that these correlations originate from coherency in the underlying neuronal activation patterns of these regions and reflect functional connectivity. Regions that show this kind of coherent functional behavior are said to form a resting-state network (RSN). Regional homogeneity (ReHo) measures the functional coherence of a given voxel with its nearest neighbors and can be used to evaluate resting-state brain activities based on the hypothesis that significant brain activities would more likely occur in clusters than in a single voxel [21]. The Kendall coeffi cient of concordance was used to measure the similarity of the time series of one voxel with that of its nearest neighbors in a voxel-wise analysis [22]. Regional homogeneity does not require the onset time of stimulus and therefore is useful for Rs-fMRI data analysis. Regional homoge-neity has been successfully used to study the functional modula-tions in the resting state in patients with Alzheimer disease [23], Parkinson disease [24], schizophrenia [25], and neuromyelitis optica [26] and in healthy aging subjects [27]. Regional homogeneity could be regarded as a measure for investigating human brain activities in the resting state. It may be helpful to understand the pathophysiology of cognitive deficits in patients with ESRD using the ReHo method, which can reflect the temporal homogeneity of neural activity. In this prospective study, we characterized and compared ReHo differences between hemodialysis patients with ESRD and healthy control subjects

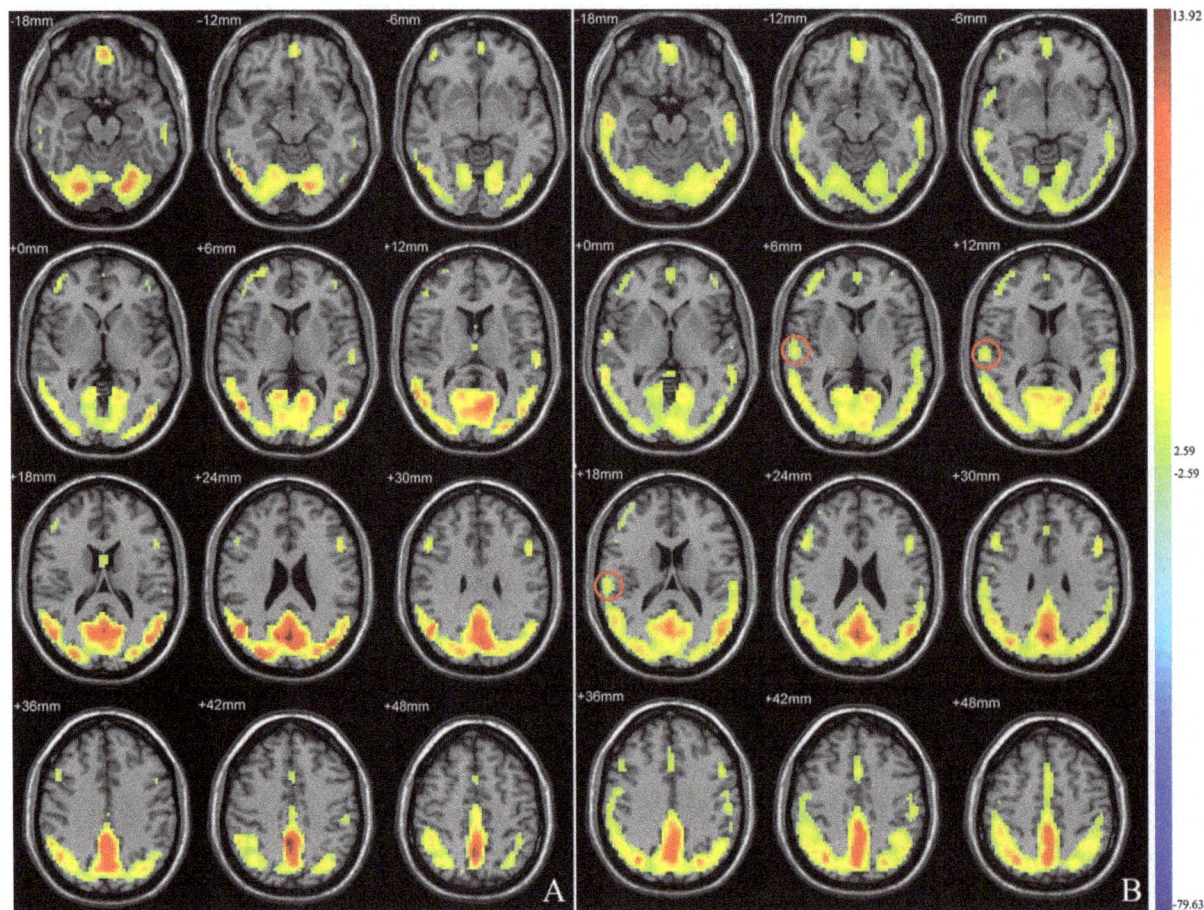

Figure 1. Mean ReHo maps within the ESRD group (A) and healthy controls (B). Left side of the images corresponds to the right side of the subjects. T-score bars are shown on the right. The images illustrate high ReHo in the default network. In the controls group but not the patient group, high ReHo was shown in the right middle temporal gyrus.

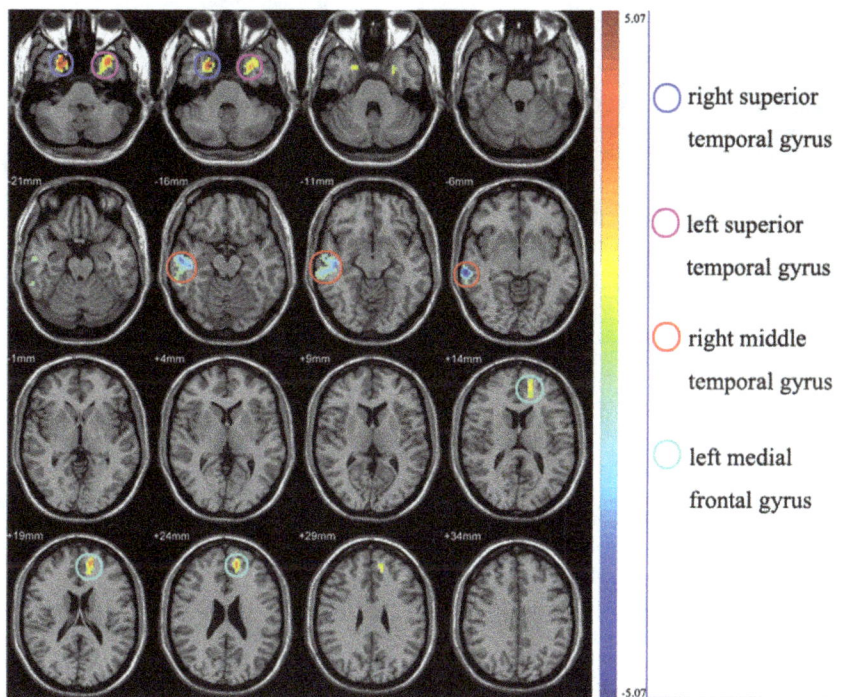

Figure 2. Maps showing statistically significant differences between the ESRD group and the control group. The Patients with ESRD showed a significant ReHo increase in the bilateral superior temporal gyrus and left medial frontal gyrus (warm colors), but a decrease in the right middle temporal gyrus (cold colors) (n = 20, corrected $P<0.05$).

using Rs-fMRI to understand the effect of ESRD on brain function.

Materials and Methods

Subjects

This prospective study was approved by the Research Ethics Review Board of the Institute of Mental Health at the Guangdong No. 2 Provincial People's Hospital. Written informed consent was obtained from all subjects. For this hospitalbased prospective case-control study, we recruited 23 patients with ESRD from the renal transplantation department at our hospital and 20 healthy volunteers with normal renal function between August 2011 and July 2012. To avoid possible confounding effects, all participants were younger than 50 years. They were excluded if they had a history of diabetes, alcoholism, drug abuse, psychiatric disorders, or major neurologic disorders (severe head injury, stroke, epilepsy, or visible lesions). Conventional MR images were interpreted by an experienced radiologist (J.Z.T) with 20 years of experience in neuroradiology who was blinded to whether the images were from the patient group or the control group. Subjects with brain lesions at conventional T1 or T2-fluid-attenuated inversion recovery (FLAIR) MR imaging were excluded. Three patients, whose T2-FLAIR MR images showed abnormal hyperintensities, were excluded because the imaging evidence suggested infarcts, one of the exclusion criteria. The final study population included 20 patients with ESRD (15 men, 5 women) and 20 healthy controls (15 men, 5 women). All patients were diagnosed with renal failure by GFR less than 15 mL/min/1.73 m^2, and underwent regular hemodialysis. Each subject completed a questionnaire before MRI examination, including age, sex, years of education, duration of hemodialysis and Mini-Mental State Examination (MMSE).

Imaging studies

MRI data were obtained using a 1.5T MR scanner (Achieva Nova-Dual; Philips, Best, the Netherlands) in the Department of Medical Imaging, Guangdong No. 2 Provincial People's Hospital. Each subject lay supine with the head comfortably fixed using a belt and foam pads. During Rs-fMRI, subjects were instructed to close their eyes and remain as quiet as possible and to not think of anything systematically or fall asleep. The conventional imaging sequences including T1-weighted images and T2-FLAIR images were obtained for every subject to detect clinically silent lesions. Rs-fMRI data were acquired using a gradient-echo echo-planar sequence sensitive to blood oxygenation level dependent (BOLD) contrast. The Rs-fMRI acquisition parameters were as follows: repetition time (TR) = 3,000 ms, echo time (TE) = 50 ms, flip angle = 90°, field-of-view = 230×230 mm^2, matrix = 64×64, and total volumes = 160. A total of 33 axial slices of 4.5 mm thickness were collected with no intersection gap. In-plane resolution was 3.59×3.59 mm^2. Each Rs-fMRI scan lasted 8 minutes. After the examination, all participants were asked questions to verify the degree of their cooperation.

Data preprocessing and regional homogeneity calculation

The imaging data were preprocessed mainly using a MATLAB toolbox called Data Processing Assistant for Resting-State (DPARSF [28]; http://restfmri.net/forum/DPARSF) for "pipe-line" data analysis of Rs-fMRI. DPARSF is based on statistical parametric mapping software functions (SPM8; http://www.fil.ion.ucl.ac.uk/spm) and REST software [29]; http://resting-fmri.sourceforge.net). For each participant, the first 10 time points were discarded to avoid transient signal changes before magnetization reached steady-state and to allow subjects to become accustomed to the fMRI scanning noise. The raw data were corrected for

Table 1. Demographic and clinical characteristics of ESRD and control groups.

Characteristic	ESRD group(n = 20)	Control group(n = 20)	t value	P value*
Age(y)	37.1±8.6	38.3±6.5	−0.499	0.621
Sex#				1.000
male	15	15		
female	5	5		
Education(y)	12.0±2.9	12.9±3.2	−0.938	0.354
No. of cigarettes/day▲	13.5±9.2	16.7±12.6	−0.325	0.768
Duration of dialysis(mo)$	10.7±6.4	NA		
MMSE score	29.2±0.8	29.5±0.8	−1.189	0.242

Unless otherwise indicated, data are mean±standard deviations.
NA = not applicable. MMSE = Mini-mental status examination.
* P values are two sided.
#For sex composition, $\chi^2 = 0.000$ and $\nu = 1$.
▲There were two patients in the ESRD group and three persons in the control group with a history of smoking.
$There were 17 inpatients in the ESRD group.

acquisition delay between slices and for the head motion (a least squares approach and a 6 parameter spatial transformation). Subjects with head motion exceeding 1.5 mm in any dimension through the resting-state run were removed. Following the motion correction, all data were spatial normalized to the Montreal Neurological Institute (MNI) template (resampling voxel size = 3×3×3 mm^3). Subsequent data preprocessing included removal of linear trends and temporal filtering (band pass, 0.01 to 0.08 Hz) to remove the effects of very low-frequency drift and physiological high frequency respiratory and cardiac noise for further ReHo analysis [18].

The ReHo calculation procedure was the same as that reported in a previous study [21]. Briefly, this is accomplished on a voxel-by-voxel basis by calculating Kendall's coefficient of concordance (KCC) [22] for a given voxel time series with those of its nearest 26 neighbors.

$$W = \frac{\sum (R_i)^2 - n(\overline{R})^2}{\frac{1}{12}K^2(n^3 - n)}$$

where W is the KCC among given voxels, ranging from 0 to 1; R_i is the sum rank of the with time point ($R_i = \sum_{j=1}^{k} r_{ij}$ where r_{ij} is the

rank of the ith time point in the jth voxel); $\overline{R} = ((n+1)\,k)/2$ is the mean of the R_i; k is the number of time series within a measured cluster (27, one given voxel plus the number of its neighbors); and n is the number of ranks (n = 150 for this study). The KCC value was calculated to this voxel, and an individual KCC map was obtained for each subject. To reduce the influence of individual variations in the KCC value, ReHo maps normalization was preformed by dividing the KCC among each voxel by the averaged KCC of the whole brain. The resulting data were then spatially smoothed with an 8-mm full-width at half-maximum (FWHM) Gaussian kernel to reduce noise and residual differences in gyral anatomy.

Statistical analysis

Two-sample t-tests were performed to assess the differences in age, duration of education and number of cigarettes smoked per day between Patients with ESRD and healthy subjects. Mann-Whitney U tests were used to analyze the differences in sex between the two groups. Pearson correlation coefficient was used to analyze the association between ReHo values and the duration of hemodialysis in the patient group. Analyses were conducted using software (SPSS, version 13.0; Chicago, Ill, USA), and a P value less than 0.05 (two-tailed) was considered statistically significant.

Table 2. Brain regions with abnormal ReHo in patients with ESRD compared with control subjects.

Brain area	No. of voxels	Side	Mean Reho value Control group	ESRD group	Brodmann area	x	y	z	Peak t value
Superior Temporal gyrus	35	R	−0.440±0.062	−0.329±0.076	38	24	9	−39	5.071
Superior Temporal gyrus	42	L	−0.366±0.074	−0.243±0.101	38	−33	12	−42	4.594
Middle Temporal gyrus	132	R	0.099±0.049	−0.033±0.072	21	66	−30	−6	−5.018
Medial Frontal gyrus	53	L	−0.239±0.058	−0.145±0.082	9	−12	48	21	4.052

L = left, R = right, MNI = Montreal Neurological Institute.

A second-level random-effect one-sample t-test ($P<0.01$, with False Discovery Rate (FDR) correction) was performed to show the ReHo results with in each group. To explore the ReHo differences between Patients with ESRD and healthy subjects, a second-level random-effect two-sample t-test was performed on the individual normalized ReHo maps in a voxel-by-voxel manner by taking age and years of education as confounding covariates. Significant differences were set at the threshold of a corrected cluster level at P less than 0.05. Threshold correction was performed by using a program (AlphaSim; Analysis of Functional NeuroImages, http://afni.nimh.nih.gov/afni/) that applies Monte Carlo simulation to calculate the probability of false positive detection by taking into consideration both the individual voxel probability threshold and cluster size [30]. Using this program, a corrected significance level of P less than 0.05 was obtained by clusters with a minimum volume of 1998 mm^3 at an uncorrected individual voxel height threshold of $P<0.01$. This enabled the identification of significant changes in ReHo in the Patients with ESRD compared with the controls. The parameters were as follow: individual voxel P value = 0.01, 1,000 simulations, FWHM = 8 mm, and whole brain mask.

Results

After exclusion of three patients with hyperintensities on T2-FLAIR images, we found no other abnormality in morphology or signal intensity on T1-weighted and T2- FLAIR images. The mean age of the patients and healthy controls was 37.1±8.6 years (range, 19–49 years) and 38.3±6.5 years (range, 28–49 years), respectively. Three subjects in the ESRD group were outpatients, we could not collect the duration of hemodialysis of them. The mean duration of hemodialysis for the patient group (n = 17) was 10.7±6.4 monthes. There were no significant differences in age, sex, years of education and number of cigarettes smoked per day between patients with ESRD and control subjects (Table. 1). The mean ReHo maps with in each group are shown in Figure. 1, illustrating high ReHo in the default network. In the controls group, high ReHo in the right middle temporal gyrus was shown, but this was not found in the patient group. Compared with the control group, the Patients with ESRD showed a significant ReHo increase in the bilateral superior temporal gyrus ($P<0.05$, AlphaSim corrected) and left medial frontal gyrus ($P<0.05$, AlphaSim corrected), but a decrease in the right middle temporal gyrus ($P<0.05$, AlphaSim corrected) (Table. 2, Figure. 2). There was no significant correlations between ReHo values and the duration of hemodialysis in the ESRD group. No significantly different score was found between patient and control groups, all subjects had normal MMSE scores (≥28).

Discussion

The ReHo is a data-driven method, which assumes that a given voxel is temporally similar to its neighbors. It measures the ReHo of the time series of the regional BOLD signal. Therefore, ReHo reflects the temporal homogeneity of the regional BOLD signal rather than its density. As the BOLD signal of fMRI may reflect neural activity [31], abnormal ReHo is possibly relevant to the changes of temporal aspects of neural activity in the regional brain. Therefore ReHo may detect the brain regions with abnormal activity.

We found ReHo values in patients with ESRD to be significantly increased in the bilateral superior temporal gyrus and left medial frontal gyrus, but decreased in the right middle temporal gyrus. Interestingly, all of the brain areas with significant ReHo changes were located in the temporal and frontal lobes,

which are closely related to the memory and cognition. Our findings are similar to those of many previous brain imaging studies in pre-dialysis patients. Using Tc-99m ethylcysteinate dimer brain single photon emission tomography, Song et al found that prior to beginning dialysis patients with chronic kidney disease have significant hypoperfusion in the right superior and middle temporal gyrus and inferior frontal gyrus [32]. In their previous study using F-18-fluorodeoxyglucose positron emission tomography, they found that several voxel clusters had significantly decreased cerebral glucose metabolism in patients with chronic kidney disease who had not started dialysis, including the prefrontal cortex, superior temporal gyrus and middle temporal gyrus [33]. Kim et al reported that depressive mood and anxiety factors were negatively correlated with regional cerebral blood flow in bilateral superior temporal gyrus, right middle temporal gyrus and left superior frontal gyrus [34]. Thus, all of them cannot reflect the baseline directly as resting-state studies can.

Recently, Xue Liang et al did a similar research to us. They used Rs-fMRI with ReHo algorithm to investigate the pattern of spontaneous neural activity in patients with ESRD. In their study, they found both MNE (minimal nephro-encephalopathy) and non-NE (non-nephro-encephalopathy) patients show decreased ReHo in the multiple areas of bilateral frontal, parietal and temporal lobes [35]. These results have a few difference to ours. It may be relate to the small sample size. Whatever, the differences in ReHo indicate a poor level of coordination and a disorder of communication among neurons in the brain region [21]. These changes in ReHo suggest an abnormality in the resting-state brain function of patients with ESRD and may be early signs for the development of uremic encephalopathy or dialysis encephalopathy.

The temporal and frontal regions are considered as important components of human default-mode networks [15,17,36], and have been shown to exhibit mild cognitive impairment (MCI)-related structural and functional abnormalities [37,38,39,40,41]. James et al reported that hemodialysis patients have a high prevalence of mild cognitive impairment (MCI) despite normal global cognitive function [42]. MCI is a transitional state between normal cognition and the earliest clinical features of dementia. MCI is likely under-diagnosed but highly prevalent in dindividuals with ESRD [43,44,45], and Murray et al described MCI in nearly 64% of hemodialysis patients [46]. In the present study, we found that patients with ESRD have normal global cognitive function (MMSE score >25), but that does not mean that these patients are free of MCI. The greatest defect in our research was that we did not assess the MCI in patients with ESRD.

In our study, there was no significant correlation between ReHo values and the duration of hemodialysis in the ESRD group. This finding may indicate that the significant change in ReHo values relates to ESRD itself but not hemodialysis.

Some limitations of our study are worth mentioning. First, we did not discriminate between neuronal versus vascular effects on changes in ReHo values in patients with ESRD. Second, the sample size in this study is relatively small, and thus the results of the current study may no be representative of ESRD in general. Third, the lack of MCI examinations in our sample is the most serious drawback of our study. Fourth, we did not collect follow-up Rs-fMRI data after renal replacement. In future studies, examinations should include not only fMRI but also arterial spin labeling perfusion imaging, electroencephalograms and other measures to discriminate between neuronal versus vascular effects on changes in neural activity in patients with ESRD. More attention also needs to be paid to mental test and serial changes in neural activity after renal replacement therapy in Patients with ESRD.

In conclusion, we found significant change in ReHo values in patients with ESRD in brain areas located in temporal and frontal lobes, which are closely related to the memory and cognition. The abnormal spontaneous neuronal activity in those areas may be the neural mechanisms underlying the cognitive impairment in patients with ESRD, and suggested that an abnormal ReHo value in certain brain areas may be a potential biomarker to detect the early cerebral ReHo changes in hemodialysis patients with ESRD.

Author Contributions

Conceived and designed the experiments: GJ HS. Performed the experiments: CL HS WZ. Analyzed the data: YQ XL JT. Contributed reagents/materials/analysis tools: HS SS. Wrote the paper: HS.

References

1. Glaser GH (1974) Brain dysfunction in uremia. Res Publ Assoc Res Nerv Ment Dis 53: 173–199.
2. De Deyn PP, Saxena VK, Abts H, Borggreve F, D'Hooge R, et al. (1992) Clinical and pathophysiological aspects of neurological complications in renal failure. Acta Neurol Belg 92: 191–206.
3. Brouns R, De Deyn PP (2004) Neurological complications in renal failure: a review. Clin Neurol Neurosurg 107: 1–16.
4. Tzamaloukas AH, Agaba EI (2004) Neurological manifestations of uraemia and chronic dialysis. Niger J Med 13: 98–105.
5. Kimmel PL, Thamer M, Richard CM, Ray NF (1998) Psychiatric illness in patients with end-stage renal disease. Am J Med 105: 214–221.
6. Fazekas G, Fazekas F, Schmidt R, Kapeller P, Offenbacher H, et al. (1995) Brain MRI findings and cognitive impairment in patients undergoing chronic hemodialysis treatment. J Neurol Sci 134: 83–88.
7. Savazzi GM, Cusmano F, Musini S (2001) Cerebral imaging changes in patients with chronic renal failure treated conservatively or in hemodialysis. Nephron 89: 31–36.
8. Suzuki M, Wada A, Isaka Y, Maki K, Inoue T, et al. (1997) Cerebral magnetic resonance T2 high intensities in end-stage renal disease. Stroke 28: 2528–2531.
9. Kim CD, Lee HJ, Kim DJ, Kim BS, Shin SK, et al. (2007) High prevalence of leukoaraiosis in cerebral magnetic resonance images of patients on peritoneal dialysis. Am J Kidney Dis 50: 98–107.
10. Kamata T, Hishida A, Takita T, Sawada K, Ikegaya N, et al. (2000) Morphologic abnormalities in the brain of chronically hemodialyzed patients without cerebrovascular disease. Am J Nephrol 20: 27–31.
11. Agildere AM, Kurt A, Yildirim T, Benli S, Altinors N (2001) MRI of neurologic complications in end-stage renal failure patients on hemodialysis: pictorial review. Eur Radiol 11: 1063–1069.
12. Hsieh TJ, Chang JM, Chuang HY, Ko CH, Hsieh ML, et al. (2009) End-stage renal disease: in vivo diffusion-tensor imaging of silent white matter damage. Radiology 252: 518–525.
13. Chiu ML, Li CW, Chang JM, Chiang IC, Ko CH, et al. (2010) Cerebral metabolic changes in neurologically presymptomatic patients undergoing haemodialysis: in vivo proton MR spectroscopic findings. Eur Radiol 20: 1502–1507.
14. De Luca M, Beckmann CF, De Stefano N, Matthews PM, Smith SM (2006) fMRI resting state networks define distinct modes of long-distance interactions in the human brain. Neuroimage 29: 1359–1367.
15. Greicius MD, Krasnow B, Reiss AL, Menon V (2003) Functional connectivity in the resting brain: a network analysis of the default mode hypothesis. Proc Natl Acad Sci U S A 100: 253–258.
16. Gusnard DA, Raichle ME, Raichle ME (2001) Searching for a baseline: functional imaging and the resting human brain. Nat Rev Neurosci 2: 685–694.
17. Raichle ME, MacLeod AM, Snyder AZ, Powers WJ, Gusnard DA, et al. (2001) A default mode of brain function. Proc Natl Acad Sci U S A 98: 676–682.
18. Biswal B, Yetkin FZ, Haughton VM, Hyde JS (1995) Functional connectivity in the motor cortex of resting human brain using echo-planar MRI. Magn Reson Med 34: 537–541.
19. Cordes D, Haughton VM, Arfanakis K, Wendt GJ, Turski PA, et al. (2000) Mapping functionally related regions of brain with functional connectivity MR imaging. AJNR Am J Neuroradiol 21: 1636–1644.
20. Fox MD, Raichle ME (2007) Spontaneous fluctuations in brain activity observed with functional magnetic resonance imaging. Nat Rev Neurosci 8: 700–711.
21. Zang Y, Jiang T, Lu Y, He Y, Tian L (2004) Regional homogeneity approach to fMRI data analysis. Neuroimage 22: 394–400.
22. Kendall M GJ (1990) Rank correlation methods. Oxford, England: Oxford University Press.
23. He Y, Wang L, Zang Y, Tian L, Zhang X, et al. (2007) Regional coherence changes in the early stages of Alzheimer's disease: a combined structural and resting-state functional MRI study. Neuroimage 35: 488–500.
24. Wu T, Long X, Zang Y, Wang L, Hallett M, et al. (2009) Regional homogeneity changes in patients with Parkinson's disease. Hum Brain Mapp 30: 1502–1510.
25. Liu H, Liu Z, Liang M, Hao Y, Tan L, et al. (2006) Decreased regional homogeneity in schizophrenia: a resting state functional magnetic resonance imaging study. Neuroreport 17: 19–22.
26. Liang P, Liu Y, Jia X, Duan Y, Yu C, et al. (2011) Regional homogeneity changes in patients with neuromyelitis optica revealed by resting-state functional MRI. Clin Neurophysiol 122: 121–127.
27. Wu T, Zang Y, Wang L, Long X, Li K, et al. (2007) Normal aging decreases regional homogeneity of the motor areas in the resting state. Neurosci Lett 423: 189–193.
28. Chao-Gan Y, Yu-Feng Z (2010) DPARSF: A MATLAB Toolbox for "Pipeline" Data Analysis of Resting-State fMRI. Front Syst Neurosci 4: 13.
29. Song XW, Dong ZY, Long XY, Li SF, Zuo XN, et al. (2011) REST: a toolkit for resting-state functional magnetic resonance imaging data processing. PLoS One 6: e25031.
30. Forman SD, Cohen JD, Fitzgerald M, Eddy WF, Mintun MA, et al. (1995) Improved assessment of significant activation in functional magnetic resonance imaging (fMRI): use of a cluster-size threshold. Magn Reson Med 33: 636–647.
31. Logothetis NK, Pauls J, Augath M, Trinath T, Oeltermann A (2001) Neurophysiological investigation of the basis of the fMRI signal. Nature 412: 150–157.
32. Song SH, Kwak IS, Kim SJ, Kim YK, Kim IJ (2009) Depressive mood in pre-dialytic chronic kidney disease: Statistical parametric mapping analysis of Tc-99m ECD brain SPECT. Psychiatry Res 173: 243–247.
33. Song SH, Kim IJ, Kim SJ, Kwak IS, Kim YK (2008) Cerebral glucose metabolism abnormalities in patients with major depressive symptoms in pre-dialytic chronic kidney disease: statistical parametric mapping analysis of F-18-FDG PET, a preliminary study. Psychiatry Clin Neurosci 62: 554–561.
34. Kim SJ, Song SH, Kim JH, Kwak IS (2008) Statistical parametric mapping analysis of the relationship between regional cerebral blood flow and symptom clusters of the depressive mood in patients with pre-dialytic chronic kidney disease. Ann Nucl Med 22: 201–206.
35. Liang X, Wen J, Ni L, Zhong J, Qi R, et al. (2013) Altered pattern of spontaneous brain activity in the patients with end-stage renal disease: a resting-state functional MRI study with regional homogeneity analysis. PLoS One 8: e71507.
36. Buckner RL, Andrews-Hanna JR, Schacter DL (2008) The brain's default network: anatomy, function, and relevance to disease. Ann N Y Acad Sci 1124: 1–38.
37. Bookheimer SY, Strojwas MH, Cohen MS, Saunders AM, Pericak-Vance MA, et al. (2000) Patterns of brain activation in people at risk for Alzheimer's disease. N Engl J Med 343: 450–456.
38. Dickerson BC, Salat DH, Bates JF, Atiya M, Killiany RJ, et al. (2004) Medial temporal lobe function and structure in mild cognitive impairment. Ann Neurol 56: 27–35.
39. Dickerson BC, Sperling RA (2008) Functional abnormalities of the medial temporal lobe memory system in mild cognitive impairment and Alzheimer's disease: insights from functional MRI studies. Neuropsychologia 46: 1624–1635.
40. Hamalainen A, Pihlajamaki M, Tanila H, Hanninen T, Niskanen E, et al. (2007) Increased fMRI responses during encoding in mild cognitive impairment. Neurobiol Aging 28: 1889–1903.
41. Wang Z, Nie B, Li D, Zhao Z, Han Y, et al. (2012) Effect of acupuncture in mild cognitive impairment and Alzheimer disease: a functional MRI study. PLoS One 7: e42730.
42. Post JB, Jegede AB, Morin K, Spungen AM, Langhoff E, et al. (2010) Cognitive profile of chronic kidney disease and hemodialysis patients without dementia. Nephron Clin Pract 116: c247–c255.
43. Sehgal AR, Grey SF, DeOreo PB, Whitehouse PJ (1997) Prevalence, recognition, and implications of mental impairment among hemodialysis patients. Am J Kidney Dis 30: 41–49.
44. Pereira AA, Weiner DE, Scott T, Chandra P, Bluestein R, et al. (2007) Subcortical cognitive impairment in dialysis patients. Hemodial Int 11: 309–314.
45. Kurella M, Chertow GM, Luan J, Yaffe K (2004) Cognitive impairment in chronic kidney disease. J Am Geriatr Soc 52: 1863–1869.
46. Murray AM, Tupper DE, Knopman DS, Gilbertson DT, Pederson SL, et al. (2006) Cognitive impairment in hemodialysis patients is common. Neurology 67: 216–223.

25

Mapping End-Stage Renal Disease (ESRD): Spatial Variations on Small Area Level in Northern France, and Association with Deprivation

Florent Occelli[1]*, Annabelle Deram[1,2], Michaël Génin[3], Christian Noël[4,5], Damien Cuny[1], François Glowacki[1,4,5], on behalf of the Néphronor Network[5¶]

1 EA 4483, Université Lille Nord de France, Faculté de Pharmacie de Lille, Lille, France, 2 Faculté Ingénierie et Management de la Santé (ILIS), Loos, France, 3 EA 2694, Université Lille Nord de France, Faculté de Médecine pôle Recherche, Lille, France, 4 Service de Néphrologie, Hopital Huriez, CHRU de Lille, Lille, France, 5 Réseau Néphronor, Hôpital Huriez, CHRU de Lille, Lille, France

Abstract

Background: Strong geographic variations in the incidence of end-stage renal disease (ESRD) are observed in developed countries. The reasons for these variations are unknown. They may reflect regional inequalities in the population's sociodemographic characteristics, related diseases, or medical practice patterns. In France, at the district level, the highest incidence rates have been found in the Nord-Pas-de-Calais region. This area, with a high population density and homogeneous healthcare provision, represents a geographic situation which is quite suitable for the study, over small areas, of spatial disparities in the incidence of ESRD, together with their correlation with a deprivation index and other risk factors.

Methods: The Renal Epidemiology and Information Network is a national registry, which lists all ESRD patients in France. All cases included in the Nord-Pas-de-Calais registry between 2005 and 2011 were extracted. Adjusted and smoothed standardized incidence ratio (SIR) was calculated for each of the 170 cantons, thanks to a hierarchical Bayesian model. The correlation between ESRD incidence and deprivation was assessed using the quintiles of Townsend index. Relative risk (RR) and credible intervals (CI) were estimated for each quintile.

Results: Significant spatial disparities in ESRD incidence were found within the Nord-Pas-de-Calais region. The sex- and age-adjusted, smoothed SIRs varied from 0.66 to 1.64. Although no correlation is found with diabetic or vascular nephropathy, the smoothed SIRs are correlated with the Townsend index (RR: 1.18, 95% CI [1.00–1.34] for Q2; 1.28, 95% CI [1.11–1.47] for Q3; 1.30, 95% CI [1.14–1.51] for Q4; 1.44, 95% CI [1.32–1.74] for Q5).

Conclusion: For the first time at this aggregation level in France, this study reveals significant geographic differences in ESRD incidence. Unlike the time of renal replacement care, deprivation is certainly a determinant in this phenomenon. This association is probably independent of the patients' financial ability to gain access to healthcare.

Editor: Gianpaolo Reboldi, University of Perugia, Italy

Funding: This work was supported by Agence de Biomédecine, Renal Epidemiology and Information Network (www.soc-nephrologie.org/REIN/); Conseil Régional Nord, Pas de Calais, DRESTIC (www.nordpasdecalais.fr/jcms/c_5001/accueil); and Université Lille 2 Droit et Santé, ED446 (http://edbsl.univ-lille2.fr/). The funders had no role in study design, data collection and analysis, decision to publish, or preparation of the manuscript.

Competing Interests: The authors have declared that no competing interests exist.

* Email: florent.occelli@univ-lille2.fr

¶ Membership of the Néphronor Network is provided in the Acknowledgments.

Introduction

In developed countries, the burdens of End-Stage Renal Disease (ESRD) and Renal Replacement Therapy (RRT) were continuously growing and now stabilize since the early 2000s. In sharp contrast, incidence rates are still growing in developing countries [1–4]. At the scale of a country, strong geographic variations in the incidence of treated ESRD have been observed [5–13]. In metropolitan France, the crude incidence rate of RRT also varies widely, from 80.4 to 238.6 per million inhabitants (pmi) in 71 districts in 2006–2007 [14]. Rates were highest in the northeast and south and lowest in the west and east. In 2008–2009, it varies from 85.8 to 225.5 pmi in 85 districts, with higher rates in northeast and southern France and lower rates in the western part [15].

The reasons for these variations remain elusive. They may result from inter-regional variations in the population's sociodemographic characteristics [6,10,15–17], from other related diseases such as diabetes and cardiovascular diseases [8,15,18–20], or merely reflect differences in the timing of dialysis initiation [14,21] and geographic distance from healthcare facilities [22].

On a smaller scale, the spatial variability of treated ESRD and its relationship to risk factors has also been assessed for US counties or census tracts [23–28], UK wards [22] and Australian postcodes [17]. There is no such equivalent in France. Such a

Table 1.

	Mean	SD	Min	Q1	Median	Q3	Max
Number of patients	27	26	2	12	21	32	219
Total crude incidence (pmi)	158	53	38	124	157	186	432
Men crude incidence (pmi)	187	72	0	144	182	230	424
Women crude incidence (pmi)	130	61	0	89	123	169	439
Smoothed SIR	0.96	0.20	0.66	0.81	0.92	1.07	1.64
Townsend index	0.00	3.71	−6.01	−2.91	−0.97	2.82	10.80
Diabetic nephropathy (%)	27.5	11.7	0.0	20.0	27.6	33.3	75.0
Vascular nephropathy (%)	24.4	12.5	0.0	16.7	23.7	32.0	100.0
eGFR (ml/min/1.73 m²)	9.05	1.46	5.59	8.05	8.92	9.84	14.40

spatial approach, made at the scale of homogeneous populations over a territory with similar health practices, may provide an improved knowledge of ESRD patterns, allowing an explanation to be found for these disparities. Such an outcome would then lead to a better understanding of environmental assumptions [29–31].

The French Renal Epidemiology and Information Network (REIN) is a national Chronic Kidney Disease (CKD) registry, which lists all patients who initiated ESRD treatment since 2002, and is currently available in 22 regions of metropolitan France [32]. Among these, the Nord-Pas-de-Calais, a small region with 4 million inhabitants, has the highest ESRD incidence, with a standardized rate of 207 new cases pmi in 2012, as opposed to 154 new cases pmi for all of France [33]. The homogeneous healthcare access (median travel-time to dialysis units: 15 min, and>45 min for only 0.46% of the patients [33]), the large number of cases and the associated population density make the geographic situation of this region quite suitable for the study of disparities in ESRD incidence in small areas, and their correlation with sociodemographic status, as well as the quality of environmental media.

The aim of this study was to analyze the spatial variations of ESRD incidence over small areas, and to analyze the correlation between geographic variability and social discrepancies (assessed using the Townsend deprivation index). The study focuses on the Nord-Pas-de-Calais, for the period between 2005 and 2011.

Materials and Methods

Study area and sources of data

The Nord-Pas-de-Calais region has a surface area of 12 481 km² with approximately 4 033 000 inhabitants, including both rural, industrial and urban regions. The region's 170 cantons (a French small administrative unit) were used to represent distinct spatial units. These are referenced by the National Institute of Statistics and Economic Studies (INSEE), and in 2009 had an average population of 23 725 (extremes ranging from 4 991 to 226 827) and an average surface area of 73 km² (extremes ranging from 2 to 258 km²).

Cases were defined as all incident patients requiring RRT registered in the REIN registry (patients were registered on the first day of RRT) in the Nord-Pas-de-Calais region, from January 2005 to December 2011 [34]. For the purpose of this study, all patients were grouped into cantons according to the postcode of their residence, determined at the time of their first RRT. They were ranked by sex and 5-year age group. The following characteristics of the patients were also collected: primary kidney disease, number of visits to a nephrologist in the year preceding treatment, estimated Glomerular Filtration Rate (eGFR) by Modification of Diet in Renal Disease (MDRD) formula at the time of dialysis initiation [35].

Demographic and socioeconomic data were extracted from the 2009 national population census, provided by the INSEE. The population data was also ranked by sex and 5-year age groups. For the Townsend deprivation index calculation, the 2009 French census output area file was matched to each patient's canton of residence. The score was computed from 4 census variables: percentages of non-owner-occupied households, unemployment, household overcrowding, and absence of access to a motor vehicle [36].

Ethics Statement

This study was conducted in accordance with Commission Nationale de l'Informatique et des Libertés (CNIL) and Comité consultatif sur le traitement de l'information en matière de recherche dans le domaine de la santé (CCTIR).

Crude incidence (pmi)

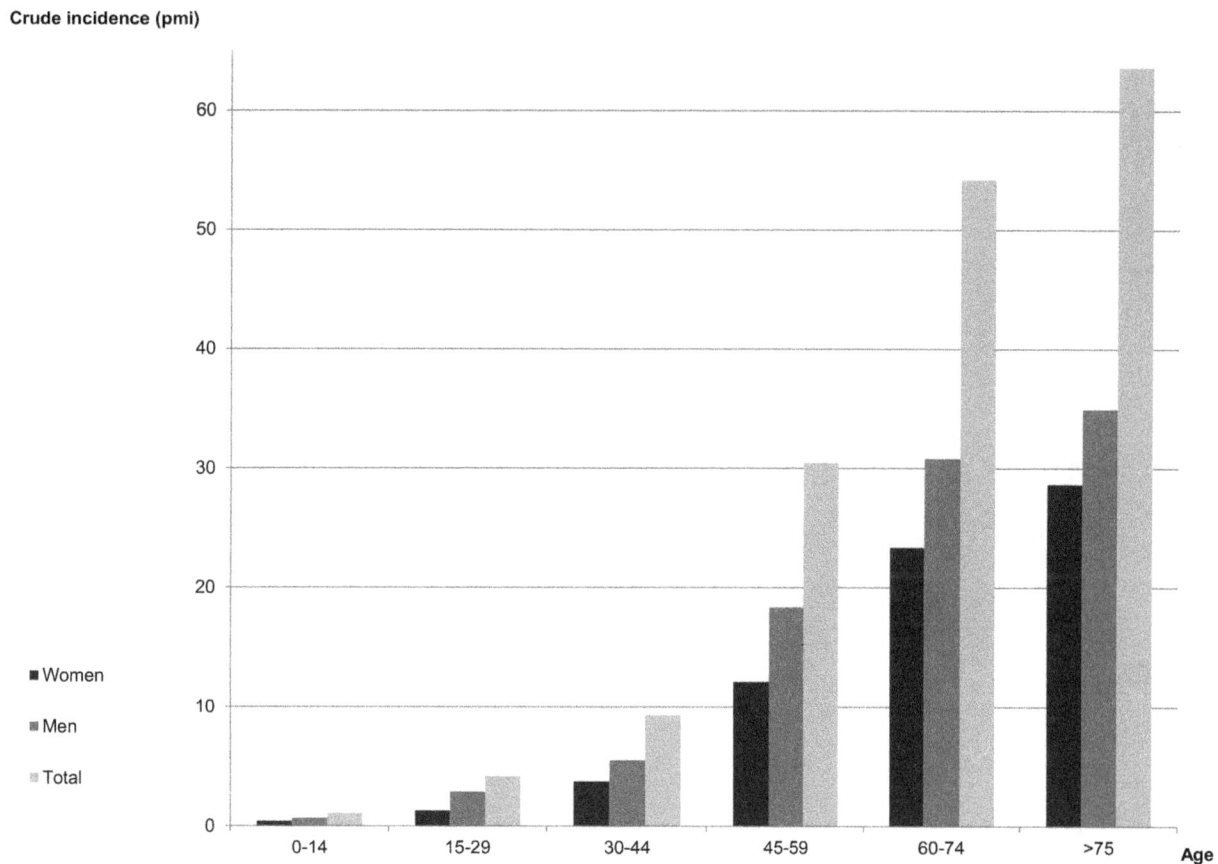

Figure 1. Crude incidence rate of ESRD (pmi) by age and gender.

Statistical analysis

Incidence rates and deprivation index. Firstly, the male and female crude incidence rates were estimated for the 170 cantons, by means of direct standardization. Crude incidence is the number of new patients divided by the total population at risk during the study period. The SIR, defined as the ratio of the number of observed cases to the expected number of cases, computed using indirect standardization, was then determined for each canton. Notice that the SIR is the maximum likelihood estimate of θ_i, the true relative risk (RR) associated with canton i. Significant SIRs have a 95% credible interval, which does not contain the value 1. The method used to calculate the incidence rate denominators assumed the population in a given canton to remain constant over the study period.

On the basis of our registry, the proportion of cases with diabetic and/or vascular nephropathy was calculated for each canton. The Townsend index for each canton was classified into quintiles, with the first quintile (Q1) corresponding to the least deprived cantons, and the fifth quintile (Q5) corresponding to the most deprived cantons.

The Pearson correlation was used to assess the correlation between the logarithm of the SIR and the eGFR.

Spatial analysis. The centroid of each canton, defined by its geographical center (longitude and latitude), was used for the spatial analysis. In order to take the instability resulting from low frequencies and spatial autocorrelation effect into account, the SIR was smoothed using the hierarchical Bayesian model with three levels, proposed by Besag et al. [37]. At the first level, the observed

number of cases in the ith canton θ_i is assumed to be Poisson distributed,

$$O_i \sim P(\theta_i e_i)$$

with a mean $\theta_i e_i$, where θ_i is the RR associated with canton i, and e_i, the expected number of cases, considered as constant and calculated by means of indirect standardization. At the second level the logarithm of θ_i is modeled as the sum of two random effects, the first, U_i, corresponding to the unstructured spatial heterogeneity and the second, V_i, describing the correlation between the neighboring cantons (sharing a common boundary):

$$\log \theta_i = \beta_0 + U_i + V_i,$$

where β_0 corresponds to overall level of the RR across the study region. The random effect U_i is distributed as a normal distribution of null mean and variance σ_U^2:

$$U_i \sim N\left(0, \sigma_U^2\right)$$

and the random effect V_i is modeled using the conditional autoregressive (CAR) model:

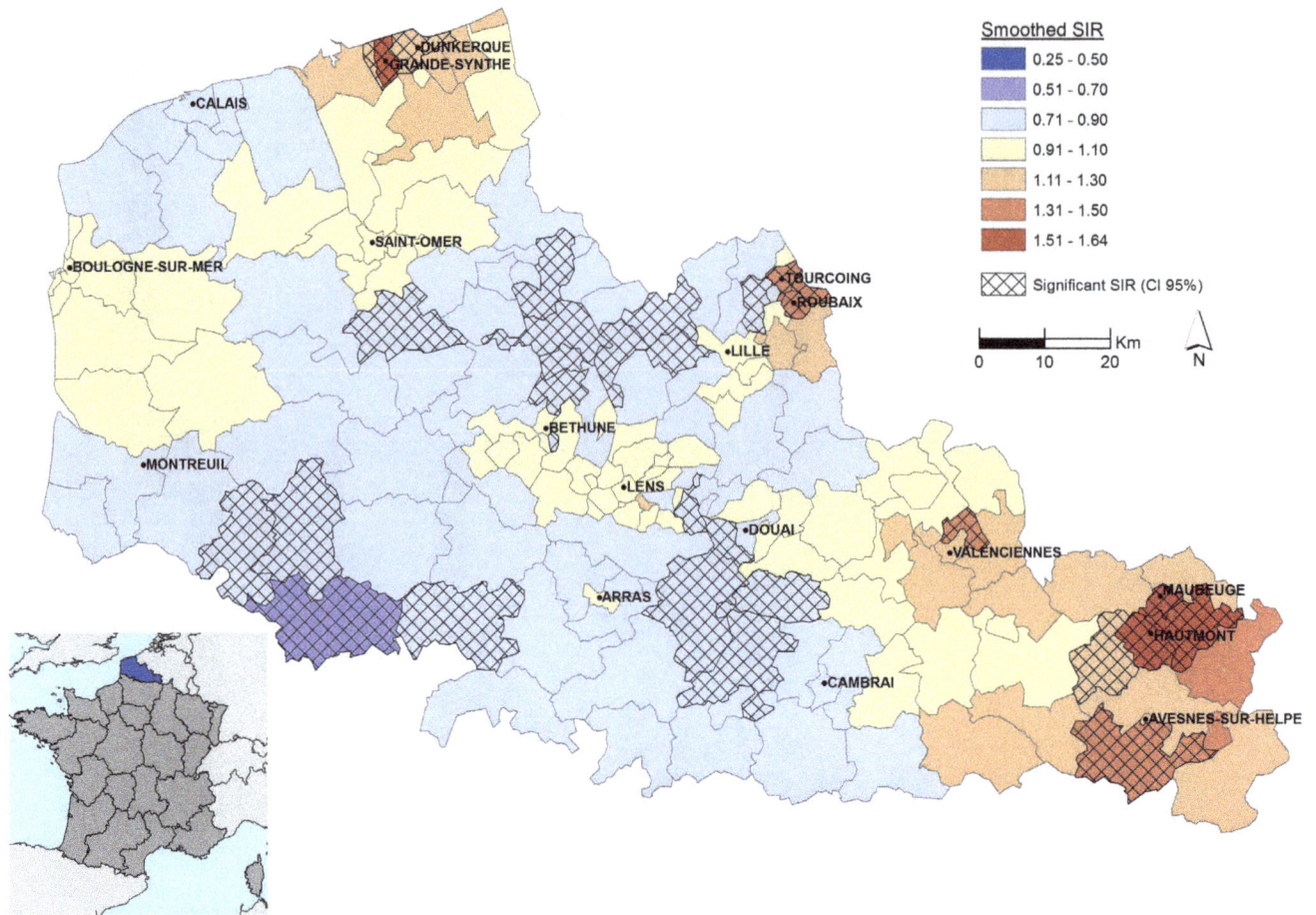

Figure 2. Smoothed SIRs of ESRD by cantons, 2005–2011.

$$\left(V_i / V_j = v_j, i \neq j\right) \sim N\left(\frac{\sum_{j \neq i} w_{ij} v_j}{\sum_{j \neq i} w_{ij}}, \frac{\sigma_V^2}{\sum_{j \neq i} w_{ij}}\right),$$

where $w_{ij} = 1$ if the canton i and canton j are adjacent and 0 otherwise. At the third level, the variances of the two random effects U_i and V_i, σ_U^2 and σ_V^2, have a non-informative gamma prior distribution as suggested by Bernadinelli et al. [38].

In order to analyze the association between ESRD and the deprivation index, the quintiles of the latter were introduced at the second level of the hierarchical model as follow:

$$\log \theta_i = \beta_0 + U_i + V_i + x_i' \boldsymbol{\beta},$$

where x_i corresponds to the vector of covariates and $\boldsymbol{\beta}$ the vector of the associated coefficients. In order to take into account the quintiles of the deprivation index, we introduced four dummy variables $x_j, 1 \leq j \leq 4$ corresponding to the second, third, fourth and fifth quintile. The first quintile has been taken as reference. Each β_j has a non-informative normal prior distribution as suggested by Lawson et al. [39].

The models were fitted using Markov Chain Monte Carlo methods with 25 000 iterations, following a burning step involving

5 000 iterations. All of the calculations were made using the WinBUGS Software [40], and the maps were produced using the ArcGIS 10.1 software (http://www.esri.com). All statistical analyses were considered significant at the 0.05 type 1 error.

Results

The study included 4 597 patients (57.2% men and 42.8% women), who began an RRT between 2005 and 2011 in the Nord-Pas-de-Calais. The overall crude annual incidence rate was 163 pmi for both sexes, 193 pmi for men and 135 pmi for women. Strong disparities were observed over the 170 cantons, ranging from 38 to 432 pmi for both sexes combined, and from 0 to 424 pmi for men and 0 to 439 pmi for women (Table 1). As expected, the crude incidence rate increases sharply with age, and males have a relatively higher proportion of ESRD incidence (Fig. 1). The median age of incidents is 69 years for men, 72 years for women, and 71 years for both sexes combined.

The smoothed SIRs vary among cantons, from 0.66 to 1.64 (Table 1), and there is a significant spatial variability of SIR within the Nord-Pas-de-Calais region (Fig. 2). There are four areas with significantly high incidence rates. In the South-East, Maubeuge, Hautmont and Avesnes-sur-Helpe are rural cantons, were SIRs are respectively 1.64, 95% CI [1.32–2.01], 1.50, 95% CI [1.18–1.88] and 1.39, 95% CI [1.05–1.79]. Northern part of Valenciennes (SIR: 1.38, 95% CI [1.12–1.68]) is more urbanized and includes several industrial activities. The Agglomeration of

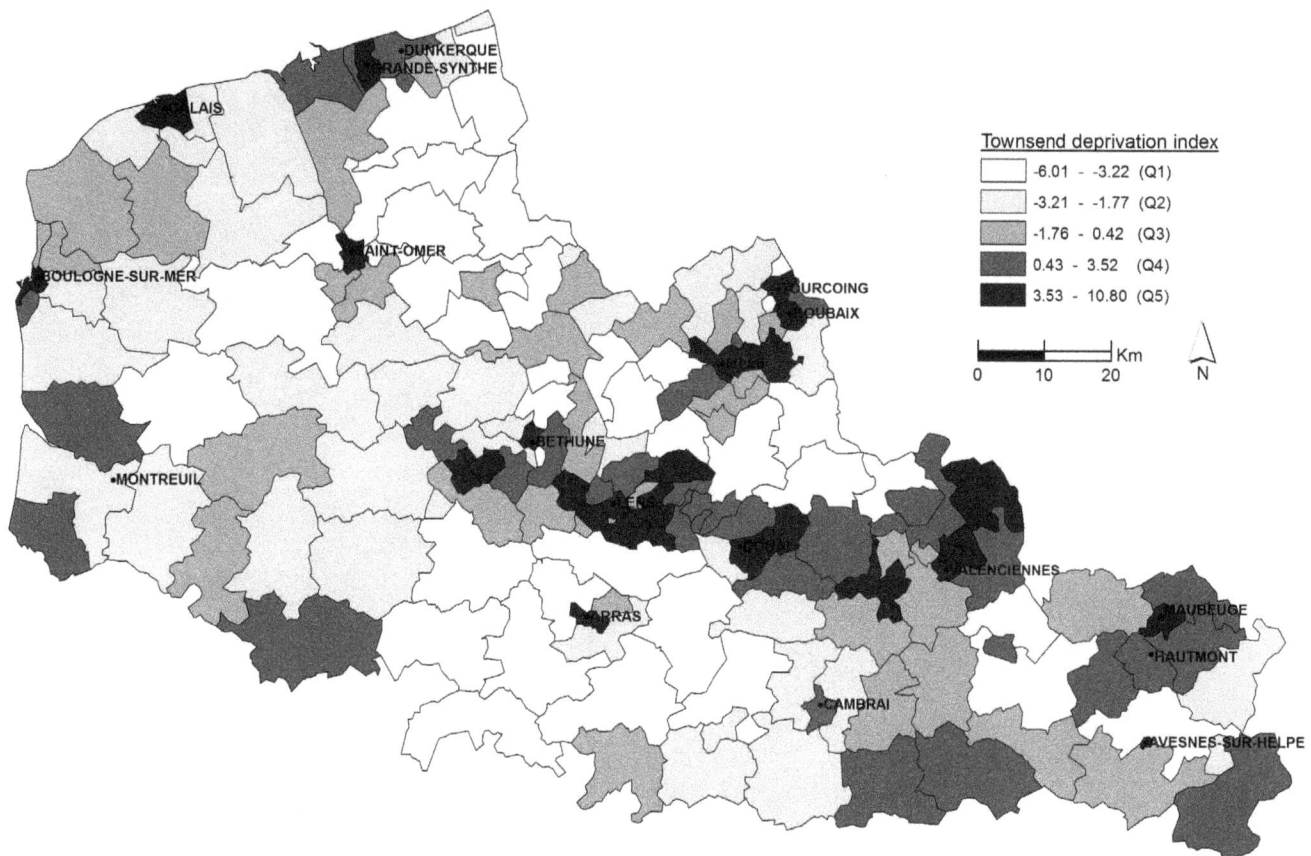

Figure 3. Spatial distribution of Townsend deprivation index by cantons, 2009.

Roubaix, Tourcoing and Wattrelos (1.48, 95% CI [1.26–1.73], 1.32 95% CI [1.13–1.54] and 1.33, 95% CI [1.07–1.63] respectively) is a densely populated urban area (≈230,000 inhabitants). In northern, SIRs are respectively 1.55, 95% CI [1.18–2.01] and 1.27, 95% CI [1.10–1.47] in Grande-Synthe and Dunkerque, which are important industrial zones, surrounded by a densely populated urban area (≈220,000 inhabitants). Three areas with significantly low incidence rates are observed. They mostly include rural areas, such as in South-Western region (SIR: 0.66, 95% CI [0.46–0.89]).

Before assessing the relationship between deprivation and these spatial disparities, the influence of early referral dialysis was examined. Early dialysis initiation was determined by measuring the median eGFR for each canton (Table 1). Although it is significant (p<0.05), the Pearson coefficient (R = 0.23) indicates a very weak positive correlation with the smoothed SIRs.

Disparities are observed in the proportions of diabetic or vascular nephropathy occurring in the different cantons within the region (Table 1). These are not correlated with the smoothed SIRs. The RR is 1.31, 95% CI [0.87–1.97] for diabetic nephropathy and 0.98, 95% CI [0.65–1.48] for vascular nephropathy.

The Townsend deprivation index varies strongly within the region (Table 1, Fig. 3), and there is a significant correlation between smoothed SIRs and the Townsend index quintiles. With Q1 taken as a reference, the relative risk (RR) of RRT was assessed for each level of deprivation (Fig. 4). Higher levels of deprivation are associated with an increase in RR: 1.18, 95% CI [1.00–1.34] for Q2, 1.28, 95% CI [1.11–1.47] for Q3, 1.30, 95%

CI [1.14–1.51] for Q4 and 1.44, 95% CI [1.32–1.74] for Q5. In addition, the residential Townsend index attributed to each collected case was compared with late referral, estimated by means of the number of visits to a nephrologist in the year preceding treatment. No correlation is found (p = 0.66).

Analysis of the geographic patterns of the smoothed SIRs, adjusted to the Townsend covariable, still reveal three areas of significantly high risk in the north and south-east of the region, in the Lille metropolis and the agglomerations of Roubaix, Tourcoing and Wattrelos. Two significantly low-risk areas are also observed in the south-west of the region and the area between Saint-Omer and Lille (Fig. 5). The corresponding smoothed SIRs vary among cantons, from 0.66 to 1.69.

Discussion

In this study, significant spatial disparities in ESRD incidence are revealed in the 170 cantons of the Nord-Pas-de-Calais region of France. Although such disparities have recently been observed among districts, they had never been seen at this spatial resolution in France. These results are consistent with variations observed at similar scales in other countries [6,17,22,28].

Several factors were analyzed, in an attempt to explain this phenomenon. It should be noted that any ecological correlations were made at the level of geographical areas, and not individuals. As a consequence, although causality cannot be assumed, etiological hypotheses can be proposed [41].

In France, Couchoud et al. [14] found that the intensity of healthcare has a substantial impact on RRT incidence at the level

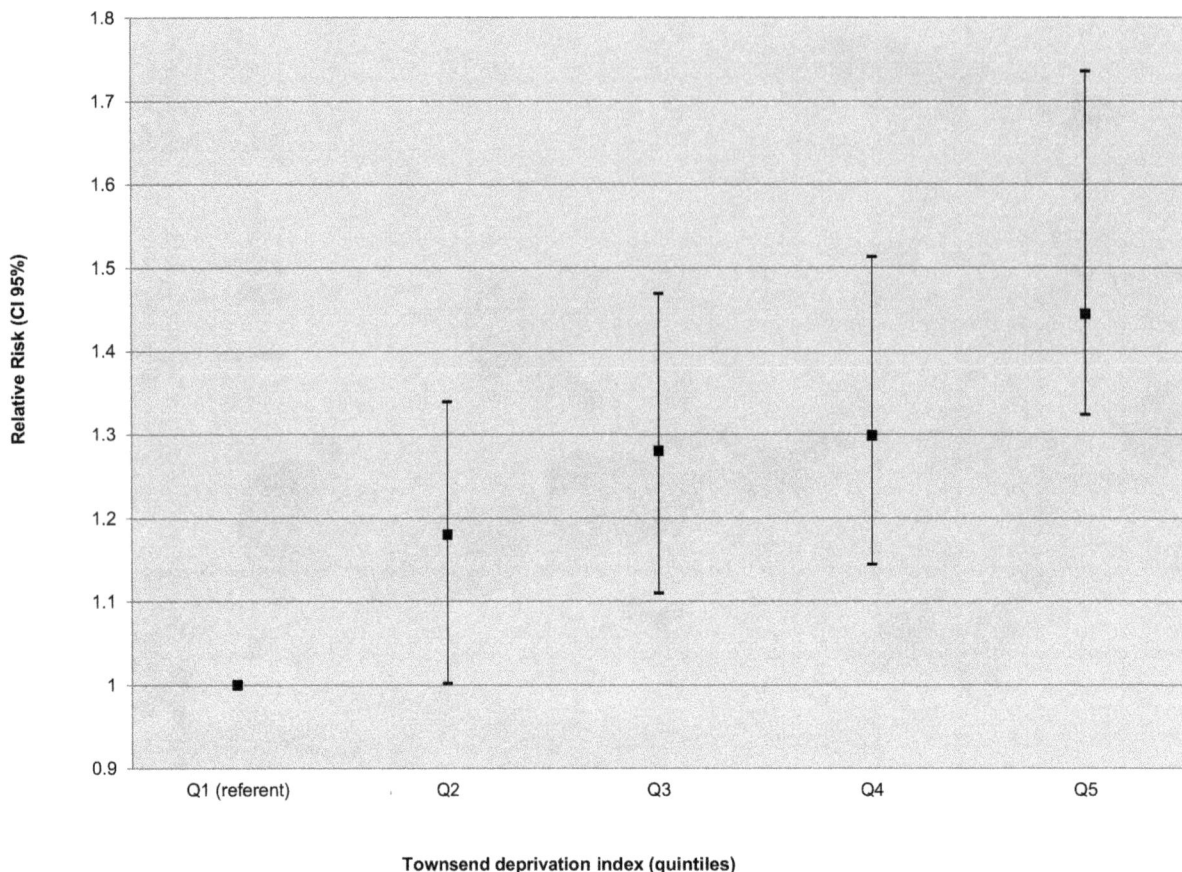

Figure 4. Relative risk (95% credible interval) of ESRD by Townsend quintile.

of individual districts. Concerning the Nord-Pas-de-Calais region, a significant, but weak association was found between the median eGFR and the smoothed SIRs. Earlier timing of dialysis initiation has a negligible contribution to spatial disparities in the incidence of ESRD within this region. This result confirms the presence of uniform medical practice throughout this territory.

The spatial heterogeneity of ESRD is not related to the incidence of diabetic or vascular nephropathies. This result means that cantons with high incidence rates are not associated with an overincidence of diabetic or vascular nephropathies. The cases developing such CKD were not the cause of the observed phenomenon. However, several studies have identified ecological relationships between RRT incidence and the prevalence of diabetics or cardio-vascular diseases [8,15,18–20]. As no data was available concerning the prevalence of these diseases at the scale of each canton, the present study data was used as a proxy, to determine the proportion of diabetic and vascular nephropathies in each canton.

On the other hand, deprivation is clearly associated with a higher ESRD incidence, and wealth with a lower ESRD incidence. These findings are consistent with results observed on a larger scale in France, since Couchoud et al. [15] revealed a positive relationship between 82 districts, whatever the socio-economic factors used. The patterns shown here are similar to those found in other studies, which focused on deprivation indicators over larger heterogeneous geographic areas. Caskey et al. [42] identified a correlation between RRT incidence and a country's macroeconomic factors, such as gross domestic product

(GDP) per capita, percentage of GDP spent on health care, and dialysis facility reimbursement rate relative to GDP. Although Ward et al. [16] highlighted a greater incidence of ESRD in patients living in Zoning Improvement Plan (ZIP) areas with a lower composite socioeconomic score, this trend was not uniform for all primary renal diseases. In the case of US counties, the incidence rate of treated ESRD has been shown to be inversely related to the level of income [25]. For similar, highly homogenous small area units, Grace et al. [17] recently found a decreasing incidence of RRT with increasing area advantage in Australia. In the UK, deprivation is found to be a determinant of geographical variations in RRT, between wards or enumeration districts [6,43]. Furthermore, Volkova et al. [28] have revealed a strong correlation between incidence rates and neighborhood poverty, corresponding to populations living below the poverty level, for the case of the census tracts of Georgia, North Carolina, or South Carolina. Although the Townsend index is criticized for its urban view of deprivation, it is nevertheless widely used. Furthermore, some recently developed indexes have been shown to be strongly correlated with this one [44,45].

In agreement with other studies, the assumption is made that deprivation is an obstacle to prevention, and that it supports the progression of CKD to ESRD [15,16]. To substantiate this hypothesis, the influence of late referral from collected cases was assessed, by determining the number of visits to a nephrologist during the year preceding treatment. There was no significant correlation between this number and the Townsend index. Patients who were treated later do not live primarily in

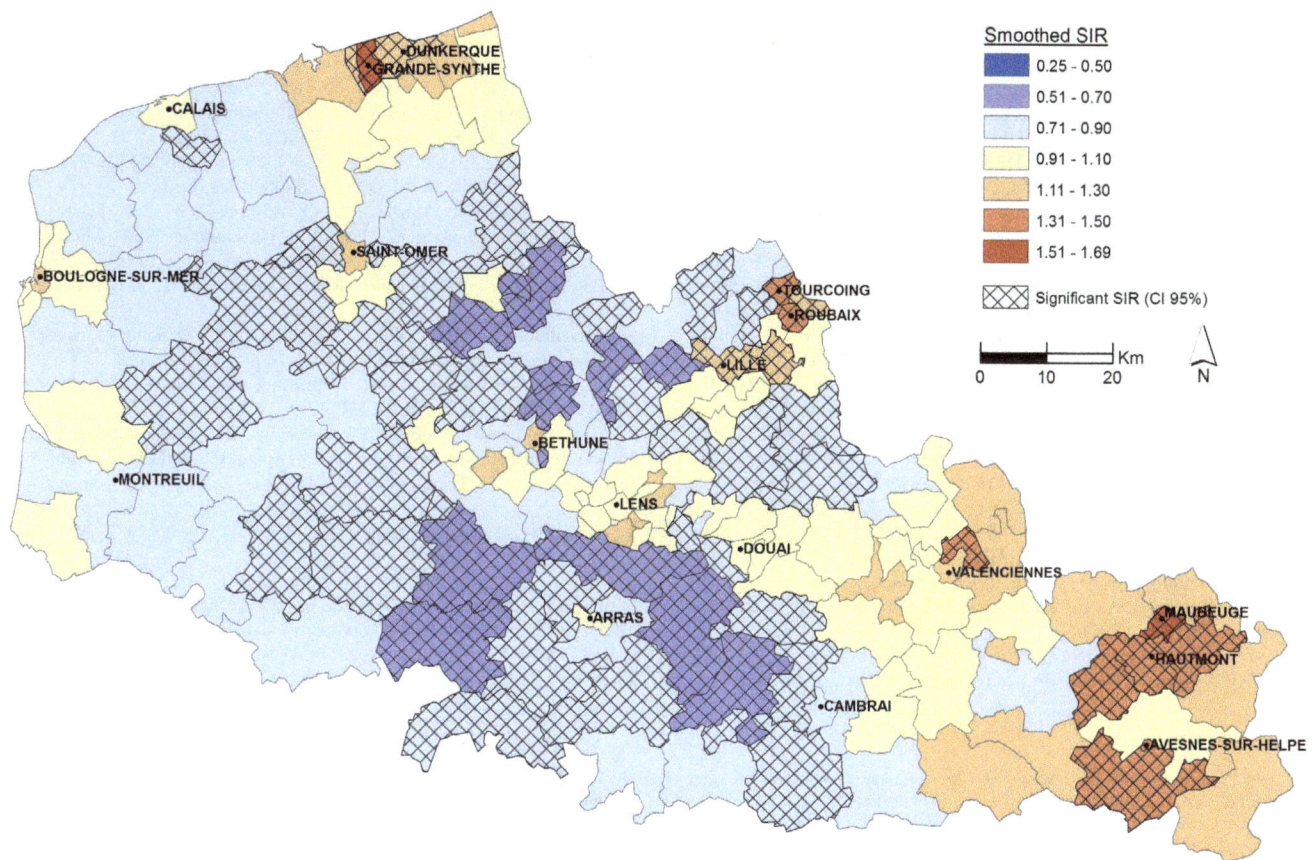

Figure 5. Smoothed SIRs of ESRD by cantons, 2005–2011, adjusted to the Townsend index covariable, 2009.

disadvantaged townships. Moreover, in France, access to health-care and medical insurance coverage does not discriminate against poverty. The medical or hospital fees associated with CKD treatment are also completely covered by public health insurance. It is thus possible that the correlation between deprivation and ESRD incidence is not related to an individual's financial capacity to access healthcare. Other more relevant factors associated with deprivation, such as health literacy, acculturation or trust in healthcare providers, could explain these variations. This is supported by Lora et al. [46], who report that lower levels of health literacy and acculturation are associated with differences in knowledge, attitude, and behavior, that may contribute to a poor outcome in patients with CKD.

In this paper, it is shown that SIR mapping can be used to highlight global spatial heterogeneities in ESRD incidence. Although this method is needed to reveal spatial patterns of interest, it cannot detect significant atypical spatial and space-time clusters in terms of ESRD incidence. Spatial and space-time scan statistics [47,48] should thus be used to test for the presence of ESRD clusters, and to identify their location in space and time.

When the SIR map is adjusted to the Townsend covariable, areas of significantly high incidence still exist. These are not explained in the present study. Other etiological assumptions such as environmental contamination should be assessed in the future. As it includes industrial, urban and agricultural territories, the Nord-Pas-de-Calais region is suitable for such a study. This should be conducted at the level of small areas, to avoid a dilution of the spatial variations characterizing nearby, heterogeneous popula-tions.

Conclusion

In developed countries, significant variations in ESRD inci-dence are observed over small areas [6,17,28]. The present study shows that this is also the case in France. Within the Nord-Pas-de-Calais territory, which has homogeneous healthcare provision, this phenomenon can be partially explained by deprivation. However, since access to healthcare is universal in France, and in the case of serious illnesses such as ESRD, this access is not affected by an individual's financial well-being, other deprivation-related factors may explain the observed correlation. Moreover, these disparities are not related to a specific type of medical practice, related to the initiation of dialysis. The SIR can be used as a geographic tool, for decision-making in the management of dialysis units and the definition of prevention campaigns at local scales. Even when the deprivation factor is taken into account, spatial disparities in ESRD incidence remain, suggesting that environmental factors such as suspected heavy metal still play a significant role [29–31]. We plan to investigate this aspect in future studies.

Acknowledgments

Nephonor network regroup all the Nephrologists working in the Nord-Pas de Calais area. We particularly grateful each of them for their contributions to this study: Larbi AAZIB[a], Abdelkader BENZIANE[a], Roseline M'BARGA[a], Guillaume BONNARD[b], Guillaume BURDA[b], Evelyne MAC NAMARA[b], Anderson RATSIMBAZAFY[b], Amina SKALLI[b], Lucie WAJSBROT[b], Pierre BATAILLE[c], Stephane BILLION[c], Alexan-dra BOTTE-NOËL[c], Maïté DAROUX[c], Rafik MESBAH[c], Irina SHAHAPUNI[c], Milad SHENOUDA[c], Pascal WHEATLEY[c], Mustapha AL MORABITI[d], Aderrahim EL AMARI[d], Bernard PAINCHART[d],

Gérard CARDON[e], J-Philippe HAMMELIN[e], Florence MOULON-GUET[e], Matthieu REBEROLLE[e], Imad ALMOUBARAK[f], Raymond AZAR[f], Laura MOUSSALIEH[f], M.Xavière VAIRON-CODACCIONI[f], Toufik BOUBIA[g], Véronique BOUBIA[g], Jean-Louis BACRI[h], Jonathan DESPREZ[h], Dominique FLEURY[h], Delphine LABATUT[h], Céline LEBAS[h], Nathalie MAISONNEUVE[h], Philippe VANHILLE[h], Laurence VRIGNEAUD[h], Amaury BEN HENDA[i], Nasser HAMDINI[i], René CUVELIER[j], Isabelle DEVRIENDT[j], Ann karolien VANDOOREN[j], Alexandre DUFAY[k], Marlène GOUBET[k], Thomas GUINCESTRE[k], Hervé LE MONIES[k], Aline TALASZKA[k], Marie FRIMAT[l], Antoine GARSTKA[l], Francois GLOWACKI[l‡], Brigitte GOSSET[l], Tiphaine GUYON-ROGER[l], Marc HAZZAN[l], Celia LESSORE DE STE FOY[l], Arnaud LIONET[l], Christian NOEL[l*], Dominique PAGNIEZ[l], Francois PROVÔT[l], Nasser HAMDINI[m], Maxime HOFFMANN[m], Géraldine ROBITAILLE[m], Elisabeth SEMJEN[m], Reynald BINAUT[n], Franck BOURDON[n], J-Philippe DEVAUX[n], Lili TAGHIPOUR TAMIJI[n], Maud DEHENNAULT[o], Annie LAHOCHE[o], Valérie LEROY[o], Robert NOVO[o], Anne VAN EGROO[o], Daniel LOUVET[p], Gilles MESSIER[p], Luc DELVALLEZ[p], Christian LAMOTTE[p], Jacques LEBLEU[p], Richard READE[p], J-François BONNE[q], José BRASSEUR[q], J. Dominique GHEERBRANDT[q], Paule HARDY[q], Corinne LEMOINE[q], Hassen ADDA[r], Bouchra CHLIH[r].

[a] CH d'Arras, Bd Besnier 62022 Arras, France
[b] CH de Béthune, rue Delbecque 62408 Béthune, France
[c] CH de Boulogne, Allée J Monod 62321 Boulogne/mer, France
[d] CH de Cambrai, 516 avenue de Paris 59400 Cambrai, France
[e] CH de Douai, route de Cambrai 59570 Douai, France
[f] CH de Dunkerque, Av L Herbeaux 59240 Dunkerque, France

[g] CH de Fourmies, 1 rue de l'Hôpital 59611 Fourmies, France
[h] CH de Valenciennes, Av Desandrouins 59322 Valenciennes, France
[i] CH de Maubeuge, 13 Bd Pasteur, 59600 Maubeuge, France
[j] CH de Mouscron Av de Fécamp 7700 Mouscron, Belgique
[k] CH de Roubaix, Bd Lacordaire, 59056 Roubaix, France
[l] CHRU de Lille, Rue Polovnski, 59037 Lille, France
[m] Clinique de La Louvière, rue de La Louvière, 59800 Lille, France
[n] Clinique Du Bois, Av M Dormoy 59000 Lille, France
[o] Hôpital Jeanne de Flandre 2 Av O Lambret 59037 Lille, France
[p] NephroCare Maubeuge, Allée de la Polyclinique 59604 Maubeuge, France
[q] Polyclinique de Bois Bernard, Rte de Neuvireuil, 62230 Bois Bernard, France
[r] Polyclinique Vauban, 10 Av Vauban 59300 Valenciennes, France
* Past coordinator and founder of the Nephronor network
‡ Actual coordinator of the Nephronor network (Email: Francois. GLOWACKI@CHRU-LILLE.FR)

Furthermore, we gratefully acknowledge the outstanding technical support of Hasna Camara, Sebastien Gomis and the staff of the Nephronor network.

Author Contributions

Conceived and designed the experiments: FO AD MG CN DC FG Néphronor Network. Performed the experiments: FO AD MG DC FG. Analyzed the data: FO MG FG. Contributed reagents/materials/analysis tools: FO CN FG Néphronor Network. Wrote the paper: FO AD MG DC FG.

References

1. Zoccali C, Kramer A, Jager KJ (2010) Chronic kidney disease and end-stage renal disease—a review produced to contribute to the report 'the status of health in the European union: towards a healthier Europe'. Nephrology Dialysis Transplantation Plus 3(3): 213–24.

2. Wakai K, Nakai S, Kikichi K, Iseki K, Miwa N, et al. (2004) Trends in incidence of end-stage renal disease in Japan, 1983–2000: age-adjusted and age-specific rates by gender and cause. Nephrology Dialysis Transplantation 19(8): 2044–52.

3. National Kidney andUrologic Diseases Information National (2012) Kidney Disease Statistics for the United States. NIH Publication No12–3895: 15p. Available at www.kidney.niddk.nih.gov.

4. US Renal Data System (USRDS) (2013) International coparisons. In: Annual Data Report: Atlas of Chronic Kidney Disease and End-Stage Renal Disease in the United States Volume two. National Institutes of Health, National Institute of Diabetes and Digestive and Kidney Diseases, Bethesda, MD, 2013. pp. 333–344.

5. Rosansky SJ, Huntsberger TL, Jackson K, Eggers P (1990) Comparative incidence rates of end-stage renal disease treatment by state. American journal of nephrology 10(3): 198–204.

6. Roderick P, Clements S, Stone N, Martin D, Diamond I (1999) What determines geographical variation in rates of acceptance onto renal replacement therapy in England? Journal of Health Services Research and Policy 4(3): 139–46.

7. Usami T, Koyama K, Takeuchi O, Morozumi K, Kimura G (2000) Regional variations in the incidence of end-stage renal failure in Japan. Journal of the American Medical Association 284(20): 2622–4.

8. Wimmer F, Oberaigner W, Kramar R, Mayer G (2003) Regional variability in the incidence of end-stage renal disease: An epidemiological approach. Nephrology Dialysis Transplantation 18(8): 1562–7.

9. Counil È, Cherni N, Kharrat M, Achour A, Trimech H (2008) Trends of incident dialysis patients in tunisia between 1992 and 2001. American Journal of Kidney Diseases 51(3): 463–70.

10. Hommel K, Rasmussen S, Kamper A, Madsen M (2010) Regional and social inequalities in chronic renal replacement therapy in Denmark. Nephrology Dialysis Transplantation 25(8): 2624–32.

11. U.S. Renal Data System (USRDS) (2013) Incidence, Prevalence, Patient Characteristics, and Modalities. In: Annual Data Report: Atlas of Chronic Kidney Disease and End-Stage Renal Disease in the United States Volume two. National Institutes of Health, National Institute of Diabetes and Digestive and Kidney Diseases, Bethesda, MD, 2013. pp. 215–228.

12. Gilg J, Rao A, Fogarty D (2013) UK Renal Replacement Therapy Incidence in 2012: National and Centre-specific Analyses. In: UK Renal Registry 16th Annual Report pp. 9–35.

13. Tanner RM, Gutiérrez OM, Judd S, McClellan W, Bowling CB, et al. (2013) Geographic variation in CKD prevalence and ESRD incidence in the United States: Results from the reasons for geographic and racial differences in stroke (REGARDS) study. American Journal of Kidney Diseases 61(3): 395–403.

14. Couchoud C, Guihenneuc C, Bayer F, Stengel B (2010) The timing of dialysis initiation affects the incidence of renal replacement therapy. Nephrology Dialysis Transplantation 25(5): 1576–8.

15. Couchoud C, Guihenneuc C, Bayer F, Lemaitre V, Brunet P, Stengel B (2012) Medical practice patterns and socio-economic factors may explain geographical variation of end-stage renal disease incidence. Nephrology Dialysis Transplantation 27(6): 2312–22.

16. Ward MM (2008) Socioeconomic status and the incidence of ESRD. American Journal of Kidney Diseases 51(4): 563–72.

17. Grace BS, Clayton P, Cass A, McDonald SP (2012) Socio-economic status and incidence of renal replacement therapy: A registry study of australian patients. Nephrology Dialysis Transplantation 27(11): 4173–80.

18. Muntner P, Coresh J, Powe NR, Klag MJ (2003) The contribution of increased diabetes prevalence and improved myocardial infarction and stroke survival to the increase in treated end-stage renal disease. Journal of the American Society of Nephrology 14(6): 1568–77.

19. Bell EK, Gao L, Judd S, Glasser SP, McClellan W, et al. (2012) Blood pressure indexes and end-stage renal disease risk in adults with chronic kidney disease. American Journal of Hypertension 25(7): 789–96.

20. Huang Y, Cai X, Zhang J, Mai W, Wang S, et al. (2014) Prehypertension and incidence of ESRD: A systematic Review and Meta-analysis. American Journal of Kidney Diseases 63(1): 76–83.

21. Van De Luijtgaarden MWM, Noordzij M, Tomson C, Couchoud C, Cancarini G, et al. (2012) Factors influencing the decision to start renal replacement therapy: Results of a survey among european nephrologists. American Journal of Kidney Diseases 60(6): 940–8.

22. Boyle PJ, Kudlac H, Williams AJ (1996) Geographical variation in the referral of patients with chronic end stage renal failure for renal replacement therapy. QJM - Monthly Journal of the Association of Physicians 89(2): 151–7.

23. Foxman B, Moulton LH, Wolfe RA, Guire KE, Port FK, Hawthorne VM (1991) Geographic variation in the incidence of treated end-stage renal disease. Journal of the American Society of Nephrology 2(6): 1144–52.

24. Moulton LH, Port FK, Wolfe RA, Foxman B, Guire KE (1992) Patterns of low incidence of treated end-stage renal disease among the elderly. American Journal of Kidney Diseases 20(1): 55–62.

25. Young EW, Mauger EA, Jiang K, Port FK, Wolfe RA (1994) Socioeconomic status and end-stage renal disease in the united states. Kidney International 45(3): 907–11.

26. Fan ZJ, Lackland DT, Lipsitz SR, Nicholas JS, Egan BM, et al. (2007) Geographical patterns of end-stage renal disease incidence and risk factors in rural and urban areas of South Carolina. Health and Place 13(1): 179–87.

27. Yan G, Cheung AK, Ma JZ, Yu AJ, Greene T, et al. (2013) The associations between race and geographic area and quality-of-care indicators in patients approaching ESRD. Clinical Journal of the American Society of Nephrology 8(4): 610–8.

28. Volkova N, McClellan W, Klein M, Flanders D, Kleinbaum D, et al. (2008) Neighborhood poverty and racial differences in ESRD incidence. Journal of the American Society of Nephrology 19(2): 356–64.

29. Hellström L, Elinder C, Dahlberg B, Lundberg M, Järup L, et al. (2001) Cadmium exposure and end-stage renal disease. American Journal of Kidney Diseases 38(5): 1001–8.

30. Hodgson S, Nieuwenhuijsen MJ, Elliott P, Jarup L (2007) Kidney disease mortality and environmental exposure to mercury. American journal of epidemiology 165(1): 72–7.

31. Muntner P, Menke A, Batuman V, Rabito FA, He J, et al. (2007) Association of tibia lead and blood lead with end-stage renal disease: A pilot study of african-americans. Environmental Research 104(3): 396–401.

32. Couchoud C, Stengel B, Landais P, Aldigier J-C, De Cornelissen F, et al. (2006) The renal epidemiology and information network (REIN): a new registry for end-stage renal disease in France. Nephrology Dialysis Transplantation 21: 411–418.

33. Réseau Epidémiologie et Information en Néphrologie (REIN) (2012) Rapport annuel 2012. 322 p.

34. Renal Epidemiology and Information Network (REIN) (2013) Guide de remplissage de DIADEM Informations sur la dialyse du registre REIN. 18 p.

35. Froissart M, Rossert J, Jacquot C, Paillard M, Houillier P (2005) Predictive performance of the modification of diet in renal disease and Cockcroft-Gault equations for estimating renal function. Journal of the American Society of Nephrology 16(3): 763–73.

36. Townsend P (1987) Deprivation. Journal of Social Policy 16(2): 125–146.

37. Besag J, York J, Mollié A (1991) Bayesian image restoration with two applications in spatial statistics. Annals of the Institute of Statistical Mathematics 43: 1–21.

38. Bernadinelli L, Clayton D, Montomoli C (1995) Bayesian estimates of disease maps: How important are priors? Statistics in Medicine 14(21–22): 2411–2431.

39. Lawson AB, Browne WJ, Rodeiro CLV (2003) Disease mapping with WinBUGS and MLwiN (Vol. 11). John Wiley & Sons.

40. Spiegelhalter DJ, Thomas A, Best NG, Lunn D (2003) WinBugs v. 1.4. User Manual. Cambridge: MRC Biostatistics. Unit. 60 p.

41. Wakefield J (2008) Ecologic studies revisited. Annual review of public health 29: 75–90.

42. Caskey FJ, Kramer A, Elliott RF, Stel VS, Covic A, et al. (2011) Global variation in renal replacement therapy for end-stage renal disease. Nephrology Dialysis Transplantation 26(8): 2604–10.

43. Maheswaran R, Payne N, Meechan D, Burden RP, Fryers PR, et al. (2000) Socioeconomic deprivation, travel distance, and renal replacement therapy in the Trent region, United Kingdom 2000: An ecological study. Journal of epidemiology and community health 57(7): 523–4.

44. Declercq C, Labbe E, Obein L, Poirier G, Lacoste O (2004) Inégalités socio-spatiales de mortalité dans la région Nord - Pas-de-Calais. Rapport Observatoire Régional de la Santé Nord – Pas de Calais. 105 p.

45. Havard S, Deguen S, Bodin J, Louis K, Laurent O, Bard D (2008) A small-area index of socioeconomic deprivation to capture health inequalities in France. Social Science and Medicine 67(12): 2007–16.

46. Lora CM, Gordon EJ, Sharp LK, Fischer MJ, Gerber BS, Lash JP (2011) Progression of CKD in hispanics: Potential roles of health literacy, acculturation, and social support. American Journal of Kidney Diseases 58(2): 282–90.

47. Kulldorff M (1997) A spatial scan statistic. Communications in statistics: theory and methods 26(6): 1481–1496.

48. Kulldorff M, Athas WF, Feurer EJ, Miller BA, Key CR (1998) Evaluating cluster alarms: a space-time scan statistic and brain cancer in Los Alamos, New Mexico. American journal of Public Health 88(9): 1377–1380.

Permissions

List of Contributors

Eliyahu V. Khankin, Walter P. Mutter, Hector Tamez, Hai-Tao Yuan
Department of Medicine, Beth Israel Deaconess Medical Center and Harvard Medical School, Boston, Massachusetts, United States of America

S. Ananth Karumanchi
Department of Medicine, Beth Israel Deaconess Medical Center and Harvard Medical School, Boston, Massachusetts, United States of America
Howard Hughes Medical Institute, Beth Israel Deaconess Medical Center and Harvard Medical School, Boston, Massachusetts, United States of America

Ravi Thadhani
Department of Medicine, Massachusetts General Hospital and Harvard Medical School, Boston, Massachusetts, United States of America

Anastasia Markaki, George A. Fragkiadakis
Department of Nutrition and Dietetics, Technological Educational Institute of Crete, Crete, Greece

John Kyriazis
Department of Nephrology, General Hospital of Chios, Chios, Greece

Kostas Stylianou, Kostas Perakis, Eugene Daphnis
Department of Nephrology, University Hospital of Heraklion, Heraklion, Crete, Greece

Andrew N. Margioris
Department of Clinical Chemistry, School of Medicine, University of Crete, Heraklion, Crete, Greece

Emmanuel S. Ganotakis
Department of Internal Medicine, University Hospital of Heraklion, Heraklion, Crete, Greece

Anna Reznichenko, Jacob van den Born, Martin H. de Borst, Stephan J. L. Bakker, Marc Seelen, Gerjan Navis
Division of Nephrology, Department of Internal Medicine, University Medical Center Groningen, University of Groningen, Groningen, The Netherlands

Harold Snieder
Unit of Genetic Epidemiology & Bioinformatics, Department of Epidemiology, University Medical Center Groningen, University of Groningen, Groningen, The Netherlands

Jeffrey Damman, Henri G. D. Leuvenink, Jan Niesing
Department of Surgery, University Medical Center Groningen, University of Groningen, Groningen, The Netherlands

Marcory C. R. F. van Dijk, Harry van Goor, Jan-Luuk Hillebrands
Department of Pathology and Medical Biology, University Medical Center Groningen, University of Groningen, Groningen, The Netherlands

Bouke G. Hepkema
Department of Transplant Immunology, University Medical Center Groningen, University of Groningen, Groningen, The Netherlands

Chi-Jung Chung
Department of Medical Research, China Medical University and Hospital, Taichung, Taiwan
Department of Health Risk Management, College of Public Health, China Medical University, Taichung, Taiwan

Chao-Yuan Huang
Department of Urology, National Taiwan University Hospital, College of Medicine National Taiwan University, Taipei, Taiwan

Hung-Bin Tsai
Department of Traumatology, National Taiwan University Hospital, Taipei, Taiwan

Chih-Hsin Muo
Department of Public Health, China Medical University, Taichung, Taiwan
Management Office for Health Data, China Medical University and Hospital, Taichung, Taiwan

Mu-Chi Chung
Division of Nephrology, Department of Internal Medicine, Taichung Veterans General Hospital, Taichung, Taiwan

Chao-Hsiang Chang
Department of Urology, China Medical University and Hospital, Taichung, Taiwan
Department of Medicine, College of Medicine, China Medical University and Hospital, Taichung, Taiwan

Chiu-Ching Huang
Department of Medicine, College of Medicine, China Medical University and Hospital, Taichung, Taiwan
Division of Nephrology and Kidney Institute, China Medical University and Hospital, Taichung, Taiwan

Loren Lipworth, Todd L. Edwards
Division of Epidemiology, Department of Medicine, Vanderbilt University Medical Center and Vanderbilt-Ingram Cancer Center, Nashville, Tennessee, United States of America

Robert E. Tarone, Joseph K. McLaughlin, William J. Blot
Division of Epidemiology, Department of Medicine, Vanderbilt University Medical Center and Vanderbilt-Ingram Cancer Center, Nashville, Tennessee, United States of America
International Epidemiology Institute, Rockville, Maryland, United States of America

Michael T. Mumma
International Epidemiology Institute, Rockville, Maryland, United States of America

Kerri L. Cavanaugh, T. Alp Ikizler
Division of Nephrology, Department of Medicine, Vanderbilt University Medical Center, Nashville, Tennessee, United States of America

Friso L. H. Muntinghe
Internal Medicine, Vasculair Medicine, University Medical Center Groningen, Groningen, The Netherlands

Wayel H. Abdulahad, Minke G. Huitema, Johanna Westra
Rheumatology and Clinical Immunology, University Medical Center Groningen, Groningen, The Netherlands

Jeffrey Damman, Marc A. Seelen, Gerjan Navis
Internal Medicine, Nephrology, University Medical Center Groningen, Groningen, The Netherlands

Simon P. M. Lems, Bouke G. Hepkema
Laboratory Medicine, Transplantation Immunology, University Medical Center Groningen, Groningen, The Netherlands

Thomas M. F. Connor, Daniel P. Gale, Guy H. Neild, Patrick H. Maxwell
UCL Division of Medicine and Centre for Nephrology, University College London, London, United Kingdom

D. Deren Oygar
Nicosia State Hospital, Burhan Nalbantoglu General Hospital, Nicosia, North Cyprus

Retha Steenkamp
UK Renal Registry, Southmead Hospital, Bristol, United Kingdom

Dorothea Nitsch
London School of Hygiene and Tropical Medicine, London, United Kingdom

Jing Liu, Kun Ling Ma, Min Gao, Jie Ni, Yang Zhang, Xiao Liang Zhang, Hong Liu, Yan Li Wang, Bi Cheng Liu
Institute of Nephrology, Zhong Da Hospital, Southeast University School of Medicine, Nanjing City, Jiangsu Province, People's Republic of China

Chang Xian Wang
Department of Infection Management, Zhong Da Hospital, Southeast University School of Medicine, Nanjing City, Jiangsu Province, People's Republic of China

Do Hyoung Kim, Yon Su Kim
Department of Internal Medicine, Seoul National University College of Medicine, Seoul, Korea
Clinical Research Center for End Stage Renal Disease in Korea Daegu, Korea

Myounghee Kim
Department of Dental Hygiene, College of Health Science, Eulji University, Seongnam, Korea
Clinical Research Center for End Stage Renal Disease in Korea Daegu, Korea

Ho Kim
Department of Epidemiology and Biostatistics, School of Public Health, Seoul National University, Seoul, Korea
Clinical Research Center for End Stage Renal Disease in Korea Daegu, Korea

Yong-Lim Kim
Department of Internal Medicine, Kyungpook National University School of Medicine, Daegu, Korea
Clinical Research Center for End Stage Renal Disease in Korea Daegu, Korea

Shin-Wook Kang
Department of Internal Medicine, Yonsei University College of Medicine, Seoul, Korea
Clinical Research Center for End Stage Renal Disease in Korea Daegu, Korea

Chul Woo Yang
Department of Internal Medicine, The Catholic University of Korea College of Medicine, Seoul, Korea
Clinical Research Center for End Stage Renal Disease in Korea Daegu, Korea

Nam-Ho Kim
Department of Internal Medicine, Chonnam National University Medical School, Gwangju, Korea
Clinical Research Center for End Stage Renal Disease in Korea Daegu, Korea

Jung Pyo Lee
Department of Internal Medicine, Seoul National University Boramae Medical Center, Seoul, Korea
Clinical Research Center for End Stage Renal Disease in Korea Daegu, Korea

Weiming Wang, Zhaohui Wang, Shanmai Guo, Pingyan Shen, Hong Ren, Xiaoxia Pan, Xiaonong Chen, Wen Zhang, Xiao Li, Hao Shi, Nan Chen
Nephrology Department, Ruijin Hospital, Shanghai Jiao Tong University School of Medicine, Shanghai, China

Jingyuan Xie
Nephrology Department, Ruijin Hospital, Shanghai Jiao Tong University School of Medicine, Shanghai, China
Division of Nephrology, Department of Medicine, College of Physicians and Surgeons, Columbia University, New York, New York, United States of America

Yifu Li, Ali G. Gharavi, Krzysztof Kiryluk
Division of Nephrology, Department of Medicine, College of Physicians and Surgeons, Columbia University, New York, New York, United States of America

Masato Furuhashi, Shutaro Ishimura, Hideki Ota, Marenao Tanaka, Hideaki Yoshida, Tetsuji Miura
Second Department of Internal Medicine, Sapporo Medical University School of Medicine, Sapporo, Japan

Manabu Hayashi
Second Department of Internal Medicine, Obihiro Kosei Hospital, Obihiro, Japan

Takahiro Nishitani
Obihiro East Medical and Cardiovascular Clinic, Obihiro, Japan

Kazuaki Shimamoto
Sapporo Medical University, Sapporo, Japan

Gökhan S. Hotamisligil
Department of Genetics and Complex Diseases, Harvard School of Public Health, Boston, Massachusetts, United States of America

William H. Walker, Adam M. Smiles, Rita R. Holak, Jackson Jeong, Kevin P. McDonnell
Research Division, Joslin Diabetes Center, Boston, Massachusetts, United States of America

Jung Eun Lee
Research Division, Joslin Diabetes Center, Boston, Massachusetts, United States of America
Division of Nephrology, Samsung Medical Center, Sungkyunkwan University School of Medicine, Seoul, Korea
Department of Medicine, Harvard Medical School, Boston, Massachusetts, United States of America

Andrzej S. Krolewski, Monika A. Niewczas
Research Division, Joslin Diabetes Center, Boston, Massachusetts, United States of America
Department of Medicine, Harvard Medical School, Boston, Massachusetts, United States of America

Tomohito Gohda
Research Division, Joslin Diabetes Center, Boston, Massachusetts, United States of America
Department of Medicine, Harvard Medical School, Boston, Massachusetts, United States of America
Division of Nephrology, Department of Internal Medicine, Juntendo University School of Medicine, Tokyo, Japan

Jan Skupien
Research Division, Joslin Diabetes Center, Boston, Massachusetts, United States of America
Department of Medicine, Harvard Medical School, Boston, Massachusetts, United States of America
Department of Metabolic Diseases, Jagiellonian University Medical College, Krakow, Poland

Seung Jun Kim, Hyang Mo Koo, Hyung Jung Oh, Dong Eun Yoo, Dong Ho Shin, Mi Jung Lee, Fa Mee Doh1, Jung Tak Park, Tae-Hyun Yoo, Kyu Hun Choi, Seung Hyeok Han
Department of Internal Medicine, Yonsei University College of Medicine, Seoul, Korea

Shin-Wook Kang
Department of Internal Medicine, Yonsei University College of Medicine, Seoul, Korea
Severance Biomedical Science Institute, Brain Korea 21, Yonsei University, Seoul, Korea

Beom Jin Lim
Department of Pathology, Yonsei University College of Medicine, Seoul, Korea

Hyeon Joo Jeong
Severance Biomedical Science Institute, Brain Korea 21, Yonsei University, Seoul, Korea

Laetitia Albano, Elisabeth Cassuto-Viguier
UMC Transplantation Rénale, Hôpital Pasteur, Centre Hospitalo-Universitaire de Nice, Nice, France

Justyna M. Rak, Doua F. Azzouz, Nathalie C. Lambert
INSERM UMR1097, Parc Scientifique de Luminy, Marseille, France

Jean Gugenheim
Service de Chirurgie et Transplantation Hépatique, Hôpital l'Archet 2, Nice, France
Université de Nice Sophia Antipolis, Nice, France
INSERM U526, IFR 50, Faculté de Médecine, Université de Nice Sophia Antipolis, Nice, France

Dong Ki Kim, Kook-Hwan Oh
Department of Internal Medicine, Seoul National University Hospital, Seoul, Korea

Hajeong Lee
Department of Internal Medicine, Seoul National University Hospital, Seoul, Korea
Department of Immunology, Seoul National University College of Medicine, Seoul, Korea

Suhnggwon Kim
Department of Internal Medicine, Seoul National University Hospital, Seoul, Korea
Department of Immunology, Seoul National University College of Medicine, Seoul, Korea
Kidney Research Institute, Seoul National University Hospital, Seoul, Korea

Kwon Wook Joo, Yon Su Kim
Department of Internal Medicine, Seoul National University Hospital, Seoul, Korea
Kidney Research Institute, Seoul National University Hospital, Seoul, Korea

Ho Jun Chin
Department of Immunology, Seoul National University College of Medicine, Seoul, Korea
Kidney Research Institute, Seoul National University Hospital, Seoul, Korea
Department of Internal Medicine, Seoul National University Bundang Hospital, Seongnam, Korea

Dong-Wan Chae
Kidney Research Institute, Seoul National University Hospital, Seoul, Korea
Department of Internal Medicine, Seoul National University Bundang Hospital, Seongnam, Korea

Leanid Luksha, Karolina Kublickiene
Division of Obstetrics & Gynecology, Karolinska Institutet, Karolinska University Hospital, Department of Clinical Science, Intervention & Technology, Stockholm, Sweden

Peter Stenvinkel, Juan Jesús Carrero
Division of Renal Medicine, Karolinska Institutet, Karolinska University Hospital, Department of Clinical Science, Intervention & Technology, Stockholm, Sweden

Folke Hammarqvist
Division of Surgery, Karolinska Institutet, Karolinska University Hospital, Department of Clinical Science, Intervention & Technology, Stockholm, Sweden

Sandra T. Davidge
Department of Obstetrics and Gynecology, University of Alberta, Edmonton, Alberta, Canada

I-Kuan Wang
Graduate Institute of Clinical Medical Science, China Medical University College of Medicine, Taichung, Taiwan
Division of Nephrology, China Medical University Hospital, Taichung, Taiwan
Department of Internal Medicine, China Medical University College of Medicine, Taichung, Taiwan

Chih-Chia Liang, Yao-Lung Liu, Chiz-Tzung Chang, Chiu-Ching Huang
Division of Nephrology, China Medical University Hospital, Taichung, Taiwan

Cheng-Li Lin, Fung-Chang Sung
Management Office for Health Data, China Medical University Hospital, Taichung, Taiwan
5 Department of Public Health, China Medical University, Taichung, Taiwan

Po-Chang Lin
Division of Infection, China Medical University Hospital, Taichung, Taiwan

Tzung-Hai Yen
Division of Nephrology, Chang Gung Memorial Hospital, Taipei and Chang Gung Univeristy College of Medicine, Taoyuan, Taiwan

Donald E. Morisky
UCLA Fielding School of Public Health, Los Angeles, California, United States of America.

Pamela J. Hicks
Department of Biochemistry, Wake Forest School of Medicine, Winston-Salem, North Carolina, United States of America

Nicholette D. Palmer
Department of Biochemistry, Wake Forest School of Medicine, Winston-Salem, North Carolina, United States of America
Center for Genomics and Personalized Medicine Research, Wake Forest School of Medicine, Winston-Salem, North Carolina, United States of America
Diabetes Research Center, Wake Forest School of Medicine, Winston-Salem, North Carolina, United States of America

Donald W. Bowden
Department of Biochemistry, Wake Forest School of Medicine, Winston-Salem, North Carolina, United States of America
Center for Genomics and Personalized Medicine Research, Wake Forest School of Medicine, Winston-Salem, North Carolina, United States of America
Diabetes Research Center, Wake Forest School of Medicine, Winston-Salem, North Carolina, United States of America
Department of Internal Medicine, Wake Forest School of Medicine, Winston-Salem, North Carolina, United States of America

Maggie C. Y. Ng
Center for Genomics and Personalized Medicine Research, Wake Forest School of Medicine, Winston-Salem, North Carolina, United States of America
Diabetes Research Center, Wake Forest School of Medicine, Winston-Salem, North Carolina, United States of America

Barry I. Freedman
Center for Genomics and Personalized Medicine Research, Wake Forest School of Medicine, Winston-Salem, North Carolina, United States of America
Diabetes Research Center, Wake Forest School of Medicine, Winston-Salem, North Carolina, United States of America
Department of Internal Medicine, Wake Forest School of Medicine, Winston-Salem, North Carolina, United States of America

Poorva Mudgal
Diabetes Research Center, Wake Forest School of Medicine, Winston-Salem, North Carolina, United States of America

Carl D. Langefeld
Center for Public Health Genomics and Department of Biostatistical Sciences, Wake Forest School of Medicine, Winston-Salem, North Carolina, United States of America

Ria Arnold, Cindy S-Y. Lin, Arun V. Krishnan
Translational Neuroscience Facility, University of New South Wales, Sydney, New South Wales, Australia

Virginija Grinius
Department of Nephrology Prince of Wales Hospital, Sydney, New South Wales, Australia

Bruce A. Pussell, Timothy J. Pianta
Department of Nephrology Prince of Wales Hospital, Sydney, New South Wales, Australia
Prince of Wales Clinical School, University of New South Wales, Sydney, New South Wales, Australia

Matthew C. Kiernan
Prince of Wales Clinical School, University of New South Wales, Sydney, New South Wales, Australia
Neuroscience Research Australia, Sydney, New South Wales, Australia

James Howells
The University of Sydney and Institute of Clinical Neurosciences, Royal Prince Alfred Hospital, Sydney, New South Wales, Australia

Meg J. Jardine
Department of Nephrology Concord Repatriation General Hospital and The George Institute for Global Health, Sydney, New South Wales, Australia

Marinus A. van den Dorpel
Department of Internal Medicine, Maasstad Hospital, Rotterdam, The Netherlands

Claire H. den Hoedt
Department of Internal Medicine, Maasstad Hospital, Rotterdam, The Netherlands
Department of Nephrology, UMC Utrecht, Utrecht, The Netherlands

Albert H. A. Mazairac, Peter J. Blankestijn
Department of Nephrology, UMC Utrecht, Utrecht, The Netherlands

Michiel L. Bots
Julius Center for Health Sciences and Primary Care, UMC Utrecht, Utrecht, The Netherlands

E. Lars Penne, Neelke C. van der Weerd
Department of Nephrology, VU Medical Center, Amsterdam, The Netherlands

Muriel P. C. Grooteman, Piet M. ter Wee, Menso J. Nubé
Department of Nephrology, VU Medical Center, Amsterdam, The Netherlands
Institute for Cardiovascular Research VU Medical Center (ICaR-VU), VU Medical Center, Amsterdam, The Netherlands

Renée Levesque
Department of Nephrology, Centre Hospitalier de l'Universitéde Montréal, St-Luc Hospital, Montré al, Canada

Rafid Tofik, Sophie Ohlsson
Department of Nephrology, Lund University, Lund, Sweden

Omran Bakoush
Department of Nephrology, Lund University, Lund, Sweden
Department of Internal Medicine, UAE University, Al-Ain, United Arab Emirates

Hsin-Yi Yang, Sui-Lung Su
School of Public Health, National Defense Medical Center, Taipei, TaiwanRepublic of China

Kuo-Cheng Lu
Division of Nephrology, Department of Medicine, Cardinal Tien Hospital, School of Medicine, Fu Jen Catholic University, New Taipei City, TaiwanRepublic of China

Herng-Sheng Lee
Department of Pathology, Tri-Service General Hospital, National Defense Medical Center, Taipei, TaiwanRepublic of China

Shih-Ming Huang
Department of Biochemistry, National Defense Medical Center, Taipei, TaiwanRepublic of China

Yuh-Feng Lin
Division of Nephrology, Department of Medicine, Shuang Ho Hospital, Graduate Institute of Clinical Medicine, Taipei Medical University, New Taipei City, Taiwan Republic of China
Division of Nephrology, Department of Medicine, Tri-Service General Hospital, National Defense Medical Center, Taipei, Taiwan Republic of China

Chia-Chao Wu
Division of Nephrology, Department of Medicine, Tri-Service General Hospital, National Defense Medical Center, Taipei, Taiwan Republic of China

Donald M. Salter
Center for Molecular Medicine, MRC IGMM, University of Edinburgh, Edinburgh, United Kingdom

Qiong Cao, Hong Zhang, Zhimei Zhang, Hao Xue
Division of Tissue Typing Center, Nanfang Hospital, Southern Medical University, Guangdong, Guangzhou, China

Di Xie
Division of Nephrology, Nanfang Hospital, Southern Medical University, Guangdong, Guangzhou, China

Jiangmei Liu, Jiyuan Zhou, Pingyan Chen
Department of Biostatistics, School of Public Health and Tropical Medicine, Southern Medical University, Guangdong, Guangzhou, China

Hongyan Zou, Yinze Zhang
HLA High-Resolution Confirmatory Typing Laboratory, Shenzhen Blood Center, Shenzhen, China

Cheng Li, Sheng Shen
Department of Renal Transplantation, Guangdong No.2 Provincial People's Hospital, Guangzhou, People's Republic of China

Huan-Huan Su, Ying-Wei Qiu, Wen-Feng Zhan, Jun-Zhang Tian, Gui-Hua Jiang
Department of Medical Imaging, Guangdong No.2 Provincial People's Hospital, Guangzhou, People's Republic of China

Xiao-Fei Lv
State Key Laboratory of Oncology in South China and Department of Medical Imaging and Interventional Radiology, Sun Yat-Sen University Cancer Center, Guangzhou, People's Republic of China

Florent Occelli, Damien Cuny
EA 4483, Université Lille Nord de FranceFaculté de Pharmacie de Lille, Lille, France

Annabelle Deram
EA 4483, Université Lille Nord de FranceFaculté de Pharmacie de Lille, Lille, France
Faculté Ingénierie et Management de la Santé (ILIS), Loos, France

Francois Glowacki
EA 4483, Université Lille Nord de FranceFaculté de Pharmacie de Lille, Lille, France
Service de Néphrologie, Hopital Huriez, CHRU de Lille, Lille, France
Réseau Néphronor, Hôpital Huriez, CHRU de Lille, Lille, France

Michaël Génin
EA 2694, Université Lille Nord de FranceFaculté de Médecine pôle Recherche, Lille, France

Christian Noël
Service de Néphrologie, Hopital Huriez, CHRU de Lille, Lille, France
Réseau Néphronor, Hô pital Huriez, CHRU de Lille, Lille, France

Index

www.ingramcontent.com/pod-product-compliance
Lightning Source LLC
Chambersburg PA
CBHW050438200326
41458CB00014B/4991